D1373264

Interdisciplinary

Rehabilitation

in Trauma

Interdisciplinary

Rehabilitation

in Trauma

JOHN J. GERHARDT, M.D.

Chief
Department of Physical Medicine and Rehabilitation,
Kaiser Sunnyside Medical Center, Clackamas, Oregon
Department of Physiatry
Clinical Assistant Professor in Orthopedics and Rehabilitation
Oregon Health Sciences University
Portland, Oregon

ECKHART REINER, M.D.

Medical Director, Rehabilitation Center for Trauma
of the General Accident Insurance Company
(Allgemeine Unfallversicherungsanstalt-AUVA)
Korneuburg, Vienna, Austria
Former Medical Director
of the AUVA Rehabilitation Center for Trauma
Bad Häring, Tirol, Austria

BERND SCHWAIGER, M.D.

Orthopedic Surgeon, Former Senior Staff Physician & Surgeon
AUVA Rehabilitation Center
Bad Häring, Tirol, Austria

PHILIP S. KING, M.D.

Associate Professor, Division of Orthopedics and Rehabilitation
and Medical Director, Rehabilitation Services
Oregon Health Sciences University
Former Chief, Department of Rehabilitation Medicine Services,
Veterans Administration Medical Center,
Portland, Oregon

Partial translation by Brigitte Marschall, Certified Translator, Innsbruck, Austria

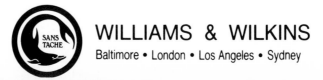

WILLIAMS & WILKINS
Baltimore • London • Los Angeles • Sydney

Editor: Kimberly Kist
Associate Editor: Carol Eckhart
Copy Editor: Shelly Hyatt Blankman
Design: Robert Och/Joanne Janowiak
Illustration Planning: Asterisk Group
Production: Raymond E. Reter

Printed in the United States of America

Library of Congress Cataloging-in-Publication Data
Main entry under title:

Interdisciplinary rehabilitation in trauma.

  Bibliography: p.
  Includes index.
  1. Wounds and injuries—Patients—Rehabilitation. 2. Physically handicapped—Rehabilitation. 3. Health care teams. I. Gerhardt, John J. [DNLM:
1. Wounds and Injuries—rehabilitation—atlases. WO 517 I61]
RD798.I57 1987   617′.1   85-20175
ISBN 0-683-03452-9

87 88 89 90
10 9 8 7 6 5 4 3 2 1

This book is dedicated to the injured and the handicapped and to the memory of our mentor and friend, University Professor Otto Russe, M.D., whose entire life was motivated by uncompromising devotion to their better care and total rehabilitation.

Foreword

Rehabilitation medicine is more than just a slogan. It has developed into an essential branch of modern medicine, a branch that is concerned with restoration of function of the human body and with the enhancement of the quality of life. The role of physicians specializing in rehabilitation is critical—to supervise the interaction of team members during its various phases of the rehabilitation process.

Rehabilitation of trauma is as old as mankind. It is, in fact, along with obstetrics, the oldest branch of medicine. H. E. Sigerist, the Swiss authority on the history of medicine, describes findings from the Stone Age (4000 to 3000 B.C.) which demonstrated bone fractures healed in good position.

Records extend from around 2600 B.C.: the Egyptian physician Imhotep, the Papyrus Smith, the first historical depiction of a leg prosthesis on a Hellenic vase, through the Vedic epoch in India about 2000 years B.C. At about 500 years B.C., the Mochica time sculptures show encased parts as limb replacements in the South American Continent. In 460 B.C., there is the Corpus Hippocraticum (the Hippocraticum collection) with preserved manuscripts dating to the 10th Century A.D. and the Ÿuan Dynasty work in the 13th to 14th centuries in Asia.

Rehabilitation as it is known today, however, evolved during World War I (1914 to 1918). Surgeons realized that their work does not end with completed surgery and the healed wound. In 1915, Professor Spitzy treated war invalids not only medically, but cared for them also for long-term needs that resulted from their injuries. He also founded the first independent Orthopedic Hospital and several schools for invalids in Vienna. At about the same time, Robert Jones and Harold Delf Gilies set up special facilities for orthopedic patients and plastic surgery, respectively.

Independent from Spitzy, Professor Lorenz Böhler achieved remarkable functional results on the Italian front during World War I from, at that time, unconventional treatment of gunshot injuries of bones and joints.

He described his approach in his "Technique of Fracture Treatment." His Field Hospital opened in 1916 in Bozen (Bolzano) was located in a trade school building. Böhler utilized the available materials and tools for functional exercises which are now utilized by occupational therapy and ergotherapy (work therapy).

Lorenz Böhler moved to Vienna after the war had ended and was able to attract the attention of the director of the Workmen's Compensation Insurance Company, by demonstrating excellent results of fracture treatments and the importance of systematic treatment and close followup. With the director's help, Professor Böhler opened the first "Accident Hospital" (Unfallkrankenhaus) on January 8, 1925, in the Webergasse in Vienna. The Workmen's Compensation Insurance extended its sphere of influence from compensation payments, welfare and prevention of accidents, to include active medical treatments beginning immediately after accidents.

It was soon widely recognized that the best primary care by physicians was the basis for successful rehabilitation. Likewise, if primary care was inadequate, rehabilitation could not be accomplished.

Today, rehabilitation is seen as a continuous process, which starts immediately after the onset of disease or injury and extends through the treatment and followup care to the final goal of reintegration into social and family life as well as work situation. In one word, "resettlement."

This book goes one step further. It is the authors' belief that rehabilitation can only be successful when a well-trained and interactive team is available to the patient. Thus, the approach of this book is to present coordinated teamwork as the crux of rehabilitation. Many of the data are based on the work at the rehabilitation center at Bad Häring in Tirol, Austria, but the techniques described can be applied by physicians anywhere. They are a living example of modern trauma rehabilitation.

Dr. Erich Frank
Medical Director
Allgemeine Unfallversicherungsanstalt
General Accident Insurance Institution
Austria

Preface

With the establishment of the first accident hospital in Vienna (see "Foreword"), a development and growth unprecedented in the field of medicine began in traumatology and trauma rehabilitation. Today, a number of modern facilities exist throughout the world. The one common bond is the significantly impaired patient, who requires the services of not only the physician but also of many other skilled health care professionals for proper management.

Individual areas of expertise overlap as they must; but, as this book demonstrates, the clinical expertise of everyone involved with the patient is at stake. A coordinated, integrated approach is neccessary to facilitate communication and to avoid conflicting messages and confusion of the patient. It is important that all team members be cheerful and capable of motivating the usually depressed patient to work with them in a positive way during perhaps the most difficult and trying period in his or her life.

Trained, knowledgeable, enthusiastic and inspiring professionals with empathy can mean all the difference in a patient whose only hope is a good mental outlook and a fulfillment of what capabilities remain after the onset of disability.

Such training and knowledge must involve the patient from the time of the accident to the time that his or her aspirations are achieved.

This volume is intended for all clinicians who work with trauma patients, including physicians, nurses, physical therapists, occupational therapists, speech-language pathologists, social workers, prosthetists-orthotists, respiratory therapists, recreational therapists, X-ray technicians and rehabilitation personnel. It will be of benefit also to attorneys, disability evaluators, insurance claim examiners, Workmen's Compensation, administrators, planning teams for health care facilities (such as hospitals, rehabilitation centers, skilled and intermediate nursing facilities), sport organizations for handicapped, home health agencies, visiting nurses' associations and voluntary organizations. The volume may be helpful to family physicians, and to some of their patients and families, as a vehicle for inspiration, motivation and exploration of available treatment and programs. Some described approaches may not yet be familiar to some practitioners.

Rehabilitation of trauma is complex and it is impossible to cover all of its aspects in one volume; but if we have contributed even in a small part to better understanding and total care of the trauma patient, it will have been worth the effort.

J.J.G
E.R.
B.S.
P.S.K.

Acknowledgments

This work is the result of many hours of preparation, planning, and action photography during regular treatment sessions, games, recreational activities, and sports, involving many individuals, providers, as well as patients, in hospitals and rehabilitation centers in Europe and the United States.

It is also the result of discussions and consultations, advice and demonstrations by many individuals and organizations who enthusiastically assisted the authors. We cannot list the names of all: Some are mentioned on this page and some in the text of this book. To all others, we would like to express gratitude and thanks, even for the smallest contribution. Each one helped our patients with acute trauma, impairment, disability or handicap in some way.

The authors extend our very special thanks to the following persons who made this book possible: Dr. Erich Frank, medical director of the Accident Insurance Institution of Austria and the entire staff and administration of Bad Häring in Tirol, Austria; Professor H. Jahna and staff at the Unfallkrankenhaus, Vienna-Meidling (Trauma Hospital); Professor Scherzer and staff at the Special Rehabilitation Center for Cranio-Cerebral Injuries in Vienna-Meidling; and Professor O. Russe (posthumous) and staff at the Trauma Department of the University Hospital in Innsbruck, Austria.

Many thanks also to the Medical Department personnel at Bad Ragaz and Clinical Valens in Switzerland, the Burn Center at Emanuel Hospital in Portland, Oregon, at Shriner's Hospital in Portland, and at the Kaiser Sunnyside Medical Center in Clackamas, Oregon.

For reviewing and helping to translate the text, we thank Dr. George Peirson, Dr. Robert Yang of the V.A. Hospital in Portland, Drs. Lieberman and B. Brown of the Kaiser Sunnyside Medical Center.

For their assistance in the preparation of this book, we thank the following persons: Evi Gründhammer, Maria Altbacher, Greta Gerhardt, Donna Holso, and Sara Walter. Sincere thanks also to Professor Artur Widra and George Peiger for their contribution to the artwork, and to the staff at Williams & Wilkins.

Contributors

Linda Allaway, R.R.T.
Chief, Respiratory Therapy Department, Kaiser Sunnyside Medical Center, Clackamas, Oregon.

Richard Altenberger, P.T.

Kiran Bhatt, M.D.
Fellow, Spinal Cord Injury Service, Veterans Administration Medical Center, Wood, Wisconsin; Assistant Professor in PM&R, College of Wisconsin, Milwaukee, Wisconsin, former Assistant Professor, University of Southern California Irvine, California, and Assistant Professor in Neurology, Oregon Health Sciences University.

Rudolf Buratti, M.D.
Senior Physician, AUVA Rehabilitation Center, Bad Häring, Tirol, Austria.

Timothy J. Campbell, M.D.
Pediatric Surgery, Portland, Oregon.

Edgar DeMar, M.D.
Physician, National Aeronautic and Space Administration (NASA), San Francisco, California; former Senior Flight Physician and Surgeon, United Airlines.

Robert Ehret, M.D.
Ehret and Sattleger Neurology and Neurosurgery Clinic, Singen, West Germany.

Maria Erlemann, R.T.A.
Senior X-Ray Technician, Trauma Department, University Hospital, Innsbruck, Austria.

Everill W. Fowlks, M.D.
Emeritus Professor in Orthopaedics and Rehabilitation, Oregon Health Sciences University; Former Chief, Department Physical Medicine and Rehabilitation, Veterans Administration Medical Center and Director of Residency Program in PM&R, Portland, Oregon.

Diana Gallardo, M.A.
Certified Feldenkrais Practitioner, Former Associate Professor in Physical Education, California State University, Pomona, California.

John J. Gerhardt, M.D.
Chief, Department of Physical Medicine and Rehabilitation, Kaiser Sunnyside Medical Center, Clackamas, Oregon, Department of Physiatry. Clinical Assistant Professor in Orthopedics and Rehabilitation, Oregon Health Sciences University, Portland, Oregon.

Signa P. Gibson, M.S., R.D.
Diet Service, Kaiser Sunnyside Medical Center, Clackamas, Oregon.

Paul Goodley, M.D.
Executive Director of the Foundation of Musculo-Skeletal Medicine, Fawnskin, California.

Scott Haetherington, D.O.
Dean and Professor of Osteopathic Medicine, Oklahoma College of Osteopathic Medicine and Surgery; Director of Osteopathic Services, Eastmoreland General Hospital, Portland, Oregon; Adjunct Professor, College of Osteopathic Medicine of the Pacific.

Jolene Heitman, O.T.R.
Portland Burn Center, Emanuel Hospital, Portland, Oregon.

Judy Henbury, R.R.T.
Former Recreation Therapist, Veterans Administration Medical Center, Portland, Oregon.

Helmut Hornof, Lt. Colonel
Teacher, Physical Education and Coach, Theresianum-Military Academy, Wiener Neustadt, Austria.

Fritz Jenkner, M.D.
University Professor, Neurosurgery, University of Vienna, Austria; Director of Pain Center, Gebietskrankenkasse Süd, Vienna, Austria.

Lawrence Jones, D.O., F.A.A.O.
Physician, Lecturer, Ontario, Oregon.

Philip S. King, M.D.
Associate Professor, Division of Orthopedics and Rehabilitation, and Medical Director, Rehabilitation Services, Oregon Health Sciences University; Former Chief, Department of Rehabilitation Medicine Services, Veterans Administration Medical Center, Portland, Oregon.

Sherry Kleier, R.N., M.S.
Director of Medical/Surgical Nursing Service, Kaiser Sunnyside Medical Center, Clackamas, Oregon.

Richard Koch, D.O., F.A.A.O.
Physician, Lecturer, Consultant, Olympia, Washington.

Cheryl Kosta, R.P.T.
Physical Therapist, Department PM&R, Kaiser Sunnyside Medical Center, Clackamas, Oregon.

Sonja Laznik, O.T.R.
Chief Occupational Therapist, AUVA Rehabilitation Center, Bad Häring, Tirol, Austria, and staff: George Peiger, OTR, Angelika Landman, OTR.

Ilse Lebic, R.P.T.
Chief Physical Therapist, AUVA Rehabilitation Center for Cranio Cerebral Injuries (Director University Professor E. Scherzer), Vienna 12, Austria; and staff.

William Long, M.D.
Medical Director, Trauma Center, Emanuel Hospital, Portland, Oregon.

Helmut Madersbacher, M.D.
Professor and Chairman, Urology Department, University Medical School, Innsbruck, Austria; and Consultant Surgeon, AUVA Rehabilitation Center, Bad Häring, Tirol, Austria.

Kenneth D. Meadows, R.P.T.
Physical Therapist, Portland Hand Surgery Center, Portland, Oregon.

Cathy Mitchell-Call, M.S.W.
A.R.T. Team, Kaiser Sunnyside Medical Center, Clackamas, Oregon.

Roger Miyaji, M.A., J.D.
Department of Legal Services, Kaiser Permanente Health Care Program, Oregon/Washington Region, Portland, Oregon.

Sue Mulligan, R.N., P.H.N.
Public Health Nurse, Home Health Agency, Kaiser Permanente Health Care Plan, Oregon/Washington Region.

Maria Mutters, R.P.T.
Senior Physical Therapist, Bad Ragaz/Valenz Rehabilitation Center (Director Wilhelm Zinn, M.D.), Bad Ragaz, Switzerland.

Peter Nathan, M.D.
Director, Portland Hand Surgery Center, Portland, Oregon.

Philip Parshley, M.D.
Medical Director, Portland Burn Center, Emanuel Hospital, Portland, Oregon.

Ann Pellegrin, M.S.W.
Coordinator, Family Services, Shriner's Hospital for Crippled Children, Portland Unit, Portland, Oregon.

Bette Perman, R.N., M.S.
Director of Nursing, Home Health Agency, Kaiser Permanente Health Care Plan, Oregon/Washington Region.

Gerhard Peter, CPO
Orthotist, Kaiser Sunnyside Medical Center, Clackamas, Oregon.

Daniel Pinter, M.S.W.
Chief, Social Services, AUVA Rehabilitation Center, Bad Häring, Tirol, Austria.

Axel Pomardi, D.D.S.
Consultant Dentist, AUVA Rehabilitation Center, Bad Häring, Tirol, Austria.

Paul Raether, M.D.
Director, Rehabilitation Services, Department of Physical Medicine and Rehabilitation, Kaiser Sunnyside Medical Center, Clackamas, Oregon.

Ken Ravizza, Ph.D.
Department of Health, Physical Education and Recreation, California State University, Fullerton, California.

Eckhart Reiner, M.D.
Medical Director, Rehabilitation Center for Trauma of the General Accident Insurance Company (Allgemeine Unfallversicherungsanstalt-AUVA) Korneuburg, Vienna, Austria, Former Medical Director of the AUVA Rehabilitation Center for Trauma, Bad Häring, Tirol, Austria.

Elle Friedman Robinson, M.A.
Counseling Psychologist, Consultant in Rehabilitation for the Disabled, Portland, Oregon, Former Certified Sexuality and Disability Educator, University of California, San Francisco, California

Martha Rushing, O.T.R.
Supervisor, Department of Occupational Therapy, Kaiser Sunnyside Medical Center, Clackamas, Oregon.

Friedrich Russe, M.D.
Senior Surgeon, AUVA Unfallkrankenhaus, Vienna 12, Austria.

Gerhard Schicht
Engineer, Consulting Architect, Portland, Oregon.

Bernd Schwaiger, M.D.
Orthopedic Surgeon, Former Senior Staff Physician & Surgeon, AUVA Rehabilitation Center, Bad Häring, Tirol, Austria.

Kay Schweickart, R.N., M.S.
Hospital Administrator, Kaiser Sunnyside Medical Center, Clackamas, Oregon.

Nita Sharp, O.T.R.
Occupational Therapist, Kaiser Sunnyside Medical Center, Clackamas, Oregon.

Blaise Scollard, M.S., C.C.C.
Speech and Language Pathologist, Kaiser Sunnyside Medical Center, Clackamas, Oregon.

Anne Smith
Secretary, Founder, Family Head Injury Support Group, State of Oregon, Portland, Ore.

Stephan Spanudakis, M.D.
Senior Surgeon, AUVA Rehabilitation Center, Bad Häring, Tirol, Austria.

Wilhelm Strubreither, Ph.D.
Clinical Psychologist, AUVA Rehabilitation Center, Bad Häring, Tirol, Austria.

Lance Tsugawa, M.S., C.C.C.
Speech and Language Pathologist, Kaiser Sunnyside Medical Center, Clackamas, Oregon, and Bess Kaiser Medical Center, Portland, Oregon.

Elizabeth Völkl, R.P.T.
Chief Physical Therapist, AUVA Rehabilitation Center, Bad Häring, Tirol, Austria, and staff: Richard Altenberger, RPT; Gabriele Berger, RPT; Theresia Barbach, RPT;

Gernot Stix, RPT; Julius Heidenwolf, RPT; Susanne Kubat, RPT; Bruno Schmiedbauer, RPT; Mathilde Netsch, RPT; Waldtraut Starke, RPT; Annemarie Juën, RPT; Herta Zwolanek, RPT; Gabriele Schmiederer, RPT; and Hubert Zoller, RPT.

William Winkler, Ph.D.
Psychologist and Sexual Therapist, Kaiser Sunnyside Medical Center, Clackamas, Oregon.

Günther Wittlinger, M.D.
Medical Director, Rehabilitation Center, Alpenbach-Walchee, Austria.

Joseph Zettl, C.P.O.
Prosthetist-Orthotist, Assistant Professor in Rehabilitation, University of Washington, PM&R Department, and Former Director, Prosthetics Research Study, Seattle, Washington.

Marcelo Zurita, M.D.
Physician and Electronic Technologist, Beaverton, Oregon.

Contents

SECTION 4
REHABILITATION OF SPECIFIC DISEASES

SECTION
1

THE FAMILY AND THE PATIENT'S VIEW

1

The Brain-Injured Patient: The Story of Brian

Anne Smith

INTRODUCTION

Anne is a single parent working as a medical secretary. She raised her four children, now 25, 23, 21 and 9, on her own, with very little and only sporadic support. Anne never resorted to welfare or public assistance. She was the co-founder and president for 5 years of the Oregon Family Head Injury Support Group, a nonprofit organization. She is now the vice-president and devotes all of her spare time to assisting families of brain-injured victims.

Anne's Description of Brian's Accident

The evening of August 27, 1977 was warm with a light rain just beginning to fall about 7:30 p.m. My son, Brian, age 15, had gone out to finish collecting from those few hard-to-reach paper route customers. "I'll be back soon" was his reply as he left—his last audible reply for 2 years.

At 8:30 that evening, I received the call every parent fears: "Your child has been in an accident and has been badly injured." The nurse on the phone said he was at the community hospital, but she was unable to tell me how badly he had been hurt—only that he had been identified from the newspaper receipt book taken from his now torn jeans. Leaving my 2-year-old child with Brian's 17-year-old sister and 14-year-old brother, I found a neighbor to drive me to the hospital. Although the drive was only a few miles, it felt like the longest drive of my life. On arrival, hospital personnel told me that Brian had been hit head on in a bicycle path by a drunk driver, that he was unconscious, and that they did not know the extent of his injuries. The one "fact" they could tell me was that if he survived for 4 hours, they would then transport him to the university hospital, which was larger. Unfortunately, we were all unaware at that time that the first few hours after an accident are the "golden hours," and that rapid and proper care at that time could have made a real difference in the overall outcome.

By midnight, Brian had survived the 4 hours, and he was taken by ambulance to the university hospital. There, everyone began frantically to work over him. A computer-assisted tomography (CT) scan showed massive intracerebral bleeding, frontal lobe damage, and brainstem injury. X-rays revealed broken bones, but few other internal injuries were found. The neurosurgeon in charge informed me that Brian probably would not live through the night and that the outlook was grim. Over the next several days, there were no changes for the better and many for the worse, and reality became very harsh. There were so many questions about head injuries, and each question had a different answer, depending on who was asked.

Financially, we were fortunate. Brian was covered by workmen's compensation because he had been on his paper route. At the time, this was actually of small comfort, but over the years I have come to be extremely grateful for this insurance.

Brian remained comatose for the next 5 months and many times I was told he probably would remain in this state all his life. Brian's brother, sister, and I rotated in shifts to provide the stimulation we thought might help this "sleeping child" to awaken—talking, reading, introducing strange or familiar smells, and most of all, just always being there. I spent many nights at the hospital in a waiting room chair, catching brief naps, because there were emergencies when Brian needed surgery and I needed to be there to sign the papers and understand the possible risks. By the time Brian's coma began to lighten, he had had 14 surgeries, some lifesaving and others corrective. I had learned more about head injuries than I had ever hoped to know. I endured the weekly hospital rounds with residents and interns taking bets for dinners and cigars as to whether Brian would survive or even regain consciousness. Seven years ago, handouts on head injury for the families were not available, nor were family support groups to offer reassurance and information. These were the longest 5 months imaginable—little change in his condition, little information, and endless frustration. These were indeed the worst of times. However, during those months of fears and many difficulties, our lives were touched by some incredible people filled with love and concern. Many were total strangers prior to the accident—the kind nurses at the hospital, therapists, and the dear janitor who always began her shift with a kiss and a song for Brian. These dear people will never be forgotten.

BRIAN'S REHABILITATION

As the coma lifted and Brian became more aware, it was time to move to a new phase of recovery: rehabilitation. We now moved into a world that was positive for the most part with so much help that we almost have been overwhelmed by it. With the transfer from the university hospital to the rehabilitation center, Brian was no longer cloistered in a small, private room. Instead, the atmosphere at the rehabilitation center was open, casual, and, most of all, very busy. Even though Brian still was unable to communicate except for a slight crooked smile, he was treated as a "real" person. Testing followed by more testing produced a game plan in which there were many participants, and Brian was the "star" of the production. After the second week, I was told by the team that Brian was making wonderful progress; casting had begun on his arms to reduce severe contractures, and a communication system was being arranged. No longer were the negatives emphasized; the positives were. Also at the end of that second week, the team said I could bring Brian home for the weekend and, if it went well, every weekend thereafter. At first, the thought of bringing my son home in this condition struck absolute terror in my heart. I thought: "I can't possibly do this." However, I soon realized that this was the very goal toward which we had been working.

The first weekend home went very well, although it certainly was a challenge. Brian needed all of his food blended because his tracheostomy tube had just been removed; he was incontinent, and he had both arms and both legs in casts. When I returned him to the center on Sunday evening, we were looking forward to the next weekend home visit. His grandparents and I were there every night to feed him "dinner." All his meals were fed through a syringe at this point. The center became Brian's main "home" for the next 8 months, and the progress was fantastic. It did not take the various team members long to ascertain that Brian had no cognitive impairment. In fact, his IQ testing was high, and there did not seem to be any short-term memory damage. He "graduated" from the crude communication system, and finally settled on a CANON communicator. This was a small device that strapped onto the arm of his wheelchair. It could be operated with one finger and had a small tape printout. Overall, Brian was progressing well in therapy.

In July, as part of his routine checkup at the university hospital, he was scheduled for another CT scan. Three days later, I received a phone call from the neurosurgeon who had been following Brian to say that the CT scan had shown a large mass. I was told that the original scan, on the night of the accident, had demonstrated the same mass; however, now it had increased in size. The neurosurgeon said that Brian must come right to the hospital for an angiogram and, possibly, surgery. This was the first I had been told of a tumor. The physician's theory was that Brian had not been stable enough to have it removed any earlier, and it would have posed one more problem for the family if I had been told of it at the time.

Brian went in the next morning for the angiogram, which showed a porencephalic cyst. On July 20, 1978, he underwent a right craniotomy, with evacuation and partial stripping of a right parietal arachnoid cyst. He returned home 4 days later to rest and recover from the latest assault to his body; he left the hospital with the resident neurosurgeon's assessment that Brian's overall prognosis was "fair." With those less-than-positive words, I prepared to reenter Brian in the center for more intense therapy. Now, the major focus was on speech; the other modalities were important, but speech took the center stage.

Fall arrived and with it came the beginning of a new school year. Brian, in his wheelchair and armed with his communicator and a wonderful smile, prepared to enter high school to begin his sophomore year. Our decision to do this was met with a terrible furor, not from the school officials and teachers, but from the psychologists and social workers with whom I had dealt. They felt Brian could not go before his peers as he now was and be expected to attend classes. Teenage years being so difficult under normal conditions anyway, why would we want to subject him to more problems? They suggested that Brian just stay at home and have a tutor. Brian, however, wanted to go and at least try. Given everything else with which he had dealt, he felt this would be relatively easy. His sister and brother were still in high school and were there to help feed him and push him to his classes. The county "tram" assisted in the transportation. Because of his fatigue level, he only attended half-days, but took regular classes. Homework was typed on the communicator, and the tiny strips of paper printouts were painstakingly glued onto regular notebook paper. His friends maintained close contact during the rehabilitation period, and he was accepted readily by his fellow students.

In the next few years, Brian had bilateral Z-plasty-lengthening and Achilles tendon-lengthening procedures; his contractures were corrected. With incredible determination, he began walking again, first with a walker and then with the aid of a cane. He had a broad ataxic gait and left-sided weakness.

His speech was slow and deliberate and those to whom he talked had to be good listeners. An obturator was made for him, and the speech pathologist and dentist who fitted Brian with this aid said it was "the best nasopharyngeal closure with the obturator in place that we have yet achieved." However, there was still a great deal of nasal emission. Even though he did breathing exercises every day, new gains were not being made to reduce the nasal air flow. Unfortunately, new testing proved the obturator was probably interfering with articulatory timing, and it was discontinued. After several consultations with a physician at the university hospital, surgery for a pharyngeal flap was performed to get better closure. The palatopharyngeal closure was very effective; however, the overall spasticity was not considered during the surgery, and Brian's temporomandibular joints (TMJs) were badly damaged. Brian now had to deal with a new problem—severe pain secondary to the TMJ dysfunction. Several procedures were tried to help the discomfort, including wiring his teeth together to rest the jaw. This only served to set back his speech therapy. One provider tried Valium, but the results of this treatment were disastrous. Rather than have further treatment in this area, Brian decided to learn to adjust to the discomfort. He has had 24 surgeries in the past 7 years.

EPILOGUE

Academically, Brian has done very well. He graduated from high school only 1 year later than he should have, and he completed all the requirements. The school was wonderful, and the teachers and special therapists made it a very positive experience for him. Brian attended 2 years at the local community college, and had three terms at a business school specializing in accounting. The department of vocational rehabilitation had tried to find work for Brian, but it was low on funding and work for the handicapped was difficult to find. We knew the right job situation would appear; in the meantime, Brian had purchased a computer and was doing some work on that at home. The great day came when in August 1985, 8 years after the accident, Brian's file was placed with a private job development company. Within 2 months he began interviews and 1 month later he was in a computer training program with Housing and Development, a Division of the Federal Government. When the training session expired, Brain was hired as a programmer 4 hours a day and 5 days a week. He is working with no absenteeism, earning a good salary, paying taxes, and making his contribution as a valuable productive citizen.

Nine years after his accident, Brian is able to walk with the aid of a cane, and his speech, although dysarthric, is easily understood. He no longer requires the use of the communicator or sign language to augment his speech. Brian's gentle nature has made the whole ordeal much easier for his family to endure. He has none of the characteristics of frontal lobe damage, and his deficits are all physical. He needs assistance with some things, but is really quite independent. He fatigues easily, and symptoms of arthritis are beginning to appear; however, he has come so much further than anyone would have dreamed, and for this we are very grateful. Figures 1.1 and 1.2 show some of Brian's accomplishments.

Head injury treatment has come a very long way since that night in 1977. Early intervention by physical therapy, occupational therapy, and speech therapy including stimulation during coma, cognitive retraining, assistance in feeding, and early communication, are done in modern acute hospitals. Families are included as part of the team, as they should be; their questions are answered and information is provided. Head injury support groups are found in any major city and act as a source of information for the families as well as an advocate for the head-injured victim. Major concerns that need attention are insurance and Social Security payments for the injured with cognitive problems, housing, transportation, and job-skill training.

Figure 1.1.

A–C. To negotiate stairs, Brian has learned to turn around and descend safely backwards.

   D. Brian enters a car.

E–F. Brian is ambulatory with a cane. His posturing is evident.

 G–I. Brian rides a bicycle safely under full control in traffic. In contrast to walking, he has practically no difficulty.

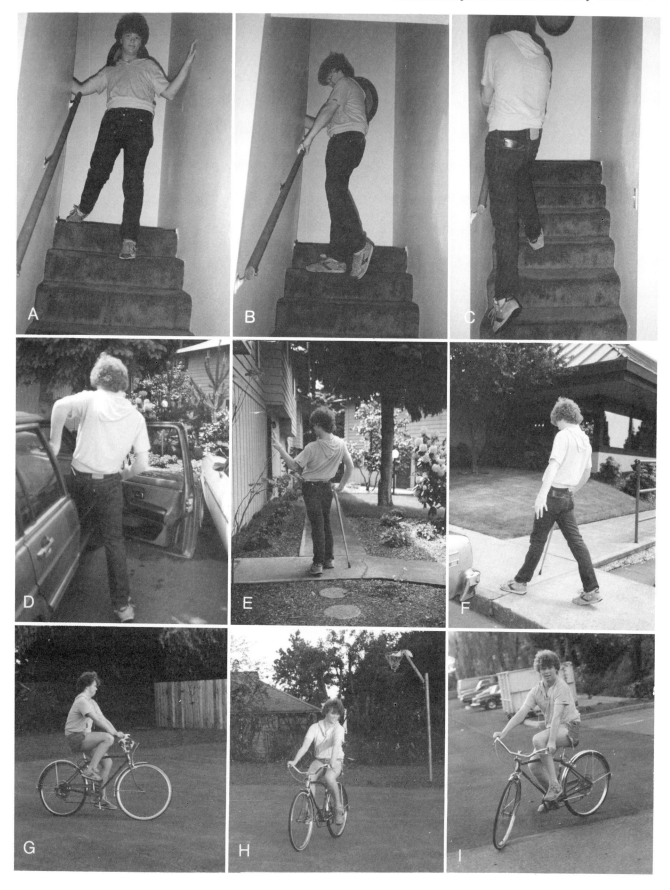

Figure 1.1.

Figure 1.2. Brian

A. Studies,

B. Inserts software in computer,

C. Operates a keyboard, and

D. Handwrites.

E. This is an example of Brian's handwriting.

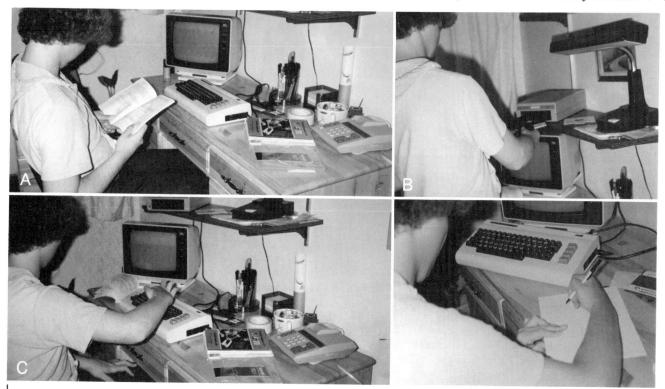

My own philosophy is just mind over matter, "if you don't mind it wont matter." All that means is if someone says, you can't do something don't believe it til you try it. Doctors despite their knowledge, only know about physical workings and not inner workings of the spirit. But its more than mind over matter it is also attitude. I even have a philosophy about attitude and that is "Attitudes arent taught, their got." You cant teach ~~some~~ an attitude, but you can pick it up throughout your life. For instance, My mom is a survior and I learned it from her I guess. Your faith is also important; Although that I dont have a philosophy about it. Its great to have that much power on your team!

Figure 1.2.

2

The Paraplegic: The Story of Elle

Elle Friedman Becker

INTRODUCTION

Elle Friedman Becker is a high-level paraplegic as a result of a horseback riding accident in 1975. During her acute hospital stay and rehabilitation period, she became very frustrated about the lack of information regarding sexuality of the female disabled and decided to correct the situation. She went back to school, studied in San Francisco, and eventually wrote the book, *Female Sexuality following Spinal Cord Injury*. She has worked as the sexuality and disability counselor at Kaiser Rehabilitation Center in Vallejo, California, as well as a vocational counselor with injured workers in Portland, Oregon. Elle earned her masters degree in counseling psychology in 1982 from Lewis and Clark College in Portland.

ELLE'S DESCRIPTION OF THE ACCIDENT

On February 25, 1975 I was involved in a riding accident. I was thrown from my horse and sustained a compression fracture of the seventh thoracic vertebra. My injury resulted in severe, permanent damage to my spinal cord, so I have no sensation or voluntary function below the level of T6.

After my injury, I had many questions regarding my sexuality. I had married my husband four years prior to my accident. Since the sexual aspect of our relationship had been, up to the time of my injury, a very integral and rewarding part of our union, I immediately became concerned about how the injury might change this.

Some of my questions have been answered completely and competently by doctors in the fields of neurology, psychology, psychiatry, and urology. However, many of my questions were left unanswered because, as I discovered, much to my consternation, there is very little information available on the subject of the paraplegic and quadriplegic female sexuality. For this reason I went to the para and quad women in my community and asked them about their lives as sexual beings. I have also sent questionnaires to women in different parts of the country.

I have tape-recorded all of the conversations, so they are as accurate as possible. All of the spinal-cord-injured women's real names have been changed; however, their life stories are true. Most of the para and quad women I talked to for the case histories in this book have learned what they know today from experimentation. Perhaps it will help a newly injured person to read what someone else with a spinal cord injury has experienced, although this should be used to supplement, not replace, sensitive, understanding and knowledgeable sexual counseling.

I share in the collective anger of many spinal-cord-injured women who labor under the destructive impact of negative labels such as "crippled," "handicapped," and "disabled." I realize that in the literal definition of the words, I must fit the description, but somehow our society has also often found these words to mean "paralyzed from the neck up," as a friend of mine would say. We are first and foremost sensitive human beings with a terrific sense of accomplishment after all of the horrible, but challenging, experiences we have been through. Second to this, I consider myself a woman, and third, a paraplegic (which is the only word I have no objection to). I hope I haven't chosen words a para or quad will find objectionable.

I can't help but cringe in my chair when the medical profession makes references to paraplegics' or quadriplegics' sexual "alternatives" as if, by implication, we cannot enjoy normal sex.

It has been demonstrated clearly by research in the fields of psychology and sociology that people with the most extensive and accurate information regarding their own sexuality have fewer emotional problems emerging from sexual conflicts. They will also make a better adjustment to life in general than those with insufficient data about sex. However, the complete lack of any extensive information regarding sexuality in the spinal-cord-injured woman is astounding. The few articles that are available rarely deal with the physical aspects of sex. If they do, it is only to mention intercourse as the only means of sexual expression and, of course, the woman is in the passive missionary position. Often they indicate a woman's sexuality is strictly related to menses, the sex act, at childbirth, with no regard for a woman's feelings. Most of the films and books I am aware of are primarily concerned with male sexuality as if we, as women, do not exist, or worse yet, are expected to completely accept the traditional passive role and not ask any questions.

DR. JOSEPH B. TRAINER INTERVIEWS FRANK AND ELLE BECKER

On May 27, 1976 Frank and I were interviewed at the University of Oregon Medical School in a class conducted by Joseph B. Trainer, M.D., where he is a Professor of Medicine and Associate Professor of Physiology. Dr. Trainer is also a Fellow with the American Association of Marriage and Family Counselors. He is well known in the northwest as the "Marriage Doctor" for his television series of the same name.

Dr. Trainer: One of the problems we have in medicine is meeting the immediate crisis of a devastating disease. This might be one of many kinds. It might be a heart attack. It might be an automobile accident with several fractures or it might be a spinal cord injury such as we are going to have today.

Spinal cord interruptions are increasingly common. We have a good many of them from the Viet Nam war and we continue to have a whole series of them from both automobile and industrial accidents.

Today we are going to program in on the humanistic aspects of medicine (which ought to be brought to bear in this problem and are *not* brought to bear very well). Technologically we do pretty well. Our accomplishment is fair. We don't restore very much function, but we keep from losing more. I think we take good medical care (technologically) of people. From the standpoint of where they are in their heads, their psyches, how they feel about what has happened to them and helping them to get over it, we do not do very well.

Elle is a remarkable creature, and I am going to have her unfold her story for you because I think it is as good a story as you will ever hear of a young person going through this kind of disaster, then finding out the way you cope with it and recuperate from it.

Frank and Elle, I think I would like you to start out by telling us about your marriage. How long have you been married?

Frank: We have been married for 5 years in . . . June? (Laughter).

Dr. Trainer: See, he passed the first test. He remembers more or less when his wedding anniversary is. I did mine on New Year's Eve and it makes it easier since you are celebrating, no matter what. How was your marriage before all of this came along?

Frank: Our marriage was fantastic. We had many communication problems, but everything was going well for us.

Dr. Trainer: Was the communication problem an early problem that you were gradually going through?

Frank: We were on our honeymoon for about a year and then we started having the communication problems. I had a tendency to internalize anxiety and not speak up. This created a lot of tension in our relationship.

Dr. Trainer: I think that is one of the gender differences between males and females. The female expects to settle her problems verbally and the male does not; therefore, there is trouble in most households because she wants to talk about it and that is the last thing he wants to do. You usually find the male in the bathroom for a long time under these circumstances. (Laughter).

How did you manage it?

Frank: In the bathroom.

Dr. Trainer: So, how were things going 2 years ago? You had been married for 3 years. Had things stabilized pretty well?

Elle: Yes. I was working full time as a secretary and putting Frank through school. Frank was working part time. I also play the bassoon, write (poems and short stories), and paint, so I was busy. We were both tremendously busy. Our communications had improved a great deal. Another activity I enjoyed was horseback riding.

One winter day I came home from work and decided to go riding. It was staying daylight longer, so I still had time to ride. Frank had prepared dinner, but I was so eager to go riding that I didn't eat my supper. I rode a friend's horse out in the open country by Newberg, Oregon. I rode for an hour or so and when I was almost home, within a hundred yards of the barn, my horse started to buck violently. I may have been dragged and then I was thrown into a tree in the orchard near my friend's house. When I was thrown I sustained a compression fracture of the sixth thoracic vertebra.

Dr. Trainer: How long ago was that?

Elle: About fourteen months ago. I'm twenty-three years old now. I was twenty-two years old when I broke my back. My husband is twenty-nine.

Dr. Trainer: Were you knocked out at that time?

Elle: Yes.

Dr. Trainer: What is the first thing you remember? Do you remember riding the horse?

Elle: Yes, prior to the bucking episode. After that, everything is blank.

Dr. Trainer: That usually happens whenever you are knocked out. You have an amnesia for the immediate period prior to the accident. Incidentally, memory can sometimes be brought back through hypnosis. This has been done in order to obtain legal evidence and it is admissible evidence.

So when did you wake up? What do you remember next?

Elle: I don't remember the ambulance ride or being in various hospitals. When I woke up there were big bouquets of flowers all over and I thought, "Oh, my God. I've died."

I had no idea where I was or what had happened. Then I took a good look at my surroundings and started noticing things sticking up between the flowers, one of which was the I.V. bottle. I was lying in an electric circle bed (a special bed designed to turn a person over with minimum movement) and realized I was in a hospital. There wasn't anybody around when I woke up. My family was there, but they weren't in my room and there wasn't a nurse or anyone present to help me get my bearings as to where I was and what had happened. I didn't find out what had happened for an extended period of time.

So two days after my injury I wondered what was going on and yet I was not told my prognosis for 2 weeks. My family was told right away and that put them in a terrible position.

Dr. Trainer: Well, what happened next then?

Elle: I thought about not being able to move or feel my legs because I wanted to get up out of bed and leave the hospital. I wanted to get out of there and I couldn't. About the third of fourth day after my injury I decided, "Well, in a couple of days I'll just get up and walk out of here. I'll be all right." I had not accepted my paraplegia yet. From denial I went into a very severe depression.

Dr. Trainer: When did that depression first hit you?

Elle: I was hurt February 25, 1975. According to the writing I did while hospitalized it was the latter part of

March, because at that time I wrote "I wish I were dead." Along with the depression I had a great deal of anger. My anger was directed at everybody and everything within my room (since that was the only place I ever was). I took it out on my family. I took it out on my husband. I threw things. I swore. It was so frustrating being unable to do anything about it. This is something Frank and I were talking about earlier today that he has experienced too.

Dr. Trainer: That you couldn't do anything about it?

Frank: Right. I've always poo-poohed people who said they had times of depression. I've never experienced anything like it in my life. I felt so helpless. I hassled doctors because I was overprotective. I was in the hospital day and night supervising the physicians, which they didn't appreciate at all. (Laughter).

Dr. Trainer: You went through a period of time where you felt you were really out of it. You were kind of psychotic over this whole thing. How long did that stage last?

Elle: About 3 months.

Dr. Trainer: Can you remember any of it? What feelings did you have then?

Elle: Vulnerable; really upset. So upset that my "wonder, wonder land" was much more preferable than reality.

Dr. Trainer: Your imagination began to work in different directions?

Elle: Very definitely. I went through a lot of emotional turmoil and suffering that could have been made easier for me to deal with; not eliminated because I had to go through the grief cycle (process of adjusting to the disability: denial, shock, depression, anger to acceptance). There isn't any way around that, but as soon as I had the proper medical professional people and the proper drugs to help me it was somewhat easier.

Dr. Trainer: But you went for 2 or 3 months without anybody giving you any personal support at all, or sitting down and talking with you about how you felt and how the prospects were.

Elle: Yes.

Author's Note: Except for my urologist at that time. He was the sweetest, kindest man I have ever had the privilege to meet. My whole family was (and is) extremely fond of him. He saw me nearly every day and we spent a great deal of time talking. He helped me very much. Also, my family gave me a tremendous amount of support. They were with me constantly during my entire hospitalization.

On April 17, 1975 (nearly 2 months after my injury) I was finally able to consult a psychiatrist. I had been having severe emotional disturbances and thoughts of suicide since the first part of March. I was not counseled very much at all by my psychiatrist, but was given several major tranquilizers; one of which helped stabilize my erratic emotional state.

Dr. Trainer: I am going to come over to sex now, because that has some relation to this class. When did you first start having sexual urges then?

Elle: I didn't have the opportunity until I went home on leave for the weekends from the rehab center. I went to rehab May 6, 1975. (A nursing note from April 19, 1975 read, "Sexually frustrated," written by an RN.)

My attitudes improved when I went to rehab. One of the first people I met there was a young paraplegic woman. She was my roommate. She left the next day, but that night I saw her come wheeling into our room and transfer into bed. At that time I was in a full Milwaukee brace (a back brace which runs from the hips to the chin designed to stabilize the spine) and I couldn't do very much for myself, so I was just flabbergasted at how much she could do for herself. Her level of injury was very similar to mine. My attitude improved to the point that I was communicating with my husband again.

I should add here that when I was in the hospital I wasn't communicating with my husband at all. I didn't want to see him, because of the way I felt about myself. I didn't understand how anybody else could love me. I didn't love myself. I couldn't understand that he still wanted me, so I was doing everything in my power to put him out of my life.

Dr. Trainer: Could you feel that, Frank?

Frank: Oh, definitely. She would just literally drive me out of her room.

Dr. Trainer: How did you feel you were going to survive that?

Frank: Well, I knew I could survive the injury, but I didn't think I could survive being driven out of her room and out of her life.

Dr. Trainer: Okay, so now you begin to recover and you start to accept or think about Frank again. He looks better than he did. As soon as you looked better to yourself, he looked better.

Elle: Right.

I came home from the rehab center and, sure, I knew how to manipulate my wheelchair. I knew how to dress myself. I could make a transfer, but there was one area that I was unsure about and that was sex. I wanted to feel close to my husband. I had been sleeping with him for nearly four years when all of a sudden I was just picked up in the middle of my life and put someplace else; so I couldn't sleep with him, couldn't live with him and couldn't be with him. I missed him. Sex was traumatic the first several times. I knew I wasn't going to have any sensation, but somehow *actually* not having any sensation (and because I never verbalized my fears, concerns, and worries) made sex a negative experience. That hurt my self-esteem because I had finally come to the point where I was starting to feel good about myself. I was starting to feel confident again, starting to appreciate and value the function and sensation that I do have. The negative sexual encounters were a setback.

The following are excerpts taken from the notes I wrote while hospitalized:

I wish I were dead! (March 24, 1975)

Hold me,
and tell me I should not be afraid
of the darkness. (No date)

Now,
Frustrated
Sad
Lonesome. (No date)

Plans for Wed. and home.
Future, school? (June 3, 1975)

Dr. Trainer: Can you remember who approached who about this? She must have seemed fragile to you, Frank, when you got her home. This fragility is something that you impose on anybody who has a sickness. You don't know what you can do. So you're scared to approach her. Were you able to say, "Hey, I'd like to have you?"

Elle: Well, I didn't feel very sexy in a full Milwaukee brace.

Frank: I think Elle was the assertive party in the first few episodes. Not that I didn't want to. Three months is three months, but she was in the brace and I didn't have that great an understanding of the injury. The furthest thing from my mind was to hurt her in any way.

Dr. Trainer: How did it work out when somebody finally got up enough nerve to make a maneuver in here someplace? She made the maneuver. She sort of assaulted you.

Frank: That's right. It was wonderful.

Dr. Trainer: This must have been a great relief to finally break through that barrier.

Elle: It was. I cried the first several times because of the lack of sensation but after a period of time and a lot of experimentation sex once again became enjoyable for us. We opened our communications to the point that we would tell each other, "Yes, I like that," or, "No, I don't like that. That really turns me on." We experimented with varieties of sexual expression and ways I could move. I didn't think it would be possible for me to achieve orgasm. I though the only way I could enjoy sexual activity was from the enjoyment I gave Frank. However, we have found it is possible for me to reach a climax of sexual excitement.

Dr. Trainer: 95% of this is in between your ears. Much of the sensory input comes from the special senses. You like the sight of the person. You like their smell. You like the sound of their voice. You like the way they taste. Those are sexual inputs.

Also, they were exploring each other and responding to each other. They were trying this and trying that. I suspect you stroked her face and tickled her ears.

Frank: Sensate focus.

Dr. Trainer: Frank, how did you find this? How long did it take you to relate to a new body, which is really what you had to do?

Frank: Well, it was tough at first. As Elle mentioned, she was very disappointed. There was a lot of difference between knowing she didn't have sensation and then *feeling* she didn't have sensation. It was terrible for me. It seemed like all of the pleasure had gone out of it for me, because as she stated, she was multiorgasmic before. That was an ego trip for me. I enjoyed her enjoyment. This was gone and it bothered me. So I almost tended to not even approach sex for awhile after those first initial experiences.

Then one night we came home and she was in her chair. I bent over and kissed her. We'd had a few drinks. We were just fooling around. Then she just convulsed. I was stimulating her breasts, touching her all over and she had an orgasm. It was just fantastic.

Dr. Trainer: A real blaster?

Frank: Yes. I kept thinking, "Oh, no. This really can't be." Even though people had told us orgasm was possible. I asked her, "Was that an orgasm?" She said, "Yes!"

Elle: I started crying again.

Frank: She ran in and called her friend. (Laughter).

Dr. Trainer: Now, you all remember to do that. If you have a good orgasm, call a friend. (Laughter).

Frank: Then she got off the phone and she said, "Gee, I forgot all about you." But really, it was quite an experience.

Dr. Trainer: I gather the friend was one in a similar situation?

Elle: Yes. Remember the woman I first met when I went to rehab? Well, we had talked about sex and we decided, "Well, I guess it isn't possible for us to have an orgasm." We had talked about why we enjoyed sex, so I just wanted to let her know that maybe it was possible after all.

Dr. Trainer: Isn't that great though? That she should think of her friend at such a time? Greater love hath no man.

Frank: Right. So that started our awareness and from there on it has been just like before.

Dr. Trainer: So it's built back up?

Elle: Yes. I finally came back to where I was emotionally and how I was adjusted before my injury.

Dr. Trainer: Except you are probably better off than you were before because you did explore, get acquainted, and talk openly to each other, which most couples never do. By this time you might have been planning a divorce.

Elle: That's possible.

Frank: I suffered from performance anxiety for awhile in our relationship before the accident. I was always trying to keep up with Elle's level of sexuality. I just couldn't handle it. She'd be saying, "Well, it's been five minutes." I've lost that totally. We have become closer and more sexually aware now. It's so different. We are not genitally focused anymore. We are not the passive, awaiting, exploitable vagina and the rigid penis. We're beyond that now and it is a wonderful thing.

Dr. Trainer: So you have gotten to the ultimate stage of being together and of having a sexual relationship that reflects the head to head intimacy you have accomplished. And it took a disaster to do it.

Figures 2.1 through 2.4 show Elle's skills.

Figure 2.1. Elle utilizes her household skills.

    A. Setting the table.

B–C. Getting dishes and cooking supplies in the pantry. Note that shelves are at wheelchair heights.

D–E. Opening refrigerator and getting food. Note that the range is at wheelchair height and allows easy access. Space for leg rests is underneath the range.

    F. Preparing food in the microwave oven; note that the lightweight tray has a thick insulating cork plate to prevent burns. Elle is anesthetic below T7 level.

G–H. Elle enjoying her meal.

    I. Rinsing dishes.

J–K. Opening and loading the dishwasher.

    L. Vacuuming.

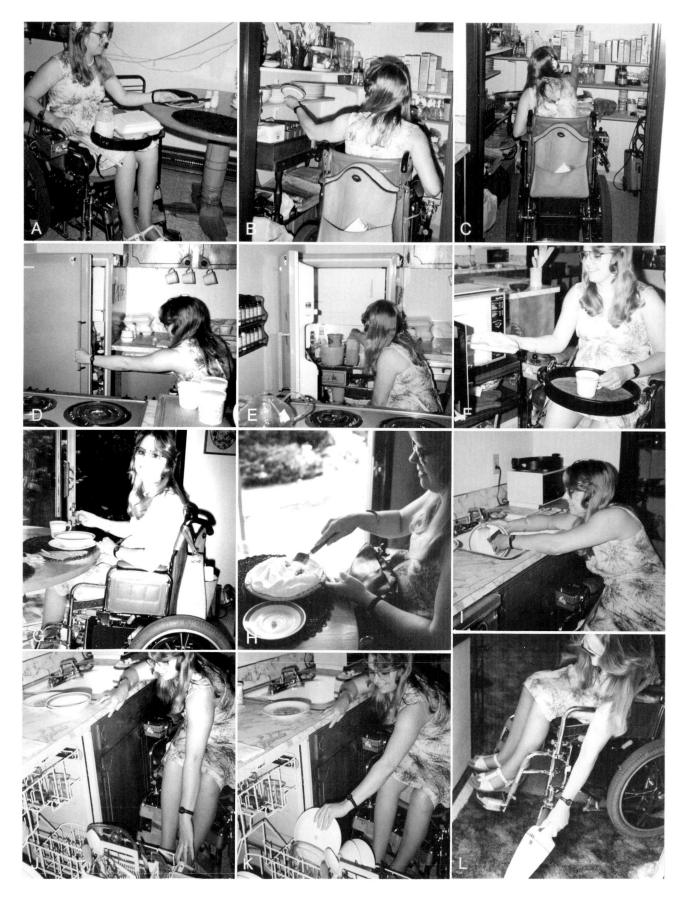

Figure 2.1.

Figure 2.2. Elle's apartment is adapted to her needs.

A–B. A decorative braided rope on the doorknob helps to close doors from wheelchair.

C–D. She opens her sliding doors.

E–F. A table close to the door on the in- and outside are helpful for placing trays, baskets, etc. while opening or closing doors.

   G. Locks on all doors have to be at wheelchair height.

H–K. The door latch at the laundry room of the apartment complex has been modified and a ramp provided, which enables her to push door open with one hand. Opening door on the way out creates no problems.

   L. She loads the washer. To retrieve laundry from the bottom of the washer, she uses an extender tongue.

  M. She retrieves laundry from the dryer.

  N. She folds laundry on a proper height table placed adjacent to the dryer.

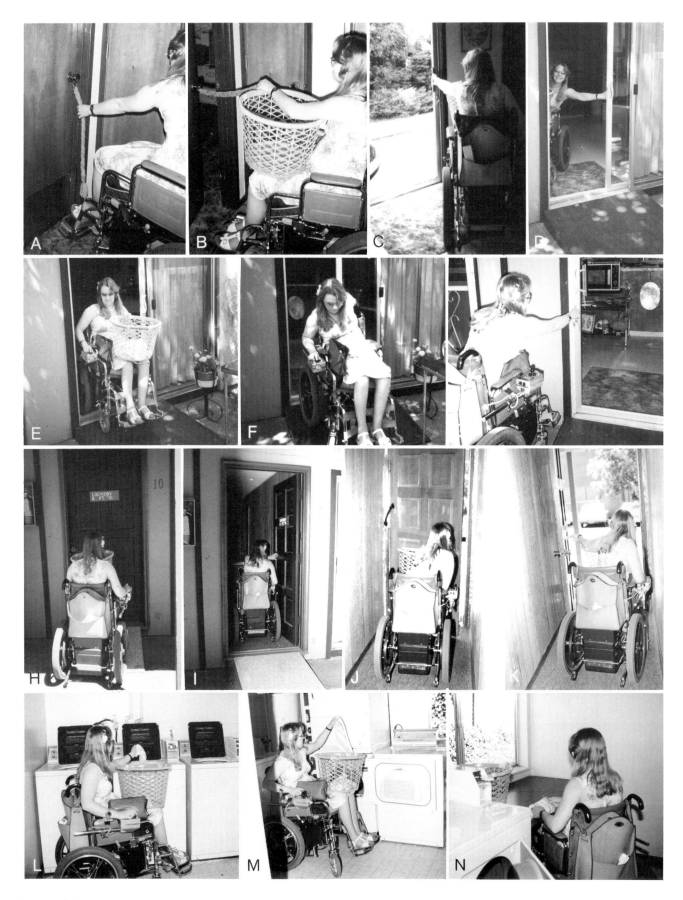

Figure 2.2.

Figure 2.3.   Elle keeps in touch with the hospital.

A–C. Arriving at acute hospital for counseling.

D–E. Counseling and interacting with a trauma patient who is on absolute bedrest.

   F. Interviewing and counseling a family member.

   G. Charting.

   H. Discussing her progress and approach with the charge nurse.

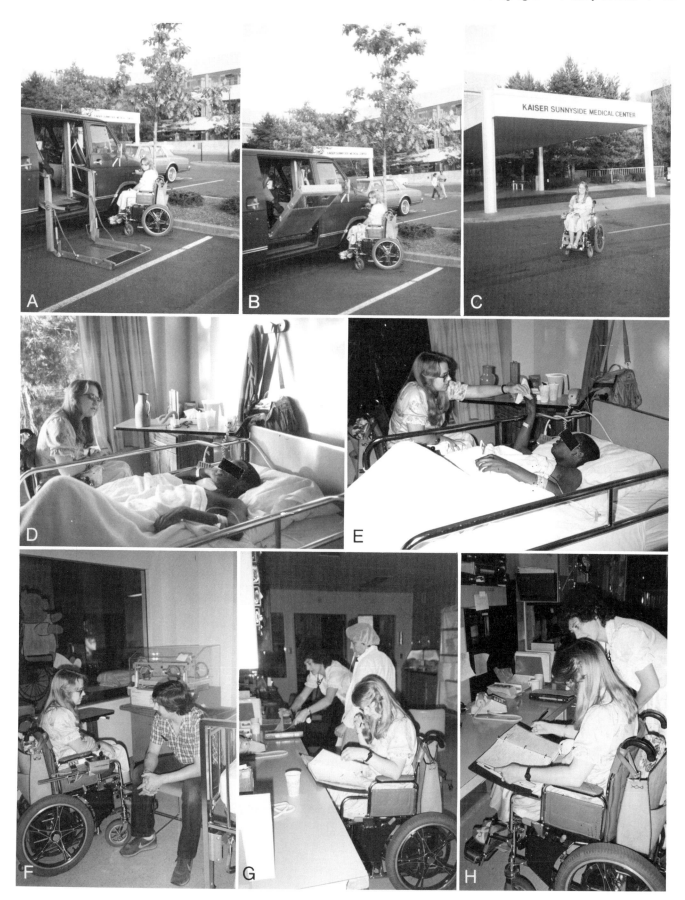

Figure 2.3.

Figure 2.4. Elle maintains her everyday activities.

A. Visiting with neighbors.
B. Getting mail.
C. Pulling curtain with cord, which is attached with a small hook to a wheelchair-high shelf in easy reach.
D. Switching light or power on and off using an extender.
E. Retrieving books from a bookshelf.
F. Studying or reading.
G. Making and receiving phone calls on a cordless phone.

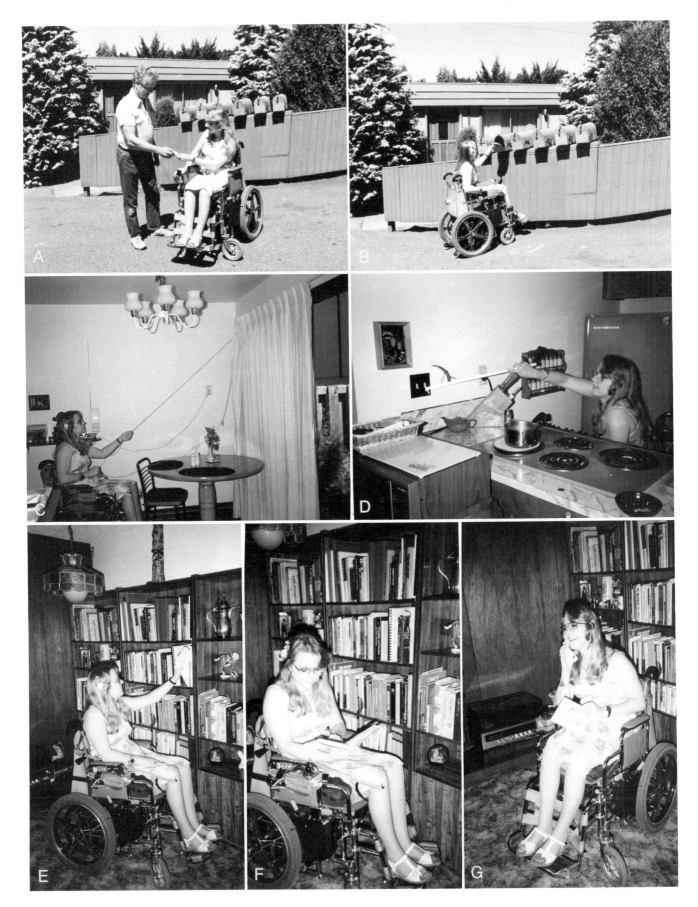

Figure 2.4.

3

The Amputee: The Story of Helmut

Lt. Col. Helmut Hornof, translated by Greta Gerhardt and Cathy Hilger

INTRODUCTION

Helmut Hornof is a 48-year-old colonel, physical education teacher, and sports officer at the Theresianum-Military Academy in Wiener Neustadt, near Vienna, Austria. He was treated in 1983 (11 years after his accident) for phantom pain at the Bad Häring Rehabilitation Center. He is still active in competitive sports for the handicapped as well as in general contests. His activities include downhill and cross-country skiing, track and field (50-m and 400-m running; 500-m obstacle course, 1,000-m cross-country racing, shot-put, discus, javelin, and long jump), horseback riding, fencing, rifle shooting, swimming (diving, 10, 50, 100, 200, and 800 m) water-skiing, windsurfing, skydiving, mountain climbing, tennis, and table tennis. He teaches gymnastics (floor exercises, horizontal bar, parallel bar, Nissentrampoline and minitrampoline) and placed fifth in the pentathlon at the first Olympics for the handicapped in 1976 in Toronto. In 1979, he became Austrian champion in this event.

HELMUT'S DESCRIPTION OF THE ACCIDENT

On a rainy October evening in 1971, I was driving my car on a highway in Austria. Suddenly, out of the darkness, many lights appeared directly in front of me! I tried desperately to stop, but my attempt was unsuccessful, and I found myself involved in a four-car collision. Although I was shaken, I was unhurt and able to get out of my car and use my flashlight as a warning device for oncoming motorists.

The rainy darkness added to the already confused scene, and apparently contributed to my wandering off the safety shoulder and onto the highway proper, where I was struck by a car going in excess of 100 km/65 mph. The impact lifted me and threw me onto the pavement with such force that it shattered both my legs and left me with a concussion and contusion of the brain. Unconscious and with multiple wounds, I was rushed to a nearby community hospital.

HOSPITALIZATION

In anticipation of septic conditions, bilateral above-knee amputations were scheduled. My wife, however, had a different idea. As a laboratory technician, she was aware of the existence of other options, and when notified of the accident, insisted that I be transferred to the trauma hospital in Vienna where such alternatives could be better evaluated. There, a below-knee amputation was performed only on the right leg. In an attempt to save the left leg, pins were put into the bones and the leg was placed in a cast and put into traction. After intensive- and progressive-care stations, isolation wards, numerous I.V. fluids, and transfusions, the pain finally subsided.

Six more weeks in traction and a cast would follow before my first attempt with "cast and crutches." The first trip to the bathroom "on foot" was a most memorable event.

My guitar music helped me and my roommates pass the time. Somehow it seemed to ease, at least temporarily, our depression and to make our pain and problems more bearable.

REHABILITATION

At the end of 3 months, I was transferred from the trauma hospital to a rehabilitation center, where specific treatments began and a temporary prosthesis was fitted. Here, practice with crutches ended in an effort to master stairs.

All of my concerns were now directed to my left leg. There was no stability of the fracture or signs of callus formation. "What will I do if the fracture does not heal?" "Will there be another amputation?" "As a bilateral amputee, what will happen to my job?" "Will I have to settle for a desk job?" "What if I cannot settle for something less?" These and a thousand other questions tormented me as I analyzed my "future" from my hospital bed. Although I had recovered from the brain injury, my leg was refusing to heal.

The stump opened and drained after much weight bearing. The left leg still did not heal, necessitating my return to the trauma hospital for bone grafting and shortening of the fibula. After removal of stitches, another cast was applied. "Will this be the last one?" I could not "smell" this one any longer.

Six months had passed since that rainy October night, and healing still was not complete. All the bed rest and inactivity resulted in a prosthesis that no longer fit. I tried again to exercise. My efforts on the parallel bars were met with praise by the caring staff, and yet I was unable to share the nagging concerns about my leg.

Knowing that He has been called upon by much greater problems of human suffering, I began to question my own dialogue with God—a dialogue that seemed especially selfish in light of a fellow patient and young paraplegic who referred to my disability as "skin abrasions."

After what seemed like an eternity, the cast was removed. I was allowed to bear weight, a sign that my leg was preserved. It was weak because of the long inactivity in casts and incomplete peroneal nerve paresis, and it was 3 cm (1¼ inches) shorter. It looked like a stork's leg, and the knee and ankle were stiff—but WHO CARED? I COULD BEAR MY WEIGHT—HOORAY!

With full speed, I headed back to the rehabilitation center with a new therapy plan: knee bender, knee extender, underwater therapy, gait training, gymnastics, games in a sitting position, and, finally, swimming. What ecstasy that after 1 year, I could submerge my entire body underwater. The days were too short to satisfy my drive for training. Spring and summer passed, and finally I was able to run 400 m. What an exhilarating feeling of success! My training program was expanded to include carpentry, woodworking, basketweaving, and ceramics. My discharge from the center was imminent, and although I was elated, I was at the same time filled with anxiety. How would I be accepted by society? Would I be pitied? Would I be fit enough to satisfy the employment requirements for a high school physical education teacher?

In the interim, I accepted a temporary position at the Theresianum Military Academy. It required developing and operating a modern pentathlon at the military center. Funds for this project needed to be generated and required much public relations work on my part. Continuous community support necessitated numerous personal appearances of myself and of the team. Nagging questions returned—could I do it? Was I ready? Once accepted, the challenge soon found the team proving itself in international competitions. My personal rehabilitation, however, was less successful. My stump broke down. The use of crutches again symbolized to me, if not to the world, that I was indeed an invalid. I saw myself as less than perfect, and therefore, as inferior.

More hospitalization and surgery, a stump revision, and a new prosthesis followed as did a new impetus to regain former levels of competence. I started to ski and eventually worked as a ski instructor. What a joy when my students were unable to detect that I was an amputee. I began to race—outracing, in fact, many able-bodied competitors. I completed the 500-m obstacle course with all 20 obstacles and the 2.4-km test run (15 sec under the required time limit), and I placed fifth in the modern pentathlon (horseback riding, fencing, rifle shooting, swimming and cross-country run). There would be no more limits for me. My rehabilitation successes had secured my reemployment as a sports officer and coach at the military academy, where I continued to compete with both the able and the disabled. I no longer view my artificial limb as a handicap. It had become instead an integral and natural part of my body.

EPILOGUE

I credit my recovery to many things. My wife, whom I had married just 2½ months before that fateful October eve, has always been my emotional, mental, and physical support. Her original insistence on the trauma hospital saved my legs and, I personally believe, my life.

Our son, now 11 years old, has experienced all the ups and downs that growing up with a handicapped father involves. This has instilled in him an empathy with the disabled that has made us all proud. Other family members, friends, caring hospital staff, the rehabilitation team, including the physical education teachers, friends, the many roommates—all have contributed to who I am and where I am today. Without such support systems, recovery would be minimal at best.

I am enthusiastically living my life. I'm trying to work at my best to teach, to motivate, to love, and to help my students understand the purpose of life. To my fellow handicapped, I am trying to be an inspiration—to show them the meaning of all suffering, as well as the way to a better, productive, and happy life in spite of their handicap. Personally, I experience each day as a precious gift from God. For that gift, I am most grateful.

Figure 3.1 shows Helmut's achievements as an amputee.

Figure 3.1.

A. Helmut races before the accident and
B. As an amputee.
C. At age 47, he places first in his age group and fourth in overall rating in the 5- and 10-kilometer International Cross-Country Ski Race for Handicaps.
D. Skydiving.
E. He leads a group of new amputees for gait exercises only days after his long leg cast was removed from the left leg.
F. He downhill races after the amputation.

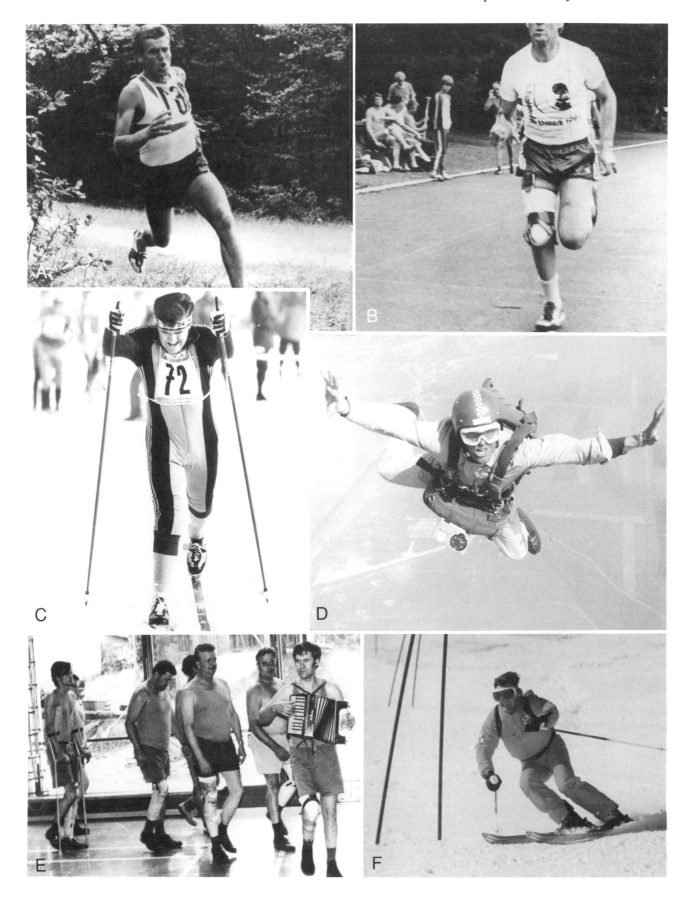

Figure 3.1.

SECTION

2

ORGANIZATIONAL AND PERSONNEL ASPECTS

4

Administration in a Rehabilitation Center

Everill W. Fowlks, M.D.

A successful rehabilitation center must integrate both administrative and medical services. Economic planning and decision making are just as vital as medical services to the functioning of a rehabilitation center.

A brief review of the background of rehabilitation centers will enable a better understanding of the administrative needs of the centers of today. World War II produced large numbers of severely disabled soldiers. Although great advances were being made in orthopaedics and neurosurgery for the treatment of the acutely disabled and injured, it soon became apparent that special centers were becoming necessary for the long periods of recovery of these patients. The armed services developed such centers at their major hospitals. However, space became limited, and many patients were transferred to the Veterans Administration (VA). To accommodate the influx of patients, the VA set up rehabilitation units in their major medical centers, which were integrated with the medical schools.

With the needs now faced by many of these new patients, the medical centers were very short of trained physical medicine and rehabilitation therapists. To meet these needs, the VA arranged the transfer of therapists being discharged from the armed services. This resulted in securing certified therapist personnel, among whom were a few physicians who had been trained during the war at the three major centers that were staffed by members of the Society of Physical Therapy Physicians. With this nucleus of physicians, the first training centers for physical medicine and rehabilitation were set up in the VA and in medical schools.

The smaller rehabilitation centers that were not adjacent to or affiliated with medical schools failed to plan adequately for the future. These centers attracted qualified therapists and physicians who had an interest in rehabilitation, but who lacked the proper administrative background. Within a period of 3 to 5 years, the grants awarded to these centers expired and they were forced to close for lack of funds. On the other hand, there were centers that did have fully qualified medical and administrative personnel, and they were able to expand because they had planned methods for obtaining funds after the original grants had expired.

It soon became apparent that at these centers, the physiatrist as medical director or chief of service would need administrative help. Centers began searching for specially trained therapists who had shown interest in becoming executive assistants or coordinators. These individuals would be responsible for the administration of the centers, working under the physiatrist. These coordinators had several duties:

1. They worked out an organizational scheme (or table) to show the interrelationships of the physiatrist with the coordinator, the consultants, the center and the outpatient clinics. These schemes were illustrated graphically and presented to the medical director-physiatrist for approval.
2. They prepared budgets for the center that were analyzed and from which 1- and 5-year plans were drawn. These plans considered salaries, consultant fees, equipment needs, costs of utilities, rental or building payments, custodial care, cost-of-living adjustments, and a contingency allotment. They reflected the present financial status and methods to be considered for obtaining future funding and grants. Lists were made of organizations that might be helpful to the center in its effort to fund itself presently and in the future.
3. They worked with the clinic personnel on a daily basis to keep the clinics running smoothly and within budget, and reported their findings weekly to the physiatrist in charge in order to discuss any problem areas.

In larger centers, the position of manager or administrator was established to take full charge of administrative matters of the center in close cooperation with its medical director. The coordinator would now become part of the medical-administrative management team. It would be up to that team to manage the center and develop plans for the future.

In the rehabilitation centers of today, coordinators have many additional duties:

1. They set up programs of preventive maintenance for all equipment and initiate early repair of any malfunctioning equipment to prevent large repair bills later. Any equipment needing extensive repairs is reported to the management team for consideration of repair or replacement according to the team's best economical judgment and available funds. Purchases are approved after standard bidding procedures are followed.
2. They propose special clinics and boards after consulting with clinical personnel regarding needs. They notify administrative consultants far enough in advance for them to prepare their reports.
3. They prepare the center for inspection by review boards, such as the Joint Commission of Accreditation of Hospitals.
4. They arrange weekly meetings between the physiatrist and the clinical personnel to assure quality care. At these meetings, intra- and interdepartmental relationships may be considered. Reports by the various members on literature in their official

journals make the personnel aware of newer developments and of the need for continuous medical education and research.

5. They develop plans for future education and research in the center. A budget should be developed for each clinic and the physiatrist to promote these plans, and to provide for attendance at the national specialty organizations and local seminars. The budget should consider the purchase of additional equipment and supplies necessary to develop a research study and protocol.

6. They arrange meetings with the consultants to determine if there are needs that are not covered in the 1- or 5-year plans. At the end of the fiscal year, a general meeting of all personnel should be called to determine how well both plans have served the needs of the clinics and the patients' care. The 1-year plan can be subjected to alterations at this time to make the subsequent 1-year plan better. The 5-year plan can also be reviewed and, if necessary, altered to meet its goals. The findings of this meeting should be presented to the management team for consideration and approval.

7. Each year, they should update the table of organization so that it reflects changes in both the clinical and consultant staffs and provides insight for changes in budget proposals.

The administration in a freestanding rehabilitation center has to understand and implement all aspects that are inherent in a modern bureaucracy, including legal safeguards and liabilities. Its responsibilities include financing, facilities and structure, staffing and contracts, equipment, organization of departments (e.g., payments and collections, personnel, payroll, medical records, stenography and telecommunications, insurance, housekeeping, maintenance, and engineering) and committees (e.g., utilization, safety, infection, and planning), short- and long-term forecast, and budget. It also has to facilitate integration of services with the community at large and its resources. Superior administration and business-like management are key elements for sound and economical delivery of quality medical care, and can even become essential to the survival of a rehabilitation department or center.

5

Rehabilitation in the Acute Care Hospital

John J. Gerhardt, M.D.

Rehabilitation of trauma, to be effective, must start on the day of admission. It is best done in specially designated trauma centers in which a *multi*disciplinary team is not only available but trained to work in a *inter*disciplinary, well-coordinated fashion. Traumatology has become one of the most important specialties in Europe; in the United States, it is just evolving on a larger scale basis. The analysis of failures or poor outcomes in trauma treatment points again and again to insufficient training of physicians in this area; poorly organized management; and the lack of qualified personnel, proper facilities, and adequate equipment. This is occurring in spite of the presently available knowledge of the medical, organizational, and rehabilitation principles necessary for comprehensive management of trauma, with the final goal of full social and vocational integration of the trauma victim.

Studies in Europe have shown that insufficient X-ray control in fracture casts is often the cause of complications (initially well-reduced fractures that slipped in the cast with corrections attempted too late—leading to additional damage of tissue or deformity).

In addition to their main activities (see Chapter 7), all team members need to be familiar with specific acute measures necessary at admission in order to be able to assist the acute team, and then to follow the patient in intensive care, progressive care, and the ward. Russe (1950) described the management of the trauma patient on admission to the acute hospital: "The triage and prioritization of patients is best done by use of the emergency categories scheme of Gögler. The priorities for treatment can change rapidly, however, as the patient's condition changes." The emergency categories of Gögler are:

1. Severe shock (massive external or internal bleeding), respiratory insufficiency, acute traumatic elevation of intracranial pressure, and extensive burns
2. Injury to intestinal or genitourinary tract without large hemorrhage, open craniocerebral injuries (open depressed skull fractures), transection of limb, injury of large vessels (reconstruction), and eye injuries
3. Open fractures and dislocations
4. Closed fractures and dislocations, lacerations, limited burns, and nerve injuries
5. Most severely injured, moribund with hopeless prognosis, and most cases of cardiac arrest with circulatory collapse

Figure 5.1 shows the equipment used in the management of these patients.

TREATMENT IN THE ACUTE HOSPITAL

The procedure for treating patients in an acute care hospital involves several steps:

1. Upon receiving notice from the site of an accident or ambulance, the complete acute treatment team in the hospital should be activated immediately to receive the patient. At least a surgeon or trauma surgeon and two registered nurses should be present. With patients in shock, there also should be an anesthesiologist with an additional nurse; with comatose patients, a neurosurgeon, X-ray and lab technicians should be present; and in all cases, other personnel must be on standby alert.
2. Measures initiated by rescue and ambulance teams should be continued (see Fig. 5.2). These measures include maintaining open airways, breathing, circulation, and using treatment for shock.
3. Clinical evaluation and documentation should be made regarding the patient's state of consciousness, respiration, and circulatory status. The status of injuries to the head, thorax, abdominal cavity, genitourinary organs, spine, and extremities should also be recorded and a neurological evaluation made.
4. There should be a laboratory evaluation, including complete blood count (CBC), hemoglobin (Hb), hematocrit (Hct), red cell count, white cell count, and thrombocyte count; Quick test; PO_2; PCO_2; Na-bicarbonate; base excess; PTT; SGOT; CPK; α-S-amylase; blood type and cross match; arterial blood gases (from the femoral artery), and chest X-ray.
5. In cases of multiple trauma, where the patient is in coma, an electrocardiogram (EKG) should be done and the central venous pressure determined; other procedures should include a neurosurgical evaluation; traumatology evaluation; routine X-rays, including a skull X-ray, (anteroposterior [AP] and lateral), cervical spine (AP and lateral), chest X-ray (AP with control of central venous catheter) pelvis X-ray, an angiography; CT scan as indicated; X-rays of any parts that have clinical symptoms of injury to bones or ligaments; abdominocentesis, if there is any suspicion of intraabdominal injury; and an indwelling catheter, except when the patient is bleeding from the urethra or when a bilateral anterior pelvic ring fracture is present. In these cases, an excretory urogram (I.V. pyelogram) should be done first. If catheter urine is bloody, a retrograde cystography, with 500 cc iodized contrast media, and an I.V.P. should be done first. Tetanus toxoid (Tetanol) and tetanus antitoxin (human) (Tetagam) should be given simultaneously.
6. Concomitant with diagnostic measures, therapy should be implemented. Treatment of shock, respiratory insufficiency, and

metabolic disturbances should be instituted. The restoration of blood volume can be done with colloid and crystalline solutions, but if the Hct is below 30, or Hb 10 or less microfiltered, whole blood should be given. This is done by the anesthesiologist, who also monitors and modifies it according to lab follow-up tests.

Treatment for Specific Injuries

Respiratory Insufficiency

With dyspnea and respiratory rate of 30/min and PO_2 less than 50 mm Hg (50 Torr) intubation and artificial respiration should be applied; O_2 content and PEEP should be regulated according to blood analysis results.

Chest Injuries

In tension pneumothorax, anterior upper thoracocentesis should be performed immediately (without X-rays) to release pressure; otherwise, all medicosurgical measures such as Bülau drainage and thoracocentesis should be done *after* emergency chest X-rays have been taken. If skin emphysema is a problem, multiple applications of thoracic drainage or anterior mediastinotomy should be performed. For craniocerebral injuries, neurological and neurosurgical evaluations should be made. There should be frequent controls, with exact progress notes of the patient's level of consciousness and pupillary size and reaction. If there is bleeding from the nose or ear, differentiation for liquorrhea must be done.

Abdominal Injuries

The most valuable single measure in suspected intraabdominal bleeding is the abdominocentesis and peritoneal lavage. It is done about 3.5 cm (1½ inches) below the umbilicus. The needle is inserted through an abdominal skinfold; the skin then is picked up with both hands by the assistant and lifted a minimal 7.5 cm (3 inches). One liter of solution (Ringer's lactate) should be introduced into the abdominal cavity, and the returning irrigation solution collected in multiple samples for comparison. Increasing blood content indicates progressive hemorrhage. The irrigation catheter should be left in place for 48 hr. Laparatomy should not be delayed.

In cases of *intraperitoneal rupture of the urinary bladder*, the bladder should be surgically exposed, and the rupture sutured and extraperitonealized. Kidney ruptures and ureter lesions immediately must be managed surgically. The injured urethra can be reconstructed primarily, or a suprapubic fistula can be created and final repair done 3 to 6 months later.

In *open fractures*, X-rays should be taken through the emergency dressing or the air splint. Removal of the dressing should be done just prior to definitive treatment in the operating room.

In *spinal cord injury*, the level of anesthesia and hypoesthesia should be determined and marked on the skin. Neurosurgical and traumatological diagnoses, including full spine X-rays, tomography and spine CT scans, should be obtained. If decompression is done, simultaneous stabilization is important. Attention to the skin, bladder, bowel, positioning, and rotation must be given.

INDICATIONS FOR EMERGENCY PROCEDURES

1. *Craniotomy.* After localization of intracranial hematoma
2. *Thoracotomy.* Performed if progressive hemotothorax is present after drainage or bleeding from drainage is more than 1 liter/hr
3. *Laparotomy.* If abdominocentesis is positive, or there are signs of diaphragmatic rupture via contrast filling of displaced stomach with soft nasogastric (NG) tube (angiographin or other absorbant iodine contrast media); during laparotomy, all intra- and extraperitoneal organs, such as urinary bladder, ureters, kidneys, pancreas, spleen, and liver, to be inspected and treated as necessary
4. *Incomplete progressive spinal cord injury.* Posterior decompression and stabilization as well as laminectomy to remove bony fragments; also recommended, osteosynthesis, with plates through the vertebral arch

Figure 5.1.   The Shock Room is used for admission, diagnostic evaluation, and emergency treatment of severely injured patients.

   A. In the shock room, the ceiling-mounted X-ray tubes have rails that allow movement across the room in both directions. Tubes have telescoping suspension for up and down motion and a turning radius of 360°.

   B. The anesthesia and resuscitation equipment, C-arm, and image intensifier are in proximity.

C–D. Movable transportation and a X-ray table with a C-arm and pedestal (donkey) are used. (see Chapter 16.)

   E. A pedestal (donkey) programmed exposure device is extremely helpful in the shock room as it avoids guessing or calculations of X-ray exposure settings, saves time and allows the production of acceptable X-rays under the most trying conditions.

   F. At the entrance to shock room, note the wide door, medicine cabinets, and ample storage space for supplies.

   G. Special traction beds are used in special trauma intensive care units.

Photos are courtesy of the trauma department at the University of Innsbruck and University Professor Dr. Otto Russe.

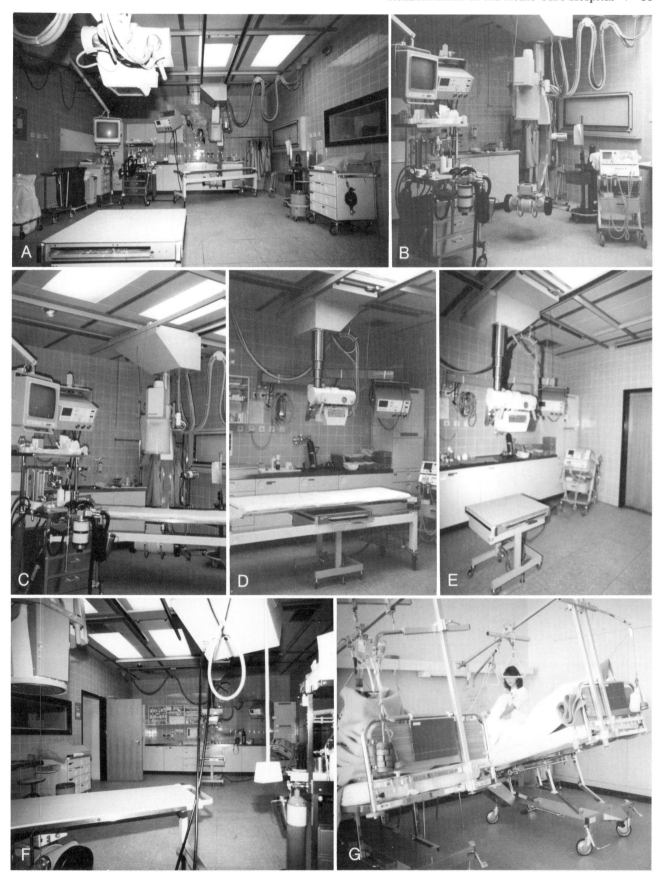

Figure 5.1.

5. *Genitourinary organs.* Kidney rupture and ureter lesions; require immediate surgery
6. *Open fractures.* Surgical treatment within 6 hr necessary; primary stabilization with osteosynthesis if general status permits (closed fractures: treatment according to general and technical requirements); follow-up treatment in specially equipped intensive care unit

The optimal treatment of the trauma patient is only accomplished if there is an uninterrupted sequence of life-saving and rehabilitation measures applied by informed and trained team members at the scene of the accident, during transportation, and continued until definitive treatment in an adequate hospital with a well-trained rehabilitation team and adequate facilities can be given. (Figs. 5.2 through 5.8).

Following the treatment in the acute hospital, long-term rehabilitation patients should be transferred to rehabilitation centers dedicated to the care of special injuries such as burns, craniocerebral-injured, spinal cord-injured, amputee patients, and others. After extensive rehabilitation, most accident victims can return home and to gainful occupations.

Figure 5.2. Treatment in the intensive care unit.

A. The patient should receive nursing care, feeding, respiratory care, and suction.
B. While a nurse applies tracheostomy care, the physical therapist is applying a passive motion through full range of the lower extremity.
C. Vibration massage should be done to loosen up mucus, and this should be followed by cough assistance.
D. Next, the patient should do breathing exercises using a tube.
E. Hand exercises often are also needed.
F. Arm-shoulder exercises are beneficial to patients in traction.

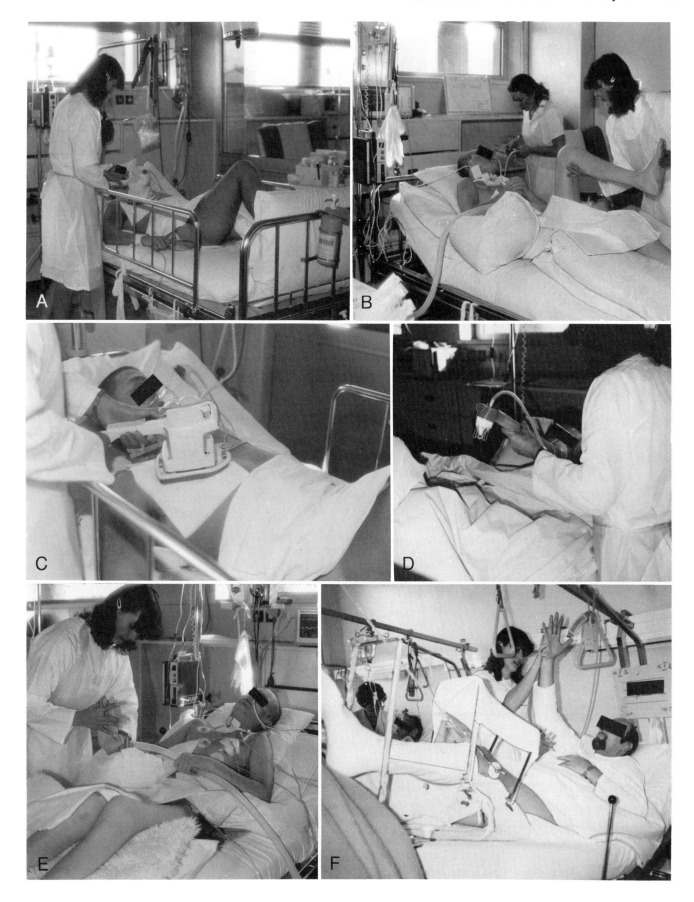

Figure 5.2.

Figure 5.3. Specific exercises in the intensive and progressive care units are vital to prevent secondary disabilities.

A–B. Knee exercises involve active-extension with the assistance of a pulley and gravity flexion.
  C. Patients can strengthen specific muscles through weighted exercises.
  D. Patients can increase knee flexion by exercising on the Böhler's knee bender apparatus.
  E. Hip-knee exercises are done on Böhler's "mountain climber" (Bergsteiger) apparatus.
  F. Quad-strengthening exercises can be done by using an arm pulley.
  G. Isokinetic exercises involve the use of Cybex apparatus.
H–I. Continuing passive motion (CPM) can be started in the recovery room while patient is still anesthetized.

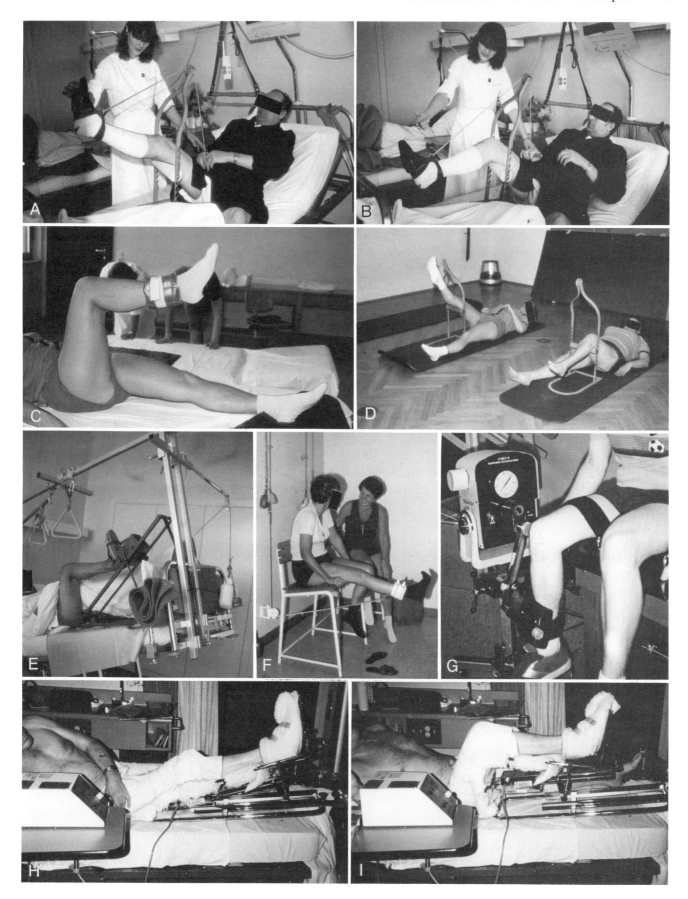

Figure 5.3.

Figure 5.4.

A–F. Bed exercises are necessary for nonambulatory patients with vertebral fractures. All joints of noninvolved extremities are exercised actively with assistance or passively as indicated.

G. Resistive exercises are used for lower extremity exercises postinjury and postsurgery of the hip.

H–I. Shoulder exercises are used for patients who are immobilized in a cast for multiple injuries, including wrist fracture and tendon repair.

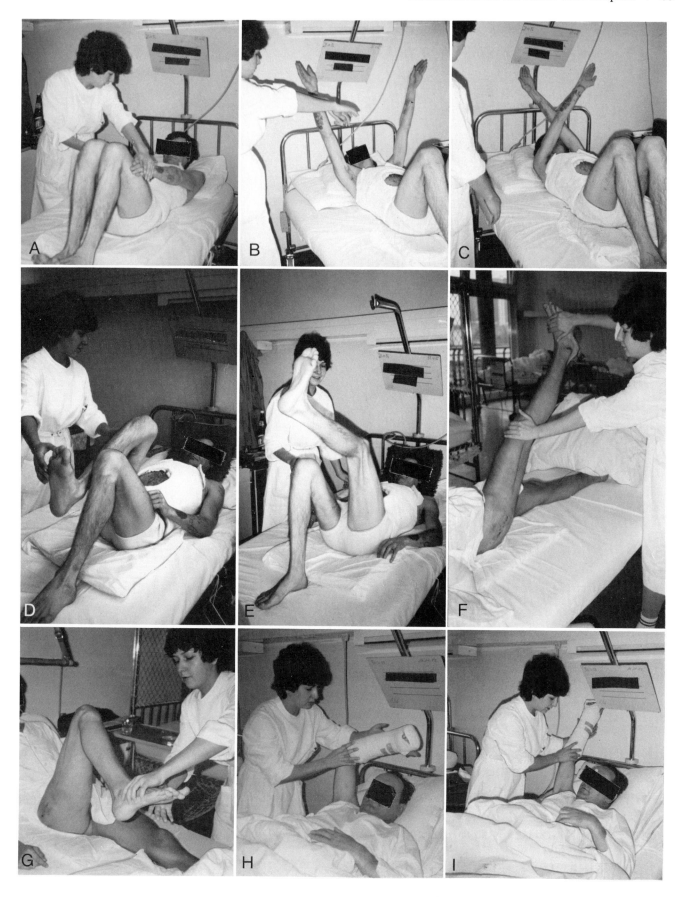

Figure 5.4.

Figure 5.5.

  A. Rehabilitation of patients with vertebral fracture requires special procedures. The vertebral fracture must be reduced immediately under local anesthesia injected into the hematoma.

  B. As early as few days after reduction, the patient is able to ambulate and to start gentle activities in the gym.

C–G. Progressive exercises on the ladder and rings in the gym can be carried out following the reduction of a vertebral fracture. The fracture should be immobilized in a Böhler's plaster of Paris hyperextension corset.

H–J. Floor exercises should be done on a mat.

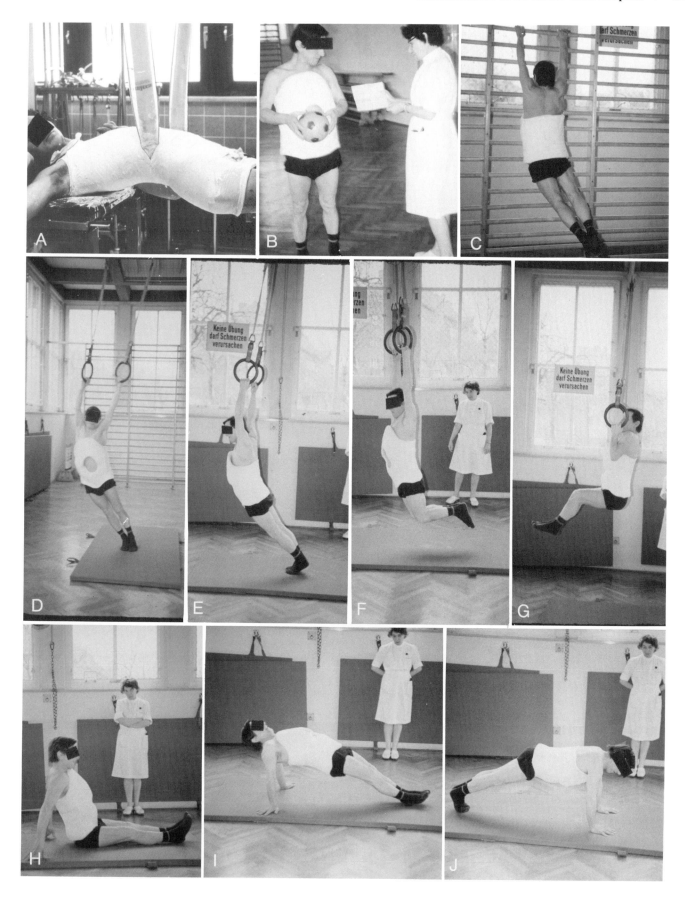

Figure 5.5.

Figure 5.6. Various group exercises are useful in rehabilitation.

A–B. While one patient practices independently, the therapist instructs other patients in mobilization and stretching exercises.

C. Instruction in active-extension exercises of trunk.

D. Group exercises in outpatient setting.

E–H. Shoulder exercises in ambulatory patients with plaster of Paris casts on upper extremities.

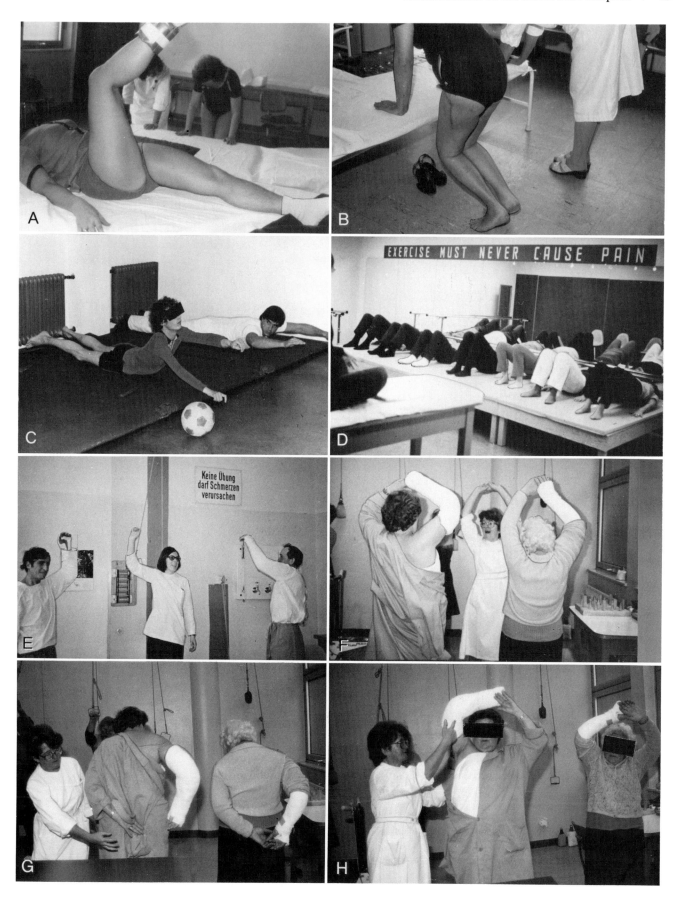

Figure 5.6.

Figure 5.7. Group exercises are extremely helpful as a treatment modality because patients learn from each other, compete, and experience no boredom.

A–D. Foot exercises and ambulation can be done with patients on crutches or canes.

   E. Here, a women's group exercises on mats with the assistance of sticks. (In the United States, redaptor stick exercises developed by Dr. Nashelsky are used.)

   F. Here, a men's group exercises on mats while the therapist corrects any faulty patterns that occur.

G–H. Women's and men's groups exercise in a gym. Assistive devices, such as clubs, balls, and stridex, are used.

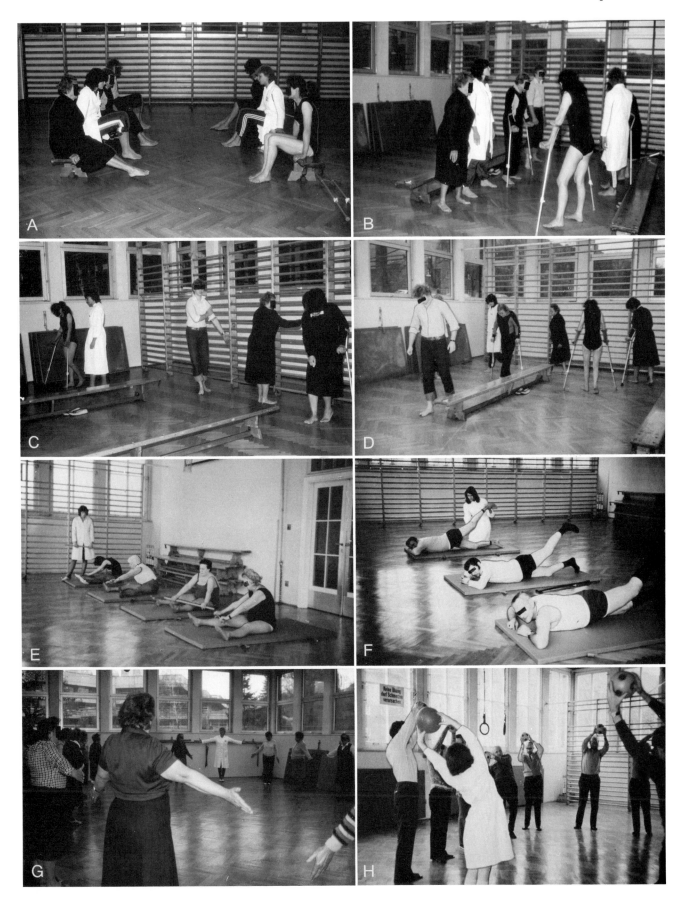

Figure 5.7.

Figure 5.8. Pool exercises can expedite the recovery of trauma patients.

A–B. Ambulation in water can include ascending and descending stairs.
    C. Flexion extension exercises of lower extremities should be done while the patient holds onto a bar.
    D. Underwater massage is helpful.
E–H. Pelvic traction is done in a tub and countertraction by a Glisan sling.

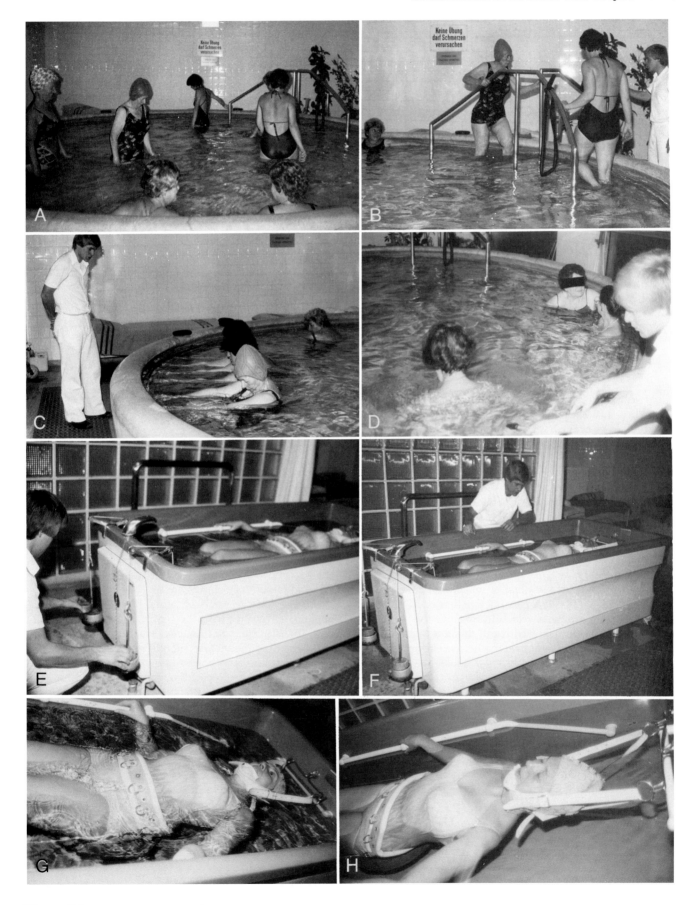

Figure 5.8.

6

Rehabilitation of Pediatric Traumatic Injuries

Timothy J.Campbell, M.D., and Ann Pellegrin, M.S.W.

HOSPITAL CARE

The principles of the management of the pediatric trauma patient are the same as for adults. The "ABC"s ("airway," "breathing," and "circulation") are the primary consideration in the initial evaluation and treatment of the pediatric trauma patient. Nevertheless, there are some physiological and psychological differences between the two groups of patients. The smaller size of the patient in the pediatric age group produces some potentially difficult technical problems in airway management and circulatory access.

Control and management of the airway is of primary importance. Intubation of the compromised airway may be difficult. The oral cavities of infants are small proportionately, and the glottis is more anterior than in adults, which tends to make intubation more difficult. Furthermore, the trachea is very short, only 5 cm in the infant and 7 cm at 18 months of age. Therefore, care must be taken to avoid inserting the endotracheal tube too far and intubating the right main-stem bronchus. Radiographic confirmation of endotracheal tube position is mandatory. The best guide for selecting the proper size endotracheal tube is to select the tube of the size of the patient's fifth finger or external nares.

A major pitfall in the evaluation of infant's and children's ventilation is related to pneumothorax. Because children's chests are relatively thin and hyperresonant, breath sounds are transmitted readily, and auscultation alone may miss a significant pneumothorax. The best clinical guide is to observe the chest for equal movements bilaterally. All children suffering from major trauma should have a chest X-ray as part of the initial evaluation to rule out pneumothorax, hemothorax, rib fractures, pulmonary contusions, or widened mediastinum.

Assessment, access, and maintenance of the infant's and children's circulation is critical for a successful outcome in major trauma.

Children's vital signs may change as they grow older (Table 6.1). Regardless of age, assessment of the peripheral circulation may be done by capillary refill. Access to circulation often presents a most vexing problem. If percutaneous peripheral venous lines cannot be established quickly, then a cut-down should be done. The preferred site for venous cut-down (in order) are: the greater saphenous vein at the ankle, the antecubital vein at the elbow, and the cephalic vein at the wrist or forearm. Central lines, if possible, should be used only for monitoring.

Table 6.1.
Vital Signs of Children

Age	Pulse	Blood Pressure	Respiration
Infant	160	80	40
Preschooler	140	90	30
Adolescent	120	100	20

Table 6.2.
Intravenous Fluid Used in Children

Child's Weight	Fluid Requirements
First 10 kg body weight	100 cc/kg/24 hr
Second 10 kg body weight (10–20 kg)	50 cc/kg/24 hr
Every kilogram over 20 kg	20 cc/kg/24 hr

Arterial and venous cut-down in the groin can be done in the patient who has major hypervolemic shock with peripheral circulatory shutdown.

Once venous access is obtained, the amount of intravenous fluid varies with the weight of the patient (Table 6.2). If the patient is in shock, a bolus of 20 cc per kilogram of Ringer's lactate should be given quickly. If no response occurs, another bolus should be given. If there is still no response, operative control of bleeding is almost always required, and type O negative blood should be started if type-specific or cross-match blood is not available. Packed cells should be given in 10 cc per kilogram bolus. If acidosis is present in the face of a PCO_2 of less than 40, sodium bicarbonate can be given, using the formula: milliequivalents of sodium bicarbonate is equal to the weight of the patient in kilograms $\times$ 0.3 $\times$ base deficit.

Children have a great amount of surface area per weight and thus become subject to hypothermia more readily than adults. Thus, great care should be exercised in the care of the pediatric patient to maintain a normal body temperature. Overhead warmers, warmed I.V. solution, and warm blankets should be used to avoid hypothermia.

Pediatric patients, in particular, are scared of unfamiliar surroundings. The receiving area for the pediatric patient, if possible, should be bright and cheery and have some pediatric decorations, such as pictures of animals or cartoon characters on the walls. Furthermore, the personnel caring for the patient should not wear masks to obliterate their facial appearance because this can lead to increased anxiety on the part of the children.

With appropriate concern to the environment and gentle care and handling of the patient, as well as aggressive treatment of life-threatening injuries, children respond beautifully and will have excellent survival following major traumatic episodes.

CARE AT THE REHABILITATION CENTER

Rehabilitation programs for children involve multidisciplinary teams representing the fields of not only medicine but also physical, occupational, and speech therapy; special education; nursing; social services; and child life, psychiatric, and psychological services. Other departments also are consulted as the need arises.

When a referral is received, an outreach visit is made by a physician, registered nurse, and physical therapist. An assessment is made of the child's suitability for the rehabilitation program. Prior to the actual admission, a tour of the facility is offered to the family. This allows them to meet with the staff and helps reduce their anxiety and fear of the unknown.

The child is admitted for a 2-week evaluation period, during which time team members assess the child's degree of functioning in the areas of mobility, self-care, cognitive ability, psychosocial interactions, education, physical abilities, and parent/sibling relationships.

At the end of the second week, team members meet to present their evaluations, and to determine the need for inpatient versus outpatient rehabilitation care. During the next week, daily schedules of activities are set up for the child and recorded in a notebook, which is given to the patient. Short- and long-term goals are formulated, and discharge planning commences. Each team member is responsible for an initial assessment, which is recorded on the patient's chart. Subsequent contacts are documented and may include changes in the goals and objectives; progress in therapies; new developments in treatment, and coordination with other disciplines, family, and community agencies.

At the weekly team/family meeting, a problem list is established and updated. A copy is recorded on the patient's medical chart. Discharge goals are formulated with input from the family and are discussed with the child. These goals are then put in the child's notebook. Thus, the notebook becomes a record of the rehabilitative process for the patient as well as for parents.

At an appropriate stage in the process, day and weekend passes are considered. This allows the family and staff to ascertain how the child will function in the home setting, and what modifications may be needed to accommodate the child's disabilities. Before a pass is issued, the parents must meet with the individual team members to observe therapies and nursing care. A list of questions relating to the child's ability to function in the home is given. Any questions or concerns are discussed at the next weekly meeting and modifications to discharge or therapy goals may be made.

As the child achieves the discharge goals, a meeting is set up with the family and appropriate community agencies (e.g., public school staff and counselors). This facilitates a smoother transition into the community and provides other caregivers with relevant information. Discharge summaries are written by the team members; these may include information on home programs in physical and occupational therapies, a nursing care plan, or community resources. The summaries are explained to the parents prior to the patient's discharge, and, with the parent's consent, copies are sent to the appropriate community agencies. A questionnaire evaluating the rehabilitation program is given to the family, and any suggestions for changes are considered by the team.

After the patient's discharge, follow-up care is provided at the outpatient clinic. The child and parents are seen by the physician; physical, occupational, and speech therapists; and the social worker. Any recommendations or changes in treatment are discussed with the family at this time. Outpatient followup must continue on a regular basis, and family members should be encouraged to contact rehabilitation team members if they have any questions or concerns.

7

The Rehabilitation Team

Eckhart Reiner, M.D.

Successful rehabilitation depends not only on a coordinated approach but also on good cooperation among team members from various medical and allied health specialties.

From the time that an accident occurs, it is helpful if all persons involved are knowledgable in first-aid and life-support procedures. A coordinated approach in removal of the severely injured patient from the accident site as well as in techniques of transportation often determine the final extent of disability. This chapter discusses separately the team at the accident site, in the general hospital, in the special trauma hospital, and in the rehabilitation center.

THE ACCIDENT SITE

Even at the accident site, several persons must work together to avoid further injury to the victim. First, there is the victim him- or herself, who, if not severely injured or unconscious, must *warn other traffic* and *call for help*. Next, if there are any individuals (laypersons) who are with the victim, they must *render first aid* at the site. If the victim is unable to move, then his or her removal and *correct positioning* require the intervention of special persons, e.g., an ambulance physician, police, or rescue team, who know the techniques of first aid.

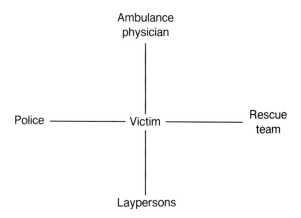

Certain procedures must be followed by these special persons in ensuring the victim proper care. For optimal positioning, first aid, and transport to the hospital, the following aspects must be considered: 1) the preservation of life; 2) the avoidance of pain and complications; 3) whether shock treatment is warranted; and 4) the prevention of additional injuries or shock. The decisions as to which hospital should receive the victim and whether the hospital should be informed by telephone or radio in advance about the kind of injury must be made at the accident site. Also, the hospital should be informed (if possible, in writing) about any medication given to the victim at the accident site or during transport. (The family should be informed of the accident as soon as possible by legal authorities or by the hospital and data should be obtained in regard to the patient's past history, medication, habits, etc.

A GENERAL HOSPITAL

Team members at a general hospital (one that has no special department for trauma patients) must work together closely. The victim should be admitted to such a hospital only if adequate treatment can be given there (e.g., for patients with an abdominal injury, vascular lesion, or eye injury) or if prolonged transport would be contraindicated. In either case, after emergency care is given, the patient should be brought by helicopter to a special hospital that has the capacity for providing the appropriate treatment, e.g., the reimplantation of extremities, or care for paraplegia, or severe craniocerebral trauma, when the interaction of team members is crucial.

THE TRAUMA HOSPITAL

At the trauma hospital, the number of team members grows. Because of its special staff and equipment, this type of hospital is prepared not only for early management, but also for the definitive treatment and management of the severely injured (e.g., amputees and paraplegics), from immediate postsurgical treatment to the delayed definitive prosthetic fitting. Although the preservation of life, shock treatment, surgical interventions, and conservative therapy are all important considerations, in the trauma hospital, medical therapy must always be at the center of attention. Rehabilitation by team members must start immediately. These members include physical and occupational therapists (for positioning, respiratory therapy exercises, and measures for prevention of contractures and decubiti), as well as social workers (to provide information about social law, to contact authorities, to help the family, etc.) The interaction of all of these elements is complex.

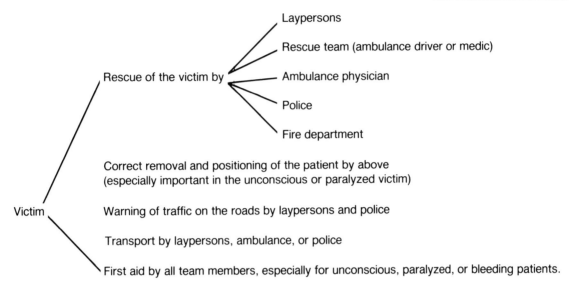

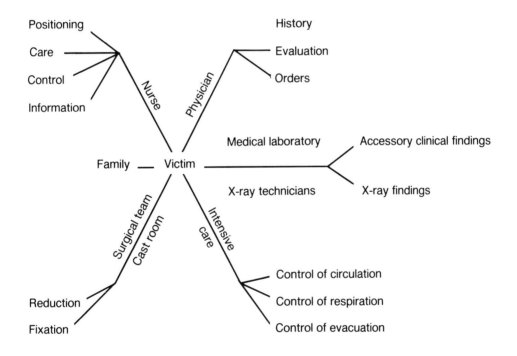

The therapy that is started after admission includes rehabilitation planning from the very beginning. This is very important when considering, for example, a surgically treated brachial palsy, with all the consecutive therapeutic measures, or a surgically stabilized vertebral fracture with spinal cord lesion. Especially in the latter, faulty positioning can lead to various kinds of contractures that require extremely lengthy treatment at best and can cause permanent secondary disability. The introduction and maintenance of an indwelling catheter for a long period of time may lead to a paraurethral abscess, with subsequent urethral fistula; this would require tedious urological treatment. Both complications would considerably impede the routine program at the rehabilitation center and cause major delays. The same is true in case of a decubitus ulcer, which develops quickly but heals slowly.

When the severely injured patient has regained consciousness at the intensive care unit, he or she needs gentle general care, which includes attention to psychological needs. Empathy, understanding, and adequate training are required of the personnel. Patients, especially if they are elderly, often wish for the comforting words of a clergyman. Such words may not only offer the patient the consolation of religion, but also may motivate him or her to cooperate with the team. From the very beginning, the patient should feel that the staff is not only concerned about the present medical situation, but also about him or her, as an individual with anxieties and needs. This

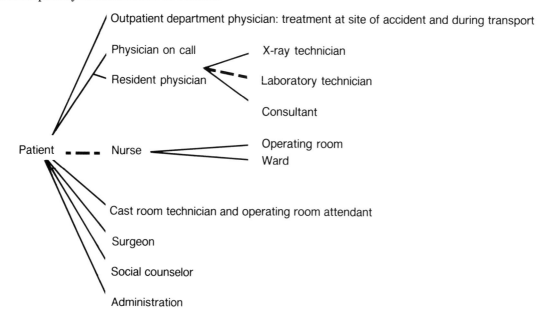

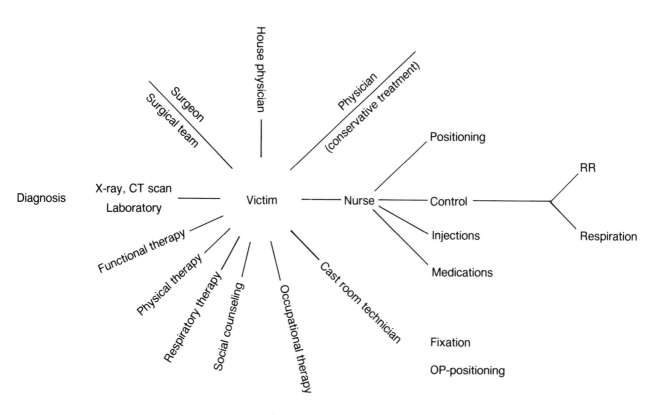

cannot be achieved by the physician alone, who usually is pressed for time, but requires the help of all team members.

THE REHABILITATION CENTER

At the rehabilitation center, it is essential that individual treatments are well coordinated, and this makes team cooperation especially important. Team members must be trained adequately, and each member also should be familiar with the tasks of the other members. To achieve

this, the team of every ward should meet once a week and report on the patient's problems, needs, and progress, as well as on organizational matters on the ward. A well-functioning information flow in vertical and horizontal directions is essential for successful rehabilitation. For all activities, the patient must be in the center; he or she is the focus and the most important member of the team.

The team in the rehabilitation center consists of many members, each of whom is equally important. Each member, in turn, takes the lead, according to the progress of

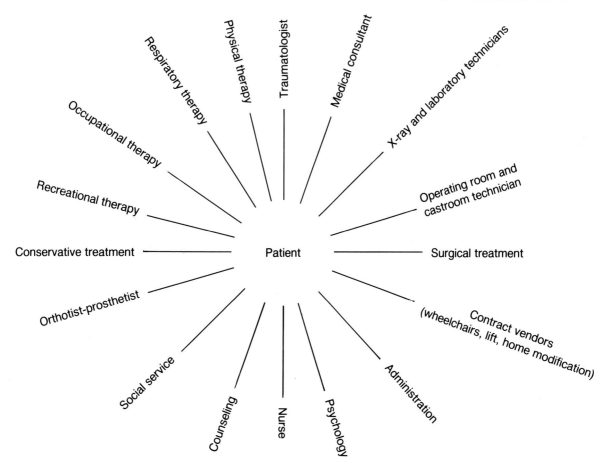

the patient undergoing rehabilitation. Once medical measures are successful, vocational and social problems may arise; the appropriate team member might be essential in helping to plan and organize the severely disabled patient's future. The *physician*, usually a physiatrist or traumatologist, by virtue of his or her education, experience, and responsibility for the patient, is the head of the team. He or she is assisted by *nurses*, who independently organize the routine care of the patient and who, along with the physician, are responsible for the special care of the patient. From the admission and beginning of treatment, special attention must be given to the prevention of complications, such as decubitus ulcers, joint contractures, urinary tract infections in patients with micturition difficulties, venous thrombosis, periarticular calcification near the large joints, and psychological problems arising from the awareness of permanent disability. This is where the *physical therapist, social worker, psychologist*, and if necessary, *speech pathologist* start their activities. In this first phase of rehabilitation, the *laboratory technician, X-ray technician, surgical nurse*, and *operating room attendants* are also important team members. In addition, long-term patients often require dental evaluations and treatment. These problems are discussed in different chapters.

When the patient can leave his or her bed and mobilization or ambulation is started, ambulation aids, such as walkers, forearm or axillary crutches, canes, wheelchairs, prostheses, orthoses, splints, corsets, or orthopaedic shoes,

often are required. The orthotist, prosthetist, and orthopaedic shoemaker can procure these aids or fabricate them according to the instructions and prescriptions of the physician. Since a physician cannot be familiar with all branches of medicine, he or she should consult specialists of other departments when necessary. The most frequently called consultants are the internist, urologist, neurologist, and orthopaedist. Occasionally, the general surgeon, neurosurgeon, plastic surgeon, gynecologist, opthalmologist, otorrhinolaryngologists, dermatologist, radiologist, and psychiatrist are also called.

The vocational counselor and the social worker not only take the social and vocational history, but also keep in touch with the disabled person's employer and with the appropriate authorities (among them, the employment office and the department of vocational rehabilitation). It frequently will be necessary to plan future accommodations with the patient and his or her family, to talk about vocational retraining, and to carry out social training. In order to give the patient the maximum mobility possible, he or she should be given the chance to obtain a driver's license for the handicapped as well as to modify his or her car, according to the disability.

In general, the rehabilitation center has three teams:

1. *The medical team on the ward.*
2. *The medical team of the center:* Consists of the physician and the supervisors of the individual therapies; solves the

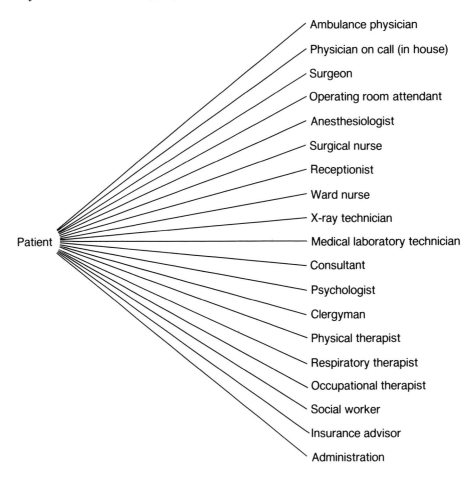

organizational problems of therapies that may arise and gives direction for comprehensive and coordinated delivery of treatment

3. *The sociomedical team*: Not only includes vocational counselors and social workers, but also members of the local unemployment office or representatives of insurance carriers; makes decisions far beyond the patient's stationary phase of treatment and influences his or her whole future, vocation, living accommodations, and social activities; is necessary to enable the severely disabled patient to live a life of fulfillment in a well-organized environment after his or her discharge

Figure 7.1 shows the overall functions of these teams.

CONCLUSION

Trauma can be simple or complex, involving one organ or many, one system or multiple systems. There can be profound physiological as well as psychological respon-

Figure 7.1. The rehabilitation team is responsible for many crucial activities.

A. Airways and breathing are restored by one team member at the accident site, while others alert an ambulance and prepare for the victim's removal.

B. The team assists during the helicopter transport.

C. The team ensures proper transfer of an accident victim with possible or probable injury to the spine (including cervical spine in craniocerebral injuries) into and from an ambulance.

D. The team in the shock room carries out simultaneous evaluation, tests, and emergency treatment.

E. The team assists in a critical care (intensive care) unit.

F. Nurses team at the progressive care unit.

G. An informal care conference is held by the minirehabilitation team in an acute care hospital.

H. A large rehabilitation center needs to be staffed by a complete team.

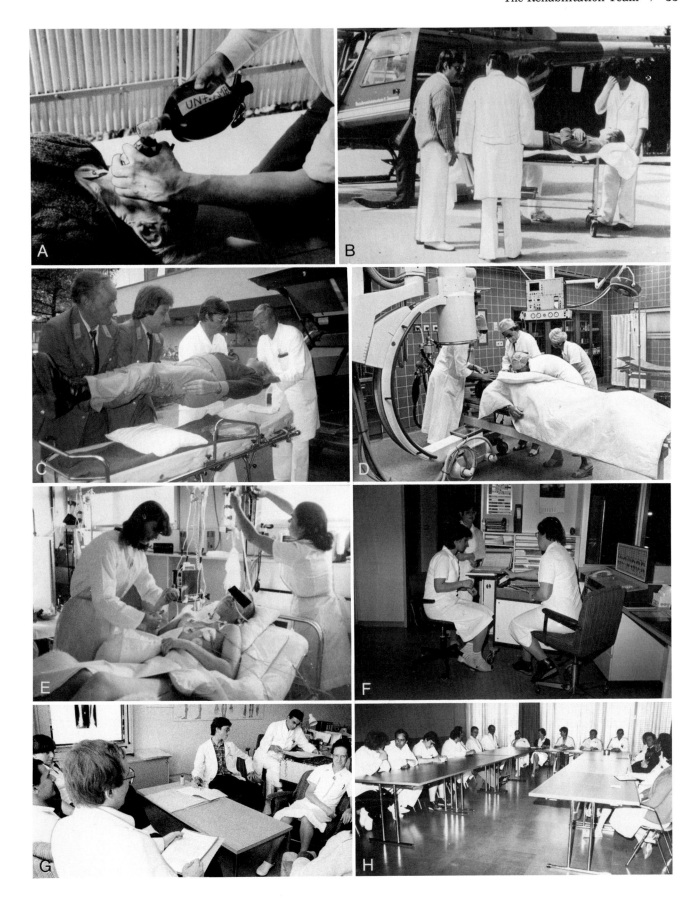

Figure 7.1.

ses. By rapid intervention, many lives can be saved and prolonged morbidity prevented. This is best done by an interdisciplinary team approach in a preplanned and co-ordinated manner.

The composition of the team varies with time and place, from the team at the accident site, to the acute hospital, to the most sophisticated trauma rehabilitation center. The authors wish to emphasize not only the importance of a "multidisciplinary" team but its "interdisciplinary" coordination and cooperation.

Each team member is familiar with the area of expertise of the other member, applying the necessary measures of his or her own special field, as well as enhancing and supporting the work of the other team members toward the victim's total comprehensive care. This can affect not only the immediate results of the team effort, but the final outcome and level of disability.

The team concept with the necessary multiple personnel may seem expensive and perhaps superfluous, but no single specialty can deliver all the diagnostic and therapeutic measures to save lives, shorten morbidity, prevent secondary disabilities, and lessen the extent of permanent disability to allow the victim reintegration into society, including resumption of gainful occupation.

Seen in this perspective, the interdisciplinary teamwork approach is the most effective from the medical-social point of view and the most cost effective by any standards.

8

The Organization of Therapy

Eckhart Reiner, M.D.

In the acute and long-term rehabilitation centers for trauma (for example, see Fig. 8.1), most patients undergo a variety of treatments. As shown in Table 8.1, these include services such as physical therapy, hydrotherapy, occupational therapy, and prosthetics/orthotics. Psychology, work therapy, social services, athletics, and sports for the disabled also are useful in treating trauma patients. A central organization of therapies is required so that

1. Patients become oriented as to the rehabilitation process.
2. A schedule can be established whereby a patient can be located during therapy hours.
3. Proper utilization of a therapist's time and therapeutic facilities can be controlled.
4. A patient's therapy record can be checked daily to determine his or her participation and compliance.
5. New admissions can be scheduled and adequately integrated into the therapies according to individual needs.

As the daily prescriptions for therapy are established, a treatment card for each patient should be filled out (see Fig. 8.2) and this schedule represented schematically in a weekly timetable (see Fig. 8.3). Each therapist should receive this every Monday morning. The schedule shows which therapist administers therapy to which patients, on which day of the week, at what time, and in which place. In this way, weekly prescriptions can be added easily to obtain monthly or quarterly totals and the quarterly sums to annual totals. This provides both the physician and the administration with solid information as a basis for negotiation, capital expenditure, hiring of staff members, and overall budget planning for the following year. The annual reports also provide objective statistical data for scientific studies.

How is therapy organized? After the patient has been admitted to the appropriate ward and has been assigned a room by the nurse, the secretary records the personal data of the patient. The physician proceeds to make a routine physical examination. The medical examination starts with a history, which should not only include information regarding the accident, but also any previous and present underlying diseases or previous injuries that might be significant for rehabilitation; particularly diseases reducing exercise tolerance or physical performance of the patient, such as heart disease, lung disease, or vascular disease; or diseases requiring special diet, such as diabetes, renal disease, or gout.

The findings should be recorded in the format of an expert evaluation and assessment. The therapy, either surgical, nonsurgical, or combined, is based on this assessment. The order of therapeutic measures must be determined. For every therapy not administered by the doctor him- or herself, a prescription is written. This prescription should include the kind of therapy and the number of applications. Diagnosis and precautions must be stated. Medication and orthotic or prosthetic devices are also prescribed. Each patient should then be discussed in the medical team conference; the attending physician reports patient's problems to the team and presents suggested further therapy, such as psychological, social, and vocational therapy. Special nursing care may also be discussed. After the evaluation of X-rays, laboratory tests, and other diagnostic procedures, a specific rehabilitation program should be established for each patient. Every therapist should become familiar with the program and understand the integrated and comprehensive rehabilitation effort. Weekly departmental conferences with the entire participating team encourages proper assessment and clarification of problems. Rehabilitative measures can then be tailored to the patient's individual needs. A good and successful outcome of the entire rehabilitative process is secured by dedicated and well-coordinated teamwork.

Figure 8.1.

A. Accident hospital Vienna 20 was founded in 1925 by Professor Dr. Lorenz Böhler.

B. The oldest rehabilitation center of the General Accident Insurance Company is Allgemeine Unfallversicherungsanstalt (AUVA) in Klosterneuburg near Vienna; from 1939 through 1959, a special department of the Accident Hosptial in the Webergasse was under the direction of Böhler; it became an independent institution in 1960 for the treatment of gait impairment and amputees; a most modern rehabilitation center is presently under construction.

C. An accident victim is admitted to the shock room.

D. The rehabilitation center at Bad Häring in Tirol, Austria, opened in 1973 as the main rehabilitation center for Western Austria. It is designed for treatment of all accident patients, such as spinal cord injury, craniocerebral injuries, amputees, and other patients with impairment of locomotor apparatus. At present, it is the most modern center of the AUVA system.

E. The newest accident hospital is Graz-Algerdorf, which opened in 1981.

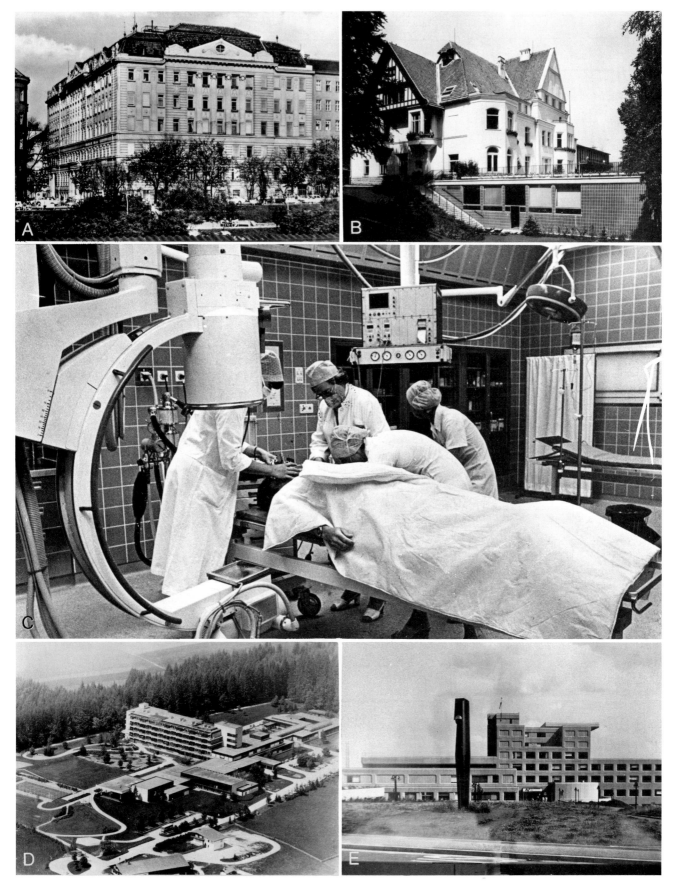

Figure 8.1.

Table 8.1.   Codes for Modalities, Activities, Prosthetics, and Orthotics

Physical Therapy

1.   Breathing exercises
2.   Individual exercises
      Stump exercises
3.   Cryotherapy (ice)
4.   Group exercises
      A. Spinal (neck and back)
      B. Upper extremity (shoulder)
      C. Lower extremity (knee)
      D. Spinal cord
5.   Electrotherapy
      A. Ultraviolet
      B. Sollux
      C. Microwaves
      D. Syretherm
      E. Short wave diathermy
      F. Diadynamic
      G. Diagnostic
      H. Stimulation
      I. Surging
      J. Galvanization
6.   Gait training (for spinal cord injury patients and amputees)
      Exercises for spinal cord injury patients
      Exercises for amputees
      Exercises without orthotic devices
      Exercise with orthotic devices
7.   Physical education
      A. General exercises for the upper extremity
      A. General exercises for the lower extremity
      A. General exercises for amputees
      General conditioning exercises
      Games for spinal cord injury
      B. Games for the upper and lower extremities
      B. Games for amputees
      B. Games for spinal cord injury patients (e.g., table tennis)

Hydro- and Balneotherapy

8.   Swimming
      A. For swimmers
      B. For nonswimmers
      C. For amputees
      D. For spinal cord injury patients
9.   Movement bath
10. Walking bath
11. Medicated bath
      A. Scrubbing bath
      B. Oak bark
      C. Spruce needles
      D. Meadow hay flowers
      E. Chamomille
      F. Carbon dioxide
      G. Aerated bath
      H. Mood bath
      I. Rosemary
      J. Brine bath (salt water)
      K. Oxygen
      L. Sulphur
12. Contrast bath (foot/arm)
13. A. Stanger bath (electr)
      B. Four-cell bath (electr)
14. Underwater massage
15. Partial massage
16. Manual lymphdrainage
17. Mudpacks
18. Paraffin treatment
19. Sauna

Occupational Therapy/Ergotherapy

20. Functional occupational therapy
      A. Muscle-strengthening
      B. Mobility
      C. Motor skills, dexterity
      D. General occupational therapy
      E. Self-help training

F. Prosthetic training

G. Concentration and memory training, cognitive training

H. School substitution training

I. Audiovisual activities, photography

20. J. Household training, ADL

1. Weaving	12. Leatherwork
2. Weaving baskets	13. Needlework, sewing
3. Woodworking	14. Pin—games
4. Metal work	15. Inner-bark fibre and straw work
5. Enamel	
6. Mosaic, inlay work	16. Typing
7. Drafting, painting	17. Writing
	18. Reading, speech
8. Painting on wood	19. Knitting
9. Wire sculpture	20. Thread, twine, cord work
10. Batik, silkscreen, printing	21. Television Lab.
11. Claywork, ceramic	22. Bicycle bandsaw
	23. Standing table

21. Work therapy (manual) wood
22. Work therapy (manual) metal
23. Work therapy—gardening
24. Work therapy—electronics

Prosthetics/Orthotics

25. Orthopaedic shoes
26. BK prosthesis
27. AK prosthesis
28. Knee disarticulation prosthesis
29. Hip disarticulation prosthesis
30. Hand partial—hand prosthesis
31. BE prosthesis
32. AE prosthesis
33. Shoulder disarticulation prosthesis
34. Canes
35. Crutches
36. Wheelchairs
37. Upper extremity orthotics
38. Lower extremity orthotics
39. Spinal trunk orthotics

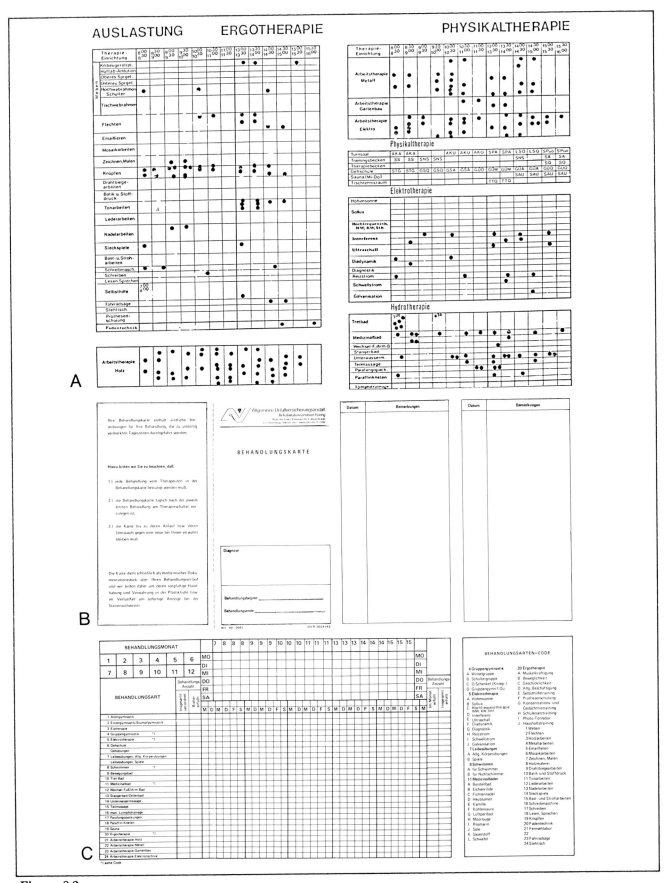

Figure 8.2.
  A. Example of schedule of various therapies.

B–C. A patient's treatment card should contain the codes of all mentioned modalities listed in
    Table 8.1 as well as schedules for the week and month and dates of actual attendance.

Figure 8.3.

A. A wall chart shows an overview of weekly schedules for all patients and therapists in all programs.

B. The wall chart schedules must match the patient's treatment card.

C. The wall chart should be updated every day.

D. The therapist's daily load schedule for one work week is shown. It should be updated every week.

E. All patients register at the desk prior to and after completion of each therapy session; the attendance and modalities are recorded on the wall chart as well as on patient's treatment card.

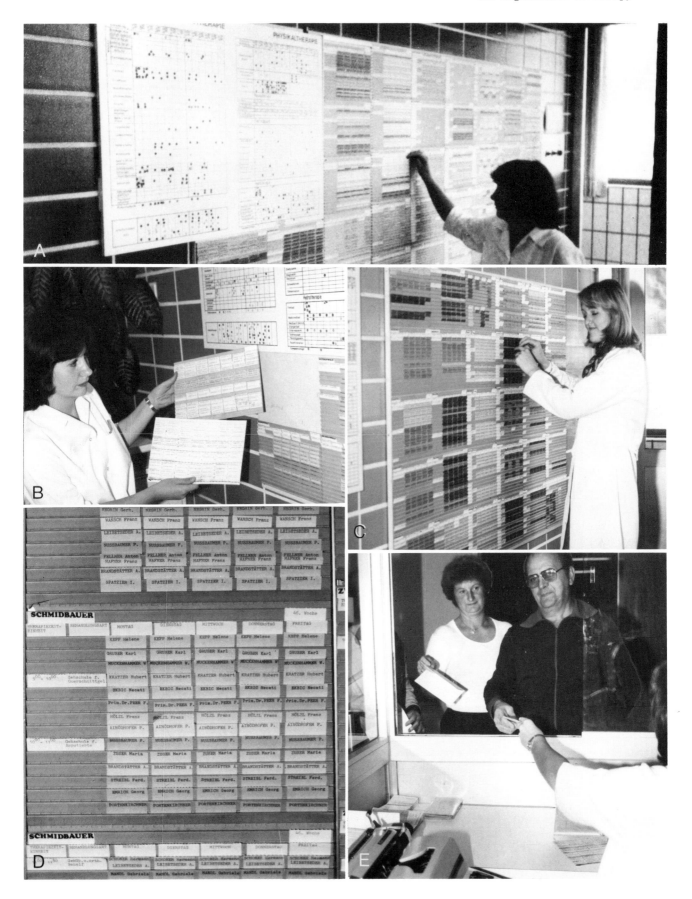

Figure 8.3.

SECTION

3

―――――

GENERAL THERAPEUTIC DISCIPLINES AND MODALITIES

9

Nursing

Bette Perman, R.N., M.S.

Trauma care is team care. The participation of nurses on the trauma team usually begins in the emergency room, continues through the critical care and medical-surgical wards; then to rehabilitation facilities; and finally, to home care. The practice of nursing in each of these areas in essence is the same, although the activities of the nurse may be vastly different. Whether the nurse is suctioning an airway, responding to pulmonary artery pressure changes, changing a sterile dressing, or teaching the patient's significant other to change the dressing, the goal is:

... to assist the individual in the performance of those activities contributing to health or its recovery (or to peaceful death) that he would perform unaided if he had the necessary strength, will, or knowledge, and to do this in such a way as to help him gain independence as rapidly as possible (Henderson, 1966, p 00).

In the emergency room, it is essential that the nurse and physician perform accurate and rapid assessments and interventions. Although the primary focus of both team members will be the support of vital life functions, the nurse also will begin to gather from the patient and his or her family information that will assist the team in the care planning process following the initial crisis.

Understanding the need for the patient to conserve energy and to minimize stress, the nurse must remain in constant attendance with the patient to reassure him or her of the surroundings and to provide information for the patient and his or her family, which the patient needs to feel safe. As the nurse is building that relationship, he or she must also systematically gather data from numerous sources and organize that data for its retrieval later.

Generally when the trauma patient leaves the emergency room, he or she is transferred to the operating room and/or the critical care setting. The critical care nurse receives the information obtained from the emergency room nurse, assesses the immediate needs of the patient in conjunction with the physician, and establishes a plan of care. At this point, information from the family or significant other is explored at greater length, and the "roles" expected by the patient, family, and health care team members are clarified.

During the critical care experience, the health care team must address vital and often unfamiliar issues with the patient and family. Issues such as artificial life support, cardiopulmonary resuscitation, and the risks and benefits of care must be explored and explained in a manner sensitive to the needs of a patient and family in crisis. The nurse must be advised closely of all information that is given to the patient and family so that he or she can assist them in understanding the information in the hours that follow. The critical care nurse must understand that individuals in crisis are limited in their ability to "hear" information; therefore, each encounter the nurse has with either patient or family must begin with an assessment of their present understanding. Clear documentation by the nurse of the patient/family understanding and their response to the crisis situation will assist all members of the trauma team in carrying out the treatment plans.

When the patient's physiological status has stabilized, he or she will be transferred from the critical care area to a medical-surgical department and the "work" of therapy, directed at maximizing that individual's independence, proceeds. The primary nurse responsible for the coordination of the plan of care should be introduced to the patient and family. The primary nurse will meet regularly with the other health care team members to assist in the evaluation of the treatment care plan and in the establishment of the discharge planning goals.

Discharge from the hospital, for some patients, also means recovery. For others, it is a change of location to an environment of rehabilitative specialists. Intensive planning and evaluation of the rehabilitation goals occur regularly. In this environment, as in the hospital, the team role of the nurse is that of coordinator, so that his or her intensive efforts at maximizing the patient's abilities do not smother or overwhelm him or her.

The trauma patient's experience moves from a life-threatening experience, to stabilization of physiological functions, to establishment of discharge goals, and finally to goals for maximum independence. The maintenance of that continuum is the goal of the trauma team; the coordination and communication of that process through systematic and interdependent problem-solving steps is the contribution of the nurse.

10

Nutrition and Diet: Nutritional Considerations of Trauma Patients

Signa P. Gibson, M.S., R.D.

Trauma patients require an assessment of nutritional needs and eating ability to prevent malnutrition during the recovery period. Traumatic injury can create hypermetabolic nutritional demands requiring specialized feeding regimes.

Response to severe trauma, such as spinal cord injury, begins with phase of elvated energy expenditure and nitrogen loss. Infection or decubiti increase the catabolic response. Following a period when energy needs and nitrogen excretion are reduced, an anabolic phase of restoration of protein and adipose tissue stores occurs.

Specific nutrient and metabolic needs of the patient should be determined by a clinical dietition. The objectives of nutritional assessment are: to calculate nutritional requirements, evaluate the patient's ability to meet the requirements, and identify patients requiring specialized nutritional care plans.

Standard nutritional assessment methods include anthropometric measures, evaluations of biochemical and laboratory data, clinical observations, and dietary evaluations. Measurable indicators of the severity of postinjury malnutrition include: height, weight and recent weight change; estimated fat and muscle mass stores compared to standard triceps skinfold and midarm muscle circumference; estimated lean body mass compared to standard urinary creatinine-height index; calculated daily nitrogen balance indicating degree of catabolism; total lymphocyte count or percentage of lymphocytes in total white blood cells; skin testing for sensitivity to common recall antigens indicating immune function; and serum albumin and calculated transferrin from laboratory analysis of the total iron-binding capacity, which indicates plasma protein.

Kilocalorie requirements should be individually adjusted above basal energy expenditure (BEE) to provide for catabolism, physical activity, fever, or malnutrition, as applicable. Energy needs may increase by 50% or more above the BEE, but overfeeding at greater than two times the BEE is generally not recommended. The Harris Benedict Equation provides a mean of estimating the BEE using sex, height, weight, and age as primary factors:

Women: BEE = 665 + (9.6 × weight [kg])
+ (1.7 × height [cm]) − (4.7 × age)
Men: BEE = 66 + (13.7 × weight [kg])
+ (5 × height [cm]) − (6.8 × age)

Protein intake following injury should be 1.0–1.5 g/kg, however energy and protein needs are interrelated. The ratio of total energy to nitrogen required during catabolism or anabolism should be approximately 150:1. Nitrogen can be calculated by dividing grams of protein by 6.25.

The Recommended Dietary Allowances provide a nutrient intake standard for vitamins and minerals. Fluid intake should be 2 to 3 liters per day if renal function is normal. Some head injuries may require fluid restrictions.

The nutritional care plan should incorporate the multidisciplinary team evaluation of appetite, gag reflex, swallowing and chewing abilities, facial paralysis, gastrointestinal tract integrity, ability to feed self, and social adjustments to the injury. Family members and the patient can assist in the team evaluation by providing baseline data regarding the patient's previous eating history, food preferences, and usual appetite pattern.

The collective data base provides the information for the dietitian to develop an individual feeding plan that is acceptable to the patient. Food selections should reflect the patient's psychological and cultural eating patterns in addition to meeting physical requirements (liquid, soft, or mechanical diet).

The eating process should be adapted to the strength and degree of the motor control of the patient. Feeding assistance, texture modifications, variety in temperature and taste, and adaptive eating utensils may encourage optimal oral intake. If the patient's appetite is depressed, small, frequent meals may be more appealing than large meals.

Nutritional adequacy may not be achieved in the hypermetabolic patient by oral intake. Enteral tube feedings may replace or supplement oral feedings. Commercial formulas are available for normal and altered functioning gastrointestinal tracts. Standard concentrations of 1, 1½, or 2 kcal/cc are available. Peripheral vein feeding or total parenteral nutrition (TPN) provides additional nutritional support for selected patients.

Patient tolerance of the nutritional care plan should be monitored continually by the dietitian and the multidisciplinary team. Body weight, daily calorie counts, nitrogen balance studies, and repeated laboratory tests provide measurable evaluation tools for assessing the patient's progress.

11

Occupational Therapy

Sonja Laznik, O.T.R., and George Peiger, O.T.R.

Over the years, occupational therapy has progressed from diversionary activities, such as making simple objects, to its present state as a comprehensive and integrated service that requires a specially trained staff. The therapist's work with a severely disabled patient runs the gamut of the patient's stay at the hospital: from the time when he or she has regained consciousness on the intensive care unit; to the patient's transfer to another ward; to the time he or she progresses to outpatient status; and finally to the final discharge.

In general, occupational therapy encompasses the following tasks:

Self-help training. Retraining and exercise for self-feeding and hygiene

Activities of daily living (ADL). Use of telephones, operation of plugs and switches, opening of letters, etc.

Homemaking training. Cooking, cleaning, washing, infant nursing, (e.g., for arm amputees, in cases of upper extremity pareses, or for persons with other disabilities)

Vocational training. Doing routine exercise activities, acquiring new skills, preparing for vocational reeducation, and work hardening

Social training. Group activities, group process sensory testing, and reeducation

Training of residual functions and compensation for lost functions. Exercise, manual skills (according to the handicap); gives the patient the experience of success and motivates him or her for active cooperation; various chapters in this volume go into detail

Fabrication of static and dynamic splints. For hand and arm and of aids for temporary use

Fabrication or procurement of definite assistive devices. Follows consultation with the nursing staff and physical and/or corrective therapists; e.g., wheelchairs, arthrodesis-wheelchair

Training of upper limb amputees. Both prosthetic training and one-hand training

When considering the great variety of tasks in which the occupational therapist is proficient, obviously there will be some overlap with the tasks of other team members. Particularly in self-help training, it is essential for the occupational therapist to communicate with the physical or corrective therapist and to cooperate with the nursing staff. For example, a person's routine homemaking activities may be possible only with mechanical aids or after physical/mechanical modifications of a dwelling. In order to achieve better mobility, that same person may need a

driver's license in order to be independent of public transportation. And, because the modern labor market offers the opportunity for qualified physically disabled workers to function in many fields, that same person may need adaptations of the workplace. If that patient has psychosocial dysfunction or craniocerebral trauma, therapy also requires close cooperation with the psychologist. Therefore, vocational rehabilitation is a field in which occupational therapy, social work, and physical therapy overlap.

The work of the team that deals with trauma patients should concentrate on the patient and should be controlled and coordinated by the attending physician. As one of the members of this team, the occupational therapist guides the patient's activities and accompanies and supports the individual on his or her way back to society, a path that the patient must help make for him- or herself. The occupational therapist can only assist and accompany the patient until he or she can function independently. Only then can the goal of rehabilitation be achieved.

It is beyond the scope of this work to discuss the different kinds of injuries separately; therefore, the following classification has been chosen:

1. Functional training of the upper extremity
2. Splinting for the upper extremity
3. Functional training of the lower extremity
4. Training of upper extremity amputees
5. Occupational therapy of patients with spinal cord injuries
6. Functional training of patients with craniocerebral injuries
7. Work therapy

It is not the intent of this classification to provide an in-depth protocol for each category, but rather to provide an overview that can be applied to an individual's own milieu. Omitted items (e.g., patients with craniocerebral injuries) are discussed in other chapters.

FUNCTIONAL TRAINING OF THE UPPER EXTREMITY

The human hand is, by its nature, able to perform a great variety of activities, with its abilities ranging from fine prehension to the power grip; from discrete sensibility to the most refined expressions of gesticulation.

If trauma to the hand results in loss of the gripping ability or of sensation, or if the hand is lost completely, the integrity of the whole person often is severely violated. Therefore, the role of occupational therapy after hand and arm injuries is clearly evident. After hand injuries, the various prehensile mechanisms must be exercised. In upper extremity injuries, the hand must be brought into the functional position. Bilateral injury compounds the problem. The complexity of arm and hand movements must be kept in mind. This requires adequate experience of the therapist, who must appropriately combine his or her training to promote power grip and tactile prehension as well as to promote skill in the routine pursuits of life, including coordination of movement.

Exercises for the hand and arm fall into several categories: (a) gripping training, (b) ADL (self-help) training, (c) general motivating exercises, and (d) sensibility training.

Gripping Training

Contracted finger joints may be loosened by working with therapy-plasticine. This material allows manifold activities, such as kneading, rolling, and forceful grasping. There are no limits to the therapist's inventiveness. The same is true when working with clay and at the potter's wheel. In addition to functional exercise of the finger joints, clay modeling stimulates the creativity of the patient. Prehension and gross grip are exercised by various media, with or without aids. The different sizes of the components of activities allow a gradual increase in the requirements on the patient's gripping skills. For simultaneous training of both hands, tying knots in macrame, plaiting, typing, and many other activities are useful (see Fig. 11.1).

ADL (Self-Help) Training

ADL training means training of self-help skills, such as bathing, eating, and dressing independently. The skill and inventiveness of the therapist in fabricating aids can facilitate these activities. Often, homemaking training (i.e., cooking, dishwashing, cleaning house, and doing laundry) may be required.

It is often important to develop communication skills, such as writing with or without a typewriter. If the function of one hand is completely lost, the patient must be retrained in maximal use of the remaining hand.

General Motivating Exercises

As the patient becomes involved in his rehabilitation program, each success he or she experiences has the effect of motivating him or her to move on and try a task that is a bit more challenging. Often this process begins in occupational therapy, when the patient succeeds at a game or produces a useful object (see Fig. 11.1).

Sensibility Training

Trauma can result in the loss of sensibility on the fingertips of the hand. When this occurs, the hand is essentially "blind" for functional use. The occupational therapist has special skills in testing sensibility to determine the appropriate time for beginning a sensory reeducation program, which improves the functional status to the maximum.

SPLINTING FOR THE UPPER EXTREMITY

Splinting an injured hand or arm may be necessary for several reasons, the most important of which are:

To immobilize it temporarily after injury to promote the healing of wounds and fractures
To prevent inappropriate positions of joints, therefore relieving tension on peripheral nerves when repairs have been completed
To use as gripping aids, e.g., an opponens splint (see Fig. 11.2), so that the hand can be in a functional position
To mobilize contracted finger or arm joints by using elastic bands

Materials used for splints are manifold. They can be divided into natural materials, like leather, cork, and metal; and synthetic materials such as Plexidur, which can be shaped under high temperatures or Orthoplast or Polyform, which can be shaped under low temperatures. These materials can be shaped directly on the hand or arm without a positive plaster case.

The following splints are commonly used:

Radial positioning splint and dorsal upper arm splint as immobilizing splints
Finger alignment splint as dynamic splint
Opponens splint as gripping aid

For the various other types of specialized splints (e.g., for peripheral nerve injuries), special publications are available.

It is essential that the fabrication of splints is left to experienced personnel and that the splint is regularly controlled by the physician and modified if necessary. For the fabrication of a positive plaster cast, in most cases the cooperation of a prosthetist is required.

FUNCTIONAL TRAINING OF THE LOWER EXTREMITY

Occupational therapy of leg injuries, as with the hand and arm, is based on functional anatomy. The occupational therapist must keep in mind both the individual joints and the interaction of several joints in routine movements, as well as the varying force factors. For training of the individual joints, the weaving loom is of particular importance (Fig. 11.3).

The following are possibilities for the operation of the weaving reed:

Training of the talocalcaneal joint. Pronation and supination of the foot
Ankle joint. Dorsiflexion and plantar flexion of the ankle joint
Flexion in the knee joint. Loom with special adapted reeds is used; the reed is adjusted by the extension (stretching) of the quadriceps femoris muscle and by the flexion of the knee joint (stretching the extensor muscles)
Hip joint movement. Usually combinations of abduction (external rotation) and adduction (internal rotation) of the hip joint

In all the exercises used with the weaving reed, required force factors can be adjusted by the predetermination of a certain amount of tension. While the leg is exercised, other joints are relieved from weight. For the simultaneous training of all leg joints, the bicycle saw can be useful.

The force factors effecting the leg can be increased by mechanical resistance of the pedals. To increase the exercise tolerance of the leg, various activities that allow the combination of work in the sitting and standing positions, such as Rya knotting and working with clay, may be useful.

When certain injuries of the knee and hip joint have resulted in severely restricted movement, exercises for self-help will have to be done. The therapy may have to provide the patient with assistive devices, such as aids for drying the foot or putting on stockings and trousers. An arthrodesis wheelchair, aids in getting up, and an elevated toilet seat may be useful. Proper shoes are also important.

TRAINING OF UPPER EXTREMITY AMPUTEES

The treatment of upper extremity amputees after the loss of a hand, lower arm, upper arm, or shoulder joint can be a great challenge to both the therapist and the prosthetist. Although it is entirely left to the prosthetist to fabricate and fit the upper extremity prosthesis and to introduce the patient to the technique of prosthetics at the beginning, it is the role of the occupational therapist to take responsibility for the choice of the prosthetic system and later to continue training the patient with his or her prosthesis. The decision as to which prosthesis is chosen is considerably influenced by the patient's vocation, recreational activities, and social needs, as well as by the condition of the stump and the level of the amputation.

Although it is certainly reasonable for a patient to desire a prosthesis that is both cosmetic and functional, it is clear that optimal cosmetics and function cannot always be achieved by one prosthetic system.

For single-arm amputees, the prosthesis generally serves as an assistive or auxiliary limb. The loss of sensory function cannot be regained by any of the commercially available systems, although devices for the solution of this problem by pressure feedback, electrostimulation of the skin, or vibration feedback are being studied.

There are several common prosthetic systems (terminal devices) for the fitting of upper extremity amputees.

Cosmetic Hand

The cosmetic hand is a nonpowered cosmetic replacement of the hand. It can accomplish some simple auxiliary functions, such as holding a telephone receiver (see Fig. 11.4). The cosmetic hand can be exchanged for working devices, such as a hook or claw.

Body-Powered Prosthesis

In such prostheses, the opening and closure of the terminal device, whether a cosmetic hand or hook type, is controlled by BOWDEN cables for opening or closing. The opposite movement is controlled by springs or rubber bands. The hook-type terminal device is more functional than a cosmetic hand.

Externally Powered Prosthesis

Myoelectrically Controlled Prosthesis. Myopotentials are taken from antagonist muscles and used for the control of finger movements. In multiple channel devices, control of pronation and supination of the hand is possible. The power for movement is provided by a battery.

Electroprosthesis. Finger movement is accomplished by switches. As in the myoelectrically controlled prosthesis, the power system is a battery.

Pneumatic Prosthesis. This prosthesis is rarely used and is of little significance.

Plastic Surgically Shaped Stump

The Sauerbruch Arm (Kineplasty). The movement of the prosthetic fingers can be controlled by pegs inserted into skin-lined tunnels below certain tendons, including the biceps tendon as well as other forearm tendons.

Krukenberg Operation. A prehensile arm is created, using the long forearm stumps by operative separation of radius and ulna; this forceps-type stump provides good function together with retained sensation. The Sauerbruch arm is rare nowadays, but the Krukenberg arm is still important to bilateral amputees, especially those who are also blind.

The goals of occupational therapy in prosthetic training are:

1. To provide information about stump care, stump remodeling, and the principles involved in the prosthetic system
2. To teach the procedure for donning and removing the prosthesis
3. To assist in prehensile training, beginning with simple gripping exercises and progressing to increasingly finer skilled movements of the prosthetic fingers, such as playing cards or writing with the prosthesis, especially for bilateral amputees
4. To develop ADL; includes training the patient to eat and drink; to operate buckles, locks, and switches; to handle coins and paper money; to use the telephone; and to drive a car
5. To provide recreational and prevocational training; to teach the use of the prosthesis in society; includes dancing and the use of the prosthesis in public means of transportation

It is essential that the patient undergo training in all five areas to reduce the probability of rejecting the prosthesis later and thereby depriving himself or herself of a functional, assistive apparatus.

OCCUPATIONAL THERAPY OF PATIENTS WITH SPINAL CORD INJURIES

Depending on the level and degree of completeness, spinal cord injury may lead to various functional losses. Therefore, the occupational therapist who works with spinal cord injured patients must be able to deal with four highly variable dysfunctions:

1. Complete paralysis of the lower extremities and portions of the trunk, with impairment of rectovesical function (*paraplegia*)
2. Complete paralysis of the upper and lower extremities and the trunk muscles, together with impairment of the rectovesical function (*tetraplegia* or *quadriplegia*)

3. Incomplete paralysis of the lower extremities and trunk, together with a more or less marked impairment of the rectovesical function, depending on the intensity of the lesion (*paraparesis*)

4. Incomplete paralysis of the upper and lower extremities and the trunk muscles, together with various degrees of functional rectovesical impairment (*tetraparesis* or *quadraparesis*)

Two basic stages of therapy apply to all four dysfunctions: (*a*) early treatment, while the patient is still bedridden, and (*b*) late treatment, starting with the mobilization of the patient.

Regardless of the particular dysfunction, the tasks of occupational therapy for spinal cord injured patients comprise five different fields:

1. Functional treatment of the handicap
2. Self-help training (see Fig. 11.5)
3. Procurement of assistive devices and wheelchair
4. Accommodation management
5. Psychological support

(Points 4 and 5 are accomplished together with the other team members.) The measure to which each of these tasks can be carried out depends on the level and completeness of the patient's lesion.

Early Treatment

Early treatment for the spinal cord injured patient should begin with a therapeutic interview while he or she is in intensive care. This will help determine their functional, vocational and avocational needs, which might be useful in later therapy.

Paraplegics who can move arm and shoulder muscles should be encouraged at this point to participate in activities such as knotting, plaiting, and leather work. Newspapers, radio, and television also are useful as recreational activities.

The training of tetraplegics who also suffer from functional losses of the upper extremities is started in the early stage by measures that enable the patient to call the nurse, to switch the light on and off, and to operate the radio and television. In addition to these activities, assistive devices, like a bed mirror or prismatic glasses, can be used to enlarge the patient's field of vision. For reading books or magazines, a reading board that automatically turns pages is available. Some patients can learn to turn pages by hand or mouth.

In both cases, even in the initial stage of treatment, it is necessary that the hand and arm be kept in the functional position. This precaution will help to avoid contractures that can interfere with an otherwise successful self-help training. The wrist must be kept in dorsiflexion and the fingers in flexion. Wearing flexion gloves (see Fig. 11.6) promotes the creation of the so-called functional hand. Also, arm muscles that are paralyzed must be kept in a relaxed position. Immobilizing splints for the arm and flexion gloves are frequently required to achieve this. In cases of flexion contractures of the elbow joint, realignment splints are required.

High tetraplegics may need assistance in feeding during the early stages. Later, they can usually eat and drink independently by learning substitute movements and with the help of various aids for holding a spoon, fork, knife, drinking cup or feeding cup with a spout.

If possible, functional training should be started from the time that the patient is still lying in bed in a lateral or prone position (Stryker frame) to later, when he or she is in a sitting position (see Fig. 11.7).

To mobilize the patient with a spinal cord injury, the physician and the physical therapist must decide together on an adequate wheelchair. The kind of wheelchair and the extent of maneuverability, the constitution of the patient (stature and weight), and applicability of the wheelchair must be taken into consideration (see Chapter 25).

Late Treatment

The later stage of treatment for patients with a spinal cord injury begins when the patient's skill level is more advanced. The goal of this stage is to increase bilateral work for the training of balance. The therapy is continued on the ward, in the rooms of occupational therapy and work therapy, and in the test apartment. Training in ADL, such as hygiene, dressing and undressing (Fig. 11.8), cleaning the apartment, and preparing meals (Fig. 11.9), is started after the patient's initial mobilization.

Activities for the Spinal Cord Injured Patient

In Bed

1. Operation of the signal for the nurse; using the switch for radio, light, and television; and using mechanical assistance as well as environment-control devices
2. Eating and drinking with aids, if necessary (e.g., wrist cuff, feeding cup with spout, plastic tube, or thickened handles for spoon and fork)
3. Gripping exercises under visual control, exercises with the magnetic rod (games); strengthening of coarse grip accomplished by resistive exercises; training of finger extension with spreading scissors (in combination with games and manual techniques); writing with the hand (with or without build-up of writing utensils to larger diameter or aid); writing with a mouth stick; using an electric typewriter (with or without an aid such as a mouth stick)
4. General motivating and functional activities, such as plaiting, painting, knot tying, weaving, or electronic work, which eventually can be combined with manual techniques

Dressing and Undressing

1. Sitting up in bed
2. Training in the neuro chair; bending forward to the toes (stretching exercises)
3. Turning over to the lateral position
4. Dressing training, first, underwear, socks, and elastic stockings; then, outerwear (during the patient's stay at the rehabilitation center, mostly the training suit); also, exercises for fastening clothes (using buttons, hooks, buckles, Velcro, and zippers; threading; and tying knots) as well as fabrication of the required aids
5. Transferring from bed to wheelchair and back with or without aids; transferring from wheelchair to toilet, out of the bathtub, into the car, and back to the wheelchair

Practicing Hygiene

1. Operating the water faucet
2. Holding the hand-shower
3. Washing with a washcloth (hands, face, trunk, genitals, and legs)
4. Brushing teeth (opening the tube, squeezing out the toothpaste, closing the tube, using a brushing aid, filling/holding the cup)
5. Manicuring (brushing, cutting, filing)
6. Shampooing hair, combing hair (using an aid)
7. Shaving (using an aid)
8. Applying makeup
9. Observing skin with mirrors for prevention of decubitus ulcers

Eating and Drinking

Another activity is preparing a meal with the necessary assistance devices.

Homemaking Training

Training in basic essential homemaking skills, first in the occupational therapy clinic; then in a model apartment; and finally in the patient's own home is another ADL skill.

General Functional Training

1. Gripping exercises
2. Plaiting (instructions, aid, and assistance by therapist or vise); application of mobile arm, also combined with gripping exercises, manual skills, and writing training
3. Weaving (at the table or wall loom, using built-up handles)
4. Nailing a picture: gluing, nailing, stringing (using an aid or assistance)
5. Writing (with the hand, using an aid or built-up handle, or typewriter); of great psychological significance for most patients because it provides a means of communication with the environment; writing, painting, and drawing, eventually can be done with the use of thickened handles, aids, or mouth rod; typewriter (manual or electric) useful for vocational rehabilitation
6. Batikking, with the assistance of a built-up handle of the brush pencil
7. Ceramics
8. Lino cutting; textile printing

In addition, working with ceramics, mosaics, leather, or in photography, maybe using an adaptation of a camera, is constructive recreation; from a psychosocial point of view, looking for motifs in nature promotes the development of a positive outlook on life. Working in an electrical, wood, or metal shop or gardening promotes the training of balance and exercise tolerance and prevocational and recreational training, as well as work tolerance training. There are unlimited possibilities, especially if the patient and therapist show inventiveness regarding the necessary assistive apparatus and adaptations. For example, for incomplete paralyses, functional training of the legs can be achieved through use of a loom, bicycle, saw, or potter's wheel.

General functional training also includes substitute schooling, if necessary, vocational training as far as possible, and memory concentration training of patients with additional craniocerebral trauma.

Other activities may involve:

Holding a book or newspaper; turning pages
Operating an elevator, switch, or plug
Opening/closing doors
Drawing open curtains
Using a telephone
Folding a letter and putting it into an envelope; opening a letter
Handling a purse or money
Opening box or can
Inserting paper in an electric typewriter
Opening and closing drawers
Locking and unlocking
Taking care of an infant
Knitting, crocheting, or embroidery

FUNCTIONAL TRAINING OF PATIENTS WITH CRANIOCEREBRAL INJURIES

Depending on the site and extent of brain damage, various kinds of handicaps can result from a cerebral injury. The broad range of defects possibly arising from craniocerebral traumas include sensory, motor, psychosocial, and intellectual impairments (e.g., hemiplegia, ataxia, gait disturbances, aphasia, mood lability, retardation). Such a range presents quite a challenge to the occupational therapist. The tasks of occupational therapy in the treatment of craniocerebral patients may be classified in several groups:

1. *First contact and motivation.* This should start as early as possible after the injury, as soon as the patient is able to cooperate.
2. *Self-help training.* This starts by explaining how to call the nurse, and how to switch the light and radio on and off as well as how to become generally oriented to the setting. This training continues with activities pertaining to personal hygiene (washing, brushing teeth, etc.). In all activities for self-help, the therapist must take care to avoid defective patterns of motion induced by the spastic increase in tone. The treatment principles of Bobath must be kept in mind (Fig. 11.10 and also Chapter 28).
3. *General measures.* Prehensile training is exercised by grip exercises and other games, mainly by using bilateral activities to improve skills, to mobilize the joints, and to increase exercise tolerance. In addition to this, social activities (recreation, movies, theater, etc.) are encouraged.
4. *Procurement of assistive devices.* These devices include non-slip support, cutting boards, safety bars in the bathroom, a tub seat, electric kitchen utensils, and a potato peeler.
5. *Training of communication skills.* By having the individual do spontaneous writing, dictation, copying and reading aloud, narration, and concentration and memory training, cerebral deficits can be diagnosed and treated systematically.
6. *Orientation in space.* This includes being able to distinguish left from right and related perceptual skills.
7. *Preparatory activities for vocational retraining (e.g., using a typewriter) or for reentry in employment (adaptations of the*

workplace). These can be implemented through a work hardening program.

WORK THERAPY

In addition to occupational therapy, which provides functional training and motivation by general activities, most rehabilitation centers also have facilities for vocational rehabilitation. To facilitate vocational rehabilitation, the occupational therapist must provide information about exercise tolerance; use of and need for assistive devices, such as prostheses (keeping in mind the need for working space) for the wheelchair-bound; and many more things. Basically, the following questions have to be answered:

1. Can the patient take up his former job after the conclusion of treatment?
2. Could an internal change of the workplace render the employee's former work possible?
3. Should vocational retraining be considered?
4. Do the after-effects of the accident prevent any further vocational activities?

Rehabilitation centers should be equipped with adequate machines or simulations to be able to answer these questions and to make prevocational tolerance tests. Apart from vocational considerations, this work can also initiate creative recreational activities for the patients.

The following workshops (Fig. 11.11) should be made available:

1. *Woodworking/carpentry.* This workshop can be utilized for various vocations (e.g., a joiner, carpenter, turner, or carver).
2. *Metal work.* This workshop could have a "smithy," welding machine, or lathe. Here, the following vocations can be tested: smith, welder, turner, toolmaker, or mechanic.
3. *Electrical work.* Simple work, like the fabrication of lamps and lights, and also more difficult work are possible. The more difficult work would include drawing circuit diagrams, making printing plates, and making workpieces by soldering. Projects could include metal detectors, alarms, ultra-high frequency receivers and many more things. In this workshop, the patient can also learn how to communicate by radio, an activity which is an excellent hobby, even for the very severely disabled.
4. *Nursery.* By cultivating a garden, the patient can regain and experience his or her relationship with nature.
5. *Other special workshops.* These may include painting or leather work.
6. *Photography laboratory.*

Figure 11.1. Functional training of the upper extremity can involve

- **A.** An overhead loom with assist
- **B.** Suspended macrame
- **C.** Therapeutic putty
- **D–E.** Dexterity—"pin-in-hole" games
- **F.** Mikado with cross-tweezers
- **G–I.** Craft activities for hand function
- **J.** Practicing tying knots, and
- **K–L.** Sensibility testing and training.

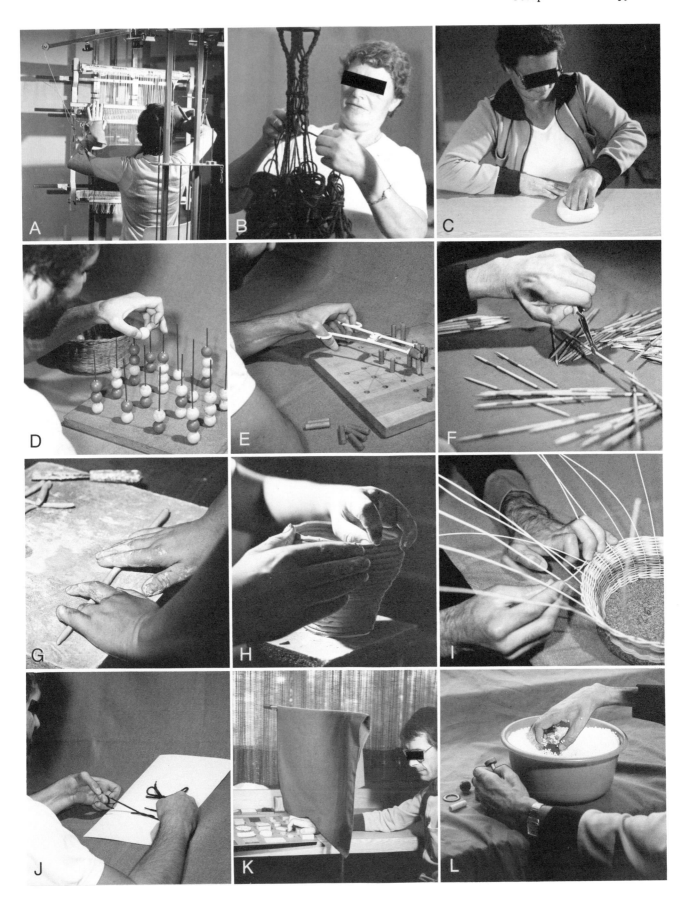

Figure 11.1.

Figure 11.2. Splinting for the upper extremity includes

A–C. Fabrication of splints
    D. Volar-forearm resting-splint with hand support
    E. Dorsal upper arm extension splint
    F. Opponens splint
    G. Splint for ulnar nerve lesion
    H. Splint for radial nerve lesion, and
    I. Dynamic splint for finger extension with outrigger.

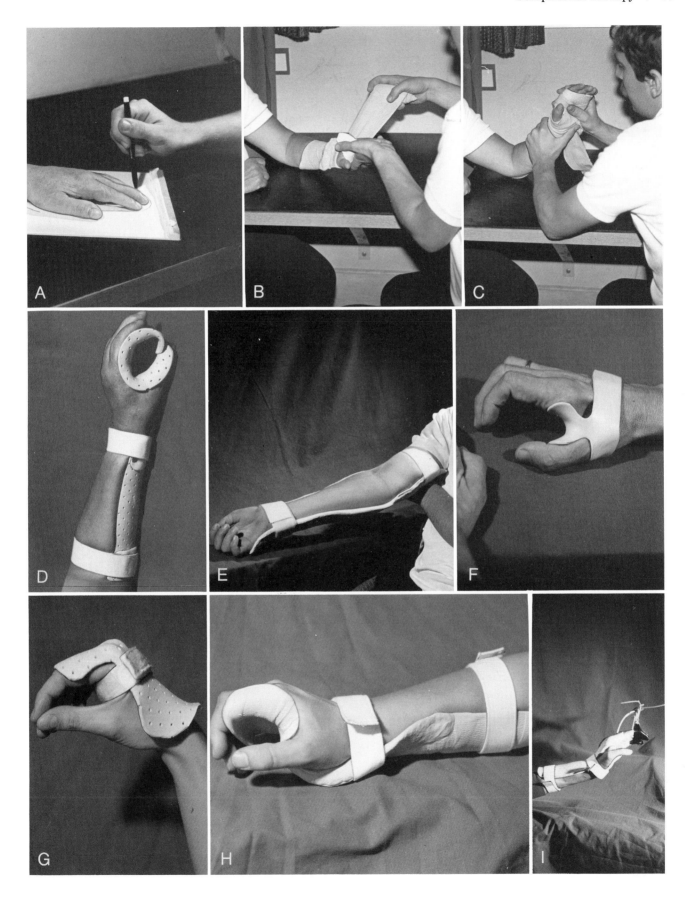

Figure 11.2.

Figure 11.3. In functional training of the lower extremity, important elements are

    A. Stress and endurance training while standing

    B. The loom with a slide for knee flexion

    C. A loom adopted for hip abduction

D–E. A loom adopted for the range of motion (ROM) of the upper ankle joint; loom adopted for the ROM of the lower ankle joint (subtalar)

    F. The bicycle saw

    G. The arthrodesis wheelchair, and

H–I. Assistive devices for dressing for patients with hip fusion.

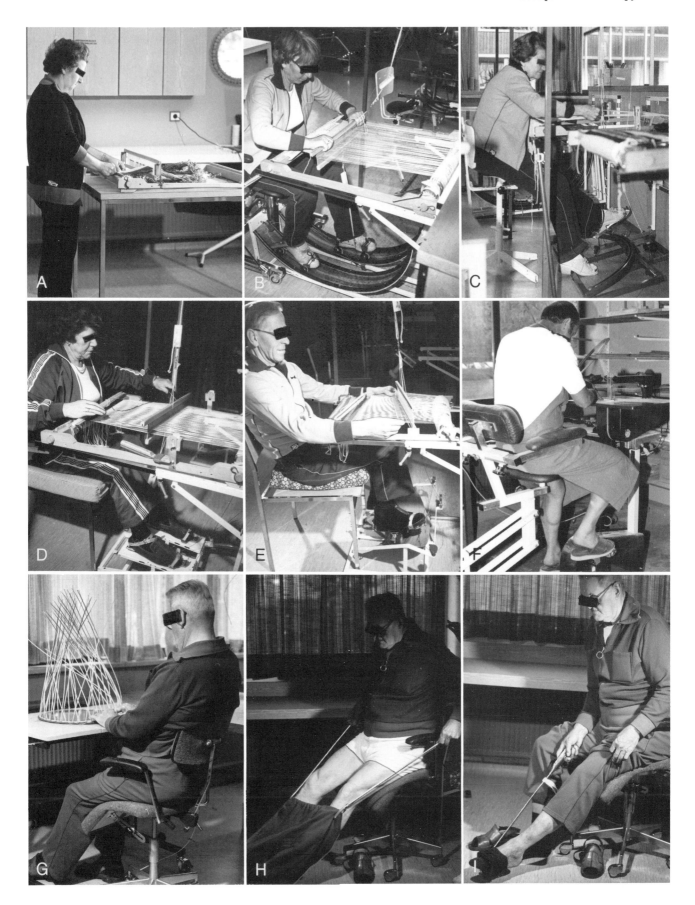

Figure 11.3.

Figure 11.4. Prosthetic training of the upper extremity amputee should include:

A–B. Full opening of terminal device; holding
   C. Penmanship
D–F. Functional training
 G–I. Self-help activities, and
J–L. Occupational training.

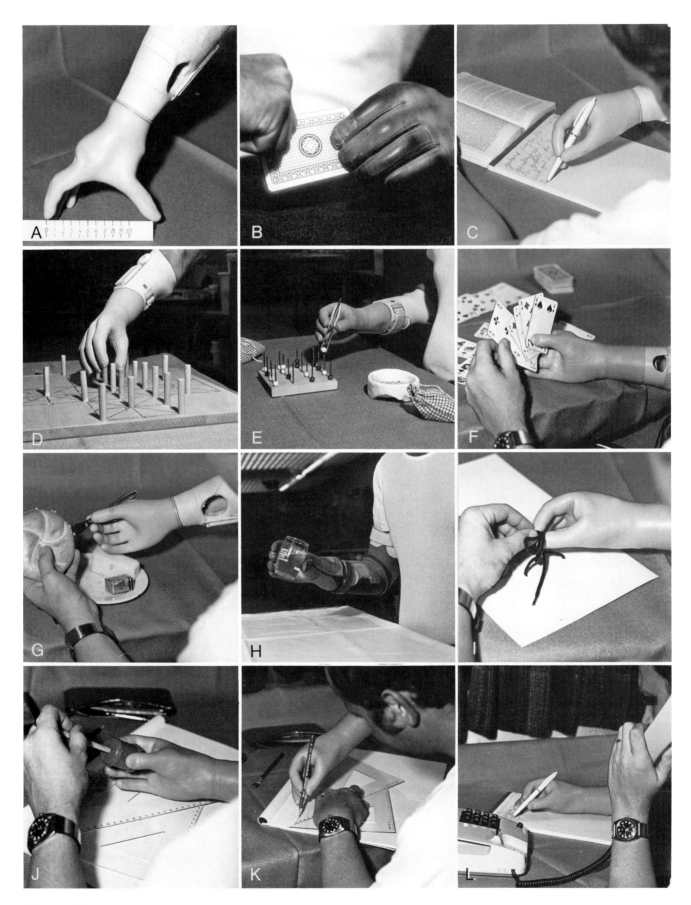

Figure 11.4.

Figure 11.5. Self-help training of the paraplegic involves

A–E. Training in cooking for paraplegics,
 F–I. Bath activities, and
 J–L. Toilet transfer.

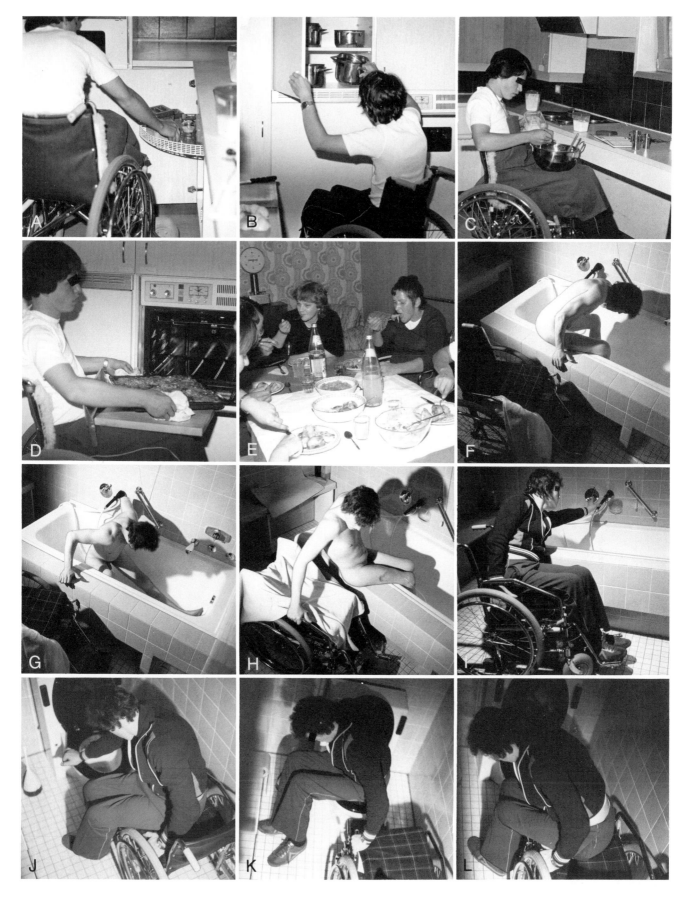

Figure 11.5.

Figure 11.6. Assistive and self-help devices for tetraplegics include

    A. Flexion glove

    B. Built-up handle (toothbrush)

    C. Button hook

    D. Handbrush with suction cups

    E. Assistive device for holding eating devices (leather, webbing, etc.)

    F. Assistive device for holding cup or glass

    G. Assistive device for telephoning

    H. Swivel arm for electric wheelchair (ball bearing feeders, etc.)

I–J. Assistive devices for writing and typing

    K. Mouthstick for typing, and

    L. Automatic page turner.

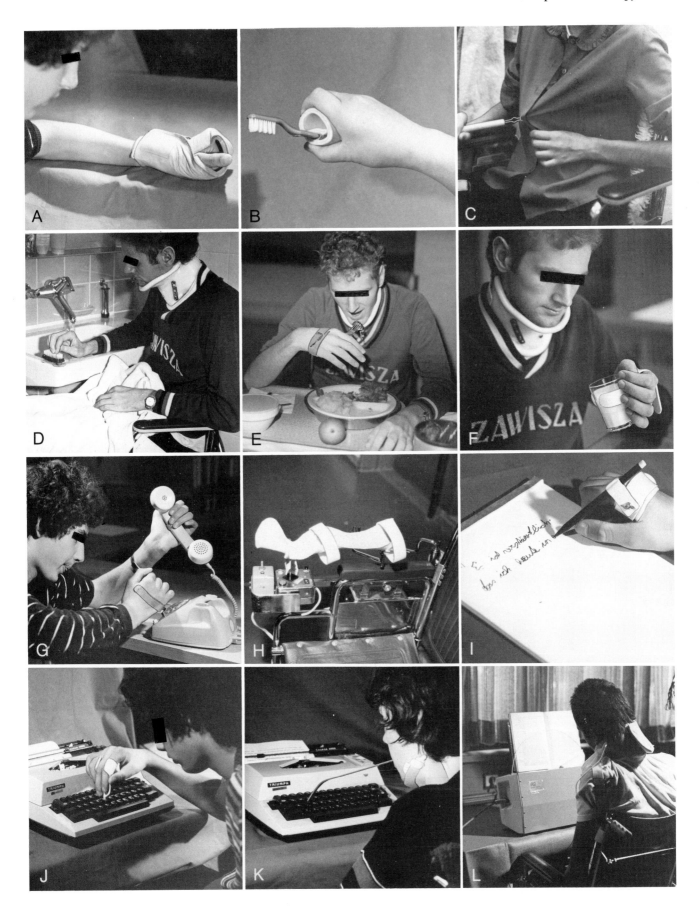

Figure 11.6.

Figure 11.7. Functional training of the tetraplegic includes

   A. Basket weaving at bedside
   B. Dexterity games (pin-in-hole)
   C. Overhead loom
D–F. Manual therapy
 G–I. Self-help training
J–K. Drawing exercises, and
   L. Teaching in a rehabilitation setting.

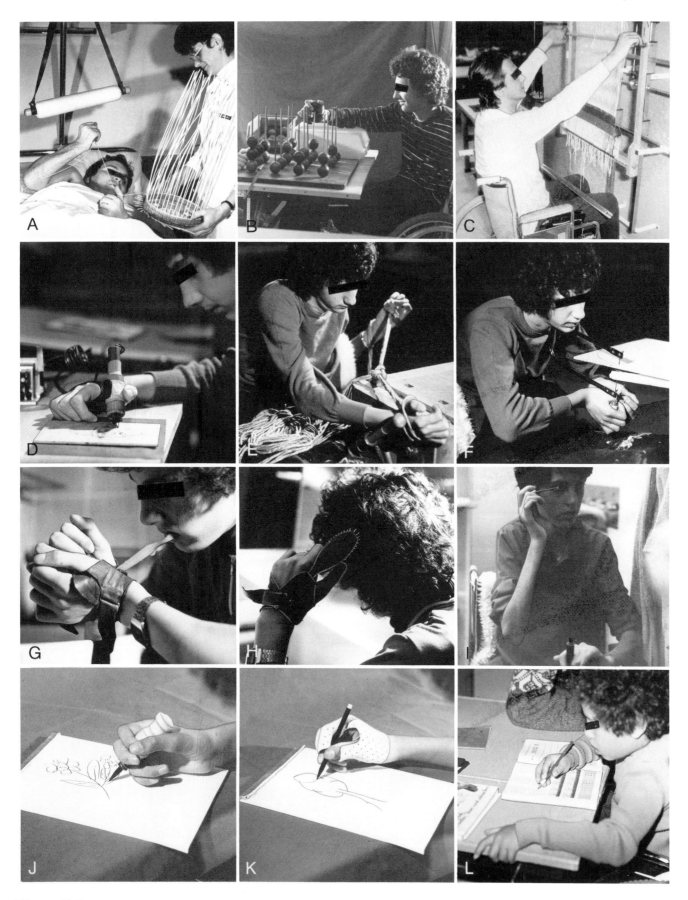

Figure 11.7.

Figure 11.8.

A–L. Dressing training for tetraplegics is part of developing ADL skills.

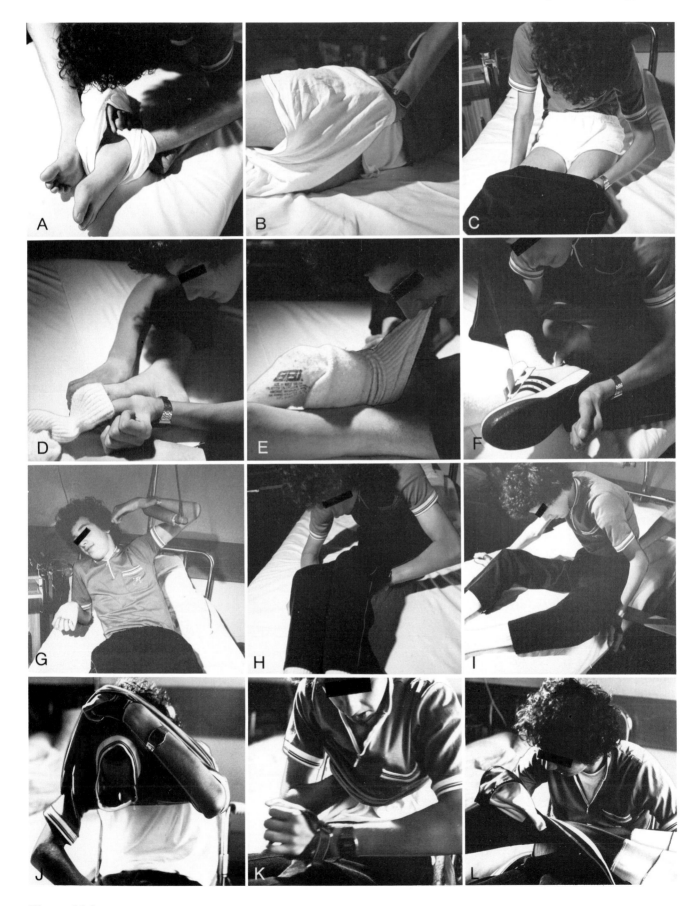

Figure 11.8.

Figure 11.9.

A–L. Training the tetraplegic homemaker is also part of developing ADL skills.

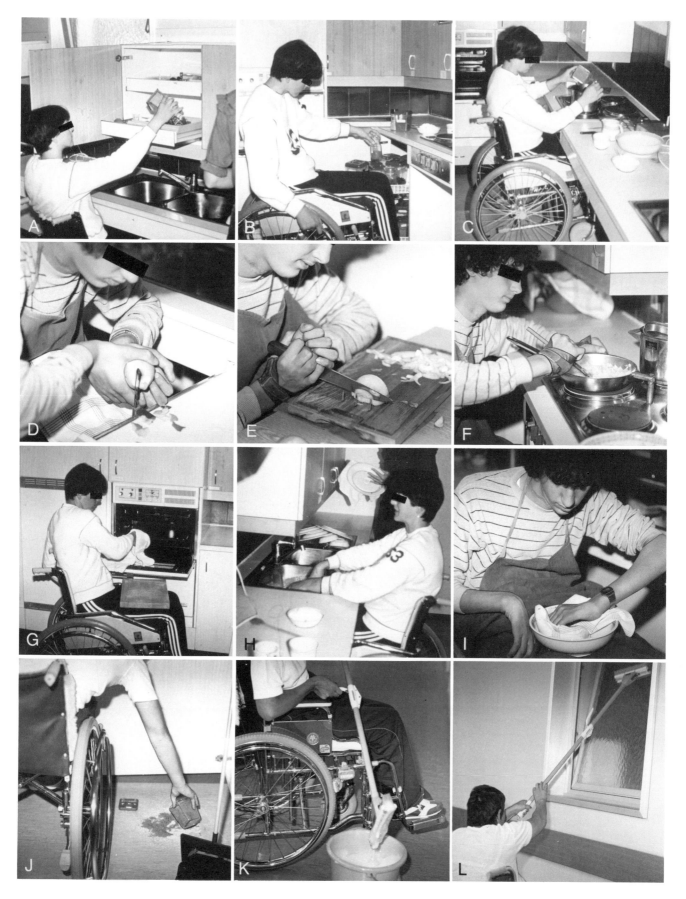

Figure 11.9.

Figure 11.10. Functional training for hemiplegics includes

A–D. Bilateral activities using Bobath techniques (e.g., dexterity games—pin-in-hole, print-ing, ball)
E–I. Dressing training
J. Shoulder abduction sling (in subluxated hemiplegic shoulder), and
K–M. Memory and perceptual training.

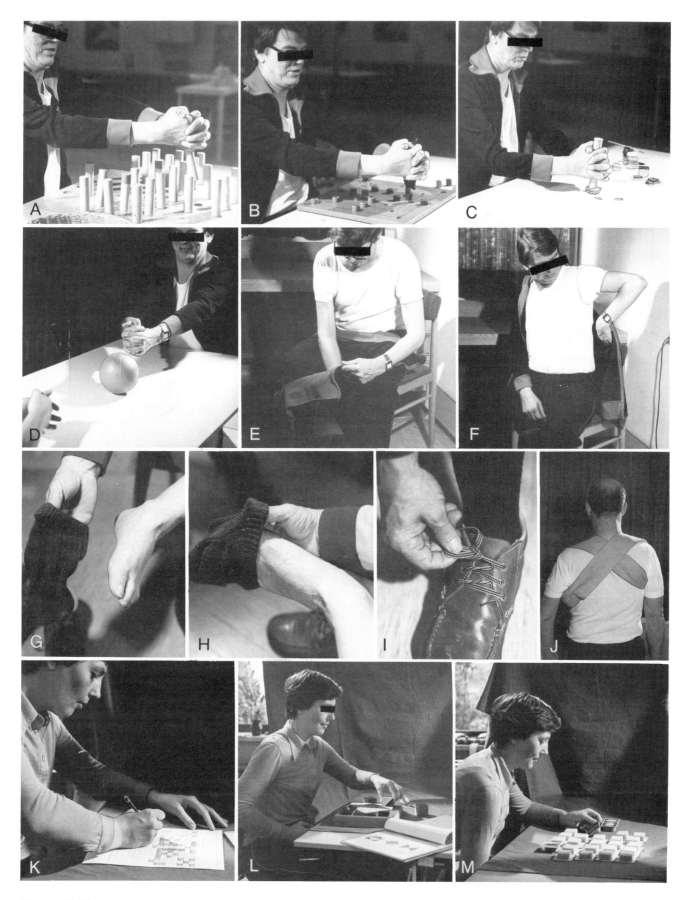

Figure 11.10.

Figure 11.11. Manual arts therapy includes

A–C. Woodworking/carpentry workshops
D–F. Metal workshops
 G–I. Electrical workshops, and
 J–L. Nursery (gardening) workshops.

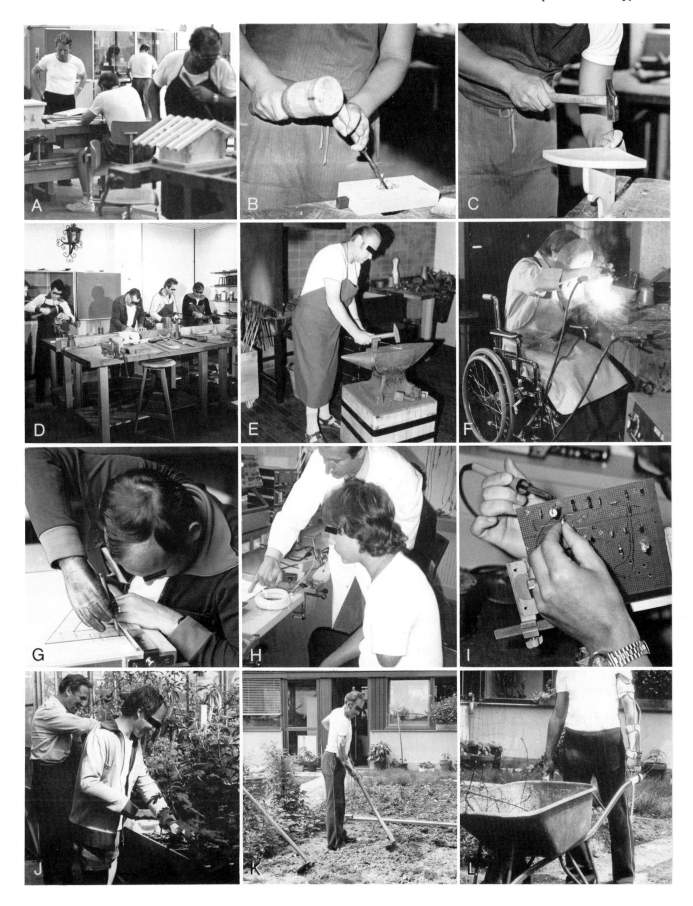

Figure 11.11.

12

Physical Therapy

This special discipline of the healing arts is particularly important for the rehabilitation of patients with traumatic conditions. This chapter is arranged according to: (a) the type of injury, impairment or handicap, and (b) the site of the injury. The first part of this chapter discusses individual exercises for the extremities. Next, a discussion of group exercises is divided according to the region of injury. Thereafter, kinetic therapy with independent active exercises and ambulation training in general grouping are discussed. Finally, modalities including electrotherapy, hydrotherapy, and massage, are reviewed. The second part of this chapter is devoted to the treatment of patients with craniocerebral injuries, amputees, and patients with spinal injuries. This arrangement is designed to enable the prescribing physician and the therapist to find the pertinent regions quickly. The atlas can also be shown to the patient and the therapeutic procedures that he or she will be receiving can be discussed using the rich pictorial material.

INDIVIDUAL TREATMENT OF THE UPPER EXTREMITY
Hubert Zoller

Before therapy is started, it is necessary to record objective findings and data. The following format has proven useful in treatment of trauma patients: (a) data regarding the accident, (b) medical case history, and (c) physical therapy evaluation. The physical therapy evaluation should consist of inspection (posture, skin, contours and bony prominences), palpatory findings (muscle tone and temperature), and functional assessment (circumferential measurements, active range of motion, passive range of motion [ROM], and firm or elastic resistance). All observations must include both sides, even if the pathology appears unilateral. Actual function, such as gait, transfer, sitting and standing balance, and strength, also should be evaluated and recorded. Short- and long-term goals can then be established in accordance with the other data.

Generally, there are three goals of therapy: 1) to improve ROM, 2) to improve muscle strength, and 3) to develop compensatory mechanisms and substitutions.

Restricted movement may be caused by: inactivity; traumatic changes of chondral, muscular, and fibroid structures (hematoma, ruptures); protective posture; or neurological deficits.

In such cases, there are two techniques for facilitating and improving the patient's ROM. The *passive* technique involves special stretching exercises. The *active* technique involves: (a) isometric contraction exercises, especially in the early stage of treatment; (b) movements under "guiding contact" with the elimination of gravity and against gravity; (c) passive, active and active-assisted exercises; (d) resistance exercises, with added stimulation by applying resistance through pushing (pressure) or pulling (traction); and (e) special exercises, such as Bobath and proprioceptive neuromuscular facilitation (PNF), which are applied in specific cases.

Muscular weakness may be caused by immobilization, paresis, or paralysis.

In these cases, three techniques are useful: (a) isometric exercises, (b) isotonic exercises (e.g., dynamic resistive exercises), and (c) isokinetic exercises (employing special equipment, such as Cybex).

In therapy for upper extremity injuries, special attention must usually be given to the shoulder joint. This joint is stabilized mainly by connective tissue structures, and therefore it is very susceptible to complications when immobilized. Contractures of the rotator cuff and muscle atrophies frequently occur. If therapy is started too late or is applied inappropriately, delayed complications occur. Frequent examples are: recurring dislocation of the shoulder, adhesive capsulitis (frozen shoulder), and traumatic or posttraumatic arthritis.

The first goal of therapy should be to develop muscle tone to prevent recurrent dislocations. Isometric contraction techniques (6 sec contraction, 3 sec relaxation) in the middle range are most often used for this purpose. A later goal should be to strengthen the deltoid, the biceps muscle, and the pectoralis major muscles. Special techniques can be applied to prevent contractures. The most effective one is the so-called *dynamic reversal movement technique*, which involves the contraction of agonists, then slow dynamic reversal to antagonists, holding, and relaxation (Fig. 12.1).

In the late stages of treatment, combined active-passive techniques are indicated. The therapist commands "contract," then "relax," and during the relaxation, slowly stretches the structures with measured force into the contracture.

Rotational movements are added to the therapy rather late. In the treatment of the elbow joint, relaxation exercises are indispensable before mobilization is started (the relaxation of the biceps muscle is especially important). After this, the extensors are strengthened by active exercises.

Manipulations are started only when there is no longer danger of redislocation or refracture. In the late therapy of contractures, active-passive techniques with longitudinal traction have proven especially successful. Further therapeutic goals are strengthening (only possible with active techniques) and the improvement of the circulation.

In the treatment of hand and wrist joint injuries, depending on the phase of the healing process, initially only isometric exercises are used in the course of treatment. Later, dynamic exercises are added (with increasing manual resistance).

INDIVIDUAL THERAPY OF THE LOWER EXTREMITY
Hubert Zoller

THE THERAPY FOR INJURIES OF THE PELVIS AND HIP

Pelvis and hip injuries include fractures and dislocations of the hip joint and femoral head, neck fractures, and fractures of the pelvis. After a thorough examination of the patient with lower extremity injuries, the therapist should determine the goals of treatment (whether to improve circulation, mobilization, strengthening, or gait pattern). If the goal is to achieve better circulation, the patient should be instructed to carry out isometric contraction exercises from the time that he or she is confined to bed. Especially by the isometric training of the gluteal muscles, a better muscular stabilization of the hip joint can be achieved. The patient can soon be allowed to perform active exercises, but resistive exercises with resistance applied by the therapist should be applied gradually. If strengthening the hip muscles is the goal, exercises in the supine and lateral starting positions are advantageous. At first, the patient should exercise against gravity only; later, against the increasing manual resistance of the therapist (see Fig. 12.2).

Partial weightbearing exercises should be started in a therapeutic pool or tank. Only when the patient no longer experiences pain and no longer uses substitution movements, should ambulation with forearm crutches start.

THE THERAPY FOR INJURIES OF THE KNEE

Knee joint injuries include dislocations; sprains; fractures of the tibial condyles; fractures of the patella; and tearing and rupture of ligaments, bursae, and menisci. There are three goals of therapy for patients with such injuries: (a) to resolve the hemarthrosis, (b) to achieve full extension, and (c) to strengthen the extensors and flexors of the knee joint.

The knee joint, one of the most sensitive joints, reacts to every disturbance by reactive hemarthrosis; this is the reason dynamic exercises are not permitted at the beginning of therapy. The combination of isometric exercises with cryotherapy has proven most favorable for the re-

sorption of intraarticular hematoma. Dynamic exercise may be started only when the hemarthrosis has disappeared. These exercises have not only a strengthening effect, but also increase the ROM. Initial exercises should be carried out in the zero position only (knee extended). Only when the knee can be held extended strongly without pain, and there are no traces of hemarthrosis, may active knee flexion be started. The patient should be instructed to contract the muscles in various positions with the hand of the therapist directing the movement (guiding contact). In case the knee joint must not yet be mobilized, the therapist should strengthen actively the hip, ankle, and foot muscles in order to prevent muscular atrophy. Static patterns should be applied against resistance with the knee joint remaining in the zero position. Active mobilization techniques are preferred. Active-passive exercises are allowed only when arthrogenous contractures are already developed.

THE THERAPY FOR INJURIES OF THE ANKLE

Ankle joint injuries include malleolar fractures of the ankle, rupture of the Achilles tendon, tearing or sprain of ligaments, and fracture dislocations. For these patients, there are four goals of therapy: to improve circulation and mobilization; to strengthen the dorsiflexors of the foot and calf muscles, to preserve muscle strength of the remaining three extremities, and to prepare the patient for weightbearing. Complications that can occur include instability, contracture, and arthrosis.

Excellent therapeutic results are achieved by cryotherapy in combination with isometric contraction exercises for the improvement of circulation. Injuries of the ankle joint may frequently cause restriction of motion. In order to prevent the loss of dorsiflexion, the therapist should start treatment by passive stretching of the upper ankle joint and the Achilles tendon. After 4 to 6 weeks, stretching by active-passive exercises is possible. The triceps surae muscle in particular may be further stretched by contraction of the knee muscles. After any kind of mobilization, the dorsiflexors of the foot should be strengthened. The triceps surae muscle (very important for gait) should be exercised and strengthened after marked improvement of the mobility of the ankle joint has been accomplished. Only then, prerequisites for optimal gait training have been established.

GENERAL PHYSICAL EXERCISES
Herta Zvolanek

In addition to individual therapy, the patient should participate in group therapy for general physical reeducation and training as soon as he or she has achieved maximum exercise tolerance. This intensive exercise program, which includes sports, is designed to help the patient meet the physical requirements of his or her future job.

In order to be able to train the injured parts of the body specifically, the patients should be divided into two main groups:

1. Patients with injuries and/or weakness and restricted movements of the lower extremities
2. Patients with injuries and/or weakness and restricted movements of the upper extremities

Each of the physical exercise group sessions should be directed toward a good general and comprehensive workout, but particularly stressing exercises for the pertinent group (e.g., exercises for the lower extremities rather than the upper extremities).

Each training session should last at least 30 minutes to allow adequate time for warm-up, main exercises (strengthening, stretching, and suppleness exercises), and cooling down (relaxation, coordination, and dexterity exercises). In this way, the sessions can provide simultaneous training of circulation and conditioning.

The sessions should include a wide variety of interesting exercises and the use of various types of gymnastic apparatus (e.g., wall bars, benches, and ropes) and hand equipment (e.g., gymnastic balls, medicine balls, bars, hoops, ropes, and clubs). Partner and group exercises (see Fig. 12.3), gymnastics with music, "circuit" training, and many kind of games have also proved successful in helping the patient take pleasure again in movement and regain confidence in his or her own abilities.

GROUP GYMNASTICS FOR THE TRUNK MUSCLES
Gabriele Berger

Patients who have spinal injuries should participate in gymnastics to strengthen their trunk muscles. Since the treatment of such injuries requires a long period of bed rest and immobilization in a corset, unavoidable muscle atrophy and restriction of motion must be handled. Therefore, the following guidelines for this treatment should be considered:

1. Strengthen the back, the shoulder girdle, and the abdominal muscles to stabilize the spine and to create a natural corset of muscles.
2. Use mobilizing gymnastics to increase the flexibility of joints and to stretch the ligaments and muscles.
3. Use exercises that change and assume various positions to facilitate the movements required in activities of daily living.

EXECUTION

The group gymnastics should last about 30 minutes and should be carried out daily. Critics of group therapy and gymnastics point out the disadvantage that these cannot possibly meet all the necessities of the individual patients. However, the fact is that scarcely any hospital can afford personnel to provide adequate individual treatment on a one-on-one basis. Furthermore, the great advantage of exercising in a group is that patients are stimulated to make greater efforts because they do not want to lag behind the others. Additional motivation is provided by the use of hand equipment such as bars, clubs, balls, medicine balls, ropes, or hoops and the use of music to provide variety, rhythm, and enjoyment during exercises. Other exercises utilize the wall bar and the bench.

STABILIZATION OF THE SPINE

Therapeutic stabilization exercises are initially extremely difficult to perform correctly. It is therefore essential that the grade of difficulty of the exercise be increased slowly in order to guarantee correct performance.

Training of the rectus abdominis and other abdominal muscles is important for the stabilization of the spine. For this exercise, the starting position is the supine position, with knees flexed and arms folded behind the neck. In the early phase of the program, the patient should lift only his or her head and shoulders. The abdominal muscles are contracted and strengthened by this exercise. Later, when the patient has developed good abdominal muscles, he or she should come up to a sitting position. Initially, the patients have the same difficulty in training the extensors of the back. This exercise starts in the prone position: the arms are elevated fully beyond the head and gently lifted up from the floor.

MOBILIZATION OF THE SPINE

Activities to mobilize the spine include all swing exercises in the standing position, with or without hand equipment. Included are the exercises that involve the tetrapod position or standing on knees as well as stretching exercises in the sitting position. In the latter, the training of the ischiocrural muscles must be included. The goal of these gymnastics is to increase the range of motion of the spine in all directions. The physical therapist must therefore choose exercises for extension, flexion, rotation, and lateral bending of the trunk.

CHANGE OF POSITION

For gymnastics of the trunk (Fig. 12.4), the following positions have proven favorable: standing, sitting, tetrapod, standing on knees, prone, and supine. Running and jumping cause extreme stress to the vertebral fracture site and should therefore be omitted from the gymnastics program.

When the patient is discharged from the hospital, he or she should have learned a simple exercise program and be able to perform it at home correctly.

KINETIC THERAPY IN WATER
Waltraud Starke

The buoyancy of water provides great advantages for kinetic therapy. In water, the human body has only one-seventh of its normal weight. Therefore, the effect of gravity is reduced significantly. Patients with paresis resulting from incomplete spinal cord injury, or with various fractures, for example, can carry out movements much more easily in water where the gravitational effect is reduced. Therefore, it is possible to devise a structured, progressive muscle reeducation and training program. Nonswimmers and poor swimmers can be given inflatable swimming wings (see Fig. 12.5) or a flotation device such as the Heidelberg collar.

Kinetic therapy in water is carried out in two ways: (a) as group therapy, or (b) individual therapy. In group therapy, patients with similar paresis or restricted movements should be assigned to the same group. The exercises, which are carried out under the supervision of a therapist, are adapted to the respective injuries; for example, paresis of the legs, for which the leg muscles are strengthened in all directions of movement by various specific exercises.

Individual therapy is required in the case of multiple contractures and for the therapy of very spastic parapleg-ics. It is carried out in a special therapy pool. For multiple contractures, it is easier for the therapist to stretch the patient in water. The lost kinesthesia of the overstretched joint can be regained better in this way. Movement is facilitated by the reduction of weight. This treatment is applied in the initial phase of therapy. When improvement has been achieved, the treatment is continued outside the pool.

Initially, the therapist must be with the patient in the pool; later, guidance and supervision of patients' pool exercises can be done from outside the pool. In cases of extremely spastic paraplegia, water of about 30°C may have a spasmolytic effect. However, some spasms can be reduced by an ice bath. It is necessary to test the patient's individual reaction before beginning treatment. As it is extremely difficult and strenuous to apply ROM exercises to patients with very severe spasms on the high mat, it is preferable to move them in water, provided that they react positively to tepid water. The patient can enter the pool independently by using a hydraulic lift, which lifts him or her in the wheelchair up to the level of the pool border.

INDEPENDENT EXERCISES
Annemarie Juën

Independent exercises are a supplement and extension of individual treatments with the physical therapists, and these should stimulate the patient's own initiative. Important criteria for independent exercises are:

1. The therapist must explain the apparatus in detail to the patient.
2. The therapist should show the patient specific exercises.
3. The patient's exercises must be monitored and adjusted regularly.

There are two positive aspects to independent exercises. First, the patient can evaluate his or her own progress by accelerating the speed of the exercises, increasing the time of exercise, and using more resistance. Second, the patient may choose the time for a rest according to his or her own judgment. There are eight examples of independent exercises using the following devices: the kneebender, the knee extender ("mountain climber"), the treadmill ergometer, the pulley block, the standard, dumbbell training, exercises at the wall bars, and the swinging frame.

KNEEBENDER

Function: To increase ROM of the knee joint; to strengthen thigh muscles
Application: For treatment of contractures, up to 90 degrees flexion
Execution: Knee flexed passively over roll by weight of leg; patient can relieve knee from weight by a pulley block; for refractory contractures, effect can be intensified by weights
Duration: 15–20 min, including pauses

KNEE EXTENDER
("MOUNTAIN CLIMBER")

Function: To strengthen thigh muscles, especially quadriceps muscle; to increase ROM of knee and hip joints
Application: For injuries of knee joint, fractures of the femur (knee contractures of more than 90 degrees and atrophy of the thigh muscles)
Execution: Weight under sole of foot is pushed up an incline; downward movement must be checked by respective muscles; patient can adjust resistance by changing height or weight and clearly can observe his or her own gradual improvement
Duration: 15–20 min

TREADMILL ERGOMETER

Function: To improvement endurance; to improve strength and speed of movement, from walking to running
Application: For injuries of upper extremity, e.g., fractures, burns
Execution: The patient is walking on the treadmill first with slow speed, then gradually increasing speed and proceeding to running; blood pressure and pulse rate are monitored in patients at risk;

electrocardiogram is attached for patients with cardiopulmonary problems

PULLEY BLOCK

Function: To strengthen upper arm and shoulder muscles; to improve flexibility
Application: For injuries of the upper extremity, e.g., fractures, burns
Execution: By moving weight up and down over pulley, patient exercises elevation/depression or abduction/adduction of shoulder joint
Duration: 15–20 min

STANDARD

Function: To strengthen lower extremity, to improve endurance, and to mobilize hip and knee joints
Application: After fractures, ligamentous or joint injuries
Execution: Patient is pedaling like on a stationary bicycle and can himself or herself determine the gradual increase of resistance and speed
Duration: 10–15 min as tolerated

DUMBBELL TRAINING

Function: To strengthen arm and shoulder muscles
Application: After any injuries of upper extremity and shoulder
Execution: Can be carried out in various positions and directions of movement; weights should be so heavy that patient must apply maximum force; weight and number of repetitions is determined by the therapist after evaluation and individually modified according to patient's condition and progress
Duration: variable (holding and repetitions)

EXERCISES AT THE WALL BARS

Function: Wall bars suitable for strengthening and flexibility exercises for both the upper and lower extremities as well as trunk and abdominal muscles
Application: After injuries to spine, upper and lower extremities
Execution: Patient stands in front of the wall bar, holds on to it and performs knee bends, then pulls himself up to standing position; various other exercises are designed by the therapist for specific injuries such as vertebral fractures in cast, etc
Duration: Varies individually

SWINGING FRAME

Function: Applied for active mobilization, passive extension of locomotor apparatus, especially axial skeleton and spine, for stimulation of respiration and circulation, and for relaxation (see Fig. 12.6)
Application: Patients with spinal injuries, especially of lumbar spine, after prolonged immobilization and for patients suffering from detrimental effects of modern civilization and stress

Execution: Patient lies on the swinging frame well balanced in prone position and by moving his arms up and down shifts the body weight causing the frame to swing up and down; frame can also be adjusted to flex and extend in the mid portion; this motion is transmitted to the spine

Duration: 5–10 min as tolerated

GAIT TRAINING IN GROUPS
Susanne Kubat

The goal of gait training in groups is to improve the patient's gait to a "normalization of gait pattern," depending on the patient's condition. At the same time, another objective is to reduce the patient's anxiety and insecurity, an aim that is positively influenced by working in groups.

There are four prerequisites that a patient must have to benefit from gait training in groups:

1. The weightbearing tolerance of the injured extremity must be sufficient, and the patient must understand and comply with his or her limitations. (Weightbearing exercises are carried out on two scales).
2. The patient's orthopaedic fittings, e.g., forearm crutches, canes, shoe supports, or splints, must meet the requirements.
3. The state of the patient's physical condition and fitness must be sufficient to enable participation without slowing the group's progress.
4. In difficult cases, the patient must undergo preliminary gait training with the therapist on one to one basis.

The patients in group gait training are divided into three performance groups: (a) those with ambulation aids (e.g., crutches or canes), and (b) those without ambulation aids. Patients who still need forearm crutches, are in a separate group and are taught the 3-point gait according to his or her exercise tolerance. As the patient's weightbearing tolerance increases, the support can be reduced gradually. When full weightbearing is allowed, the forearm crutches can be exchanged for canes until ambulation without aids is accomplished.

AMBULATION EXERCISES

Ambulation (gait training) exercises can be modified in each of the above described groups according to patients needs and capacity and may include:

Ambulation forward, backward, and sideways
Ambulation along line and floor patterns
Variation of step width: equally long, short and long steps
Ambulation with a long step of the unimpaired leg and a small step of the injured leg; change of cadence
Walking on tiptoes, heel walking, and making large steps
Walking in time, at different speeds
Walking on level ground, on a slope, in uneven ground (e.g., lawn, gravel, or sand), or forest roads, and on rough slopes
Weightbearing exercises in the standing position, standing on tiptoes and heels
Steps over obstacles, balance exercises (see Fig. 12.7)
Ambulation in stooped over and half-squatting position
Narrow-gauge ambulation, walking on a line in a heel-to-toe fashion
Walking with simultaneous arm swinging; additional arm weight is provided by holding clubs, bars, etc.

Especially important in gait training for these patients is the correction of faulty posture and incorrect gait patterns, such as limping, irregular step length or width, insufficient weightbearing, incomplete extension of the hip joint, excessive external rotation of the injured leg, incomplete, incorrect, or missing heel-to-toe phase of gait, and posture in general. The coordination of movements; proper concomitant arm swing; and the avoidance of cramping, holding, and bracing of muscles are observed and mistakes corrected.

ELECTROTHERAPY
Elizabeth Völkl

There are multitudes of different modifications of electrical currents used for patient therapy.

Currents maybe divided into galvanic (constant) currents, interrupted galvanic or pulsed currents, faradic (alternating) currents, and sinusoidal currents.

Modifications may include variations in frequencies (low frequencies: 1 to 1000 Hz; medium frequencies: 1000 to 20,000 Hz, and high frequencies: 20,000 and above Hz), variations in voltage from low voltages to high ones, and modification of wave patterns.

GALVANIZATION

Procedure

Treatment with constant direct current

Effect
Stimulates circulation and nutrition, alleviates pain, regulates the tone, and has an electrolytic effect
Indication
Neuralgia, neuritis, arthrosis, myalgia, disturbed circulation, pretreatment of flaccid paralysis
Duration
10 to 20 min
Intensity
0.1 ma/cm^2 (the patient must not experience pain)

IONTOPHORESIS

Procedure

Drugs administered through skin by use of galvanic current; drugs must be applied at appropriate electrode (anode or cathode) according to properties of their electrical charges
Effect
Accomplished by the medication introduced to the tissue through the skin (as opposed to oral or parenteral route) and depends on the medication applied
Intensity
As for galvanization, never exceeding tolerance limit

DIADYNAMIC CURRENT

Procedure

Frequency-modulated, low frequency sinusoidal pulsed current with variation of frequency intensity and duration for different physiological effects developed 1940 by French Physicist P.M. Bernard
Effect
Fast alleviation of pain, acceleration of absorption of edema, relaxation of hypertonic muscles
Indication
Injuries of supporting, stabilizing, and locomotor apparatus; peripheral nerve lesions

Intensity
Must not exceed tolerance limit
Duration:
No longer than 10 min

EXPONENTIAL CURRENT

Procedure

Triangular current (sawtooth)
Indication:
Treatment of peripheral paralyses; selected denervated muscles can be stimulated separately; muscles with normal irritability are not stimulated simultaneously
Effect:
Prevention of atrophy, preservation of residual contractile muscle fibers, enhancement of nerve healing, maintenance of circulation and nutrition of the tissue
Intensity
0.1 μA/cm^2 (μAs per square cm)
Duration:
Pulse and intervals can be calculated by I/t curve; rise between **ART** and **ART, msp. 191**
Average values:
150 ms pulse, 1000 ms interval

PULSED CURRENT

Procedure

A rhythmic increase and decrease of series of pulses, applied for muscular exercise in inactivity atrophies
Indication
Treatment and assistance in treatment of inactivity atrophies
Intensity
Variable
Effect
Muscle exercise to increase volume and strength
Duration
1 ms; triangular pulse, interval: 20 ms

INTERFERENTIAL ALTERNATING CURRENT

Procedure

Application of two carrier frequencies (3,000 to 4,000 Hz), are constant frequency, one variable with a maximum difference of 120 Hz; the intersection of two currents produced by two independent circuits generates frequency shift leading to endogenous low frequency; it was developed 1951 by Austrian Physicist H. Nemec
Effect
Well tolerated, as there is no danger of skin burn

Indication and Choice of Frequency

Upper frequency range (90 to 100 Hz): analgesia, depression of sympathetic influence, regulation of vegetative dysregulation

Lower frequency range (>0 to 10 Hz): main effect on muscle contraction, deep "massage"

Duration

6–12 min

Intensity

20 μA to 30 μA according to size of electrodes

ULTRASOUND

Procedure

In ultrasound no current reaches the patient; an AC current is converted by an oscillating circuit into resonant frequency of the crystal used, than the high frequency is transformed into high voltage current (2000–3000 volt for Quartz crystals and 200–300 v for synthetic crystals); this modified electromagnetic energy is then coupled to the crystal and causes the crystal by the so called piezoelectric effect to emit ultrasound waves which are transmitted to the tissue by a tranducer and a coupling media or submersion of the treated part and the transducer in water; (the current cable and the crystal must be perfectly sealed to prevent electrical hazards)

Effect

According to mode of action

(a) thermal: formation of thermal energy, (b) mechanical: vibrational effect by pressure and tension, and (c) physicochemical: stimulation of the intermediary metabolism, increase in the rate of diffusion

Indication

Arthropathies, vertebrogenic syndromes, ankylosing spondylitis, tendinopathies, tendonitis, posttraumatic states

Duration

1–10 min, according to technique (i.e., stationary or moving transducer)

Applications:

Direct treatment with ultrasonic waves using a coupling medium or indirect underwater ultrasonic treatment; transducer moved in small circles over site to be treated

Intensity

Depends on area treated, mode, and individual patient (e.g., obesity); 0.5 W/square cm to 2.5 W/cm^2, with submersion 0.02 to 0.1 W/cm^2

HIGH FREQUENCY CURRENTS

Procedure

High frequency currents include shortwave, microwave, and ultrahigh frequency currents, as well as thermotherapy with depth effect; the depth depends on wavelength and the choice of electrodes; (the deepest heating can be achieved by ultrasound)

Applications:

The application of these currents covers a wide range, including rheumatoid diseases of joints and muscles and organic diseases

Contraindications

Include implanted cardiac pacemakers and pregnancy. It is important that all metal objects, damp clothes, and fabrics made of synthetic fibers such as Dacron, Orlon, and nylon, are removed. As far as dosage is concerned, the patient should experience agreeable warmth

Duration

Lasts from 10 to 20 min

Infrared

Thermotherapy of superficial tissue (see Fig. 12.8)

Indications

Migraine and inflammatory processes (frontal sinusitis) rheumatism, furuncles, and carbuncles)

HYDROTHERAPY
Mathilde Netsch

Sitz baths (or *hip baths*) are used for treatment of the pelvic and gluteal areas of the body (see Fig. 12.9). Hot sitz baths bring about relief of pain syndromes, spasms, and cramps of all muscles in the pelvic and abdominal area. Neutral (body temperature) sitz baths for 15 to 30 min relax the patient and can be hypnotic.

The *four-cell bath* is a hydroelectric partial bath composed of two containers for the upper extremities and two for the lower extremities. The electrodes are built into the containers. The intensity of the current can be adjusted to the patient's condition and needs. Indications are central and peripheral pareses, multiple sclerosis, and nervous irritability syndromes. The *warm partial bath* is usually given with added herb extracts.

The *contrast bath* improves circulation. Total time is 10 to 15 min, during which alternating submersions are made in cold and warm water, starting with warm water and followed by shorter submersion in cold (cool) water. The usual ratio is 30 sec to 1 min warm, 5 to 10 sec cold.

Paraffin submersion is used in patients with injury to hands and fingers. Several dips into liquid paraffin are done to build up several layers; then, the hand is wrapped in a fleece towel. After cooling about 5 to 10 min, the paraffin is peeled off, and the patient can use it for kneading therapy. The purpose of this submersion is to apply heat as well as to strengthen.

The *medicinal bath* provides a thermal stimulus by warm water, and chemical stimulus through additives. The chemicals act on the skin and body in liquid or gaseous form.

Underwater massage is a treatment given to parts or to the entire body by underwater jets with 1 to 4 atms of pressure. It is used for relaxation of tight, "cramped" muscles and for stimulation of circulation. Its contraindications are cardiovascular disturbances, impairment of circulation, acute inflammatory processes, and severe neuralgia.

Fangotherapy is a heat modality with deep action. It is used after soft tissue injuries, dislocations, fractures, chronic inflammatory processes, and articular and nonarticular rheumatic diseases.

Wading pools and *"sand/water walkways"* (*Sandwassergasse*) are filled on one side with warm water and on the other side with cold water. The floor in both pools is filled with sand and fine gravel. The patient wades in the pools several times and performs specific foot exercises (toe walk, heel walk, eversion and inversion, and others as directed).

The *Stanger bath* is a hydroelectric bath for full body submersion. The electrodes are built into the walls of the tub. Herbal additives during the bath provide iontophoretic effects. The temperature should be 35 to 38°C. Indications for the Stanger bath are: rheumatic diseases, arthritic conditions, neuralgia, and pareses. Contraindications are all inflammatory skin conditions and any implants.

MASSAGE CRYOTHERAPY
Annemarie Juën

Cryotherapy is a modality of the application of cold as a supportive measure to active physicotherapeutic exercises. Its effects on muscle tone are, with long application, relaxation and, with short application, stimulation. It also increases muscle contractility, reduces edema and, for example, in treatment of irritable joints, controls pain. Contraindications are blood vessel pathology and circulatory dysfunction, kidney and bladder diseases, muscle diseases and replantations.

"Flake ice" is produced by a special ice machine. It is spread over a damp terrycloth towel and placed over the treated extremity (Fig. 12.10). The duration of this application varies from patient to patient.

In an *ice bath treatment of spasticity*, ice is added to a tub filled with cold water. The temperature is maintained at about 0°C (32°F). The patient takes the cold bath for about 4 min and is then rubbed dry with warm terrycloth towels. The achieved relaxation allows easier application of exercises.

In *stimulation with ice*, small circumscribed areas are treated; for example, the extensor of the elbow (triceps) is stimulated in spastic hemiparesis.

MANUAL LYMPH DRAINAGE AND MASSAGE
Mathilde Netsch

The effects of manual lymph drainage are multifold. It reduces edema and pain, is soothing, and possibly influences body defense systems. For optimal effectiveness of manual lymph drainage, exacting techniques must be applied according to each disease: the room temperature must be comfortable, the patient must be placed in a relaxed position; and there should be no disturbing noises or glaring light. The hands of the therapist should be warm; no pain should be elicited by this treatment. The time of application varies with each disease (see also Chapter 3). Absolute contraindications are: thrombosis, neoplasms, and acute inflammatory processes.

Massage is a procedure in which the tissue of the ill person is influenced by the hand of the therapist for healing purposes. The indications of massage are: postinjury conditions, muscular rheumatism, arthritic joint changes, all forms of convalescence, and regional as well as general functional disturbances.

Techniques of manual massage are: stroking (effleurage); compression (pétrissage), which includes kneading, squeezing, and friction; and percussion (tapôtement), including hacking, clapping, beating, pounding, pummeling, and vibration. The treated part should show erythema and improved blood supply; this, in turn, provides for rapid removal of waste products and facilitates the supply of tissue with oxygen and nutrients.

Contraindications of massage are: inflammation of skin and subcutaneous connective tissue, acute injuries, infectious diseases, varicosities, and high blood pressure, as well as diseases of bones and bone marrow. During pregnancy, neither superficial nor deep massage (bowels) should be performed in the abdominal area.

STUMP EXERCISES
Bruno Schmidbauer

The preservation of physical health and especially the care of the stump should be routine for every amputee, but this is not always accomplished. A considerable percentage of lower limb amputees have complaints that are secondary to a lack of functional stump muscles. The neglect of stump exercises by inactive amputees may lead to a reduction of musculature and muscular atrophy, even in otherwise good functional stumps. Exercises should be carried out regularly by the amputee. The exercises should strengthen muscles that have or have not lost their insertions by the amputation as well as all muscles in the remaining extremity (thigh, quadriceps, abductors, and adductors, hamstrings, hip extensors, and flexors). Leg muscles for plantar and dorsiflexion of the ankle should also be exercised.

The preservation of stump muscles that have lost their insertions by amputation is only possible if they are kept active by movement. This can be achieved by stump exercises described later and by exercises that utilize phantom sensations for simulated movement. In the latter, for example, the patient may simulate flexion and extension of the missing knee (see Fig. 12.11), and a below-knee amputee may simulate gripping exercises with his or her toes.

Stump gymnastics may be considered an extension of the described phantom exercises. Active therapy after the amputation starts with isometric exercises in bed. Later, the patient exercises in the therapy department: extension and flexion of the stump (flexion of the hip-iliopsoas muscle; extension of the hip-gluteus maximus muscle) and adduction and abduction of the stump (abductors—gluteus medius and minimus muscles; adductors).

These exercises are initially carried out without, and later with, applied resistance. The intensity slowly is increased. The abdominal and back muscles are also strengthened. The exercises should never exceed the threshold of pain. Excessive tension on the recently sutured skin by excess movement should be avoided.

The significance of regular muscular training was demonstrated by a study of Müller and Hettinger (1900). They found that with daily training of not more than 15 sec exerting two-thirds of maximum strength, an increase of 4 to 5 cm in circumference of stump musculature and an increase in strength of 33% could be achieved in the above-knee amputee. Perhaps the results of this study will motivate some amputees, who believe that daily stump exercise is of no benefit, to carry them out regularly.

Gait depends not only on muscle strength or atrophy; contractures of the hip and knee joints have a negative influence on the gait and endurance as well as on posture. Even during the first few days after the amputation, correct positioning of the stump is essential to promote future mobility. For example, a frequent mistake is to elevate the stump on pillows while the patient is supine in bed, or to support the above-knee stump on the handle of the forearm crutch. Both promote flexion contractures of the hip and/or knee joint. If these contractures cannot be corrected by intensive special exercises, they can have a detrimental effect on the gait pattern and can delay considerably the prosthetic fitting.

Massage can never replace active body exercise, but it is a good supplement when done by an experienced practitioner. The amputee should learn simple manipulations and include them in the daily stump exercises and stump care. Proper bandaging of the stump for shaping and shrinking is also important, especially when no rigid dressing has been applied immediately after surgery. Common mistakes include bandaging with the hip flexed and abducted and proximal constriction. Bandaging technique for the above-knee stump is shown on Figure 12.12.

AMBULATION TRAINING FOR AMPUTEES
Julius Heidenwolf

Ambulation training enables the patient to achieve the best possible ability to walk. Mobilization activities may roughly be classified in four ways:

1. Those that enhance the patient's activity, especially elderly persons and those who lack initiative and motivation
2. Those that prepare the patient for prosthetic fitting (i.e., below-knee, above-knee, and bilateral amputees)
3. Those that instruct the patient in the use of prosthetic devices
4. Those that provide anatomophysiological gait training

A systematic procedure is essential for success. Therefore, the various stages of exercise are distributed into several training lessons.

FIRST LESSON

This first stage of exercise trains the patient to remove the prosthesis (this applies to both above-knee and below-knee amputees.) The therapist must supervise the procedure to correct mistakes; at the same time, pressure areas on the stump and malalignment of the prosthesis can be identified and corrected.

SECOND LESSON

This stage involves standing and balancing exercises using parallel bars (see Fig. 12.13). It is essential that the patient can watch him- or herself and correct faulty posture. For this purpose, two mirrors should be placed in a way that the patient has both an anterior and a lateral view of him- or herself. Also during this lesson, patients should learn to apply pressure alternately on the unimpaired and the prosthetic leg. Stump and gluteal muscles should be contracted during weightbearing.

THIRD LESSON

This lesson involves ambulation exercises. It is the most difficult lesson for the patient and, in order to avoid failures, should be divided into five phases:

Phase 1 The hip is pressed to the prosthetic side. Then, while the muscles are being contracted, pressure is applied on the prosthesis. This should be repeated frequently.

Phase 2 The unimpaired leg makes one step forward and then one step back to the initial position. Pressure is exerted on the prosthesis. The patient and trainer should now try to identify pressure areas—ischial tuberosity, end of stump and insertion of the adductors in above-knee amputations; patella and end of stump in below-knee amputations.

Phase 3 Weightbearing on the unimpaired leg, contraction of the muscles and lowering of the hip on the amputated side are done. The prosthetic knee is flexed involuntarily.

Phase 4 The stump is lifted slightly; then, the leg swings forward. The trainer's instructions are to lift the stump, put down the heel, and extend the knees.

Phase 5 In this phase, long steps are made with the unimpaired leg; short steps, with the prosthetic leg.

These exercises are always performed using two crutches or two canes.

Ninety percent of all above-knee amputees take longer steps with the prosthetic limb. It is important that the prosthetic knee is always flexed behind, and not in front of, the body. The prosthetic leg should always step over an obstacle first. As a general rule: "Take two steps without a cane rather than a 10-minute walk with one cane."

GAIT TRAINING FOR AMPUTEES
Julius Heidenwolf

Gait exercises are not easy for the new amputee. Even in such a technically advanced era as the 1980s, there are still two problems concerning prosthetic fitting:

1. Anatomical-orthopaedic problems: The patient does not immediately accept the prosthesis and considers it as a foreign body.
2. Orthopaedic-mechanical problems: The prosthesis cannot perform the fine skill motor movements of the leg.

The great individual differences in age, constitution, stamina, and stump condition make it difficult to predict at which time the gait exercise program should be changed from a merely static training to a dynamic gait training. According to the experience of the author, ambulation training should start after about 3 to 4 weeks of preparatory gait training.

Among other things the patient must learn how: (a) to lie down and get up from the floor, (b) to go up and down stairs, and (c) to walk across different terrains (cross-country training, see Fig. 12.14). To lie down and get up from the floor, the patient should learn to set the unimpaired leg one step forward and, at the same time, to bend the trunk forward; next, the patient should flex the prosthetic knee joint and support himself or herself on both hands; finally, he or she should swing around to the unimpaired side and sit down on the floor. Getting up is accomplished similarly, reversing the sequence described.

To go up and down stairs requires a special gait pattern. Stairs with very low steps can be climbed as usual. If steps have the common height of 17 to 18 cm, the unimpaired leg should climb up one or two steps first and the prosthetic leg follow. Descending stairs is a little easier. The patient should put the heel of the prosthetic leg on the edge of the next lower step, move the hip forward, hold on to the handrail with one hand, and place the foot of the unimpaired leg on the same step. If the patient is able to skip the next step with the unimpaired leg, he or she can descend the stairs in a normal way. This is called the "swing gait downstairs."

Bilateral above-knee amputees can climb stairs only with somewhat straddled legs. Both knee joints must be extended. They should hold on to the handrail with one hand and use a forearm crutch on the other side. Descending stairs is accomplished in the same way as by unilateral amputees with forearm crutch on one side and the handrail on the other side.

For walking across different terrains, if the terrain is not too steep, normal walking is possible with the prosthesis. The negotiation of steeper terrain is similar to that of climbing stairs. Going uphill, the unimpaired leg should go first and the prosthetic leg follow. Going downhill is similar to descending stairs (Fig. 12.14).

TRANSFER
Waltraud Starke

PARAPLEGICS

For the paraplegic, the transfer is one of the basic skills he or she must learn to achieve independence. In the course of the rehabilitation program, transfers are practiced on the high mat following instructions of a skilled therapist. The higher the spinal cord lesion, the more difficult the transfer is for the patient.

Prerequisites for independent transfer are balance and supporting function; both must be developed, learned, and practiced.

Paraplegics initially use a sliding board for transfer (Fig. 12.15). The patient puts one end of the board under his or her buttocks and the other end on the mat. He or she then should slide slightly forward in order to avoid being injured by the wheel of the chair. Then the patient should slide on the board from the wheelchair to the mat and lift his or her legs on the mat. This can also be done the other way around; first the legs lifted on the mat, then the body. During the transfer, the therapist should stand in front of the wheelchair to assist the patient and to protect him or her if there is a loss of balance. The transfer back to the wheelchair is accomplished in the same fashion.

When the paraplegic has gained more strength and has developed good support and balance, he or she may transfer without the board. Such patients should slide slightly forward in the wheelchair and lift their body from the wheelchair with their arms to the mat, using a swinging motion.

TETRAPLEGICS

Tetraplegic injuries can be divided in two groups:

1. Triceps brachii muscle innervated and functional (lesion below C7 with C7 spared)

2. Triceps brachii muscle nonfunctional (lesion at C7 or above)

In injuries at and above C7, the transfer is more difficult because of the unstable balance. The triceps brachii muscle provides a fair supporting function of the arm and allows push-ups for transfer. Marked differences exist in transfers of a paraplegic as compared to the tetraplegic because of hand involvement of the latter. The tetraplegic must pull up his or her legs with his or her arms holding the wrists in dorsi- or volarflexion. This type of tetraplegic can also learn the transfer without the board.

Tetraplegics with spinal cord lesions at or above C7 must replace the lost function of the triceps brachii muscle by locking the elbow using a trick movement: The arms should be rotated externally and the elbow joints thrown into extension. This provides good support for the transfers. The legs are pulled back with dorsiflexed wrist joints as there is no active volarflexion. This patient will always depend upon a sliding board.

If a patient has spasms, this may be an advantage as well as a disadvantage; pure flexion or extension spasms create problems, but in proper combination, they may actually facilitate transfers.

When the patient has learned the transfer on the high mat, he or she can then proceed to practice it during self-help training. The patient can learn independent transfer from the wheelchair to the bed, to the toilet, and to the bathtub. He or she must appreciate and be motivated to learn transfers to his or her regular chair or sofa. Finally, the patient should practice transfer into and out of the car.

RANGE OF MOTION EXERCISES OF THE LOWER EXTREMITIES AND THE TRUNK
Waltraud Starke

The paraplegic patient needs maximum mobility to be independent. The ROM exercises of the lower extremities (see Fig. 12.16) keep the joints flexible in all directions of movement and stimulate circulation. Groups of muscles and tendons that have a strong tendency for contraction, such as the ischiocrural muscles and the Achilles tendon (talipes equinus), are stretched. The movement must be very gentle in order to avoid microtraumas and danger of unintentional side effects, such as periarticular calcifications (PAC).

In rehabilitation, passive ROM exercises should be started at bedside during the acute phase. The extent of movements depends on the level of the lesion. In lesions involving the lower thoracic or lumbar spine, comotion of the spine should be avoided by using a reduced ROM. If the lesion is located in the upper thoracic or cervical spine, passive movements of the extremities are allowed as usual. After the patient has been mobilized and the training on the mat has started, daily ROM exercises should be continued. Special care should be given to the dorsiflexion of the ankle joint to avoid an equinus foot deformity. The so-called "wheelchair contracture" (flexion contractures of the knee and hip joints) must be avoided because it might affect the sitting posture in the wheelchair. The patient should be told to take special care of his or her legs. As soon as possible, the paraplegic and skilled tetraplegic should be taught how, by themselves, to move their legs passively through the range. Movement through the full range is especially important in the spastic paralysis because of an increased danger of contractures. Besides, passive ROM exercises per-

formed for a longer period of time may also reduce spasms. Especially suited for this is the rotation of the lumbar spine.

The flexibility must be increased in areas of the spine that are not stabilized. If several vertebral segments are fixed, the flexibility of the spine must be replaced partly by the hip joint, which means that the hip joint becomes hypermobile. If the patient is not able to accomplish the passive movement by him- or herself as, for example, a tetraplegic at or above C7 or a patient with severe spasms or contractures, a member of the family or attendant should be taught how to do it.

After being discharged from the hospital, the patient must continue his or her daily ROM exercises at home to prevent contractures.

RANGE OF MOTION OF THE UPPER EXTREMITY
Gabriele Schmiederer

Flexibility of all joints is a prerequisite for strengthening exercises. The tetraplegic tends to develop contractures because of the loss of large groups of muscles. The following joints are especially at risk:

1. Shoulder joint—all directions
2. Elbow joint—flexion contracture
3. Wrist joint—flexion contracture
4. Finger joints—extension contracture

Passive ROM exercises must be started immediately while the patient still is in bed (provided that no contraindications exist). When the patient already has exercised on the mat, generally every treatment starts with passive movements.

SHOULDER JOINT

When moving the shoulder girdle (exclusive of glenohumeral joint), which must be flexible in all directions, special care must be given to the mobility of the scapula (see Fig. 12.17). Several muscles, such as the serratus anterior and the rhomboid muscles, can be contracted. The more normal the ROM, the better the chances for relative independence (eating, brushing hair, etc.).

Shoulder joint exercises should be carried out against resistance. The flexibility of the shoulder joint is of special importance to patients who depend on trick or compensatory movements.

ELBOW JOINT

Faulty positioning, inactivity, and neurological deficits all lead to contractures of the elbow joint, especially in

tetraplegics. An elbow joint that cannot be completely extended cannot provide optimum supporting function. A flexible elbow joint can be trained for maximal extension and flexion. If a transverse lesion has made the extension of the elbow by the triceps brachii muscle impossible, a "trick extension" must be learned.

By internal rotation and adduction of the shoulder joint, and supination of the elbow joint, the arm can be "flung" into extension. This is also possible by external rotation, abduction, and supination.

"Trick extension" of the elbow is required for the hand-wrist support, which is fundamental for the transfer from bed to wheelchair and vice versa, as well as to the toilet, bathtub, and car.

WRIST AND HAND

For the passive movement of the wrist joint, special care must be given to the dorsiflexion, as both passive and active formation of a fist is only possible with adequate shortening of the extensor tendons. Flexion must be possible in all finger joints. If this is not possible, flexion gloves must be applied for passive fist formation.

In tetraplegics, a functional hand by flinging back the wrist joint, the natural tenodesis mechanism allows for a "fist" position, which is frequently required in everyday life activities. In wrist dorsiflexion fingers are drawn into flexion, in wrist volar flexion fingers extend a fist opens.

Patients can place the thumb of one hand into opposition passively using the other hand as assistance.

SITTING UP
Theresia Barbach

The paraplegic patient who has lost certain groups of muscles because of spinal injury must once again learn how to sit in an upright position. This is accomplished under the supervision of the therapist and is included in the treatment during the very beginning of rehabilitation. According to the level of the lesion, different techniques are applied. *The paraplegic* starts with lateral sitting up: He or she turns to the side, props elbows on the floor, and extends arms. When the shoulder muscles have gained strength, he or she then can sit upright from the supine position, pulling both elbows below his or her shoulders, extending one arm after the other and straightening upright (see Fig. 12.18).

The tetraplegic with a lesion at or above C7 (without the triceps brachii muscle) must turn his or her body to the lateral position by swinging the arms, then bringing the head toward the knees with the support of the elbows, and then stretching the arm by a trick movement and linking it to the knees. The patient should swing his or her head to the side in order to get speed for the extension of the lower arm, which is accomplished by a trick movement.

The tetraplegic with a lesion below C7 (with the triceps brachii muscle intact) can learn to sit up from the lateral position according to the same principle as the tetraplegic with a lesion at or above C7, but this patient will have fewer difficulties because the triceps brachii muscle is innervated and the trick movement does not have to be used. The patient with a lesion below C7 can also learn how to sit up from the supine position as soon as his or her arms and shoulder muscles have become strong enough. The technique is the same as that of the paraplegic.

The paraplegic can learn to sit upright within a few hours of beginning to exercise. The tetraplegic often needs 2 to 3 months with daily exercises. The training can be facilitated by a high mat with a smooth surface on which it is easier to slip forward. Sitting upright is not only part of a training program but also an essential movement pattern that the patient needs to learn in order to become independent in his or her everyday life (for example, to sit upright in bed).

EXERCISES FOR HAND/WRIST SUPPORT
Theresia Barbach

The paralysis of the lower extremity makes it necessary to learn hand-wrist support because this type of support will have to replace the function of the legs.

As the sensitivity of the gluteal region is lost, the use of the correct hand-wrist support is crucial to avoid skin damage (caused by skimming over the wheelchair wheel during the transfer). Special exercises help to teach the patient the correct way of pushing himself up. The patient must have a good sense of balance. Support blocks of various heights can be used as aids (see Fig. 12.19).

There are two basic differences in approach between paraplegics and tetraplegics.

EXERCISES FOR PARAPLEGICS

As the development of the hand-wrist support requires much strength, arm and shoulder muscles must be well exercised. However, these exercises by themselves provide a good training for strength. The paraplegic should start with a support block, about 15 cm high. The patient should be instructed to put his or her head forward, round the shoulders, and press the shoulder joints downward. The patient should push him- or herself at least up to the level of the block.

Further exercises include pushing up from sitting and swinging the buttocks sideways and exercises using the oblique position of the support blocks. Once the patient masters these exercises, the number of blocks can be increased up to three pieces, which corresponds with a height of about 45 to 50 cm. Further exercises are carried out with the support blocks only on one side of the patient in order to teach him or her how to change between seats of different heights.

EXERCISES FOR TETRAPLEGICS

At or Above C7 Level Lesion

This patient initially practices the pushup without support blocks. He or she must learn how to extend his or her arms by a trick movement. It is very important for the patient to use the shoulder muscles correctly. At the beginning of the training, drawing the shoulder blades apart (*abduction*) and pressing the shoulders down (*depression*) is exercised. At the end of the training, the patient will be able to push him- or herself up a few centimeters. Thereafter, hand-wrist support exercises, using blocks of wood with specially rounded edges, should follow.

Below C7 Level Lesion

This patient can learn how to push him- or herself up in the same way as the paraplegic, but he or she will have greater difficulties due to impaired balance caused by the paralyzed hand muscles. The technique is the same as for paraplegics. With increasing strength, he or she can also master the same height of the pushups as the paraplegic.

The exercises for hand-wrist support are a preparation for effective independent transfer and for climbing into the wheelchair from the floor. Besides, it is important that the patient is able to relieve pressure on his buttocks by pushups several times a day to avoid pressure sores.

TRAINING OF BALANCE
Gernot Stix

The training of balance is of great importance in the overall rehabilitation of paraplegics. The sense of balance must be newly developed because it is now controlled by the shoulder girdle alone. For this kind of control, it is essential that the residual muscles of the trunk and the arms are brought into optimum condition by adequate exercise. They must be in better condition than those of an average healthy person.

Several training positions are used: (a) exercises in the long seat (with knees extended), (b) exercises in the short seat (the taylor seat, with or without a mirror), and the tetrapod position. All of these exercises are carried out with or without aids and with open, and later closed, eyes.

Apparatus that can be used includes: the bar, balls (of different weights), dumbbells, and support blocks. To reduce boredom during training, it is advisable also to include some kinds of sports, such as badminton or family tennis.

At the beginning of the training, the patient should sit with knees extended and try to find his or her center of gravity. At first, the patient will lean forward but, with practice, he or she will learn to straighten up and maintain a sense of balance. Later, the therapist may try to throw the patient off-balance on purpose; the patient must learn to maintain balance.

The goal of therapy, for tetraplegics as well as paraplegics, is to develop the patient's ability to sit without a backrest and to do easy work in this position.

To accomplish this goal, balance standing training should include sitting balance, using a mirror for feedback, sitting in the quadriped position, and using a ball, tilt belt (for tetraplegics), tilt belt with pads, tilt table, and parallel bars (see Fig. 12.20).

STRENGTHENING OF RESIDUAL MUSCLES
Gernot Stix

The paraplegic must develop the ability to perform all possible activities substituting remaining functional muscles for paralyzed or paretic muscles. Therefore, the remaining muscles should be strengthened as much as possible. The training of the noninvolved muscles is one of the most important tasks of the physical therapy rehabilitation of the paraplegic patient. The three main goals are: to develop strength, to develop balance, and to develop the ability to propel a wheelchair.

Training usually starts while the patient is still in bed, and is intensified when he or she is able to transfer to the mat. The therapist should emphasize to the patient the great importance of such a strenuous training program in order to ensure his or her cooperation. The patient must be convinced that the exercises are indispensable, and that they must be continued daily after the formal rehabilitation has ended.

For training without apparatus, common techniques used in physical therapy are proprioceptive neuromuscular facilitation (PNF) (Fig. 12.21) and parts of Klapp's scoliosis exercises in the quadruped position.

For training and strengthening exercises the following assistive devices have proved successful:

Medicine ball
Dumbbells
Weight for exercises on the bench
Rubber elastic bands, thera bands
Stretch springs
Compression springs

The so-called Böhler's "mountain climbers" for quad-strengthening and knee extension
Knee benders for knee flexion
Pulleys
Variety of N-K tables or modern mechanized exercisers, e.g., the Cybex system for isokinetic exercises

There are scarcely any limits to the therapist's inventiveness in designing a program for intensive training that is as diversified as possible. However, injuries and overexertion should be avoided. The tetraplegic needs flexion gloves to enable him or her to use pulleys, dumbbells, etc. The patient should be introduced to the various exercises individually. As soon as he or she has acquired adequately some experience and strength, he or she should participate in group training. The performance can further be diversified and improved by rhythmic exercises with music.

AMBULATION TRAINING FOR PARAPLEGICS
Bruno Schmidbauer

After the patient has gained sufficient strength and sitting balance, the spine is stable and he or she is ready to start intensive physical therapy, including ambulation training. Standing and walking are vital for paraplegics for the following reasons:

1. They improve circulation.
2. They ensure better urinary drainage.
3. Weightbearing and loading of long bones reduce demineralization and the possibility of fractures.
4. They prevent hip and knee joint contractures.

The training of quadriplegics starts with standing in the mechanical or electrohydraulic standing bed (tilt table) for the regaining of circulatory homeostasis. The patient is secured by a belt, and the bed is gradually tilted to the vertical position by the therapist. This is done manually or by operating the electronic or hydraulic mechanism. Patients with functional arm muscles can stand in a standing table and the quadriplegic can learn to use standing splints, which provide external locking of the knees.

Well-rehabilitated quadriplegics (below C4) should be able to pull themselves into an upright position and stand with braces between parallel bars without assistance. Most are able to stand for 30 min.

Gait training of paraplegics starts with standing between parallel bars with temporary braces (see Fig. 12.22). Subsequently, depending on the level of the lesion, the patient starts with the swing to, swing through, or 4-point-gait between parallel bars. For the swing gaits, well-developed and trained shoulder girdle, arm, and hand muscles, as well as a passive hyperextension of both hip joints, are required.

Patients with lesions below the 9th thoracic vertebra can learn the 4-point-gait since they have functional la-tissimus dorsi and quadratus lumborum muscles, which connect the shoulder girdle, the spine, and the pelvis. If the patient is capable, he or she should learn the 4-point-gait because it provides greater stability on uneven ground and narrow spaces. When the patient has achieved a good gait pattern between the parallel bars, he or she should continue ambulation with one forearm crutch and one hand on the bar; then the patient should walk with two forearm crutches.

In order to facilitate the change from the parallel bars to walking with two forearm crutches, the patient may, for a short time, walk with the reciprocal walker. It provides more security because of its 4-point support. When the patient's gait pattern has become satisfactory and his or her walking performance becomes consistent with the temporary locking devices, he or she can be supplied with a knee-ankle-foot orthosis (KAFO). This has a knee joint with a lock and a flexible ankle joint.

The gait training also includes the climbing of stairs, which the patient can accomplish with the help of the handrail and one forearm crutch (depending on the level of the lesion). Part of the training is to teach the patient how to get in and out of the wheelchair and how to sit and arise from ordinary chairs, independently and safely, with the help of ambulation aids.

All paraplegics are trained on a mat in methods for falling safely arising independently, using two forearm crutches. At the end of his or her stay in the rehabilitation hospital, the paraplegic with complete lesion (depending on the level of the lesion) should be able to walk for about 50 to 100 m (150 to 300 ft) with two forearm crutches and supporting devices; also they should be able to climb stairs and to get up from the floor independently.

SWIMMING WITH SPINAL CORD LESIONS
Bruno Schmidbauer

All paraplegics, quadriplegics, and patients with incomplete lesions should be given the opportunity for regular swimming because it improves the function of the cardiovascular system. Prerequisites for swimming are good skin condition and functional reflex action of the bladder and bowel. Swimming is an excellent training for mobility of the shoulder girdle. It relaxes the overloaded arm and trunk muscles and provides good exercise for paretic muscles in patients with incomplete transverse lesions. Furthermore, it promotes coordination and sometimes reduces spasticity. However, occasionally warm water may lead to increased spasms. A prerequisite for participation of paraplegics in swimming programs is wheelchair access to the shower, dressing room, toilets and swimming pool. Shower wheelchairs (Fig. 12.23) should also be available so that the paraplegic will be able to get onto the pool ramp and take a shower before and after swimming. Unfortunately, public pools rarely meet these requirements, and the disabled must often rely on rehabilitation centers with all the equipment for disabled sports available.

The temperature of the water should be between 28 and 32°C (80–90°F). Even these high temperatures initially may lead to signs of hypothermia, especially in patients with higher lesions. Therefore, swimming must be started carefully, the training slowly, and the patient's performance gradually increased to a competitive sports level.

Paraplegics should be lifted into the water by therapists or assistants. Quadriplegics and very heavy paraplegics can enter and leave the swimming pool with the help of electric or hydraulic lifts. Well-rehabilitated paraplegics can manage the transfer independently using a swivel rope ladder. The water should at least be 1.5 m deep (5 ft) because in shallow water, the paralyzed legs are dragged along the floor of the pool possibly causing skin damage.

At the beginning of the training, the therapist should try to acquaint the disabled patient with the new environment. When the patient feels safe and secure in the water, the backstroke (the most advantageous technique for paraplegics) can be started. Quadriplegics can use the Heidelberg collar to keep the head above water. To prevent the pelvis from sinking, the arms should be moved through the water more rapidly and pulled slightly under the pelvis; and the head should be hyperextended to keep the body's center of gravity above the pelvis. When the paraplegic has become proficient in this technique and is able to swim without the therapists assistance, he or she can (depending on the level of the lesion) turn to other swimming styles, such as the breaststroke, crawl, or butterfly stroke. As a rule, the functional abilities of the paralyzed should be utilized to the utmost by teaching various techniques.

WHEELCHAIR TRAINING
Richard Altenberger

After strengthening remaining muscles, learning adequate support techniques, and developing balance, wheelchair training can be started. This is most important in the final phase of rehabilitation. A systematic and forceful approach is needed to enable the patient to master uneven ground, architectural barriers, and obstacles, and above all, to make him or her independent in a wheelchair.

GETTING IN AND OUT OF THE WHEELCHAIR

As soon as the wheelchair driver knows how independently to transfer from the wheelchair to the floor and return to the wheelchair (see Fig. 12.24), he or she will loose the fear of falling from it. Under the supervision of a therapist, the patient should learn the correct pattern of motion and the correct reactions: taking his or her legs off the legrest and putting them beside it with knees flexed; sliding forward to the edge with his or her buttocks, put-

ting the nearer hand on the floor, and letting him- or herself fall down to the side of the wheelchair. The therapist should make certain that no part of the patient's body or clothing gets caught on the wheelchair. The transfer from the floor to the wheelchair requires more skill, strength, and coordination because a difference in level of about 60 cm (2 ft) must be overcome. The patient should start from the squat position, with the legrest of the wheelchair between his or her bent legs in an angle of about 90 degrees beside the wheelchair. The upper extremity, which is nearer to the wheelchair, should grasp the forward edge of the seat while the other arm provides support between the pelvis and knee. He or she should then push up and bend the trunk forward. This maneuver stretches the legs, extends the knees, and keeps the center of gravity low. The feet serve as the pivotal point. As the pelvis is relieved from weight, the patient will be able to pivot and sit down into the wheelchair.

At the beginning of training, the therapist should stand behind the patient and give assistance by grasping him or her at the trousers or pants and shoulders.

TILTING THE WHEELCHAIR

Before tilting exercises are started, the patient must show full control of the wheelchair on all four wheels. A great number of exercises and training devices are available to train the patient in good sitting balance in the wheelchair. Tilting means that the wheelchair is balanced on its two back wheels (a "wheelie," Fig. 12.25). It is one of the most important ways of moving a wheelchair because it enables the patient to overcome obstacles.

At the beginning of the tilting exercises, the therapist should secure the patient or the backrest of the chair with a rope. With a short quick forward acceleration of the driving wheels, the front wheels should then be lifted off the floor and the patient should try to keep his or her equilibrium while balancing on the back wheels. The proper reactions that avoid falling out of the wheelchair are practiced. When the patient falls backward, he or she must learn to pull the driving wheels back quickly with a jerk, which will bring the center of gravity forward. If the patient falls forward, he or she must quickly push the wheels forward to maintain balance. After learning to keep balance in the tilted position, tilting in motion should be practiced. The patient should drive slowly and reach far back with both hands, then grasp the driving wheels and pull them quickly forward. This manuever tilts the wheelchair, lifting the coaster wheels off the ground. The patient can then keep the wheelchair in balance on the driving wheels while riding forward.

OVERCOMING OBSTACLES
Richard Altenberger

Starting on slightly uneven ground, the patient should be encouraged to tilt his or her wheelchair but should be instructed not to tilt more than is necessary to overcome an obstacle. The following sequence of individual movements should be practiced:

1. Drive directly toward the obstacle.
2. Tilt only enough to clear the obstacle's height.
3. Place the coasters on the obstacle while moving forward.
4. Follow with the driving wheels after reaching back with both hands, bending the trunk forward, and drive over the obstacle.

For a smooth operation, harmonious, coordinated, and sequential movements are important. The more refined and controlled the movements, the better the obstacle is overcome without damage to the wheelchair or discomfort to the rider.

At the end of rehabilitation, a paraplegic should be able to master sidewalk edges up to 15 cm high (6 inches) without help. Driving down from obstacles is also done in the tilted position. The wheelchair driver should approach the edge of the obstacle, tilt the wheelchair, and glide over the edge with the back wheels of the chair. The therapist should make certain that the patient stops in tilted position immediately after the obstacle, leaning against it. This is also important for driving down several steps or stairs (Fig. 12.26).

DRIVING UP AND DOWN STAIRS

The ability to negotiate stairs or steps upward is achieved only rarely. It can only be accomplished when the lesion is low (up to about T10) in young and strong paraplegics with well-developed remaining musculature. A solid handrail is required. The patient should tilt his or her chair and place the coasters on the first step; he or she then should grasp the handrail with the nearer hand and propel and tilt the chair until the back wheels are in good contact with the stair or step. With the other hand, the patient should pull the driving wheel over the first step and, at the same time hold on to the handrail, pull up the other wheel. This process is repeated until the top of the stairs is reached.

This is the most difficult way of forward movement because it requires much strength and many skills. Descending stairs however, is much easier and can be learned by almost any paraplegic.

DESCENDING WITH HANDRAIL

To descend steps using a handrail, the patient should drive backward to the first step, grasp the handrail with the near hand, and hold the opposite driving wheel back with the other hand; he or she then should roll over the first step with both wheels while bending his or her trunk slightly forward and stop one step below. The patient must be told never to let go of the handrail in order to avoid the danger of falling.

DESCENDING WITHOUT HANDRAIL

To descend steps without a handrail, the patient should drive his or her wheelchair forward to the first step in a tilted position and slowly roll over the first stair, coming to a stop on each step. Whether the patient is ascending or descending stairs, he or she must always be accompanied by an experienced assistant.

Recent studies at the rehabilitation center in Bad Häring, Tirol, Austria and other centers have shown that much more attention must be given to the rehabilitation in the wheelchair. The patient's entire life depends on the wheelchair, and he or she deserves the best training increase independent functioning. All persons working with wheel-dependent patients should pay special attention to this aspect of rehabilitation. In an environ- ment often filled with obstacles and architectural barriers, independence is the goal that every patient in a wheelchair must achieve. The curve of a sidewalk, an inclined street, or a slope should not restrict locomotion of rehabilitation.

Figure 12.1. Individual treatment of the upper extremities includes:

A–E. Flexion, extension, abduction, adduction and rotation of the shoulder
F–G. Extension of the elbow and supination of the forearm
H–I. Dorsiflexion of the wrist, ulnar deviation of the hand, and
J–K. Extension, abduction of fingers
   L. Flexion and opposition of the thumb.

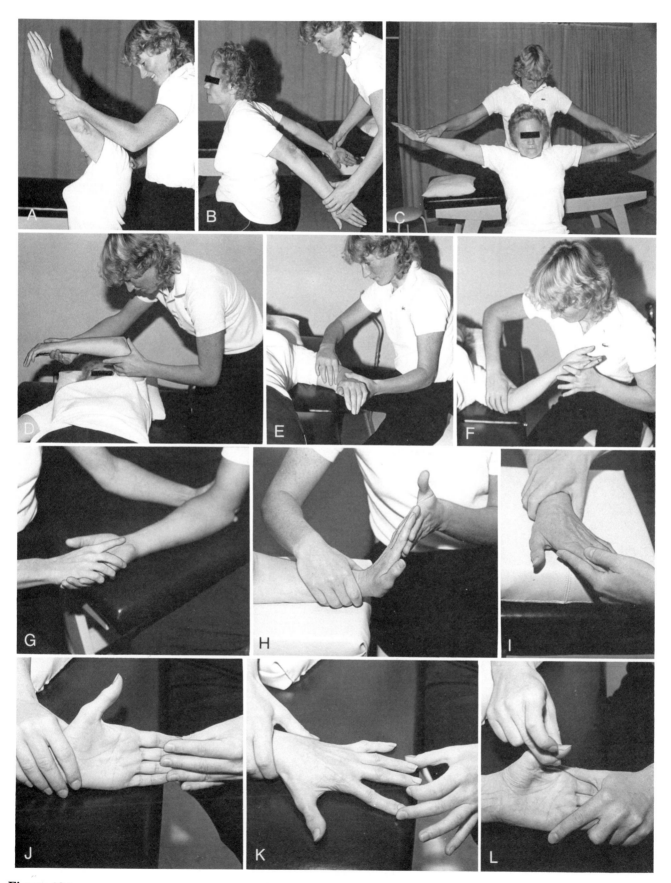

Figure 12.1.

Figure 12.2. Individual treatment of lower extremities includes:

A. Flexion of the hip and knee against resistance
B. Passive flexion of the hip and knee
C. Strengthening of the quadriceps
D. Passive knee flexion
E. Active abduction of the hip
F. Active extension of the hip
G. Passive dorsiflexion of the upper ankle joint (stretching of triceps surae)
H. Plantar flexion against resistance, and
I. Passive mobilization of the lower ankle joint.

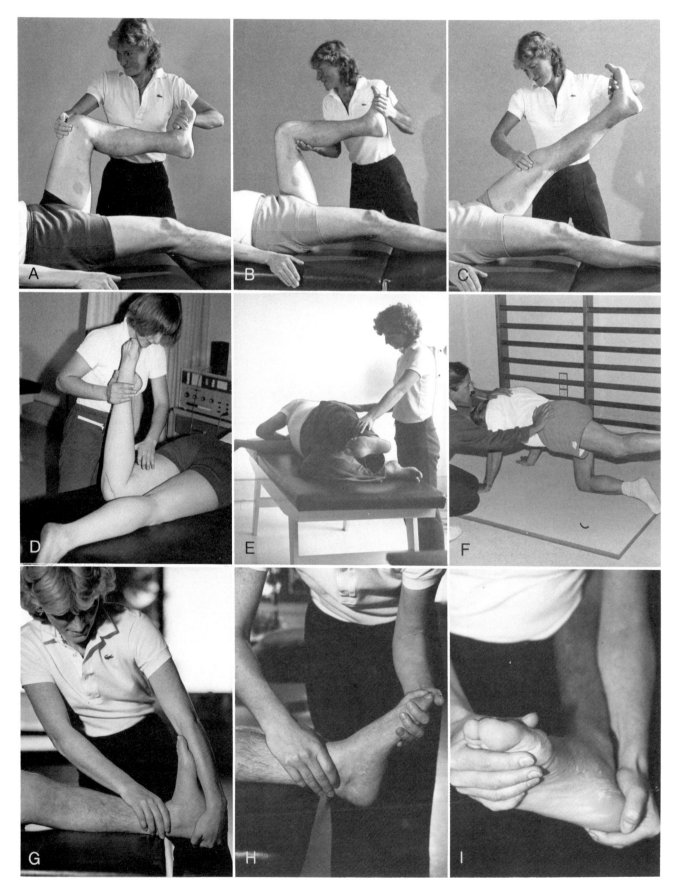

Figure 12.2.

Figure 12.3. General physical exercises

A–J. Relaxation and strengthening exercises of upper and lower extremities in groups are shown.

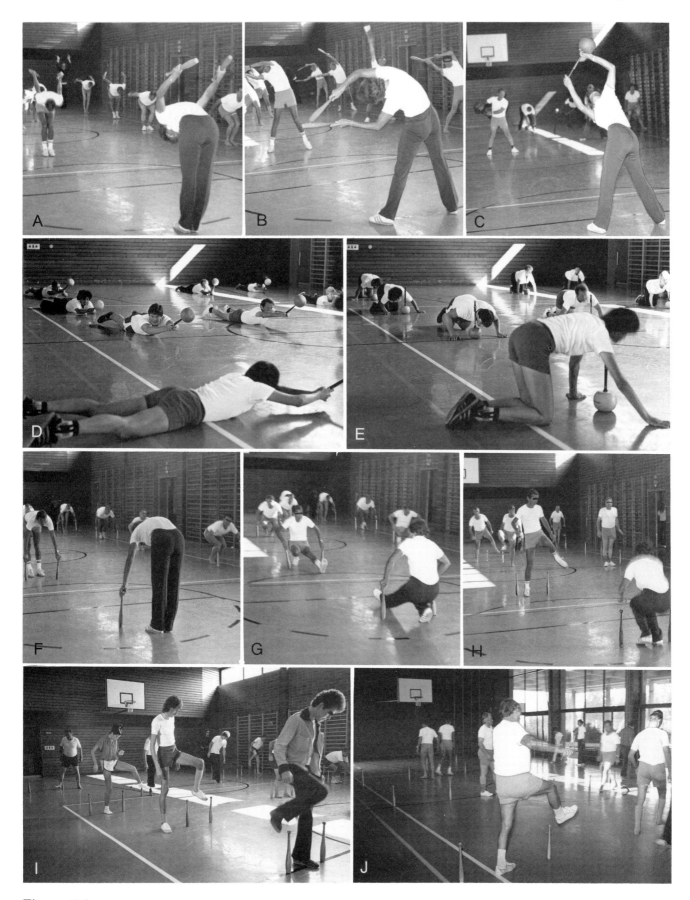

Figure 12.3.

Figure 12.4. Group gymnastics for the trunk muscles include:

A, C, G. Exercises for abdominal muscles
    B. Back extensor strengthening
  D, F. Stretching of back and hip flexors
    E. Relaxation and
    H. Swing motion
     I. After group exercises, patients assist in retrieving mats for storage.

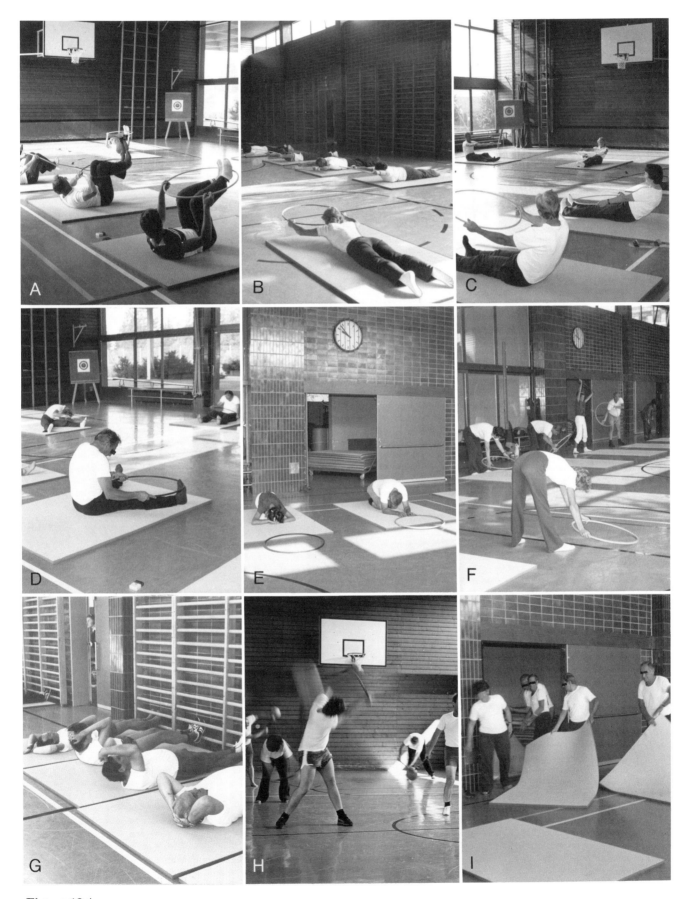

Figure 12.4.

Figure 12.5. Kinetic therapy in water involves:

   A. Life preservers and inflatable "floating wings"

B–C. Sunken area in floor with disinfectant solution through which each patient entering the pool must wade

D–E. Therapeutic pool, and

  F–I. Individual therapy in water (tetraplegia post-brain injury).

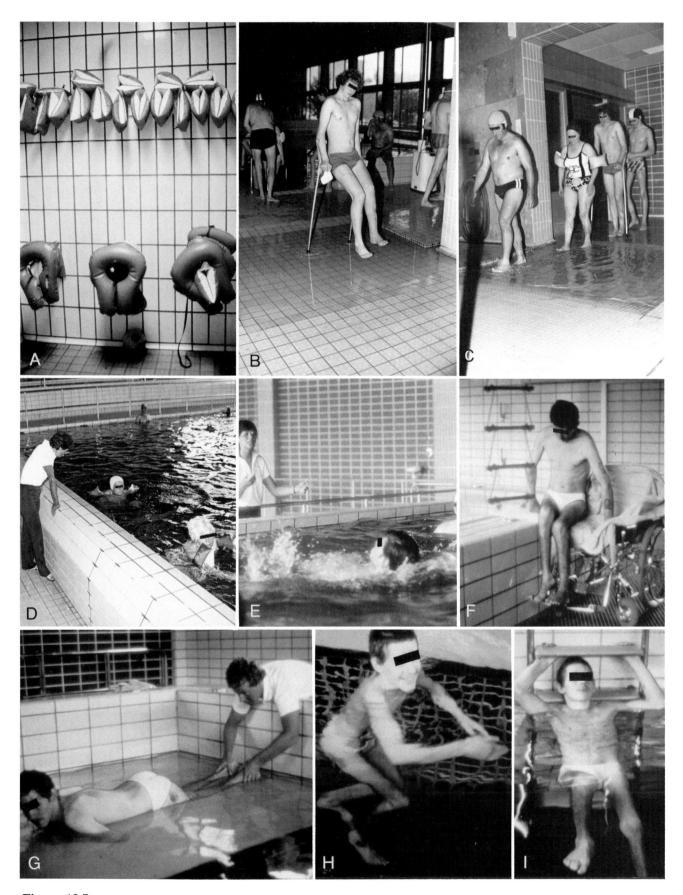

Figure 12.5.

Figure 12.6. Independent exercises include:

   A. Knee bender

B–C. Knee extender ("mountain climber")

   D. Treadmill ergometer

   E. Pulley block

   F. Stationary bicycle

   G. Bench press (dumb bar)

   H. Exercise on wall bars, and

   I. Swing frame.

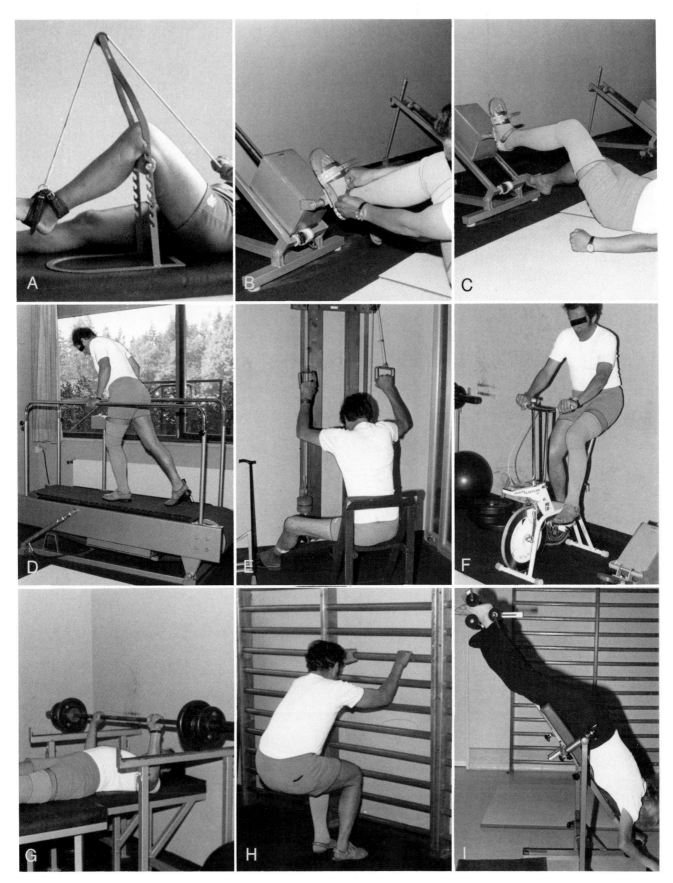

Figure 12.6.

Figure 12.7. Gait training in groups involves

A–B. Postural and gait exercises
C–F. Obstacle course, and
 G–I. Training on various surfaces.

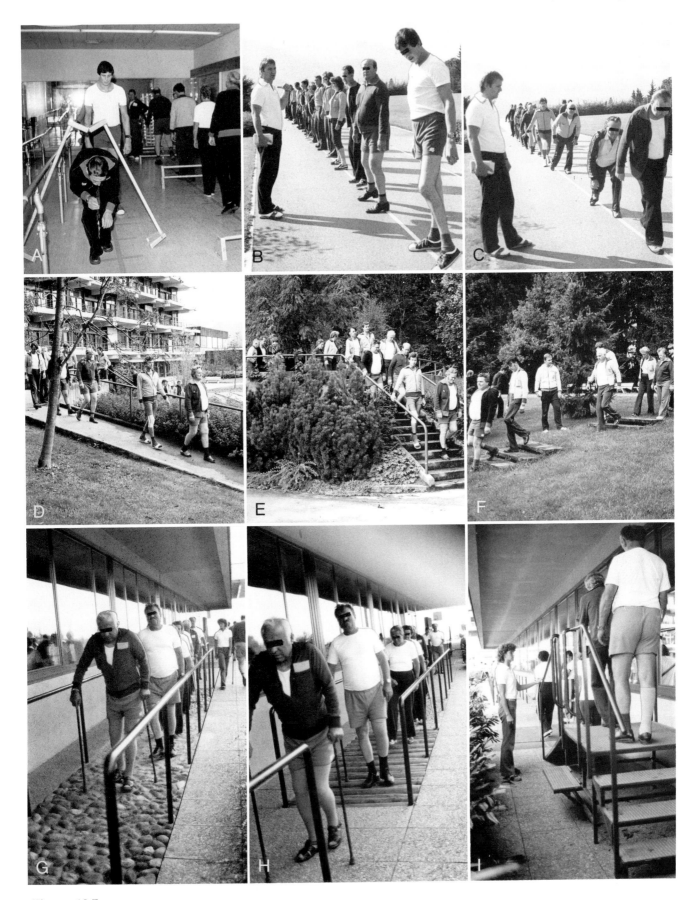

Figure 12.7.

Figure 12.8. Electrotherapy involves

    A. Infrared lamp
B–C. Shortwave, decimeter wave (high frequency therapy)
    D. Ultrasound
    E. Interference current
    F. Exponential current
    G. Galvanization
H–I. Diadynamic current, and
    J. Ultraviolet lamp.

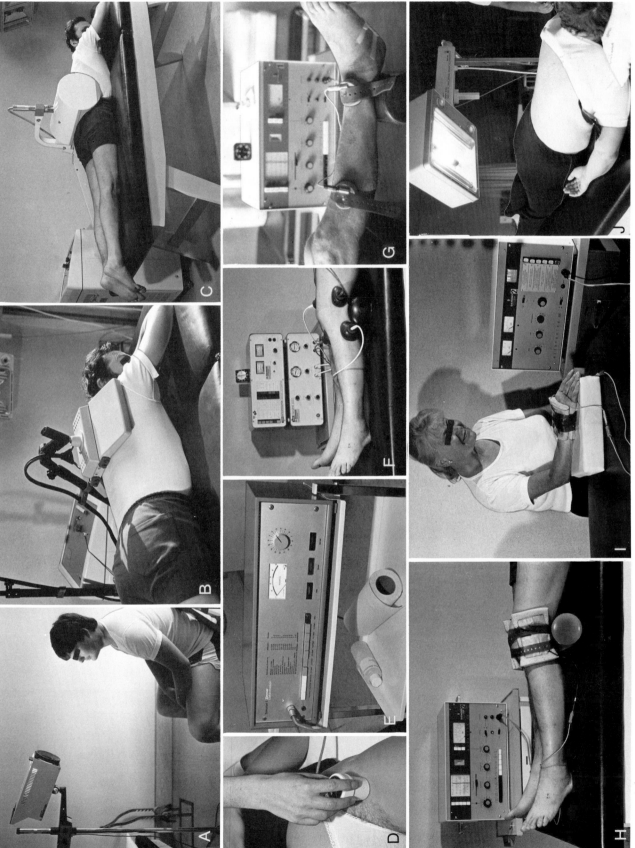

Figure 12.8.

Figure 12.9. Hydrotherapy uses

    A. Sitz bath
    B. Four-cell galvanic bath
    C. Partial submersion bath
    D. Contrast bath (warm, cold)
    E. Paraffin bath and kneading
    F. Medicated bath
    G. Underwater massage
  H–J. Fangotherapy (hot mudpack), and
  K–M. Wading pool (sand/water walkway).

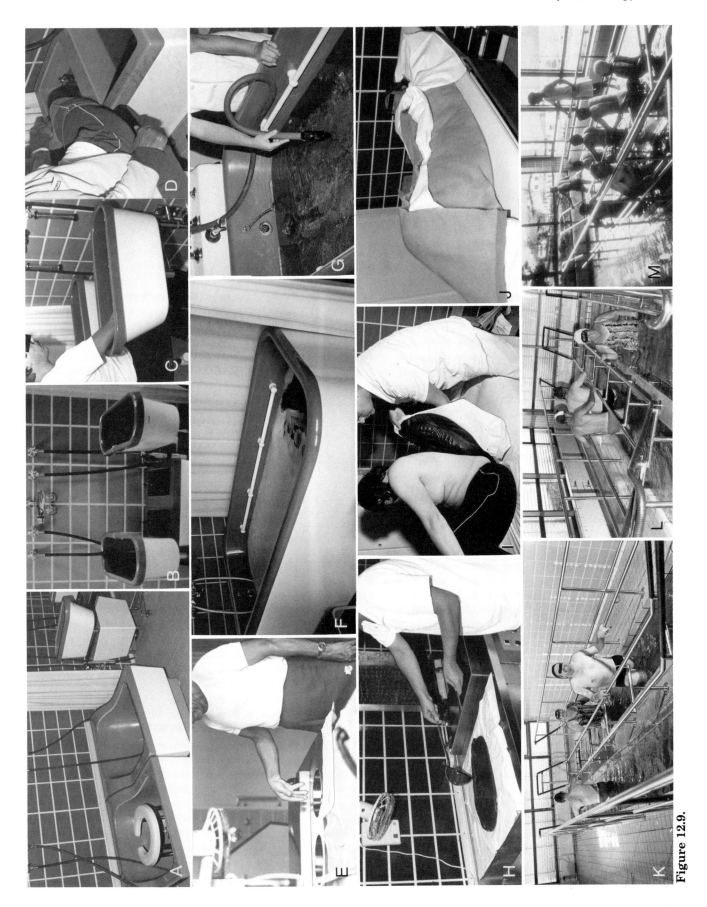

Figure 12.9.

Figure 12.10. Massage cryotherapy involves

A–B. Preparation of ice pack
   C. Treatment of contracture
   D. Ice bath in spasticity
   E. Suppression of spasticity
   F. Stimulation with ice
   G. Manual lymph drainage, and
H–I. Dry massage.

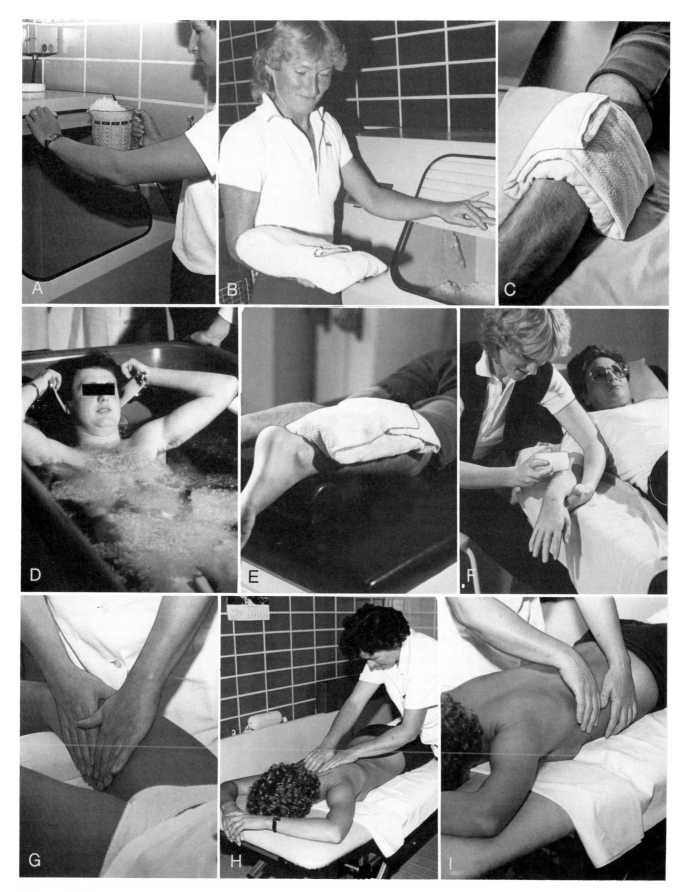

Figure 12.10.

Figure 12.11. Stump exercises include

A–C. Short above-knee stump bandaging (note: hip spica)
D–E. Below-knee stump exercises, extension and flexion against resistance, and
 F–I. Above-knee stump exercises, all movements against resistance.
J–L. Faulty positioning promotes knee and hip flexion contractures.

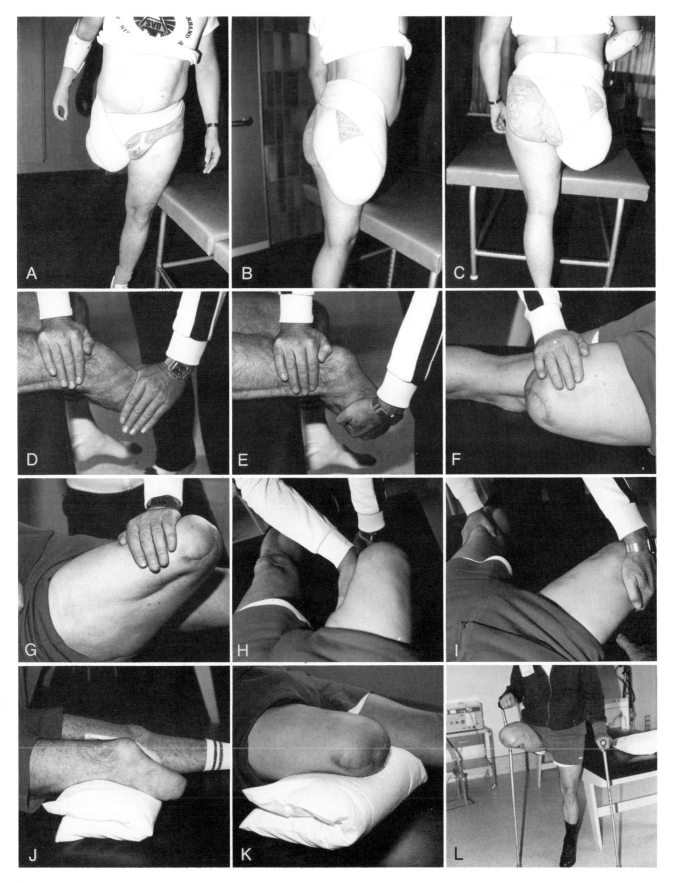

Figure 12.11.

Figure 12.12. Bandaging of an above-knee residual limb (reprinted with permission from Gerhardt JJ, King PS, and Zettl JH *Amputations: Immediate and Early Prosthetic Management.* Hans Huber Publishers, 1982, p 104).

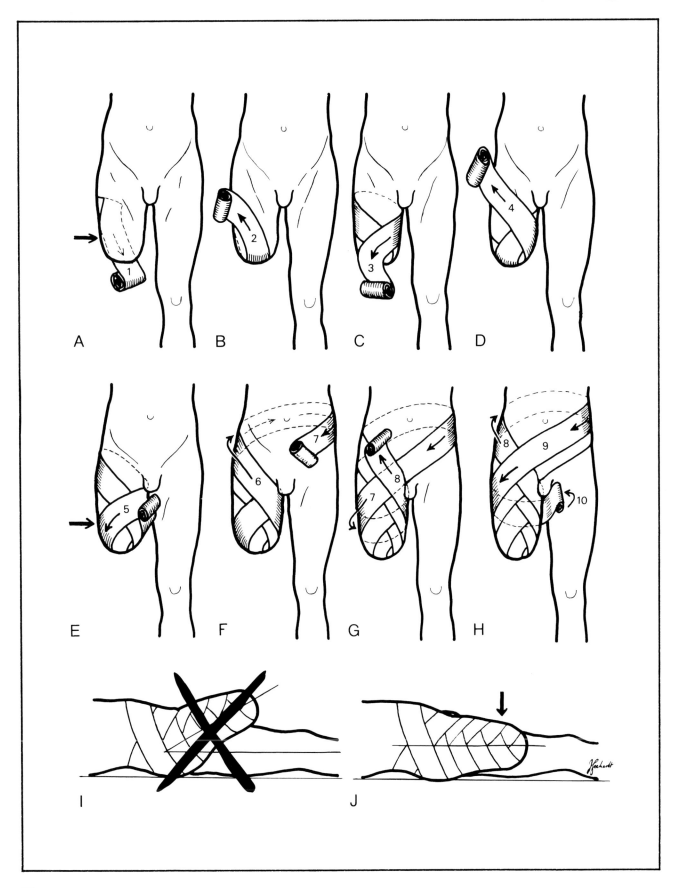

Figure 12.12.

Figure 12.13. Ambulation training for amputees involves

A–C. Standing balance and gait exercises

D–E. Gait and postural exercises, and

F–I. Indoor obstacle course training.

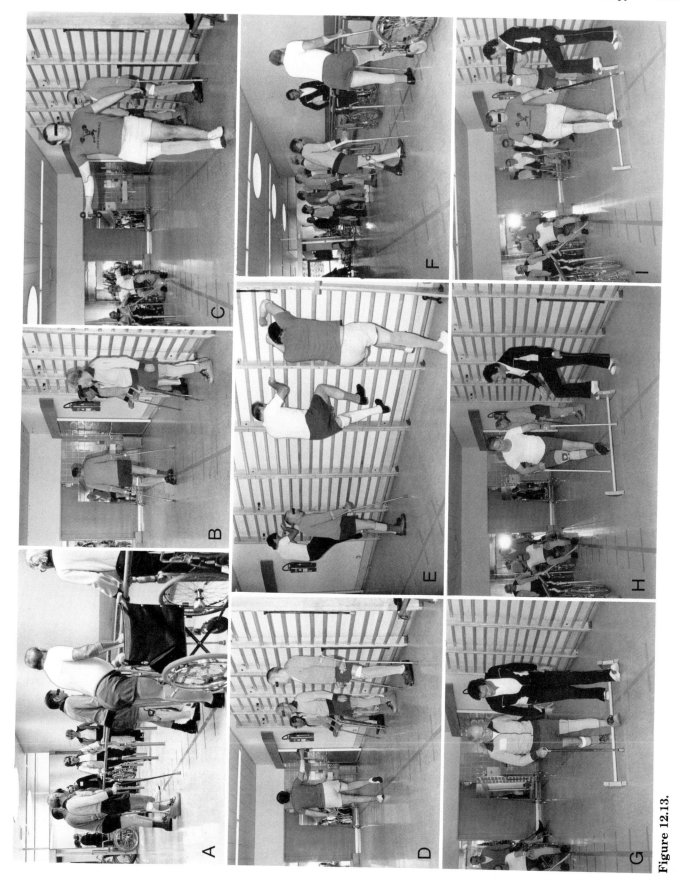

Figure 12.13.

Figure 12.14. Gait training for amputees involves

A–F. Practicing to fall down safely.

G–N. Cross-country training helps the patient to negotiate obstacles, including up- and down-hill slopes and stairs.

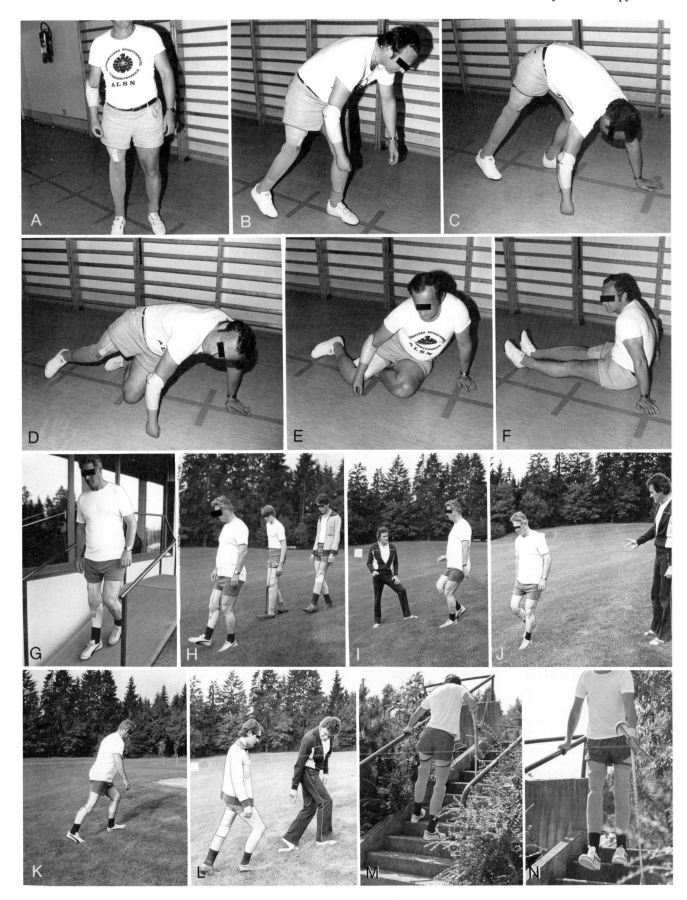

Figure 12.14.

Figure 12.15. Transfer

A–C. In paraplegia can be made from wheelchair to bed with a sliding board

D–F. In tetraplegia, from bed to wheelchair with a sliding board, and

G–J. In tetraplegia, from wheelchair to bed without sliding board.

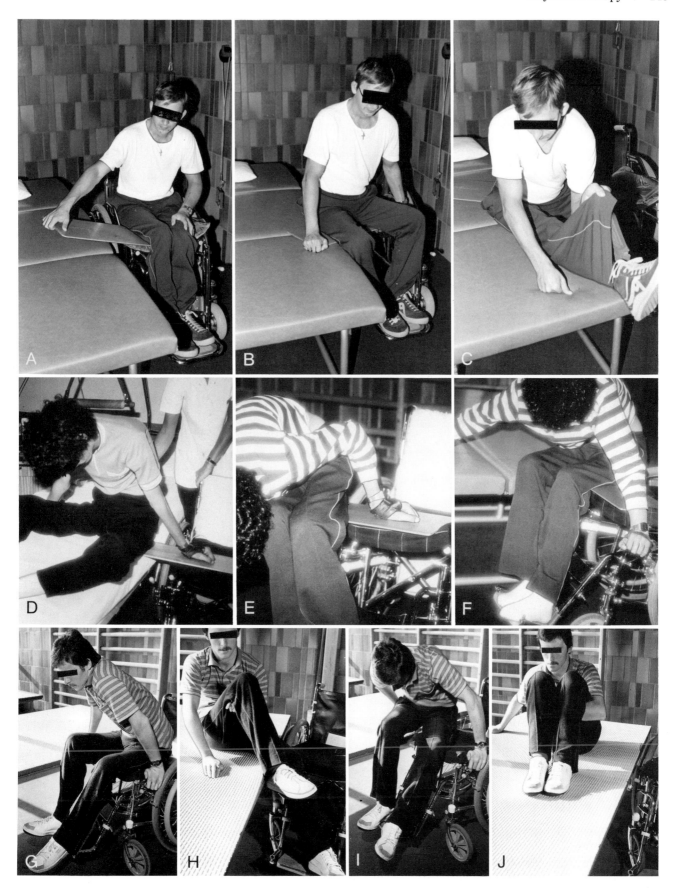

Figure 12.15.

Figure 12.16.   Range of motion exercises of lower extremities and trunk involve

    A. Abduction and flexion of the hip
    B. Stretching of the heelcords
    C. Stretching of the hamstrings (ischiocrural muscles)
D–F. Treatment of adduction and flexor spasm (gentle stretching)
G–H. Trunk flexion with legs extended, and
    I. Independent ROM exercises.

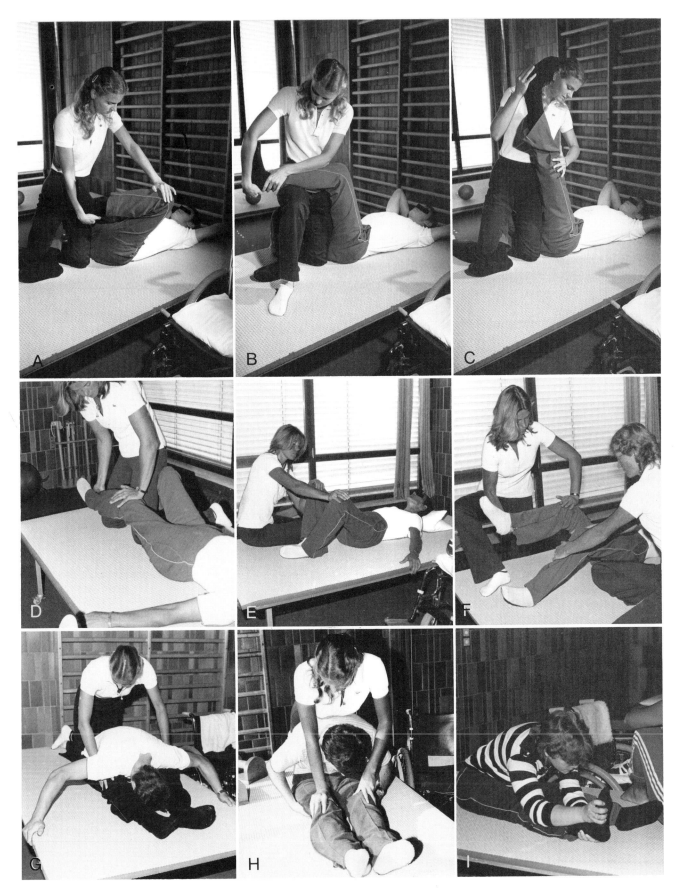

Figure 12.16.

Figure 12.17. ROM of the upper extremity includes

A–C. ROM of the shoulder

D. Strengthening of the biceps muscle

E–F. Extension of the elbow with nonfunctional triceps muscle, trick movement by external rotation of the shoulder and elbow extension by gravity

G–H. Extension and flexion of fingers

I–J. Wrist: functional hand (natural tenodesis) with dorsiflexion fingers close, volar flexion of the wrist: finger opening), and

K. Opposition of the thumb.

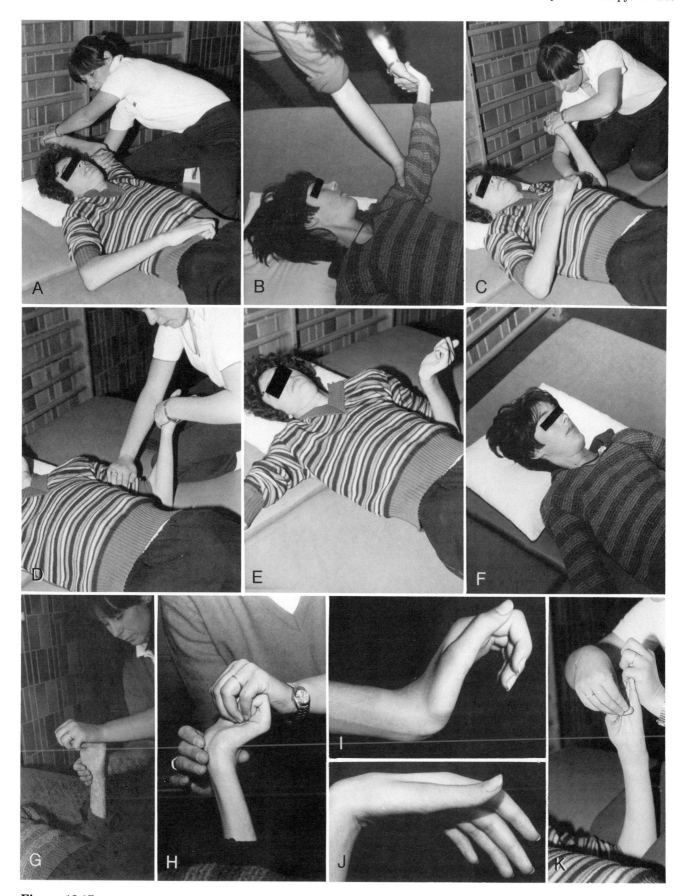

Figure 12.17.

Figure 12.18. Sitting upright for the tetraplegic with functional triceps muscles is done

A–C. From a prone position, over side to sitting position, and
D–H. From a supine position to sitting position.

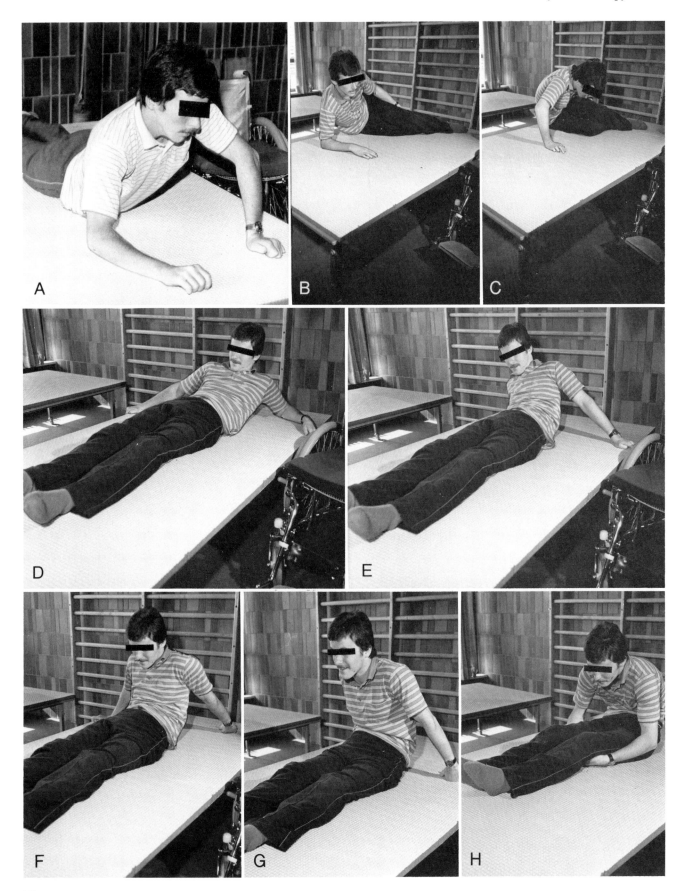

Figure 12.18.

Figure 12.19. Exercises for hand-wrist support involve

A–D. Low-level assistance devices (e.g., blocks and portable bars)
E–G. High blocks, and
 H–I. One-sided push-ups (in preparation for transfer).

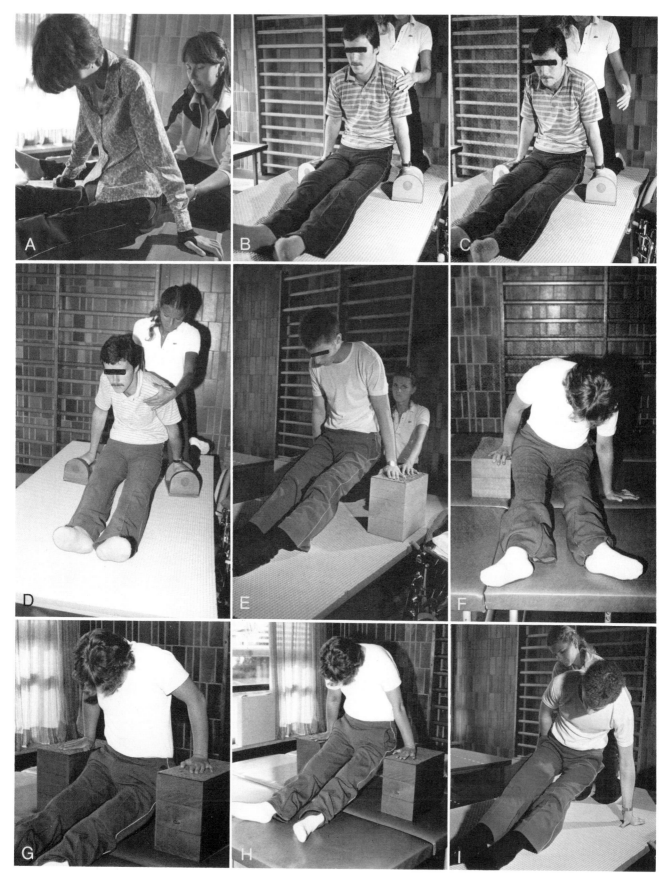

Figure 12.19.

Figure 12.20. Training of balance involves

A–B. Sitting balance in front of a mirror

C. Exercises in the quadruped position

D–F. Exercises with a ball

G. Tilt table in tetraplegia, with gradual tilt to upright position

H. Tilt bed with desk-type board attachment for activities in standing position

I. Standby frame with desk attachment, and

J. Standing between parallel bars with long leg braces.

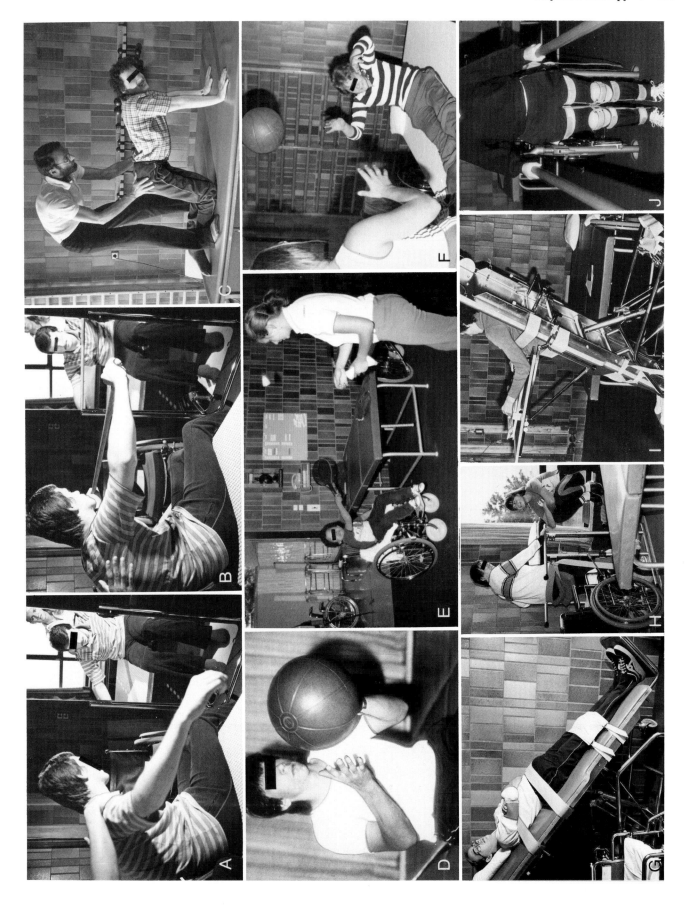

Figure 12.21. Strengthening of residual muscles can be accomplished through

A–D. Proprioceptive Neuro-Facilitation (PNF) techniques (upper extremities)

E. Upper extremity muscle strengthening with dumbbells attached to special gloves for tetraplegics

F–G. Exercising with weights (in paraplegia)

H–K. Training with fitness devices and gymnastic apparatus (pulleys, etc.).

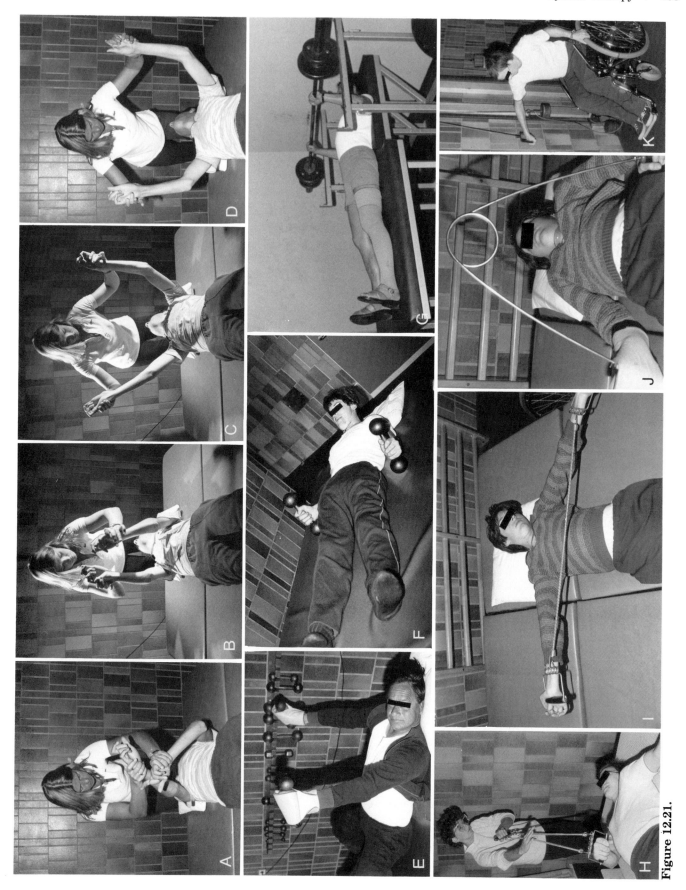

Figure 12.21.

Figure 12.22. Ambulation training for paraplegics involves

A–C. Practicing "swing-to" gait between parallel bars with long leg braces.

D–F. Practicing "swing-through" gait outside of parallel bars using parallel bar on one side and the crutch on the other.

G–H. Practicing 4-point gait with parallel bar, with one crutch,

   I. With two crutches, and

J–L. With reciprocal walker.

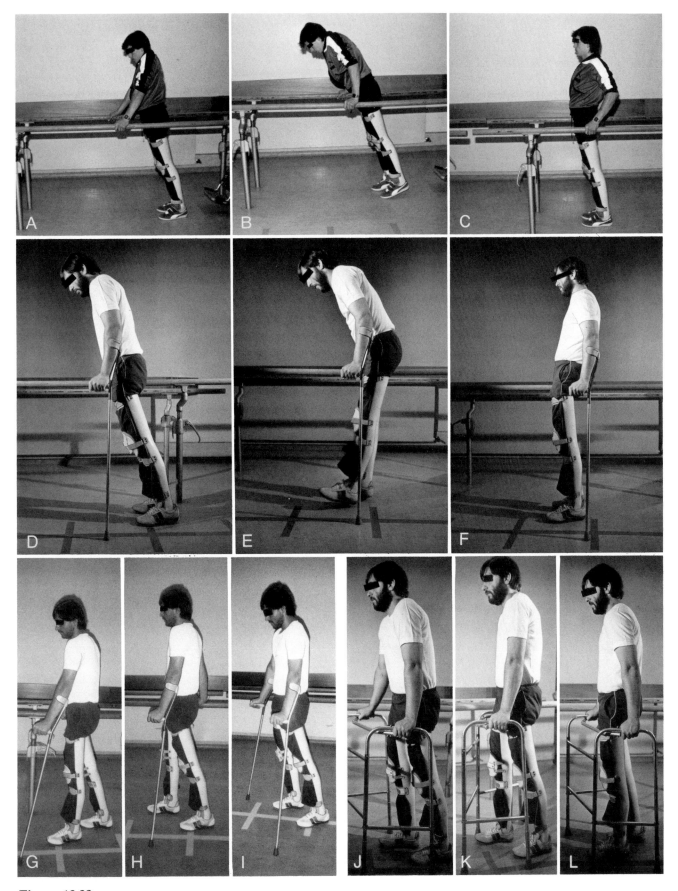

Figure 12.22.

Figure 12.23. For swimming in spinal cord injury, certain elements are necessary, including

A–B. Wheelchairs for taking showers and

C. Disinfection tub.

D–H. There are various techniques for transfer into the pool.

   I. Swimming lessons should be under the supervision of a therapist.

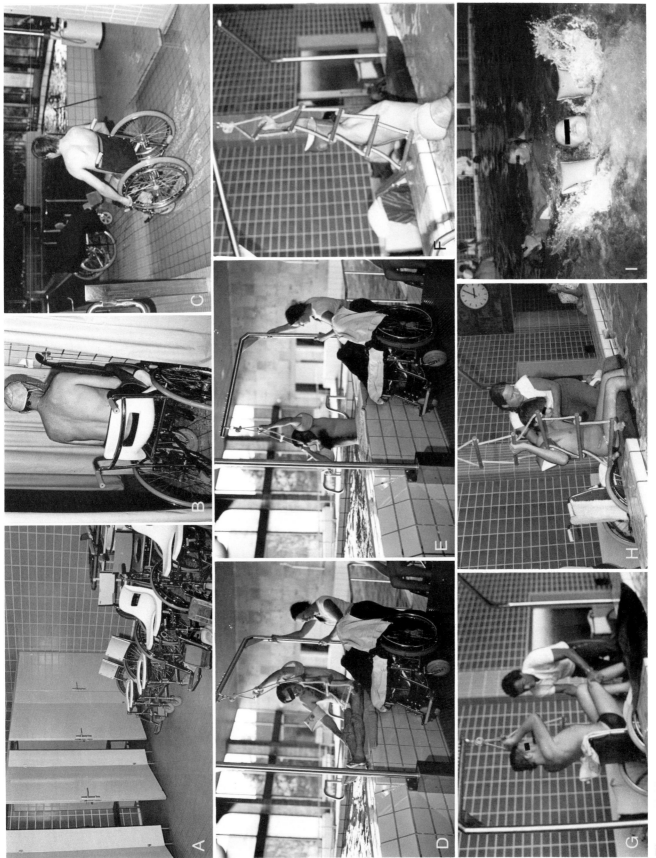

Figure 12.23.

Figure 12.24. Wheelchair training for paraplegics should involve

A–C. Transfer from wheelchair to floor
D–H. Transfer from floor to wheelchair
I–L. Practicing the wheelchair tilt ("wheelies") with and without the assistance of the therapist. When practicing the wheelchair tilt, safety ropes should be attached to the rings in the gymnasium.

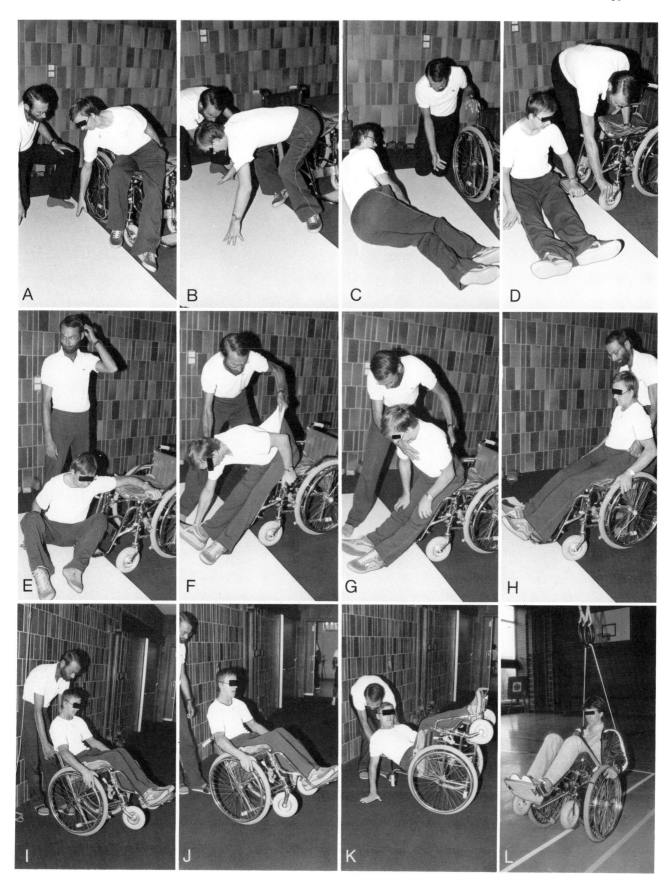

Figure 12.24.

Figure 12.25. Wheelchair training for paraplegics should involve

  A–C. Independent transfer from the floor to the wheelchair outdoors

     D. Riding the wheelchair cross-country on two wheels ("wheelies")

  E–G. Negotiating stairs in a wheelchair without use of the handrail (downward only), and

  H–I. Negotiating stairs with the use of the handrail (up- and downward).

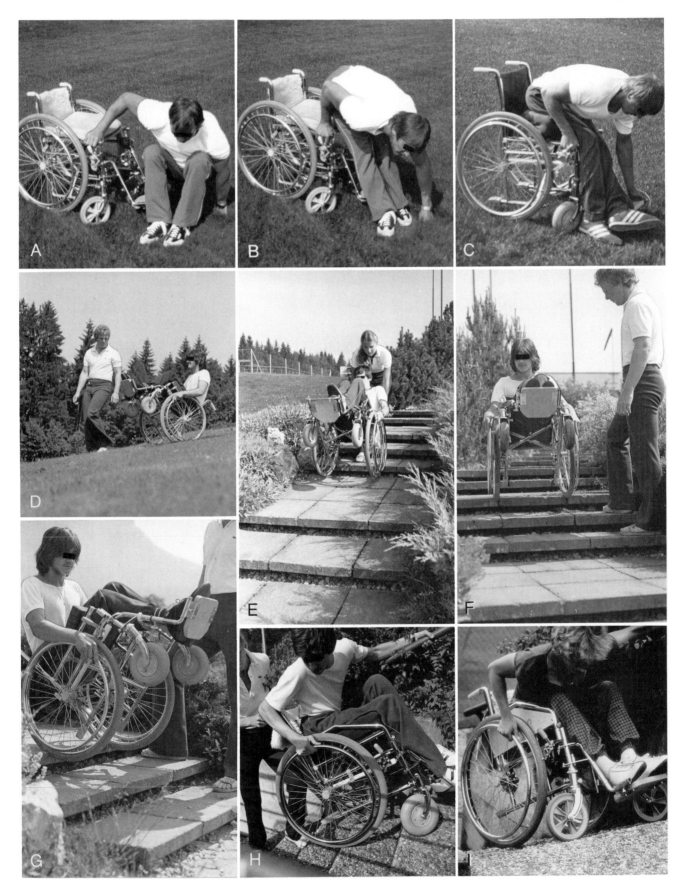

Figure 12.25.

Figure 12.26. Overcoming obstacles is helped by

    A–B. Balance and ROM exercises in a wheelchair group session in the gymnasium

    C–D. Wheelchair circuit training in the gymnasium (gates are improvised by clubs or pins), and

    E–H. Practice of negotiating steps and inclines in the wheelchair in the gymnasium.

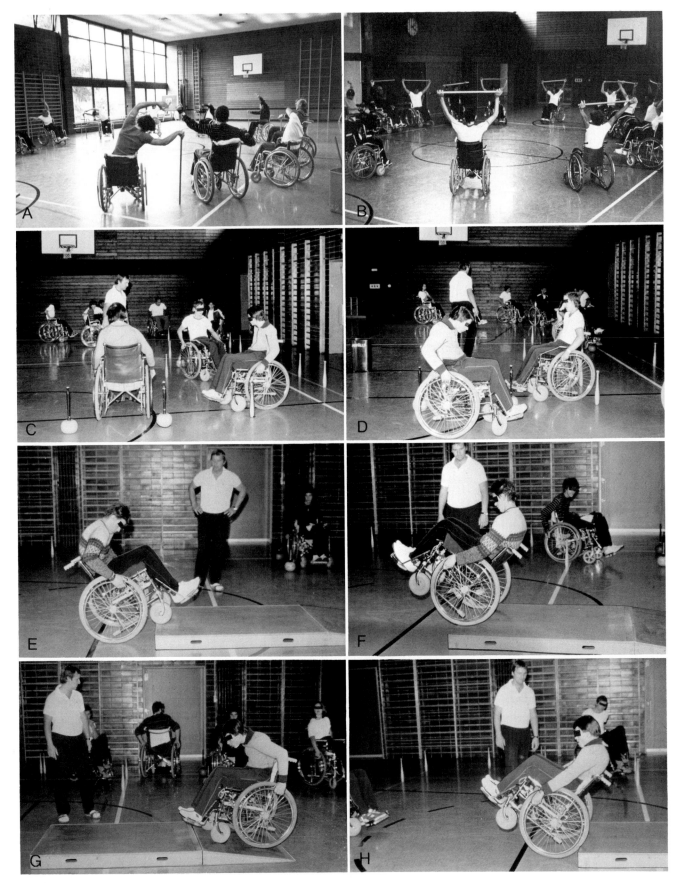

Figure 12.26.

13

Prosthetics and Orthotics

Bernd Schwaiger, M.D.

ORTHOSES

The requirements for the efficient fitting of orthoses and prostheses are: (*a*) correct diagnosis and indication, (*b*) correct and clear prescription, and (*c*) final checkup for workmanship, function, and safety.

Diagnosis and Indications

Good knowledge of anatomy and kinesiology, normal function, abnormal conditions (i.e., congenital, degenerative, posttraumatic, and imbalance, as well as deformity) and an orthotic-prosthetic background are necessary in order to make an adequate diagnosis and to prescribe orthotics and prosthetics. Diagnostic instruments include a physical examination, X-ray, podogram, and podoscope.

Indications for supports depend on the type of deformity. For example, for *plantar arches*, the highest point of the longitudinal arch support is usually below the sustentaculum tali. In posttraumatic pes planus, the distribution of weight is shifted to the plantar side of the calcaneus. The major weightbearing area must not be distal to the Chopart's joint. Support of the transverse arch should be placed proximally to the tarsal heads. The labile pes transversoplanus (unstable splay or spread foot) should be supported by metatarsal pads of different heights; the rigid (contracted) pes metatarso-planus arch is relieved by full metatarsal support (metatarsals I–V). This deformity is common in rheumatoid arthritis.

In the case of *isolated pain areas*, such as in insertional tendonitis or plantar fasciitis (calcaneal spur), *reduced weightbearing capacity of isolated areas*, or where there is a danger of *pressure sores* (e.g., metatarsal stump or anesthetic foot), special padding, with relief of specific areas built into the material of the support, can be applied. The relief concavities may be filled with soft material. Also, the pressure can be redistributed over wider areas using total contact technique, e.g., in a transmetatarsal amputation, where the support is placed under the preserved proximal diaphyses.

In the treatment of *noncontracted deformities*, supports rarely are necessary after traumatic lesions, but often are applied in children with early imbalance deformities of the foot.

Orthoses for the Foot

The technical data in prescribing an arch support should include: (*a*) the material to be used, (*b*) the type of support (scaphoid, metatarsal, partial or full heights, shapes, etc.), and (*c*) posting, wedges, degrees of incline, corrective flanges, etc.

Presently, four materials are prescribed for supports.

Aluminum (Alloys)

Partly prefabricated blanks of sheet metal are formed by embossment and are usually covered with leather (metal-leather support). The advantage of aluminum is that any shape can be achieved by embossment. Also, there is an unlimited number of correction possibilities that are inherent in making supports out of aluminum. The disadvantage of using aluminum is that a very experienced orthotist is necessary to fabricate this type of support. Indications for the use of aluminum include severe labile foot deformities because the material is easily workable and corrections are possible. Special supports made of aluminum such as the Volkmann's angle lever support (Winkelhebeleinlage), and Whitman plates (3-flange support), are very useful for specific deformities, especially in children.

Plexidur

Plexidur is a thermoplastic transparent material. The advantages of using it for supports are that it is washable, it is an absolutely self-supporting system, and it is easily formable. The disadvantages of it are that reshaping is difficult (the primary shape may be lost by heating the material again) and that no acute shaping of margins or abrupt change of planes is possible. Indications for the use of Plexidur are the plain, "everyday" support, the noncontracted splay foot, the pes transversoplanus, and the pes valgus. It also is useful after fractures of the os calcis, and it often is used in workboots because it is resistant to moisture and easy to clean.

Ortholen

Ortholen (Fig. 13.1) is a thermoplastic material. Its advantages are that it is washable and that it can be reshaped mechanically or thermoplastically. If cup-shaped, it is self-supporting. The disadvantage of its use is that it is an inherent support only when it is cup-shaped. Indications include primary or secondary pes valgus, e.g., severe and posttraumatic cases. Also, Ortholen is useful when the support must be cup-shaped. The material can be used for posting as well.

Cork-Leather Support

The cork-leather support is an ideal combination of materials for total contact support (Fußbettung) or inserts in orthopaedic shoes; it is less suitable for the correction of severe deformities. Its advantages are that it may easily be reshaped, it is lightweight, it has a cushion effect, and it wears well. The disadvantage is that it tends to gradually lose its shape and height (including torsion). Cork requires reinforcement with the right material for weight-bearing and surface cover. Also, it is not washable. Indications for the use of cork-leather support are for prefabricated blanks together with various reinforcing materials such as metal, plastic, or rubber. These supports also are ideal for total contact supports and orthopaedic shoe inserts. Major alterations of these supports are not possible.

Final Check-Up

Workmanship, function, and safety can be objectively evaluated, but the subjective statement of the patient as to symptoms and improvement of function is crucial for acceptance. The support must be modified or altered until the patient is able to wear it.

Shoe Modifications

These are orthopaedic modifications applied to commercially available shoes (Fig. 13.2). From the orthopaedic point of view, the criteria for a suitable shoe are:

1. Good mediolateral stability (solid heel counter)
2. Stable, nonflexible sole at the posterior half, but increasing flexibility toward the front part of the sole
3. Lacing that keeps the foot back and down against the heel counter, not merely holding it down
4. Enough depth for toes and the required orthosis

Metatarsal Bar or Rockerbottom Sole

Restriction or loss of the dorsiflexion in the ankle joint (such as in paralysis, arthrodesis, arthrosis, arthritis, posttraumatic deformity or other painful posttraumatic conditions of the metatarsal area) leads to disturbances of the normal gait pattern (Fußabwicklung, heel-strike foot-flat, or toe-off sequence). The metatarsal bar is a segmental component attached to the midpart of the sole, with its axis in the transverse plane; the position of the apex is determined by the prescribing physician, but is in any case placed proximally to the metatarsal heads.

Medial or Lateral Elevation by Wedges

Medial or lateral elevation by wedges (pronation and supination wedges or valgus varus posting) are rarely applied in traumatology; it is occasionally prescribed for relief of a knee compartment syndrome. In orthopaedics, it is frequently used for the gradual correction of alignment deformities, such as varus or valgus of ankle and knee in the growing child (Fig. 13.1).

Mediolateral or Anterior Widening of Heel

By the anterior extension of the medial or lateral part of the heel, the transverse axis of the foot/ankle motion (Fußabwicklung) is deflected toward the varus or valgus. Medial extension (Thomas heel) produces varus deflexion; lateral extension (reversed Thomas heel), valgus deflection.

Lateral Widening of Heel

The lateral widening of the heel (lateral flare) counteracts supination (varus) position of the foot.

Dorsal Reinforcement

This can be incorporated in a commercially available boot. Although it often is used in flaccid drop foot deformities (Heidelberger Schuh), a peroneal orthosis is preferred in such cases.

Simple Elevation of Heel

Simple elevation is used for the compensation of slight leg-length discrepancies or pain syndromes in the heel area (e.g., in insertion tendonitis and fasciitis, apophysitis, calcanei Haglund's disease).

Orthopaedic Shoes

These are shoes made by an orthopaedic shoemaker to fit the individual needs or deformities of a patient. A special shoe last must be fabricated after a plaster mold has been made. As for every orthotic aid, the prerequisites for efficient fitting are: critical and precise indication, exact prescription, and evaluation and check of the final product.

Diagnosis and Indications

Orthopaedic shoes can preserve walking ability, even in patients with severe contracted foot deformities. They prevent secondary deformities caused by imbalance. Ankle joint instability and major leg-length discrepancies can be treated conservatively with success.

Prescriptions

Details for prescription of plantar supports and materials have been discussed previously. Additional information can be found in the section on shoe modification. The sole of the orthopaedic shoes can be stiffened and posterior or lateral reinforcements can be incorporated. Orthopedic shoe inserts can be fabricated. They provide good cosmesis (stockings or socks may be worn over them); they can be incorporated into orthopaedic shoes or any suitable stock shoes (possible exception: heavy workboots).

Final Checkup

The same conditions apply to orthopaedic shoes as to supports: evaluation must be objective and acceptance, subjective.

Orthoses for Lower Extremities

An orthosis substitutes for lost function of the locomotor system. This definition (Fig. 13.3) differentiates it from a prosthesis and from other orthopaedic aids.

The main indications in traumatology for the use of orthoses are central and peripheral neurological lesions with paralyses and the reduced weightbearing capacity of a limb as a result of instability or fracture. Orthoses are classified according to function: (a) weightbearing orthoses, and (b) supporting orthoses.

Weightbearing Orthoses

For limitation of weightbearing of the leg, orthoses with patellar tendon bearing features (PTB suspension system) are used. They are made of thermoplastic materials, with a molded proximal cuff; lateral uprights with or without an ankle joint, an ankle joint with double adjustable stops, or dorsiflexion assist, as indicated. The foot part should be made in sandal form out of thermoplastic material or molded leather.

For the relief of weightbearing of the entire lower extremity, an *ischial bearing seat* is required. The standard version of this orthosis has an ischial seat, lateral uprights and a knee joint with Swiss locks or a drop lock. A Thomas splint as a temporary weightbearing device can be used. Without weightbearing, the foot hangs free; for partial weightbearing, models with variable spring-loaded pressure relief are available. In selected cases, molded thermoplastic components (e.g., ischial seat socket and thigh and calf shells) can be used for construction.

Supporting Orthoses

Below Knee (AFO). Below-knee supporting orthoses are used for stabilization of the distal part of the leg, ankle joint, and tarsal area of the foot. In most cases, two uprights with a proximal calfband made of thermoplastic material and a molded shell, with or without an ankle joint, are used. The foot part is constructed from thermoplastic material or molded leather.

Knee (KAFO). The main indication for the use of knee supporting orthoses is posttraumatic ligamentous instability. Side joint with proximal and distal bands provide lateral stability. Polyaxial knee joints, positive knee locks, and extension assist devices are available.

Hip/Knee (HKAFO). Side joints with bands made of molded thermoplastic shell constructions are used for above knee supporting orthoses. A great variety of prefabricated components for the knee, ankle, hip, and other types of joints allow individualized fitting. For paralyzed patients (e.g., paraplegics and hemiplegics), orthoses with pelvic shells and various simple and complicated hip joints are commercially available.

Orthoses for Patients with Paresis or Paralysis

Ankle/Foot Orthoses (AFO). For peroneal nerve lesions, AFO include a variety of types, e.g., splints, spring-loaded AFO, and molded thermoplastic shells.

KAFO and HKAFO

Lightweight custom-made models of thermoplastic material are used. Some materials have inherent elasticity to permit ease of donning and doffing of the appliances. Most common are shell-type constructions; stabilization of the ankle in these constructions is provided by medial and lateral extension of the shell. A large variety of prefabricated units allows individualized construction of orthoses for patients with spinal cord lesions of traumatic and non-traumatic etiology (myelomeningocele).

Splints

In both orthopaedics and traumatology, splints are utilized for a wide range of indications. Depending on the primary purpose, splints are classified as *immobilization*, *corrective splints*, or *dynamic splints*.

Plaster of Paris is used for provisional or temporary splints because it is inexpensive and easy to handle. Thermoplastic material also is used to make splints. Low-temperature thermoplastics can be molded directly to the limb or body after reheating in a warm bath. Mechanical reshaping and simple thermoplastic corrections are possible. Because of these mechanical properties, the material is used for many kinds of upper extremity splints (Fig. 13.4).

Thermoplastics like Resur, Ortholen, or Plexidur can only be molded at higher temperatures; special heating plates and ovens are necessary. Mechanical reshaping is accomplished easily, but thermoplastic reshaping is more difficult than with low-temperature thermoplastics. Strength and durability are superior, however, so high-temperature thermoplastics are widely used for lower limb orthoses.

The most frequent indications for splints in orthopaedics and traumatology include postoperative immobilization, night and rest splints, and positioning splints for the prevention of contractures.

General precautions that should be taken are the use of adequate padding where required, inspection of skin, monitoring of circulation, and close follow-up.

Trunk Orthoses and Braces

Supporting braces for the cervical spine are available in various forms for posttraumatic and postoperative fixation of the spine and for temporary application for patients with degenerative cervical, cervicooccipital, and cervicobrachial complaints (Fig. 13.5).

Braces (most commonly, plaster of paris stabilizer cast) are used for the conservative treatment of vertebral fractures and for primary postoperative treatment. For maximum mobilization of higher parts of the spine, the brace must extend to the neck and, in some cases, must include the head. For the adequate immobilization of lower parts of the lumbar spine, a component with a hip joint can be added.

A polyurethane corset (neofract) may be constructed of polyurethane foam with layers of duplex stockinette. A zipper is incorporated that allows quick removal of the brace for skin inspection and care as well as physical therapy.

Frame braces, such as the Taylor-Knight type, have been used in traumatology for the conservative treatment of vertebral fractures and for postoperative immobilization. Two active braces for the orthopaedic treatment of scolioses are the Boston and the Milwaukee braces.

Body corsets and flexion jackets include a variety of types that are available for chronic recurrent lumbalgia of degenerative and/or traumatic etiology.

All of the braces and corsets discussed in this section bring short-term relief of pain, but prolonged or permanent use can lead to hypotrophy of back and abdominal muscles, which in turn leads to an aggravation of the original symptoms and signs. This can render the patient dependent on the brace.

Braces and similar aids of this design, therefore, are intended only for short-term application until the symptoms are reduced or absent. Treatment is then followed with active exercises for the strengthening of back *and* abdominal muscles.

PROSTHESES: FOR LOWER EXTREMITY AMPUTEES AT DIFFERENT LEVELS

For patients who have had toes amputated, shoes usually are fitted with a total contact arch support, and in the case of multiple loss of toes, filling material is incorporated (see Fig. 13.6). Particularly after the loss of the second toe, a well-fitting component or Hallux-valgus splint is recommended. Multiple amputations of toes require sole reinforcement with a steel shank and a low metatarsal roll.

Metatarsal amputations are also fitted with a total contact arch support and filling material. Shoe modifications may be necessary (see Fig. 13.7). Correct molding of the longitudinal arch, so that weightbearing is largely through the lower part of the calcaneum, is important to provide relief for the tarsal joints and the ends of the stumps.

For *Lisfranc's amputations*, well-balanced functional stumps can be fitted with shoes.

It is important that the tarsal stump is positioned in a positive and, if possible, almost physiological calcaneal angle (25°). To achieve a functional gait, there must be functional dorsiflexion of the ankle.

Common prosthetic fitting is with a cork-leather bootie, with tongue, in a high-top shoe (either commercially available or custom made).

For *Chopart's amputations*, the few cases of balanced Chopart's stumps can be fitted with slipper-type shoe inserts. Chopart's stumps in unfavorable positions must be fitted with prostheses, usually with the PTB system. But even then, pressure problems are quite frequent.

Operative correction may become necessary, using the method of Maurer (triple arthrodesis) or Pirogow-modifications, as described by Spitzy and Guenther (1900). Figure 13.6 shows Chopart's stumps in position, with a failure of partial or stopper-type problems. The X-ray reveals malposition and identifies potential pressure areas in the region of the end of the stump.

Special prostheses are used after corrective fusion of the hindfoot (triple arthrodesis).

The construct is by lamination cast-resin technique, with PTB system and customized SACH-foot.

For *prosthetic fitting of below-knee stumps*, three basic systems are used.

1. *PTB system.* The oldest principle of weightbearing; 40% of weightbearing distribution over patellar tendon and 60% over tibial flare; suspension provided by a suprapatellar strap, elastic sleeve, or thigh-lacer
2. *Kondylen-Bettung-Münster (KBM) system.* Total contact socket; includes weightbearing mainly over patellar tendon and medial flare of the tibial condyle, but also over lateral aspect of tibial bulge to provide counterpressure (Fig. 13.7); should provide sufficient relief for hamstring tendons (ischio crural); high medial and lateral supracondylar wings provide lateral stability (formerly, usually rigid with wedges; now, mostly flexible and casted); occasionally, soft inserts (e.g., Tepeform, Kemblo, Nickelplast; in some cases, also leather, silicone, or PPT) used; is standard fitting for below-knee amputee (with the exception of extremely short stumps); applicable to all age groups; its advantage is that without the thigh-lacer, atrophy of quadriceps muscle can be avoided
3. *Prosthese tibiale supracondylienne (PTS) system.* Uses same weightbearing principle as the KBM, plus supracondylar suspension; used mainly for extremely short stumps (Fig. 13.8)

A resin lamination technique for hard sockets is used for the construction of the prostheses. It is fabricated over soft liners, and a foot unit is attached. Alignment of the prosthesis is done according to the type of foot used. Generally, alignment of the foot is in slight valgus. The increased equinus position improves security (which is important in elderly patients) but impairs gait pattern. More stability is also achieved by anterior shift of the foot.

For *prosthetic fitting of knee disarticulations*, the resin amputation technique is used for the socket (see Chapter 26 for details about the stump). Three types of sockets are used: an anterior opening with a groove and tongue cover, an anterior opening with a hinged cover, or a flexible laminated cast-resin socket with soft insert (Botta system). No ischial seat required.

Knee disarticulation joints are available with multiaxial constructions. The center of rotation is above the joint. The joints are available with or without a lock (e.g., Otto Bock 3R21, 3R23). These joints are used together with below-knee pylons (modular design) and foot units, according to individual requirements.

As an alternative, medial and lateral joints (as used in orthotics) can be laminated into the socket. This is especially recommended for the prosthetic fitting of children under 10 years of age, as no prefabricated units are available for this age group.

Above-Knee Amputations: Fitting and Prosthetic Construction Aspects

In contrast to all other amputation levels of the lower extremities, the above-knee stump, regardless of length has no direct skeletal control over the prosthesis (Fig. 13.9). The movement of the bony stump is transferred to the prosthesis only through a layer of soft tissue of variable thickness. (This occasionally is called stump "pseudarthrosis.") Control of a prosthesis is progressively more difficult with increasing shortness of the stump. An ischial seat is necessary for every above-knee stump. (For surgical details about above-knee stumps, see Chapter 26.)

Every above-knee prosthesis consists of four components: (a) above-knee socket with ischial seat, (b) knee joint, (c) shank unit, and (d) foot. Apart from the above-knee socket, which is formed according to individual requirements, these components are almost exclusively prefabricated units. The particular choice among the various systems available depends on the age and general condition of the patient and how the prosthesis will be used in the future.

Alignment devices are used dynamically to adjust to the individual according to his or her needs.

Reference Points

Weightbearing Line. The centroidal axis, an important criterion for the construction of the prosthesis, is drawn through an imaginary or calculated weightbearing point. As this point is not well defined and cannot be determined in the static position, different theories and systems have emerged. The stump is correctly aligned, when the plumb line dropped from the trochanter intersects the center of the femoral head, through the middle of the ankle and foot (TKA line).

Knee Axis. The farther the knee axis lies behind the weightbearing line, the greater the stability against flexion in stance, but the greater the effort required to initiate swing phase. Multiaxial knee joints offer varied alternatives (see below).

Below-Knee Units. These are made from various materials, mainly hard foam, wood, polyester resin (laminated units or modular), pylon systems, and a soft foam cosmetic cover that can be added. Advantages of the below-knee units include that they are lightweight, that they are constructed easily, and that alignment changes to fit individual needs can be provided easily. The disadvantage is the high price.

Foot Center and Foot Axis. Reference marks for the suggested alignment of every foot type are provided by the manufacturer. Anterior displacement of the foot center from the indicated midposition and slight plantar flexion will result in increased stability of the knee joint. The disadvantage is greater resistance to achieve midstance, and the toe-off phase. The longitudinal axis of the foot is commonly aligned in 15° of the external rotation in relation to the midline (sagittal plane).

Prefabricated Prosthetic Units

Above-Knee Socket. Currently, above-knee sockets usually are made of plastic. The advantage of this is that they are lightweight, washable, and break-resistant. Occasionally, wood sockets are fabricated in special cases, such as for patients who are allergic to plastic. Wood is nonallergenic and comfortable, but no exact duplication is possible and therefore, the prosthetist must be highly skilled. Also, wood splinters easily.

The form of the cross-section must be chosen individually. If at all possible, total contact (distribution of weight to all parts of the surface) should be used. The ischial seat should be horizontal and the medial wall of the socket

should not be too low in order to prevent soft tissue bulge and chafing of the skin. There should be high socket brim lines for anterior support with bulge over the Scarpa's triangle and adequate relief for the adductor tendons. The height of the anterior wall is also determined by the flexion in the hip joint. For the suction socket, the valve spring should be at the medial distal aspect of the socket to facilitate removal of the application stump sock.

Knee Joints. Numerous knee-joint constructions are available (Fig. 13.10). They include:

1. *Knee joints with lock or without a lock.* Knee lock provides stability for amputees with muscle weakness and instability. They can be constructed single or double axis.
2. Knee joints without a lock are used in all other cases. Friction knee joints can be provided with single or polycentric axis and different friction mechanisms, mostly mechanical, to provide stability at various angles of flexion under weightbearing conditions; these joints are used mainly for elderly and frail patients who are inactive.
3. *Knee joints without friction.* Multiple axis, or polycentric, knee joints, which usually are used for modular constructions; provide stabilization in the stance phase through heel strike, foot flat, and toe-off, and provide smooth motion in the swing phase; and also allow anterior placement of the knee joint axis, which is more functional. Single axis knee joints are less expensive.

Knee Joints with Hydraulic Components. Knee joint constructions with a braking effect and/or hydraulic control of the swing phase are available. Occasionally, they are used with lock mechanisms. The advantage of this type of unit is that there is relatively good control of the swing phase with smooth gait pattern. However, it also has increased weight, is higher priced, and is not trouble-free in arctic or tropical climates.

The "Physiologic" Knee Joint. This type of joint is produced by the Austrian manufacturer Striede. Anatomically shaped components resembling the natural joint are connected by adjustable leather straps, which imitate major knee ligaments. The Striede knee is a simple, relatively problem-free, and very functional knee joint. It requires, however, proper training of the amputee in its use. This service is provided by the manufacturer. Patients are admitted for a 1- to 3-week training program after they receive their new above-knee prosthesis. A great number of commercial units are available. The authors recommend the use of models that are familiar to the available prosthetist, but an open mind toward new developments and innovations should be kept.

Prosthetic Foot. In general, two versions are available. The *prosthetic foot without an ankle joint* is called the solid ankle cushion heel (SACH) foot. The SACH foot is a standard foot unit that is simple and durable. There are no ankle joints, but instead, a compressible posterior wedge of various densitites. The front part of the foot is made of flexible polyurethane (Pedilian). The combination of both simulates gross function of the ankle and foot and enables the patient to achieve an excellent gait pattern. Newer developments incorporate a spring into the foot which absorbs energy during early phases of gait and releases it during the push off phase, thus providing the amputee with additional energy. It is especially effective in amputee sports. An example is the Seattle Foot described later. The *prosthetic foot with an ankle joint* is available in various models. They can be made of rubber, of metal with rubber bumpers, and have a hydraulic ankle or knee-ankle control (hydrocadence). There are also two- and four-way ankle joints (Otto Bock, Greisinger, etc.).

The cosmetic design of the above-knee socket and foot (e.g., Botta) is possible but not done routinely. The below-knee prosthesis should correspond in shape with the unimpaired leg. This is sometimes difficult, especially when the stump has a great deal of redundancy. Adequate shaping of the below-knee units, knee disarticulation, and above-knee prostheses should always be considered. For endoskeletal system with pylons, a foam cover should be applied. New feet are available with precarved ankles and toes. Final shaping is done by skilled prosthetists.

PROSTHESES FOR UPPER EXTREMITIES

In upper limb prostheses, the proper placement and positioning of the terminal device, which substitutes for hand function, should be the primary consideration in fitting (Fig. 13.11). This becomes increasingly difficult with higher amputation level and with increased impairment or loss of sensory feedback.

Prostheses of the upper extremities require one of two power sources for operation:

1. Body-Powered Prostheses: Movement is accomplished mechanically using unimpaired muscles of the body. Muscle power is transmitted by Bowden cables to the prosthetic mechanism. (For example, the neck can be used to move the elbow or activate the terminal device, i.e., hand or hook.)
2. Externally Powered Prostheses: These prostheses have been applied in the past in patients with bilateral amputation and congenital deformities.

Externally powered prostheses include pneumatic prostheses, which use CO_2 gas as a power source. Today, they are used only occasionally for elbow control. Another example is myoelectric prostheses, which are most commonly applied today; movement is provided by small, efficient electromotors (Fig. 13.12). The efficiency of the prosthesis depends on its coordinated and sequential control.

Many actions of the body are for controlling the prosthetic components. There are many advantages to this as often unnoticed, precise physiological signals are elicited by the appropriate muscles. Their action potentials are picked up by the surface electrodes located in the socket or over other appropriate muscles, electromyographically amplified and used to operate and to control the motor-driven prosthetic components—mainly, the terminal device and elbow unit (Fig. 13.13). Besides classification according to the number of channels, the following functional categorization can be utilized in the myoelectric prostheses.

1. On/off control—mechanical or electronic switches are the simplest form of control
2. Proportional control—control of the electromechanical unit accomplished proportionally to parameter (e.g., the myoelectrically transmitted control signal); makes the velocity of movement of the prosthesis (e.g., the functional hand) continuously variable and an optimal form of control
3. Step-up control—less complicated than the proportional control; e.g., in step controlling an electromechanical hand prostheses; a strong or weak muscular contraction produces a defined strong or weak grasp of the prosthetic hand

Prosthetic Fitting of Various Amputation Levels

Finger Amputations

In most cases, cosmetic gloves are provided. After amputations of the thumb, in select cases, an artificial sheet metal post is constructed to oppose the fingers and make the hand more functional.

Amputations in Metacarpal and Carpal Regions

Nonfunctional cosmetic prostheses may be used. In functional prostheses, due to the stump length, the prosthetic fitting must be a cosmetic compromise; the hand unit is fixed by a posteriorly displaced bayonet lock. The opening of the socket on the volar side of the distal stump (the so-called "open end" prosthesis) provides for additional sensory feedback. The hand units are usually metal hooks with mechanical control and are very useful for hard manual work. Various different implements can also be attached to the prosthesis. Finer skilled activities are accomplished without a prosthesis, respectively with the opposite hand.

Wrist Joint Disarticulations

In the socket, adequate embedding of the bulky end of the stump makes a supracubital suspension dispensable.

Terminal Devices (Hand Components)

There are different terminal devices on the market; some in the form of a hand; some in different shapes of hooks; and some with adapters for all kinds of tools, such as hammers and pliers. Some are very functional and others purely cosmetic.

Body-Powered Functional Devices. *Voluntary-opening terminal devices* (Einzughand) are opened by operating a single cable. Closure is passive by springs or rubber bands, which are placed under tension during the opening phase. Voluntary opening devices are used widely as they are practical, do not require much care, and are efficient and effective in that their use can be learned quickly by the amputee.

In *voluntary closing devices* opening is provided by spring action, closing by pulling the cable. Releasing tension at the moment of adequate pressure or grasp of the terminal device locks the terminal device in place. A following pull on the cable unlocks the device and relaxation of the tension finally allows the hook to open again. These devices are more difficult to operate but provide graded prehension.

Externally Powered Functional Devices. Presently, most of the commonly used upper extremity prostheses in Europe are myoelectrically controlled electromechanical devices. Hooks can be controlled by electric motors or compressed gas. The so-called adaptive hands have been developed in several centers; they allow a variable closure pressure and range of motion of the fingers, which then conform to the shape of the object grasped by the hand. They are operated by a rather complicated, computerized, multichannel proportional control system. For several reasons, these systems are not widely used.

The most frequently used device in the shape of a hand is the so-called "three-jaw" chuck hand. In the electromechanically controlled hand, the thumb meets the second and third digit in a pinching position, while the fourth and fifth digits are only dummies (nonfunctional). A hand of this type can be designed as a voluntary opening hand, with springs providing return to the three-jaw chuck pinching position.

Nonfunctional Terminal Devices. These are purely cosmetic hands, molded of different materials that try to resemble the color, form, and texture of the normal hand and skin. Some are covered by cosmetic gloves, which also come in various colors and shades to match individually the skin color of the remaining hand.

All devices come in various sizes. The fitting of the devices has to be done individually, and is best done in special centers in which physicians, prosthetists, and occupational therapists fit a relatively large number of patients and thus have the necessary experience in the best selection and individualized fitting of the devices.

All terminal devices are attached to the socket by wrist units. There is a variety of wrist components: some are threaded, some have a quick disconnect mechanism, some can be locked in different degrees of rotation, some have a continuous rotation controlled by friction, and some permit wrist flexion. Many of the units are available in different sizes and shapes to allow fitting in different age groups as well as at different levels of amputation. Rotational wrist components can also be powered electromechanically by means of batteries that are attached to a socket or—in very short stumps—incorporated in the socket. Hooks, functional or cosmetic hands can be attached to the same wrist units or adapters.

Forearm Amputations

It is common to use supracubital suspension in the prosthetic fitting of forearm stumps. The exceptions are long stumps with strong muscles in patients who do not have to perform work requiring tensile force or strain where a supracubital suspension (Munster) can provide good stability but prevents active forearm rotation. Supracubital prostheses for short forearm stumps frequently lead to a marked restriction of flexion, the prosthetic fitting is therefore accomplished in some flexion (loss of extension is functionally less important). A cable-operated split socket with step-up hinge can be used successfully. This is especially important in the short, below-elbow amputee with reduced flexion. (A regular socket is attached to the short stump and a second split socket is placed over the short socket and attached to the step-up hinges but not to the short socket. The split socket thus can move over the short

socket and increase flexion.) The sockets are made almost exclusively of cast-resin.

Elbow Disarticulations

Special elbow joint constructions are available. All require elbow hinges with a locking mechanism external to the socket.

Upper Arm Amputations

The difficulties in prosthetic fitting increase with higher levels of amputation. There is impaired or no sensory feedback, and more prosthetic components are necessary. All must be positioned and controlled to provide optimal function of the terminal device.

Socket. The socket of an above-elbow prosthesis must provide a means for suspension of the entire prosthesis as well as permit transmission of shoulder movements in all three planes, except for sockets with a shoulder cap. To allow fitting of the above-elbow stumps, (including elbow disarticulations) with sockets that do not restrict movements appreciably (sockets without shoulder clasps or shoulder caps), an angulation osteotomy of the stumps has to be done. The sockets are made almost exclusively of cast-resin. In externally powered prostheses, the myoelectrically controlled electrodes are incorporated into the shoulder cap or socket.

Prosthetic Units. For details regarding the terminal devices and hand units, see the section dealing with prosthetic fitting of forearm stumps. For elbow joints, myoelectrically powered joints are available. For routine prosthetic fitting, elbow joints with cable-operated, positive-locking mechanism and forearm assists are used. A friction-plate turntable mechanism can be incorporated for rotation of the forearm component. Very long, above-elbow stumps require outside elbow hinges.

Shoulder Disarticulations

Large shoulder caps are required, and limited active positioning is only possible by shoulder girdle muscles. The construction of the prosthesis corresponds with that of the above-elbow prostheses. Cosmetic upper extremity prostheses can be constructed from polyfoam and are held in place with straps.

Suspensions. Suspension is provided by straps and harnesses. Many designs are available. The most commonly used is the harness. The straps can be either sewn together in the back or attached to a ring. The anterior strap attaches to the socket. For heavy-duty work, shoulder saddle harnesses are prescribed.

Control Cables. Mechanical control of the prosthetic components, especially the terminal device and elbow, is provided by braided cables, which are guided through the housing that is attached to the prosthetic components by retainers. They can be compared to any modern control cable (e.g., Bowden cables) used in engineering. Similar control cable systems, such as the Fair-Lead Control System, are available.

The selection of prosthetic units from the great variety of available models must be adapted to the needs of the individual case and must take into consideration anatomical, physiological, and pathological aspects of the stump; kinesthetic sensation and pain; vocation; potential to be engaged in the patient's previous occupation; the patient's attitude toward getting a job; occupational training; attitude toward acceptance or rejection of the prostheses; and socioeconomic factors. This is one of the most difficult tasks in prosthetics.

INDICATIONS—SUMMARY

Normal hand function cannot be replaced satisfactorily with any prosthesis because the sensory and propriceptive feedback is either absent or considerably changed. These two factors make the control of the prosthesis more difficult and almost impossible without visual control. These problems are still greater when an elbow joint must also be controlled, or when the prosthetic controls must be accomplished by the shoulder girdle alone.

Practice has shown that adequate prosthetic fitting without major problems is best achieved at levels distal to the elbow. Above-elbow amputees usually use the prosthesis only as assistance for specific tasks. They will use the remaining limb for activities of daily living or any tasks they can perform one-handed. The introduction of

the immediate postoperative prosthetic fitting principle often avoids this common pattern of not using the prosthesis optimally (see Chapter 26).

The prosthetic fitting of high upper-extremity amputations is fully accepted only in cases of bilateral amputees or those with other handicaps and should be carried out at specialized centers. It is beyond the scope of this work to give details about so many technical possibilities of prosthetic fitting. However, there are some general guidelines for indications:

1. The simpler the prosthesis, the better the chance of its acceptance and use.
2. The prescription must be individualized according to the functional capabilities and needs of the amputee.
3. The acceptance and functional use of the prosthesis can be enhanced by application of the immediate postsurgical prosthetic fitting.
4. Satisfactory function, especially for the upper-extremity amputee, is best achieved when the amputation itself is performed by a surgeon who is familiar with prosthetics and the choice and fitting and when the training of the amputee is performed in a special rehabilitation center that has an experienced, well-trained, and coordinated team of specialists in medical, technological, psychological, and vocational areas.

Figure 13.1. Fabrication of an Ortholen-plastic splint.

A–C. Plaster of paris mold.
D–E. Fabrication with positive cast.
F–H. Application of heated thermoplastic material.
    I. Finished splint.

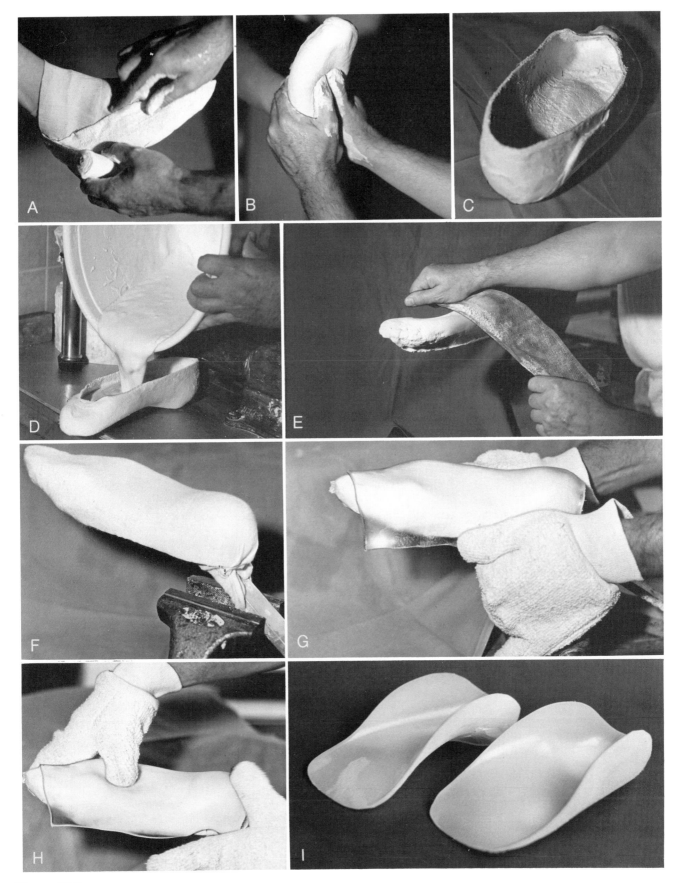

Figure 13.1.

Figure 13.2. Shoe modifications, orthopaedic shoes.

    A. Correct orthopaedic shoe with sufficient space for supports.

    B. Various kinds of metatarsal bars.

C–D. Thomas heel with lateral flex (*right*) and supination wedges (*left*).

    E. *Left shoe*: pronation wedge.

F–G. Inner shoe technique.

    H. Test shoe.

    I. Orthopaedic shoes.

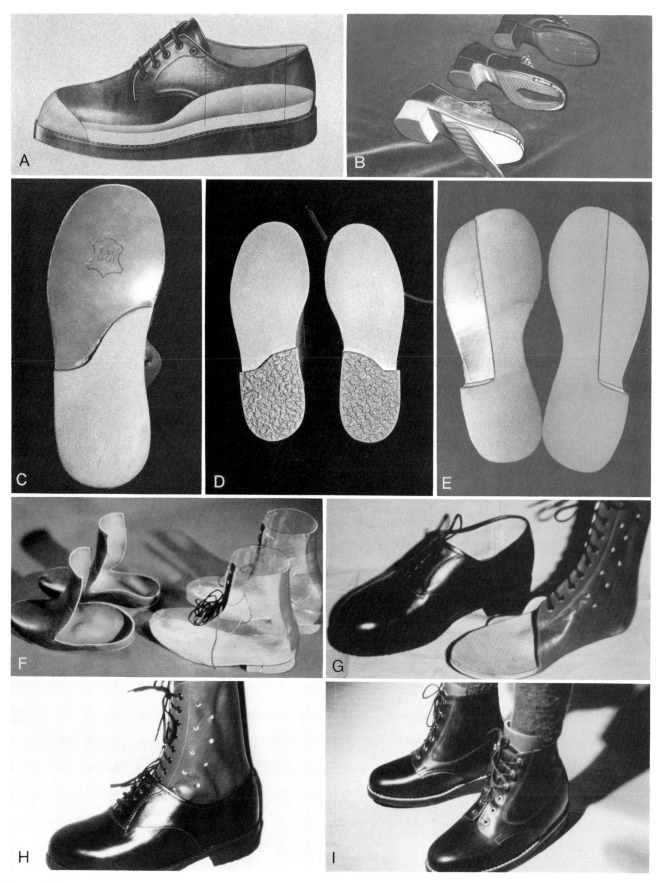

Figure 13.2.

Figure 13.3. Orthoses, apparatus for lower extremities.

A–D. Peroneal nerve orthoses.

E. Support apparatus for leg.

F–G. Knee support apparatus.

H–I. Longley support brace (Resur material for patients with paresis or paralysis).

J. Limited weightbearing splint with patellar tendon-bearing features.

K–L. Thomas splint.

M–N. Longley support apparatus, knee joint with Swiss lock, free ankle joint, molded leather sandal.

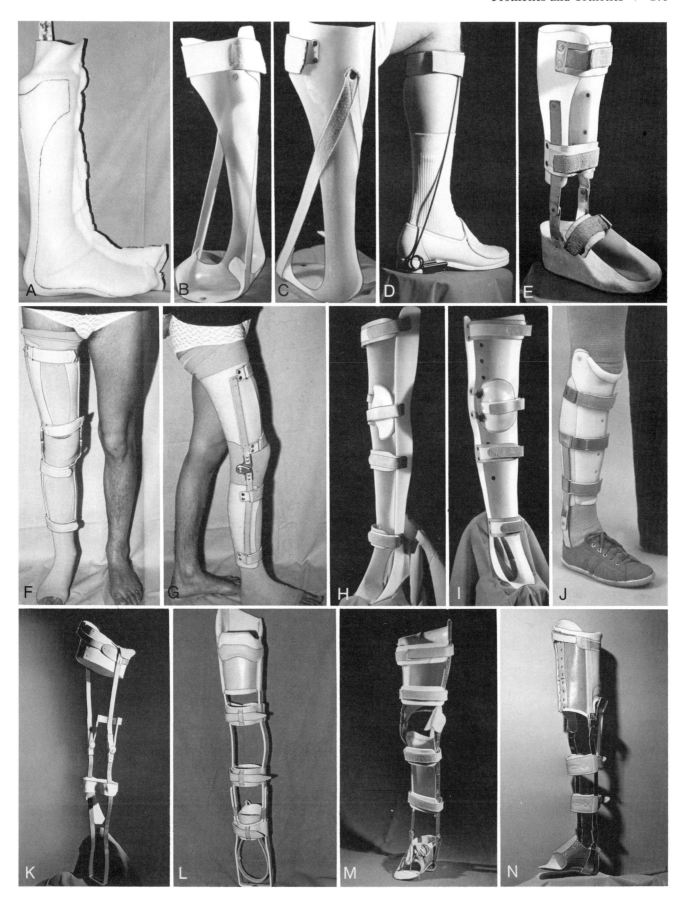

Figure 13.3.

Figure 13.4. Splints for upper extremities.

A–B. Volar forearm rest splint.
    C. Median nerve paresis splint (opponens splint).
    D. Radial nerve paresis splint (cock up splint).
    E. Ulnar nerve paresis splint (flexes MP joints).
F–G. Splint to correct ulnar deviation in the MCP joints.
H–I. Shoulder abduction splint, adjustable (airplane splint).
    J. Dynamic splint for elbow extension (Quengel).
K–M. Dynamic finger splints (Quengel).

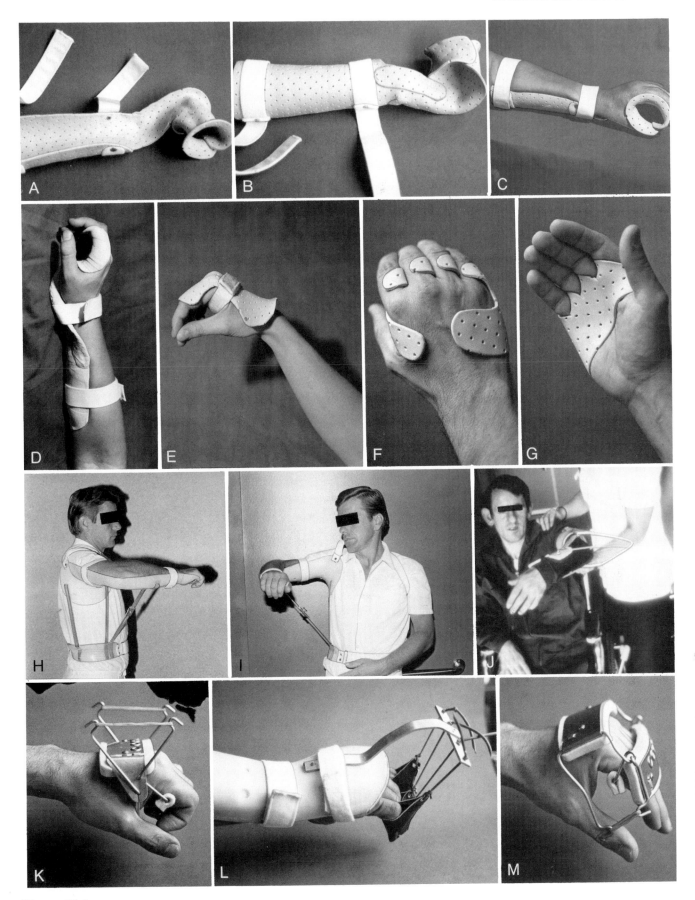

Figure 13.4.

Figure 13.5. Trunk orthoses, corsets.

A–C. Support orthoses for cervical spine.
   D. Neofract (plastic) corset.
E–F. Frame corsets.
 G–I. Various trunk-support orthoses.
J–K. Boston brace.
   L. Milwaukee brace.

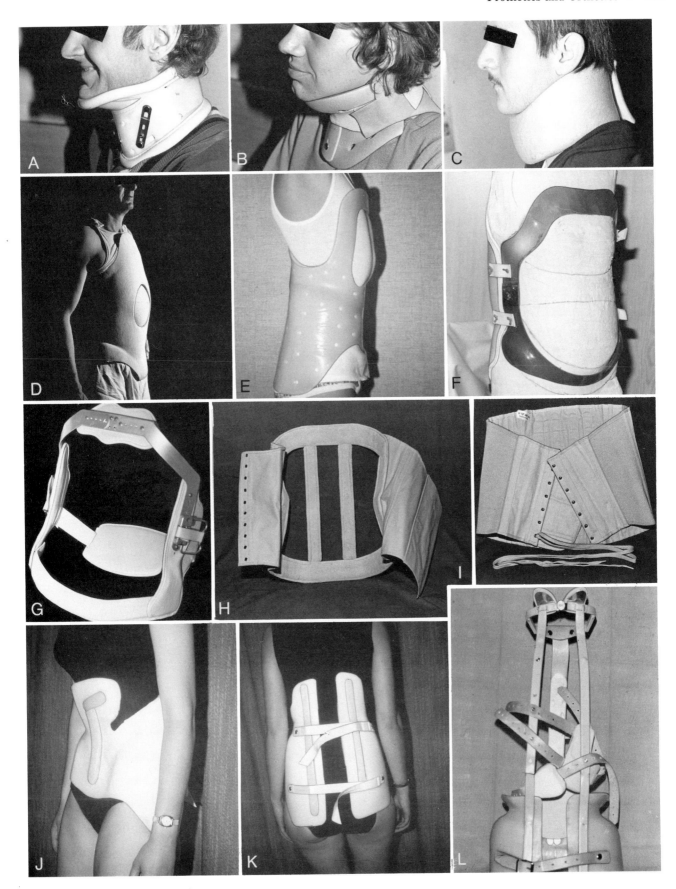

Figure 13.5.

Figure 13.6. Fitting of below-knee amputees.

A–C. Multiple toe amputations (*right*), metatarsal amputation I–II. *Left*: clinic and fitting.
D–F. Lisfranc's amputation, X-ray, clinic, and fitting.
G–I. Chopart's stump in malposition, attempt of fitting with inner shoe failed.
   J. X-ray; lateral view of corrective arthrodesis in the tarsal area according to Spitzy.
K–L. Patellar tendon-bearing prosthesis for all forms of amputations about the tarsal area.

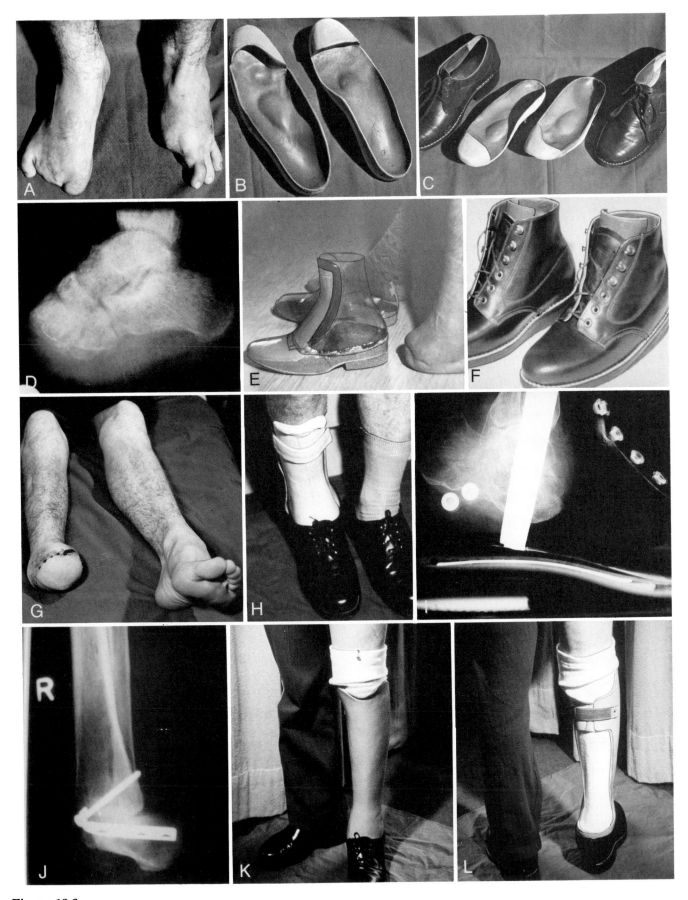

Figure 13.6.

Figure 13.7. Prostheses, lower extremity

A–D. Kondylenbettung Münster (KBM)—below-knee prosthesis.
E–H. Knee disarticulation prosthesis Otto Bock knee joint 3R21.
I–L. Fitting system of knee disarticulation according to Otto Bock (flexible socket).

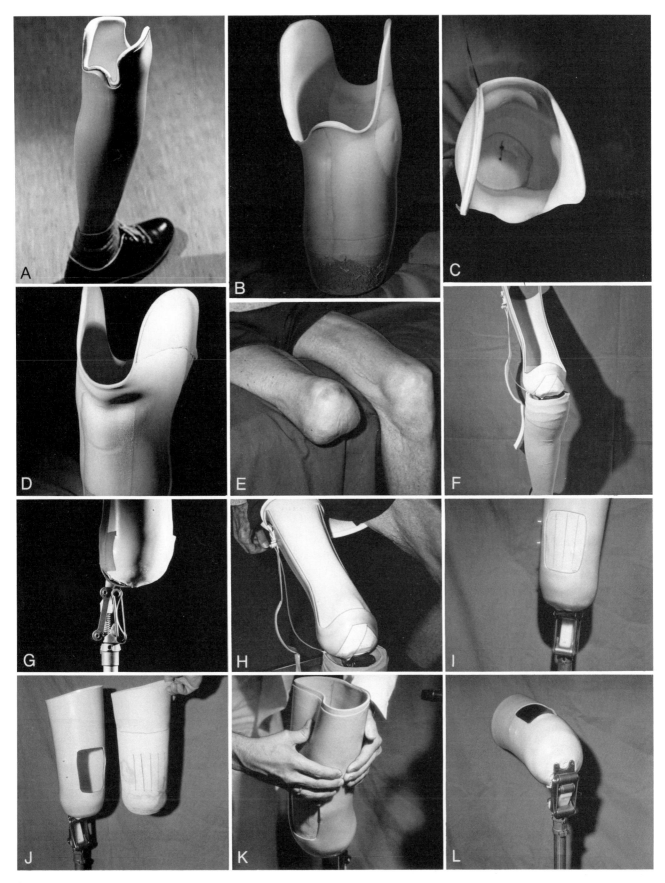

Figure 13.7.

Figure 13.8.

A–B. Patellar tendon bearing (PTB) prosthesis with external keel SACH foot for improved cosmesis about foot-ankle joint.

C. Bilateral geriatric below-knee amputee with PTB prosthesis.

D. Standard thigh cuff suspension system for PTB.

E. Cross-section of PTB prosthesis with soft insert showing total contact principles.

F. Supracondylar suspension system (wedge type).

G. PRS hard socket PTB supracondylar suspension wedge.

H. Fillauer type-rigid wedge in combination with PTB and soft insert liner.

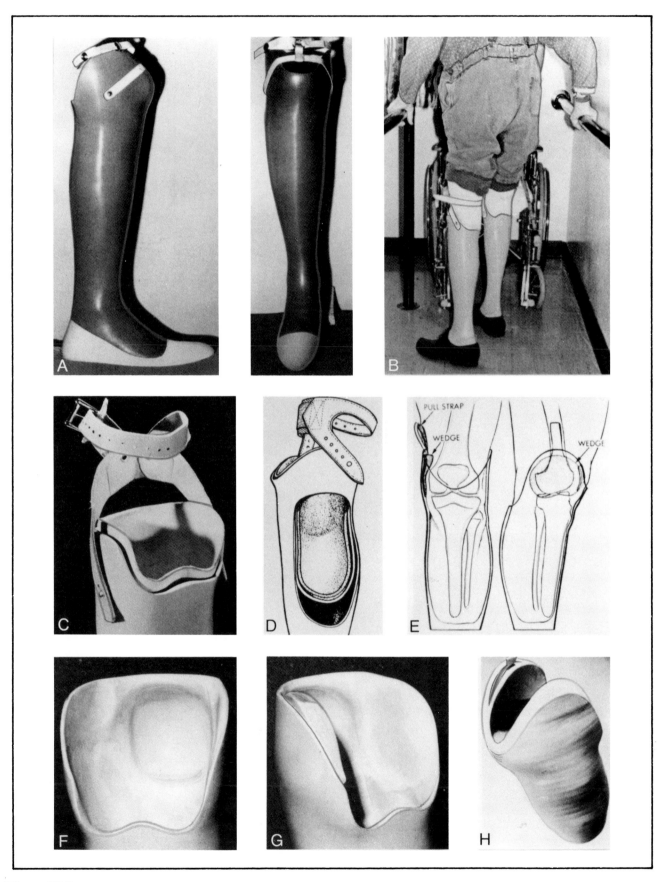

Figure 13.8.

Figure 13.8. (continued)

I–K. PTB—Prosthesis with side joints and lacer, waist belt, and hooked suspension strap.
L–N. PTB—Endoskeletal system with soft foam cover (Otto Bock system).

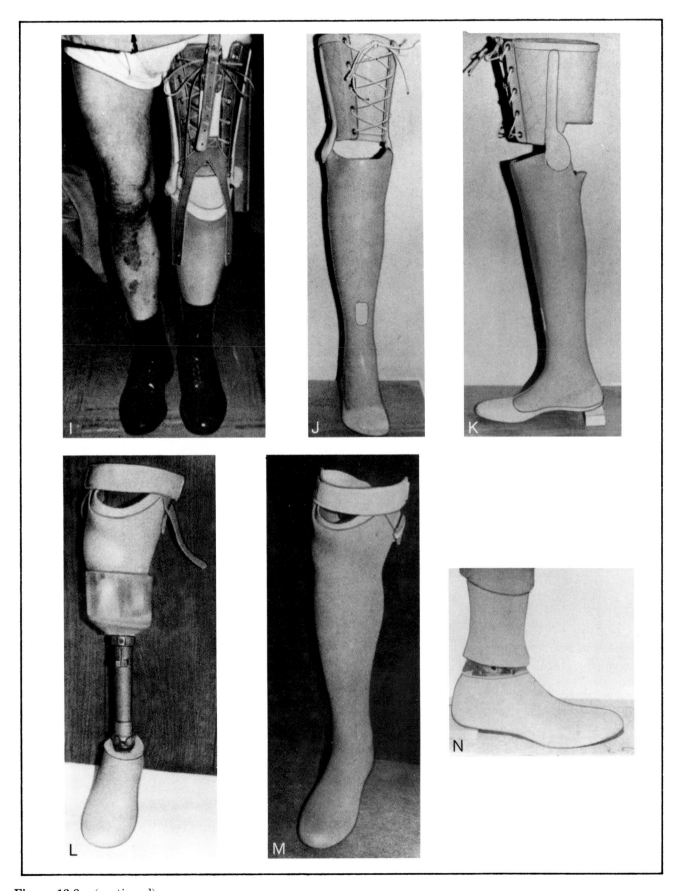

Figure 13.8. (continued)

Figure 13.9 Above-knee prosthesis.

    A. Prostheses in the gait training room.

    B. Above-knee plastic socket therapeutic training prosthesis.

C–D. Fabrication on the adjustment jig.

    E. Finished left above-knee prosthesis.

    F. Knee joint with lock after removal of cosmetic cover.

G–H. Hip disarticulation, fitting with Canadian hip disarticulation prosthesis. Above-knee amputation with above-knee prosthesis right.

 I–M. Preparation of cosmetic details according to Botta.

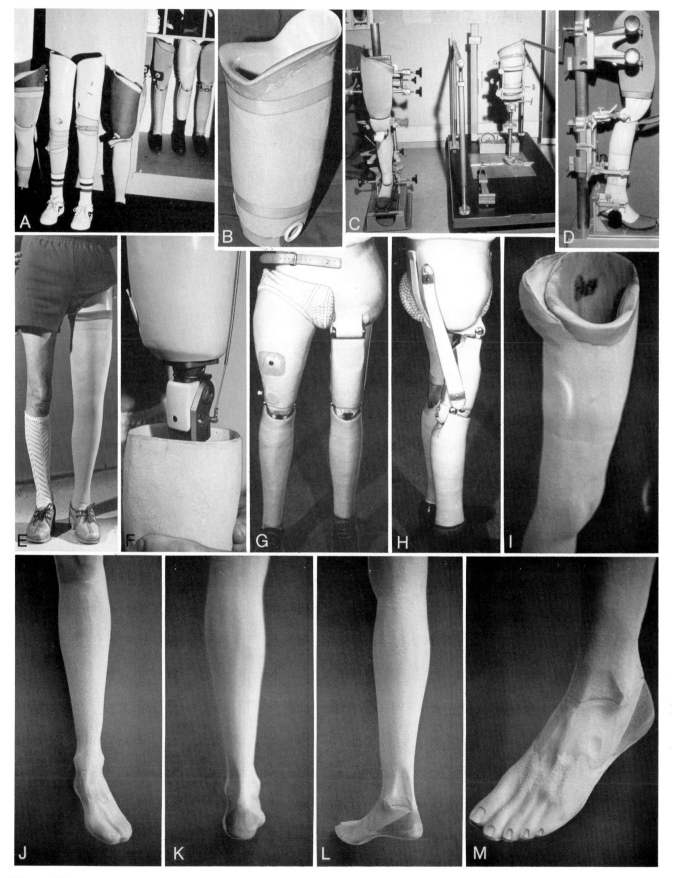

Figure 13.9.

Figure 13.10. Components for lower extremity prostheses.

   A. SACH foot (rigid).
   B. Multi-axial foot; Greissinger, 5-way Otto Bock old style.
   C. Multi-axial foot, new style (Hängelagerfuss).
   D. Knee joint, wooden component, single axis with lock.
   E. Modular system—lock knee (Otto Bock 3R17).
   F. Modular system—single axis safety knee (Otto Bock 3R15).
G–H. Wooden component, single axis safety knee (Jüpa knee).
   I. Modular system, polycentric knee joint with four-bar stabilization (Otto Bock 3R19).
   J. Modular system knee joint for knee disarticulation with four-bar stabilization (Otto Bock 3R21).
K–M. So-called "anatomical" knee- joint—system Striede.

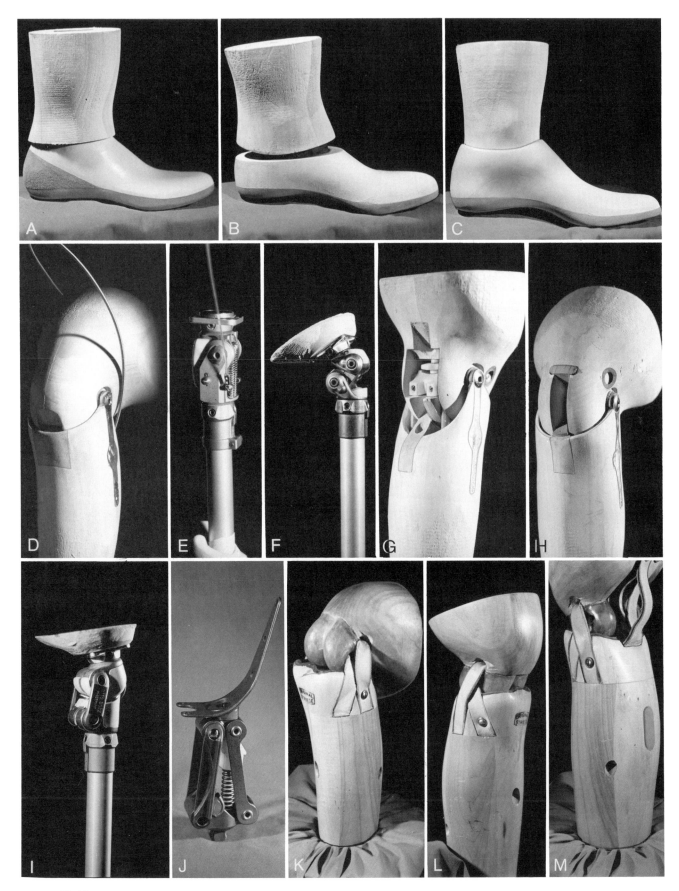

Figure 13.10.

Figure 13.11. Upper extremity prostheses.

A–B. Open-end prosthesis with hook for transcarpal amputation.

C–D. Wrist disarticulation prosthesis—myoelectric, with simple socket (no supercondylar suspension).

E–F. Below elbow prosthesis—supercondylar suspension socket.

G–I. Extremely short forearm stump fitting with step-up hinges (double socket).

J. Cosmetic hand.

K–M. Terminal devices, mechanical-single cable-hand, hook, different exchangeable terminal devices for different tasks.

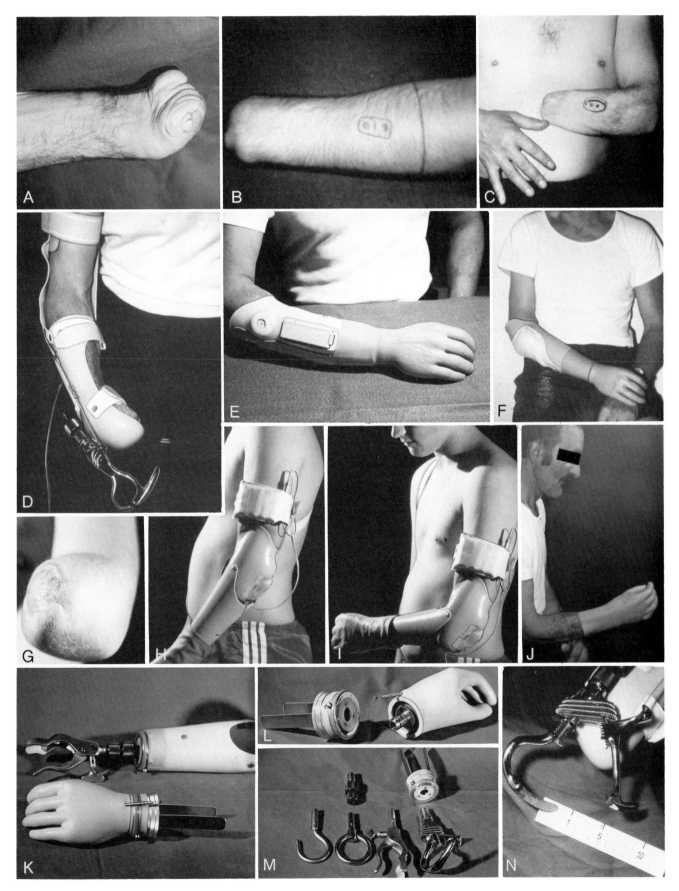

Figure 13.11.

Figure 13.12. Upper extremity prostheses.

A–B. Testing for positioning of electrodes in the myoelectric prosthesis.
  C. Myoelectric prosthesis, socket with supercondylar suspension. Electrode is clearly visible.
  D. Myoelectric prosthesis with rachet-adapter system (System Otto Bock).
  E. Myoelectric hand prosthesis, uncovered to show system.
  F. Myoelectric hand prosthesis—"electro hook" with racket adapter (Myobock system—electric Greifer with friction).
G–H. Myoelectric hand prosthesis Viennatone system (older model).
  I–J. Vienna (adaptive hand).
  K. Cosmetic aspect of a below-elbow prosthesis without supercondylar suspension of socket.

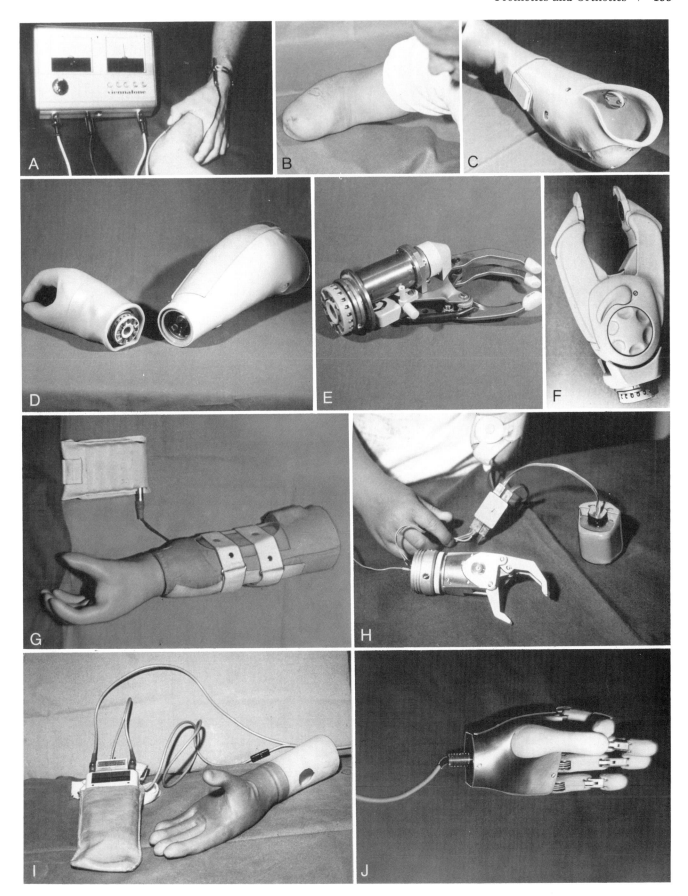

Figure 13.12.

Figure 13.13. Upper extremity prosthesis.

A–C. Above-elbow prosthesis with resin-shoulder socket, mechanical locking elbow joint and functional mechanical hand (one cable voluntary opening)

  D. Mechanical locking elbow joint (system Balser)

E–F. Above-elbow prosthesis with Balser elbow joint and myoelectric hand control; electrodes are in the shoulder socket and batteries in the above-elbow shaft.

  G–I. Bilateral above-elbow amputation fitting as described above in 13.3 E–F. (Photo courtesy of Professor Schmidt, Budrio, Italy)

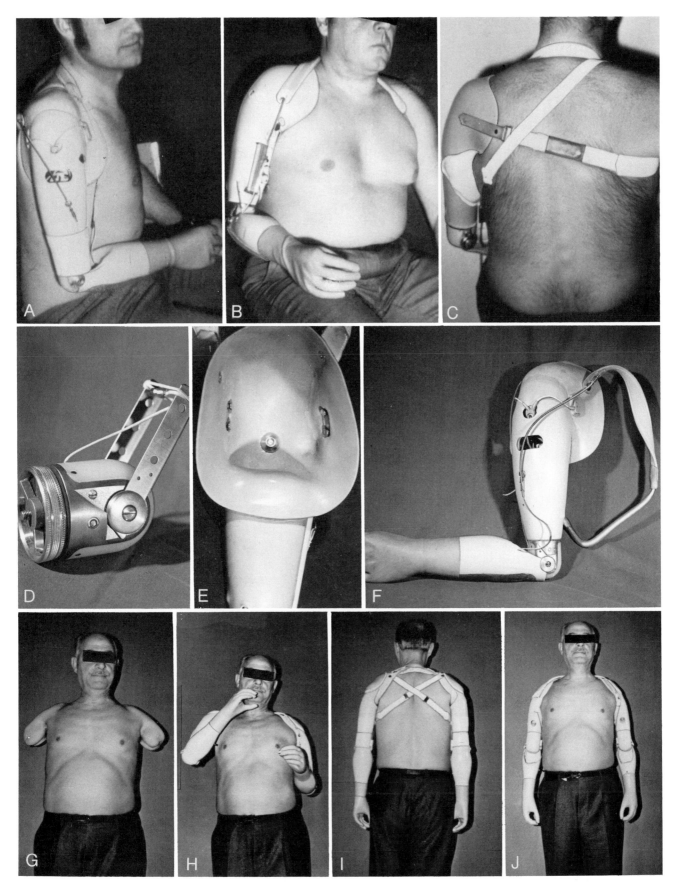

Figure 13.13.

Figure 13.14.

A. Lateral view
    1. α tibia-calcaneus angle
    2. β calcaneus-floor angle
    3. γ calcaneo-metatarsal V angle
    4. δ convergence of talus and calcaneus

B. A-P view
    δ divergence of talus and calcaneus

C. Foot in A-P view
    1. long axis of foot
    2. axis of talus
    3. navicular-cuneiform axis
    4. Lisfranc axis
    5. calcaneus axis
    6. α valgus angle between b and c
    7. β varus angle between a and c

D. Foot in A-P view
    1. α hallux valgus angle
    2. β metatarsale varum angle

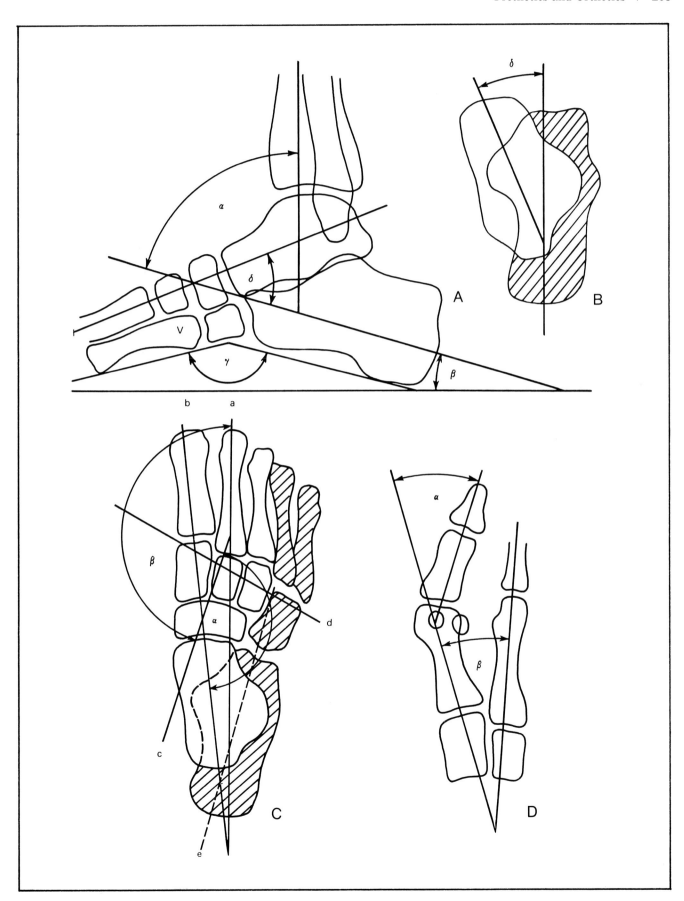

Figure 13.14.

Figure 13.15.

A–C. Syme prosthesis. Modified posterior opening with hinged trap door and Velcro closures. Exterior wood keel SACH type foot.

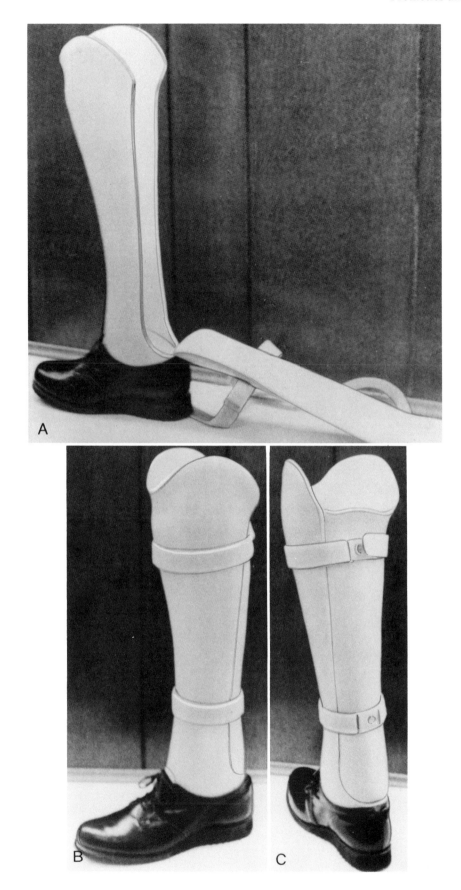

Figure 13.15.

Figure 13.16.

A–B. Syme prosthesis with medial opening for donning and doffing of prosthesis.

C–D. PRS closed Syme prosthesis with soft insert. This design eliminates customary posterior or medial openings and results in a stronger and more cosmetic design.

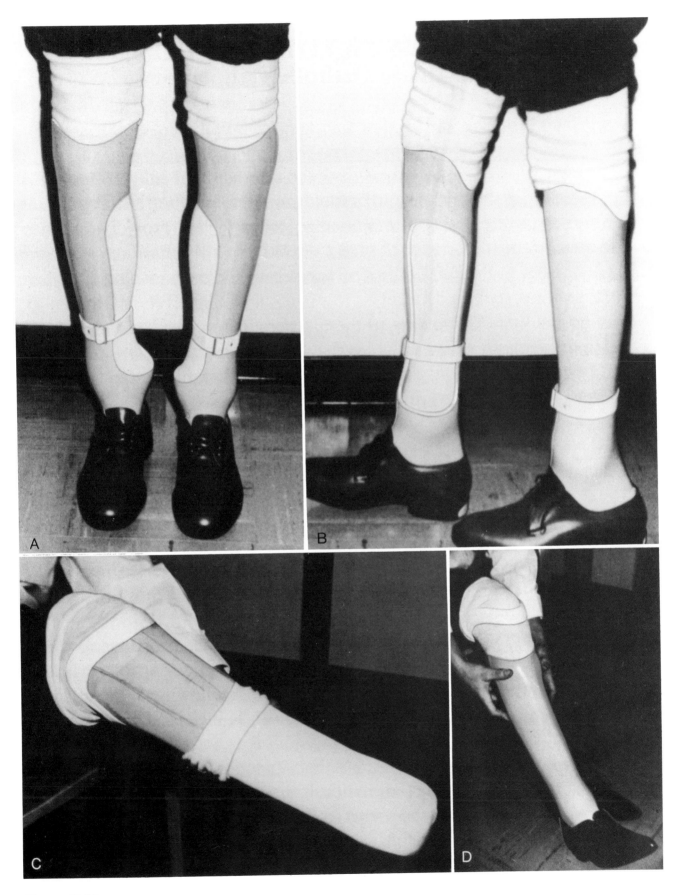

Figure 13.16.

14

The Prosthetic-Orthotic Laboratory

John J. Gerhardt, M.D.

The design of a prosthetic-orthotic laboratory is of great importance for cost-effective production and fitting of prostheses and orthoses (see Fig. 14.1).

Special considerations have to be observed in the planning of a plant of this type, especially when located in the hospital area.

There *should be an adequate fresh air supply, i.e., ventilation.* Air-conditioning, heating, filter, fire alarm, and sprinkler systems should be incorporated. In case of fire, automatic switches should activate the alarm and sprinkler systems, close all recycling air ducts, and allow 100% fresh air only to enter the area. The air supply is determined by volume of space according to codes.

There should be a special and separate exhaust system because of noxious fumes and dust produced during fabrication of modern prosthetic and orthotic appliances. There

should be exhaust ducts over workbenches and other ducts should be attached to machines that produce dust. The exhaust air should be filtered and diluted before it is allowed to enter the atmosphere. The exhaust outlets should be away from places such as fresh air intake ducts or windows to prevent reentering of the used air and exhaust fumes into the building.

Reasonable arrangements should be made to diminish the noise of machines in the production area. Noise- and dust-producing machines should be placed in separate, enclosed, and insulated rooms—in a so-called "dirty area."

The supporting floor should have adequate strength to safely withstand the weight and vibration of machines.

There should be 220 V, as well as 110 V, electrically grounded outlets in strategic areas.

There should be adequate space for the storage of materials. If possible, a separate space should be provided for each type of supply, such as leather, cloth, plastics, wood, metal parts, shoes, canes, and crutches.

This chapter was prepared courtesy of Paul Campbell, M.D., medical director of the Portland unit of Shriners Hospital For Crippled Children.

Figure 14.1.

A. The floor plan of a prosthetic-orthotic laboratory typically includes:
1. A waiting room area
2. An office for the chief prosthetist-orthotist
3. A fitting room
4. A plaster room
5. A general prosthetic-orthotic room, including workbench area, sewing area, and leather area
6. A so-called "dirty area," including band saw, grinders, sanders, and ovens
7. A separate welding room
8. A cold room for storage of liquids, plastics, glues, etc., to increase the shelf life of certain chemicals
9. A general storage area
10. A shoe storage room, and
11. A myoelectric room.

B. The evaluation and fitting rooms should divided by curtains or rigid walls as necessary. Each fitting room should have a stretcher and X-ray view box.

C. In the plaster room, note sink, trays, X-ray view box, worktable, elevated bench for taking molds, and space for chairs and stretchers.

D. An orthopaedic technician finishes a splint on a grinder.

E. An overall view of the laboratory shows the band saw, oven, and welding room in the back. Note that these are separated from the other rooms.

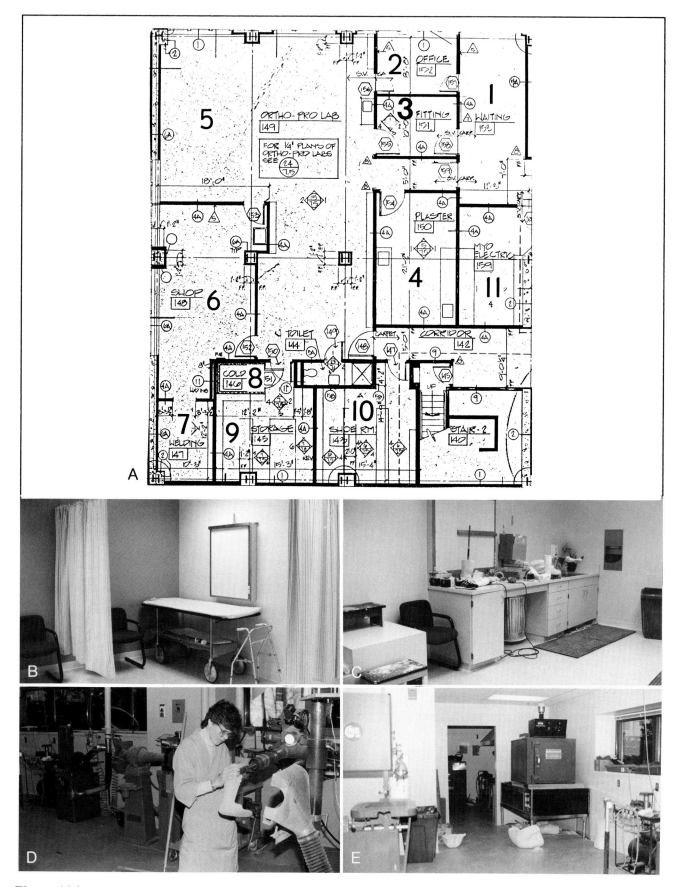

Figure 14.1.

There should be a so-called "cold room" (i.e., a walk-in refrigerated room) for liquid plastics, glues, and other chemicals to extend their shelf life.

A fitting room should be close to, but well separated from, the fabrication and waiting room area.

There should be a separate cast room or plaster room close to the fitting area where models can be taken and special fittings can be provided.

Adequate space is needed for parking wheelchairs and stretchers to prevent obstruction and hazards in any of the above areas.

A separate "myoelectric room" should be planned if fitting and service of myoelectric prostheses are being considered.

Finally, the physical plant, as well as machines, should conform to federal, state and hospital safety codes.

Figure 14.2.

A. In the general working area, note exhaust arrangements on each workbench area and
B. Mechanical workbench arrangement.
C. In the sewing area, note the different sizes of straps, Velcro straps, and different belts that can be pulled down from rolls stored in overhead cabinets.
D. A prothetist works on a leg brace.
E. The machines are in the general working area but have low noise and an incorporated exhaust system.
F. Note the heavy insulated door of the cold room.
G. Leather is stored here.

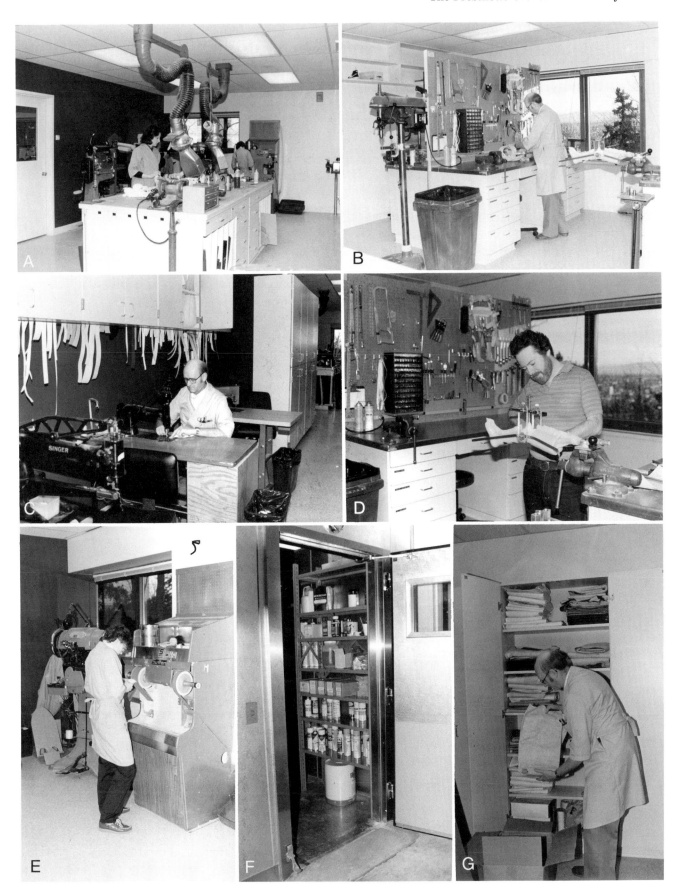

Figure 14.2.

15

Psychology

Wilhelm Strubreither, Ph.D.

Rehabilitation may be defined as helping the handicapped patient to achieve the best possible restoration of physical, psychological, social, and vocational functions so that he or she will be able to regain the optimal position in society. The tasks of the psychologist in rehabilitation are varied.

PSYCHODIAGNOSTICS IN REHABILITATION

It is essential that the rehabilitation team include a psychologist as diagnostician. An accurate diagnosis is the basis for all subsequent measures. Formal tests should be administered if they will help to plan the therapeutic program for rehabilitation. The diagnosis should lead to a psychopathological differentiation of the personality structure, and to the selection of appropriate psychotherapeutic measures. Diagnostic work-up includes, the therapeutic interview, thought exploration, history, observation, and behavior analysis based on learning theory, as well as discussion among team members. Also, a number of standardized tests and types of test equipment are available for diagnosis, therapeutic planning, and case control.

Standard Tests

Wechsler Intelligence Scale for Adults and Children (WAIS and WISC) *Hamburg-Wechsler-Intelligenztest für Erwachsene und Kinder (HAWIE, HAWIK)*

Amthauer Intelligence Structure Test
Intelligenz-Strukturtest (IST) nach Amthauer

Horn Performance Test System (detection of brain lesions)
Leistungs-Prüfsystem (LPS) nach Horn

Culture-Free Intelligence Test
Grundintelligenztest CFT-3

Raven's Standard Progressive Matrices
Progressiven Matrizen nach Raven

Wechsler Memory Scale

Viennese Dementia Test
Wiener Demonztest

Attention and Stress Test d2
Aufmerksamkeits-Belastungstest d2

Minnesota Multiphasic Personality Inventory (MMPI)

Freiburg Personality Inventory
Freiburger Persönlichkeitsinventar

Minnesota Importance Questionnaire (MIQ)

Clinical Self-Rating Scales of the Munich

Psychiatric Information System

  The Paranoid-Depression Scale (PD-S, D-S)
  The Complaint List (B-L)
  The Situation-Existence Scale (BF-S)

Psychiatrischen Informations-Systems die
  Paranoid-Depressivitäts-Skala (PD-S, D-S)
  die Beschwerden-Liste (B-L)
  die Befinlichkeitsskala (BF-S)

Questionnaire for the Assessment of Suicide Risk by Stork
Fragebogen zur Beurteilung der Suizidgefahr (FBS) nach Stork

Depression Inventory by Beck (BDI)
Beck-Depressions-Inventar (BDI)

Questionnaires for Insecurity Evaluation—The Fear of Failure Evaluation (FAF)
Unsicherheits-Fragebogen

Difficult Situations for Paraplegics

Questionnaire for the Evaluation of Psychosomatic Disturbances
Schwierige Situationinen für Querschnittgelähmte (SSQ)

Vocational Aptitude Test by Schmale
Berufs-Eignungs-Test (BET) nach Schmale

Vocational Interest Test by Irle
Berufs-Interessen-Test (BIT) nach Irle

Personality-Interests Test (PIT) by Mittenecker/Toman
Persönalichkeits-Interessen Test (PIT) nach Mittenecker/Toman

Projective Thematic Apperception Test (TAT)
Projektiven Thematic-Apperception-Test (TAT)

Rorschach Test

Wartegg's Design Test
den Wartegg-Zeichentest

Additional Tests

Allport, Vernon, Lindzey Test for Value Attitude
Carrier Assessment Inventory California Psychological Inventory (CPI)

Differential Aptitude Test (DAT)
Flanagan Aptitude Classification Test (FACT)
General Aptitude Test Battery (GATB)
Internal-External Focus of Control by Rotter (I-E Scale)
Kuder Occupational Interest Survey
Occupational Aptitude Pattern (OAP)
Specific Aptitude Test Battery (SATB)
Strong Campbell Interest Inventory (SCII)
Primary Mental Abilities (SRA)

Testing Equipment

The Vienna Determination Apparatus
das Wiener Determinationsgerät (see Fig. 15.1)

Motor Capacity Series of Schoppe
die Motorische Leistungsserie nach Schoppe

The Vienna Concentration Apparatus
das Wiener Konzentrationsgerät

The Critical Flicker Fusion Analyzer
der Flimmerverschmelzungsfrequenz-Analysator

Reaction Time Apparatus
ein Reaktionsgerät

Performance Testing Apparatus
das Leistungsprützerät

EMG-Biofeedback Apparatus
ein EMG-Biofeedbackgerät

These testing procedures should help establish a correct diagnosis. Apart from this, some of the test equipment, such as the Vienna Reaction Apparatus, are used for the diagnosis and treatment of patients with delayed reaction, disturbed mental functions, lack of drive, etc. Such a treatment leads to a general stimulation of function and is very popular among the patients.

Examination methods include test batteries. They are used, for example, to diagnose psychological deficits and changes after craniocerebral trauma, including in particular, the so-called posttraumatic organic "psycho syndrome" following the acute phase. This battery mainly explores memory, perception (especially partial disorder of visual perception), thinking, concentration, reaction, disturbances of the sensorimotor flexibility, personality, behavior, and intelligence. The tests are administered in close cooperation with the neurologist.

Another example of the application of various methods of psychological examination (combined with the collaboration of the whole team) is the Functional Disability Profile (*Funktionales Behinderungsprofil*), developed by the chief physician of St. Polten, Dr. Grabner. This battery is applied as part of the examination and follow-up of patients with craniocerebral trauma and severe physical handicap. This profile is established by the attending physician together with the psychologist, the physical therapist, and the occupational therapist.

PSYCHOTHERAPY IN REHABILITATION

Psychotherapy means treatment by psychological means. In addition to the "pure" psychological disturbances, psychogenic diseases and physical diseases accompanied by psychological symptoms are also treated by psychotherapy. Close cooperation and coordination of psychiatry, neurology, and psychology are necessary to make diagnosis and therapy profitable to the patient. Within the narrow bounds of this brief compendium, it is not possible to define the whole area of indications for psychotherapy in rehabilitation, which ranges from psychoses and psychosomatic diseases to reactive personality disorders, etc.

Apart from this, psychotherapy can deal with specific problems of rehabilitation, such as poor or no acceptance of the disability after the accident, where a change of attitude might be needed. To eliminate factors that might obstruct rehabilitation, the patient should be motivated to take initiative or an active part in the management of daily living. Psychotherapists can help persons in rehabilitation develop responsibility for themselves and others, provide extensive health education, and establish new behavior patterns on the basis of psychosocial reorientation of the patient.

After a particular case has been discussed among team members, the patient can be treated in individual or group therapy. The psychological disorder to be treated is not merely the result of the patient's physical disability and so it has to be viewed in context of his or her whole personality, social background, and environmental conditions. All of these factors need to be considered for adequate treatment.

There are many methods of treatment. These include: the utilization of: (*a*) learning theory together with social psychological, psychosomatic, and other cognitive principles; (*b*) behavior therapy; and (*c*) nondirective client-centered therapy. The method of choice may include the integration of effective elements of other kinds of therapy (e.g., the use of autogenous training and elements of client-centered therapy as components of behavior therapy, Kathathymes imaging experience, or hypnosis).

Psychologists usually spend most of their time involved in individual and group treatments, according to the symptoms and results of the evaluation and diagnosis. In addition to this, at the Bad Häring Rehabilitation Center in Tirol, Austria, a number of "semistandardized" psychotherapeutic procedures are used for the treatment of brain-injured patients, for patients with nonspecific syndromes, for social training of wheelchair patients, and for sexual counseling of patients with spinal cord injuries.

Treatment of Brain-Injured Patients

The diagnosis of an organic psychosyndrome determines the specific type of treatment for the psychological disturbance. At the Bad Häring Rehabilitation Center, new treatment methods were recently developed and applied. The treatment material corresponds with the test items, so that the disturbed functions can be specifically managed. The Vienna Determination Apparatus (see Fig. 15.2), the Concentration Apparatus, and the Performance Testing Apparatus are in frequent use. A major part of the treatment is assumed by the occupational therapist.

The treatment material is designed according to the patient's individual needs, and the methods are adapted dynamically to the individual's progress. Before the patient is discharged, another follow-up evaluation is made. This follow-up evaluation, on the one hand, controls the treatment method and allows improvements of the pattern used; on the other hand, it assesses the patient's progress. Also, an exercise program, based on this final evaluation, is developed for home practice.

Treatment of Patients with Nonspecific Syndromes

Autogenous Training (AT) and Progressive Muscular Relaxation (PMR)

Patients frequently present nonspecific syndromes, such as psychovegetative and psychosomatic disturbances, depressions, or somatic complaints with massive psychological overlay. These disturbances are mostly treated by individual therapies. (However, the patient can be taught skills to help him- or herself in these areas.)

Two types of relaxation techniques used for these patients are: *autogenous training* (AT) and *progressive muscular relaxation* (PMR) (see Fig. 15.2). These techniques differ in that the PMR is an active, physical method utilizing easy isometric contractions followed by relaxation, while the AT is a passive, slowly consolidating, vegetative autoregulation technique.

In general, both methods can be applied with psychosomatic and psychovegetative syndromes. The AT has proved useful with neurodystonia, nervousness, circulatory instability, vegetative symptoms caused by stressor, and gastrointestinal disturbances. (It may also be used as a preventive measure.) AT is especially effective with problems most frequently arising in rehabilitation centers, such as pain and insomnia. The PMR usually is indicated in muscular tonicity, posttraumatic syndromes with muscle holding and reflex bracing, tension headaches, cervical and thoracolumbar spine syndromes, hyperexcitability, hypotonia, and limited mobility. A modification of Jacobsen's PMR is the Muscular Depth Training (MDT) (*Muskulares Tiefentraining*). MDT was developed by Stocksmeier and has been successfully applied.

The methods described above are the basis for many psychotherapeutic interventions (e.g., systematic desensitization). They are all taught in small groups. AT takes at least 10 sessions and MDT takes at least five sessions to be an effective therapeutic measure. These groups are very popular among the patients, especially for those who are defensive against a psychological interpretation of their complaints, because they provide a good and harmless introduction to psychotherapy.

Social Training for Wheelchair Patients

The initial treatment of patients with traumatic transverse lesions should develop and maintain their self-image and also make them as independent as possible. This program concentrates on primary prevention and is designed to help traumatically injured patients avoid or at least reduce any impairment of their self-concept and dependence on others.

Social training includes interaction with others and systematic social experiences. These are made under the guidance of the psychotherapist, who helps the patient to assimilate and accommodate future experiences. The patient is supported in actualizing his or her concept of reality. Teaching the patient to anticipate solutions for new situations, which will occur in the future, increases self-confidence so that present goals (and wishes) can be obtained. This enables the patient to improve his or her ability to act independently and with self-confidence. This also enables the patient to achieve the following aims:

To learn how to act independently and to avoid feeling helpless in social situations that are changed, and made more difficult, by dependence on a wheelchair

To strengthen the patient's confidence in his or her ability to cope with the new situation and to avoid self-devaluation and retreat from the family and society

To improve social contact and avoid an increase in social distance to prevent isolation

Psychosocial training is patterned according to ideas of Schöler, Lindenmeyer, and Schüsler (1981) and are divided into individual treatment units, each of which concerns one of the several essential difficulties. One treatment unit comprises at least two sessions. The first session consists of group games that are designed to sensitize the patient to specific problems, to improve his or her communicative abilities, and to enable the patient to overcome basic conflicts. In the second session, possibilities for the solution of particular problem situations are worked out systematically and tried out in the form of role playing. This role playing teaches the patient new skills by giving him or her an opportunity to try new ways of thinking and behaving in a safe environment.

The sessions are held twice a week and last for about 1½ hours. Additionally once a week, the social treatment takes place in a real life situation; together, the patients and therapist go shopping, go out for dinner, visit theaters, movies, etc. Thus, the way back to "normal" living is facilitated. (This is also a good opportunity for behavior observation and analysis by the therapist.) This social program is carried out in close cooperation with the social workers; and recommendations of the whole team are considered as well. In addition, the Bad Häring Rehabilitation Center has a permanent place where team members and patients can meet informally twice a week to talk about arising problem.

Sex Counseling of Patients with Spinal Cord Injuries

This group program gives comprehensive information about various aspects of sexuality and of the physically disabled. The program consists of lectures about the medical and psychological aspects of sexuality and disability, discussions, and films. It is carried out by the psychologist together with the urologist, nursing staff, and other interested and knowledgable team members.

All of these psychotherapeutic procedures can certainly only be a supplement to the individual care of the patient.

OTHER ACTIVITIES

Biofeedback procedures are utilized increasingly. They are especially useful in treatment of conversion reactions, such as psychogenic paralyses, and other conditions. Also, a self-help program for pain management was started at the Bad Häring Rehabilitation Center because of the large number of patients with pain syndrome. This can be done in groups, informal seminars, or symposia, preferably after the participants have been introduced to AT. Therapeutic programs (especially for occupational therapy) and exercises should be designed, planned, and practiced with the goal of having the patient continue these at home after his or her discharge. Patients can also be sent to other institutions or therapists for subsequent outpatient therapy.

The personnel at rehabilitation centers should have the opportunity to participate in psychotherapy training. Every course (especially AT) should also be attended by several members of the rehabilitation team. Additionally, group discussions should be held for physical and occupational therapists as well as the nursing staff. Daily ward rounds and team conferences complete the all-important overall picture of the patient.

OUTLOOK FOR THE FUTURE

In the future, biofeedback procedures, mainly the muscle tone feedback, will be applied more frequently. Increasing numbers of patients with depressive symptoms, prompted staff of the Bad Häring Rehabilitation Center to establish a self-help program against depressive attitudes in the form of group therapy. In addition, training in hypnosis and autosuggestion also will be applied as self-controlling techniques for pain syndromes. Public relations and interaction (e.g., in schools) will be intensified. Various groups (youth groups, nursing schools, etc.) from the surrounding communities will be included increasingly in social training.

Figure 15.1.

A. In the diagnosis of the organic psychosyndrome (organically based psychosis), special testing equipment is used in addition to the achievement tests and personality tests. This equipment includes the Flicker Analyzer (Flimmerverschmelzungsfrequenz-Analysator).

B. The Vienna Reaction Apparatus.

C. The Motor Achievement Series, and

D. The Vienna Determination Apparatus.

E–F. Some testing devices, such as the Vienna Determination Apparatus, the Concentration Apparatus and the Achievement Testing Device also proved valuable in the training of organically disturbed psychic functions.

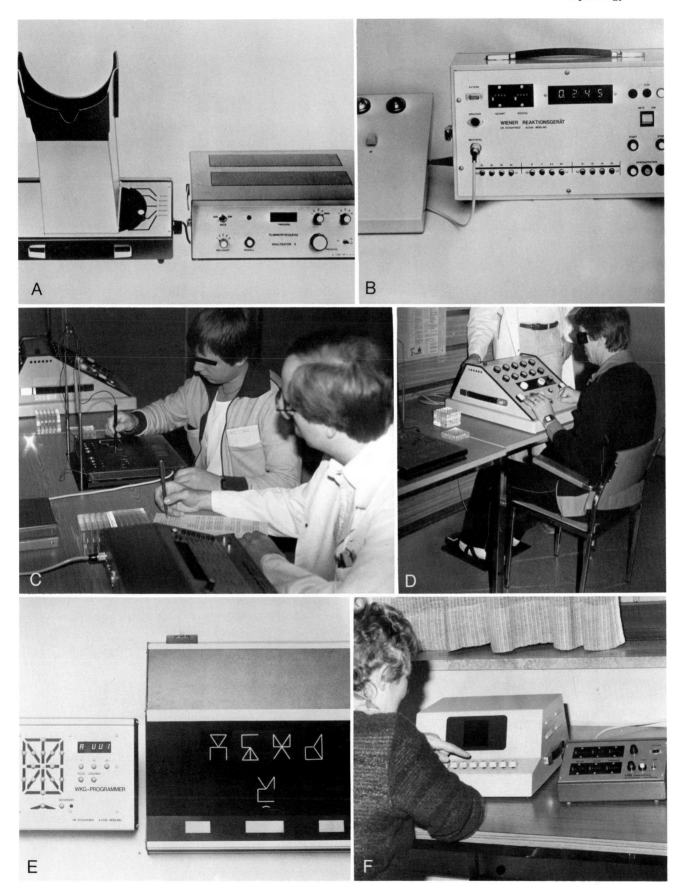

Figure 15.1.

Figure 15.2.

   A. AT in a rehabilitation center is taught in small groups. A maximum of 10 participants proved most effective. Individual sessions also are scheduled routinely. In groups, males are mixed with females and the same participants are always grouped together.

   B. After group discussions, specific exercises are applied in the group setting. Group participants at Bad Häring felt the exercises that were conducted while lying down were the most pleasant. During these exercises, a small pillow is placed under the head or a roll is placed under the neck. An additional pillow is placed under the knee to support and relax the ligaments of the extremities and the back. Blankets should always be available.

   C. Social training is suitable for wheelchair patients, especially adult spinal cord injury patients. However, other handicapped patients also participate on a regular basis in these groups. These groups should include a variety of disabilities; however, the participants should be in the same group (maximum: 10 patients). Additionally, unlike the AT group, the social training group continually receives and discharges members. In this group, the new inexperienced members learn from the more advanced members in a progressive fashion.

   D. PMR is usually started in individual sessions with simultaneous use of biofeedback equipment.

E–G. A prerequisite for any therapeutic intervention is an exact diagnosis and assessment that includes history taking, interview, observation and behavior analysis.

   H. The rehabilitation center in Bad Häring maintains a model suite, in which the patient and team members meet during their leisure time on a casual basis. This allows for a special place to discuss problems and difficulties that which do not surface during the formal therapeutic sessions.

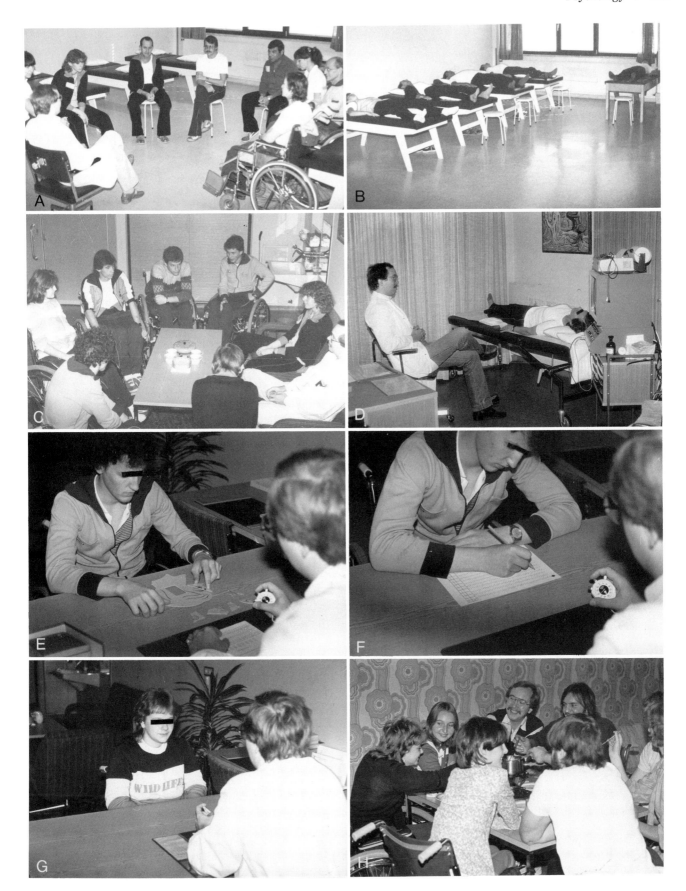

Figure 15.2.

16

Radiology in Trauma

Maria Erlemann, C.R.T.

The X-ray picture in trauma is not only a document of injury and an evaluation to aid the diagnosis and early treatment, but is also of great importance for the assessment of follow-up management and the healing process. It may lead to modification of approach, treatment methods, corrections, or revisions, and, finally, may assist in disability evaluation. For all these reasons, the X-ray must be technically perfect. It should not only show the region of immediate injury, but allow assessment of impact of injury upon adjacent areas, tissue, and structures. Angulations and displacements of bones must be shown clearly. (Fig. 16.1).

X-rays are obtained on patients who are in pain, who should not be moved, and, in many cases, who are severely injured. Sometimes splints or emergency dressings have been applied. Treatment of shock and life-sustaining activity must go on without interruption. The X-ray technician working in trauma must be specially trained to handle any of these situations, and must still be able to produce a meaningful radiograph quickly and safely.

The technician must master all techniques and positioning to avoid repetitions and time loss as well as unnecessary radiation exposure. Many of the techniques cannot be learned in school and come only with practical experience. For this reason, the X-ray technician should be assigned to the trauma department permanently rather than on a rotating basis. This is only possible where the trauma department, even a small one, has its own radiology service. There should be a complete supply of radiology equipment in the shock room, which is located close to the admitting area. A well-coordinated X-ray team must be available day and night, 7 days a week.

Assistive positioning devices, such as wood and foam wedges, foam pillows, wooden boards, split binders, and head positioning devices must be at close reach. It is important to have movable ceiling-mounted unit holders or tripods, on rails which allow anterioposterior (A-P) or lateral projections in any position so the patient does not need to be moved.

The X-ray equipment and mounting in the admission shock room should be different from a conventional X-ray department in that it should be designed to accommodate severely injured patients. Besides the ceiling mount, there should be a pedestal (usually called a "donkey"), which can be moved under the stretcher or X-ray transport table. The pedestal contains a measurement chamber with three measuring planes at which the central ray of the X-ray tube can be focused. A specific automatic exposure setting for different structures or organs is preprogrammed. The pedestal can be turned 90 degrees for horizontal views. The ceiling-mounted X-ray tube has a turning range of 360 degrees and can be moved in longitudinal and transverse directions. On top of the transportation stretcher, there should be a radiolucent pad, which can be pulled with little effort over a regular X-ray table for less severely injured patients.

For X-rays during surgery or on the ward, there are portable X-ray units available. In the operating room, there are also image intensifiers (see Fig. 16.2). A C-arm with a built-in camera for single and serial pictures is available (see Fig. 16.3).

With the portable unit, all X-rays in the average size patients, except lateral views of the spine, can be taken quite satisfactorily. If high resolution X-rays are mandatory, the patient must be moved to the X-ray department. X-rays on the ward should be limited to patients who are in traction or who cannot be moved, and other patients in the same room should be shielded.

The choice of X-ray format and size is determined not only by the tentative diagnosis but also by the positioning. For example, in wrist fractures, the elbow should be included in the first film to exclude a Monteggia fracture (distal radius-proximal ulna). In ankle or distal tibial fractures, the knee should be visible to exclude a proximal fibula fracture (Maisonneuve). In femoral fractures, the pelvis should be included to exclude hip dislocation or subluxation. It is advisable in initial pictures to choose a large format; follow-up X-rays can be smaller as indicated.

The labeling of X-rays is important to allow quick retrieval of films and minimize misfiling. The printing on the label should be read easily and should include the name of the institution; the patient's first name, middle initial, and last names; the patient's age, chart number, and accident number; the date; and whether the side X-rayed was left or right. This information is best typewritten on one line, with the film preexposed marginally ("scribor" procedure). This prevents covering up what are often important parts, which is a problem with the conventional square labeling. X-rays that are taken at the same time, upon admission for example, should be marked with a white marker in the left upper corner with the same number (e.g., **1**); the additional films should then be marked **1a**, **1b**, **1c**, etc. For example, the AP view would be **1**, lateral view, **1a**; oblique (L) **1c**; and oblique (R) **1d**. If additional X-rays of the same area are necessary, these should be marked 1', 1", etc.

Follow-up X-rays that are taken the same day (for post-surgery, reduction, etc.) should be marked **2, 2a**, etc.; later controls, **3, 3a**, etc. This allows for quick retrieval of X-rays during rounds and conferences or for retrieval of the first and last X-rays without tediously looking up dates on which the X-rays were taken. It also allows for quick and orderly filing. If X-rays are taken of the noninvolved side or extremity for comparison, the involved side should be marked with Arabic numbers; the uninvolved, with Roman numerals. If there are multiple injuries, the main parts should be marked **1, 1a**, etc and the other parts, a capital letter before the **1**. For example:

	Skull	Thorax	Forearm (R)	Ankle (R)	Ankle (L)
5/25/85	1, 1a, 1b	A1	B1, B1a	C1, C1a	CI, CIa
5/25/85	2	A2			
6/1/85		A3			

The X-rays should be stored in an envelope that contains the data (which should also be printed on the outside of the envelope and a printed X-ray report. It should also be color-coded to make correct filing and detection of misfiled folders easy. The envelope should contain the body area or part taken on a given day and the follow-up report (Fig. 16.4).

In trauma and rehabilitation centers, in addition to the chart number, the patient should receive an accident number, which allows easy retrieval of statistical data for follow-up studies on outcomes in individual patients or similar injuries.

Daily X-ray conferences in trauma hospitals, during which all X-rays of the previous day admissions and treatment are briefly discussed with all physicians present, are of great importance. These provide checks of optimal treatment methods, necessity of corrections, or additional measures to be taken within 24 hr of the accident. This also allows discussion of approaches before surgery. The X-rays are prearranged by the X-ray technician and displayed on a multiscreen viewer as follows:

1. X-rays of patients scheduled for surgery the same day: initial X-ray and control
2. X-rays before removal of hardware: initial X-ray and last X-rays
3. X-rays of new admissions: initial X-rays and postop or post-reduction views
4. X-rays of patients in intensive care
5. X-rays of follow-ups of ward patients (from day before)

X-ray conferences in long-term rehabilitation centers are held prior to closed reduction or surgery days, usually twice a week. These conferences are crucial in clarification of ambiguities and controversial views; they are a great aid in continuing education, and allow a more uniform approach to total comprehensive management of trauma patients.

Figure 16.1.

A. A child is brought to the X-ray service, located in the evaluation area of the trauma department. Note X-ray files of recent cases, which are kept in the trauma department and not in the central X-ray file room until the patient is discharged and the treatment completed.

B. The child is positioned for X-ray of the skull.

C. The X-ray label is typed.

D. In recent injury X-ray files in the trauma department, color codes facilitate filing and prevent misfiling.

E. Forms produced by the Banda Hospital Record Multiform Copying Machine with appropriate imprints are taken from the original admission sheet in less than a minute. The X-ray envelope is on the left lower side of the picture.

F. A daily early morning X-ray conference is held in the trauma department. The X-ray technician prepares films on alternators (mass film viewers) prior to the conference to enable physicians to view and discuss a large number of X-rays in a short time.

G. Professor Dr. Otto Russe, conducting the X-ray conference, discusses a patient's hand injury with a visiting professor (Dr. Ernest Burgess).

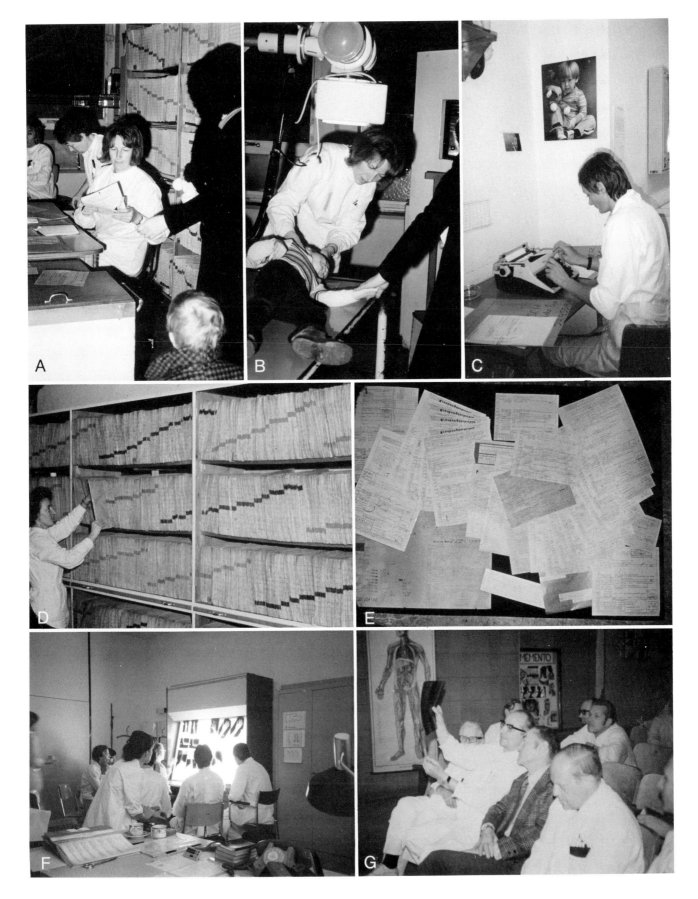

Figure 16.1.

Figure 16.2.

A–B. A calcaneal fracture is diagnosed and treated in the minor surgery room in the outpatient area of the trauma department utilizing the C-arm image intensifier.

C. X-rays of same patient are taken after reduction and fixation of the fracture.

D. A chest film X-ray is labeled.

E. The patient is positioned for a stress X-ray of the ulnar collateral ligament of the metacarpophalangeal joint of the thumb.

F. The stress X-ray shows abnormal angulation and subluxation, indicating a ruptured ligament.

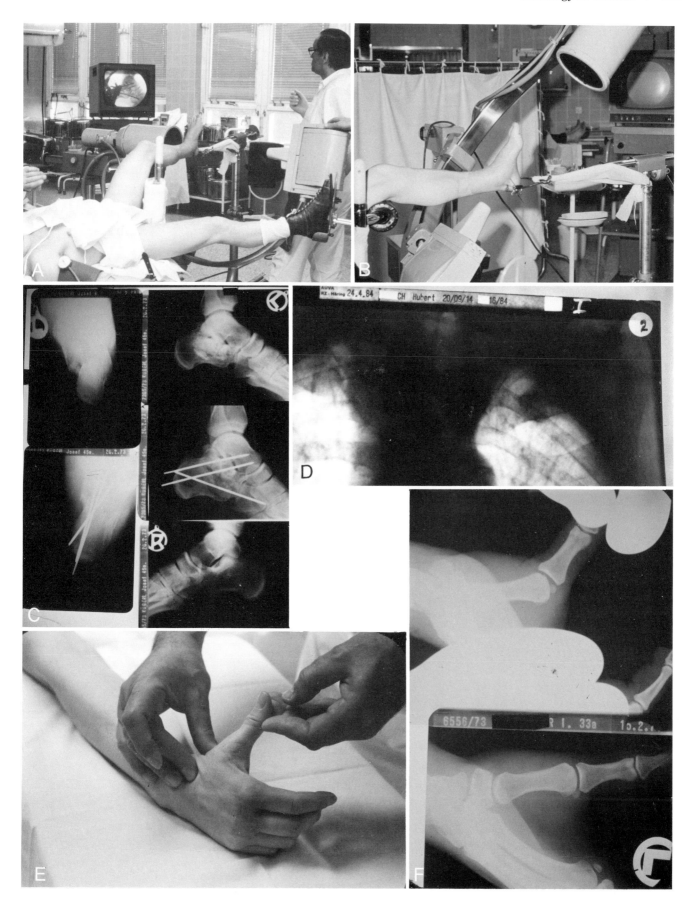

Figure 16.2.

Figure 16.3.

A–C. Accident victims with polytrauma (multiple fractures and internal injuries) are a challenge to any X-ray technician. Only technicians experienced in trauma and X-ray techniques can work fast and produce X-rays acceptable for diagnosis and treatment without delay or exposing the patient to additional stress or injury.

   D. The same patient is in the intensive care unit. X-ray rechecks have to be taken under trying conditions, working around life-support systems, traction devices, etc., without moving the patient.

   E. Plaster of Paris dressings and tractions add to the difficulties.

   F. X-ray technicians take X-rays and prepare the patient for closed intramedullary rodding of a femoral fracture, positioning two C-arms (for AP and lateral views) in the operating room.

   G. AP and cross-table lateral views are arranged in femoral neck fractures.

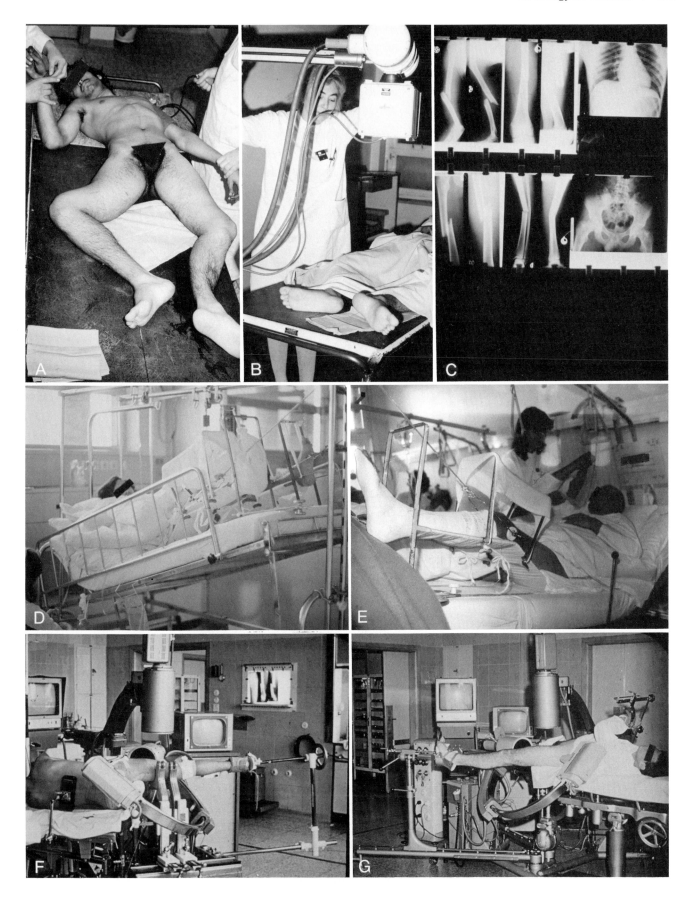

Figure 16.3.

Figure 16.4.

A–B. An X-ray of a knee (AP and lateral views) has an unobstructive identification label containing institution, date, last and first name of patient, birthdate, record number, and year; markings include left or right as well as sequential numbers. (For example, 3 for AP view; 3a for lateral view). This speeds up filing and retrieving of films immensely.

C–D. In contrast, conventional identification labels may obstruct important parts of the film.

E. On a xerography of an actual X-ray file envelope, the color coding for every day of the month is on the left side; the file number is in the corner. On the right, there is a copy of the admission record, including an initial X-ray report printed on the envelope in the admitting office by the Banda Hospital Record Multiform Copying Machine. On the left, there are the date and codes of the X-rays taken on a given day. Details of the codes on the X-ray envelopes are shown. It reads: September 28, 1985 Cervical spine (HWS-[Halswirbelsäule]), Skull A1, A1a (for AP and lateral views), Chest B1, C1, C1a (for AP and lateral). There is room for subsequent X-ray reports.

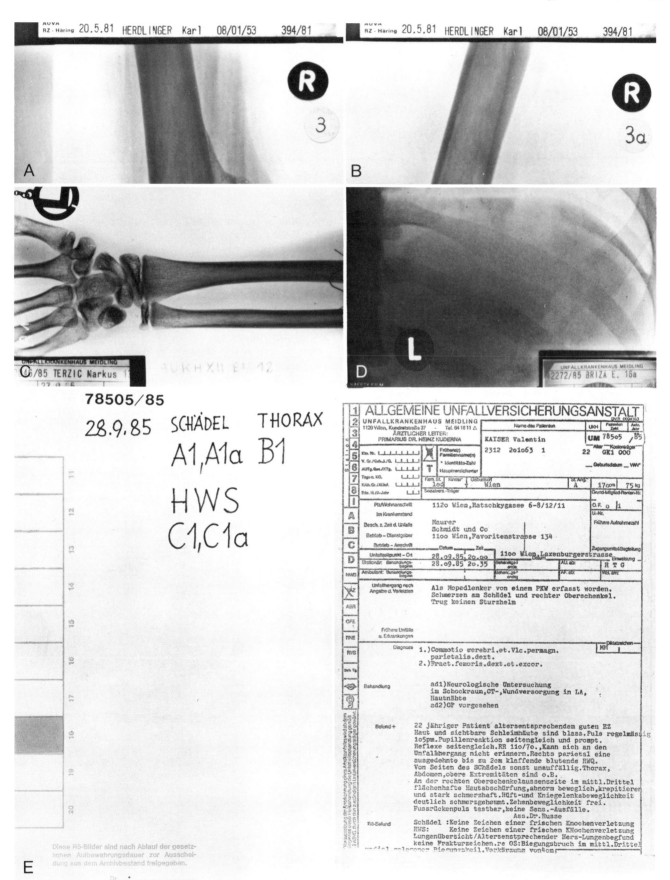

Figure 16.4.

17

Recreational Therapy

Judy M. Henbury, R.T.

The service of recreational therapy involves the application of prescribed and voluntary activities, designed to promote the constructive use of leisure time, physical well-being, and resocialization.

Therapeutic recreation utilizes recreational services for purposeful intervention in some physical, emotional, and/or social behavior to bring about a desired change in that behavior and to promote the growth and development of the individual. Therapeutic recreational activities provide challenges in a planned, coordinated, and structured manner. The activities provided should be selected carefully so that they are not only enjoyable but are also beneficial in overcoming specific problems. For example, a physically handicapped patient, such as a trauma victim, amputee, or paraplegic, participates in enjoyable activities that not only conserve and strengthen the abilities that have been affected, but that also exercise and encourage use of those facilities that have been impaired. Without an activities program, such a person would not use the impaired facilities. Withdrawal and depression might cause the patient not to want to do anything at all, thus losing even those abilities that had not been impaired.

In a physical rehabilitation hospital, the recreational therapist's role is to help the patient adjust to the period of hospitalization through therapeutic recreational intervention. A recreational therapist works closely as a team member with the patient's medical doctor, physical therapist, educational therapist, and occupational therapist. All team members participate in the many therapies that are available, and the usefulness of the recreational therapy program is contingent on the skillfulness of the treatment team. The recreational therapist utilizes the physician's medical evaluation in order to determine the appropriate activities, keeping in mind the patient's abilities and limitations. With tools ranging from those as simple as a game of cards to those as sophisticated as applying complex principles of leisure counseling, therapeutic recreators use their skills and resources to bring about results that contribute to raising the level of the individual's quality of life.

The most challenging part of the recreational therapist's job is to encourage persons to participate—to get them involved. Even the most varied and exciting activities reap no benefits if a person will not participate. It is the recreational therapist's responsibility to provide activities that present a challenge and that make persons *want* to participate and achieve. Recreational therapists can motivate, excite the will, and relight the candle of interest in life. Just as activity is the sign of life, achievement is the purpose of life. No matter how small the achievement, it brings with it dignity, self-respect, self-reliance, and a will to stay alive to achieve more.

18

Respiratory Therapy

Linda Allaway, R.R.T.

Respiratory care is of primary importance for the initial assessment of the patient to his or her successful discharge from the acute care setting. Several categories of traumatized patients require respiratory assistance, including thoracic trauma, the postsurgical, and neurological trauma patients.

Thoracic trauma may result in a wide variety of disorders that may respond to respiratory care. An artificial airway with or without mechanical ventilation may be necessary. Appropriate diagnostic monitoring and therapy intended to maintain adequate pulmonary expansion and oxygenation are essential to management of these patients. Breathing exercises with assisted cough techniques commonly are used to assist the patient to successful recovery from insults of this type.

Traumatized patients requiring general anesthesia and surgical intervention commonly display several pulmonary deficits. Alveolar atelectasis presents with changes in pulmonary volumes and an increase in the work of breathing. For trauma patients, this may be compounded by aspiration, changes in lung water, and a previous history of pulmonary disorders. Respiratory therapists are responsible for diagnostic monitoring, including bedside pulmonary function testing, arterial blood gases, oximetry, and where appropriate, transcutaneous monitoring (see Fig. 18.1). Many therapeutic modalities are available that include airway management, such as intubation; maintenance of artificial airways, including tracheostomies, by appropriate humidification; operation of gas delivery systems assuring proper oxygenation; mechanical ventilation; chest physical therapy, including postural drainage, percussion, and vibration; and breathing exercises to prevent and reverse alveolar atelectasis. Breathing exercises may become quite extensive if diaphragmatic impairment has occurred. Aerosolization of bronchodilators may be utilized to improve secretion clearance and treatment of the bronchospastic airway.

Nearly 50% of the deaths on most *neurosurgical or neurology units* are due to respiratory complications. Two basic considerations guide the respiratory care treatment plan in dealing with neurological trauma. First, the immediate neurological trauma, with resultant alteration in intracranial pressure, may be controlled by mechanical hyperventilation. Second, pulmonary complications secondary to prolonged immobilization and hypoventilation may require intervention.

Airway management may include intubation assisted by bronchoscopy to avoid compromise of an unstable cervical spine. Spinal cord injuries may present with loss of innervation to most of the muscles of respiration, and upper cervical cord lesions (C2–C3) can be expected to result in respiratory failure. Other lesions may significantly impair secondary respiratory muscle innervation. Breathing exercises aimed at the development of compensatory respiratory function of sternocleidomastoid and trapezius muscles to maintain adequate vital capacity may be used to prevent atelectasis and to allow the patient to mobilize more effectively pulmonary secretions.

Pneumonia presents a major threat secondary to retained respiratory secretions, and may be prevented by effective mobilization of secretions and maintenance of good pulmonary hygiene. Bronchial hygiene activities, such as postural drainage, percussion and vibration, need to be combined with breathing exercises to allow optimal use of functional muscles. Bronchoscopy with therapeutic assistance may be required in the removal of mucous plugs. Preexistent pulmonary disorders must be recognized and managed to avoid further complications. The oxygenation status of the patient requires continuous monitoring and careful manipulation of gas delivery systems.

In addition to the pulmonary complications of infection and atelectasis, pulmonary embolism is a major cause of both morbidiity and mortality in quadriplegics who survive initial injury. Careful pulmonary monitoring of these patients is required in their successful management. Procedures such as bedside pulmonary function testing, assessment of oxygenation by arterial blood gases, and oximetry may be required.

Mechanical ventilation must be monitored carefully by the respiratory therapist. Long-term intubation may result in permanent tracheal strictures. Tracheostomies allow for more stable airway management but are not without hazard, especially with regard to infections. Aspiration remains a threat, and careful, thorough suctioning is required. For patients with nutritional abnormalities, respiratory therapists may assist with evaluation of nutritional status with sophisticated metabolic analysis.

Long-term management requires constant vigilance and monitoring of the pulmonary status of the traumatized patient. This is surely a multidisciplinary effort among physicians, nursing personnel, and the respiratory therapist.

Figure 18.1.

A–B. The Allen test is applied prior to drawing arterial blood.
  C. Blood sample is taken from radial artery for evaluation of arterial blood gases.
  D. The arterial blood sample immediately is placed in a plastic bag filled with crushed ice.
  E. The respiratory therapist performs bedside spirometry.
  F. Aerosol therapy, along with postural drainage.
  G. Aerosol therapy and cough assistance are applied.
  H. The respiratory therapist attends a patient with craniocerebral injury.
I–J. A mechanical ventilator requires monitors.

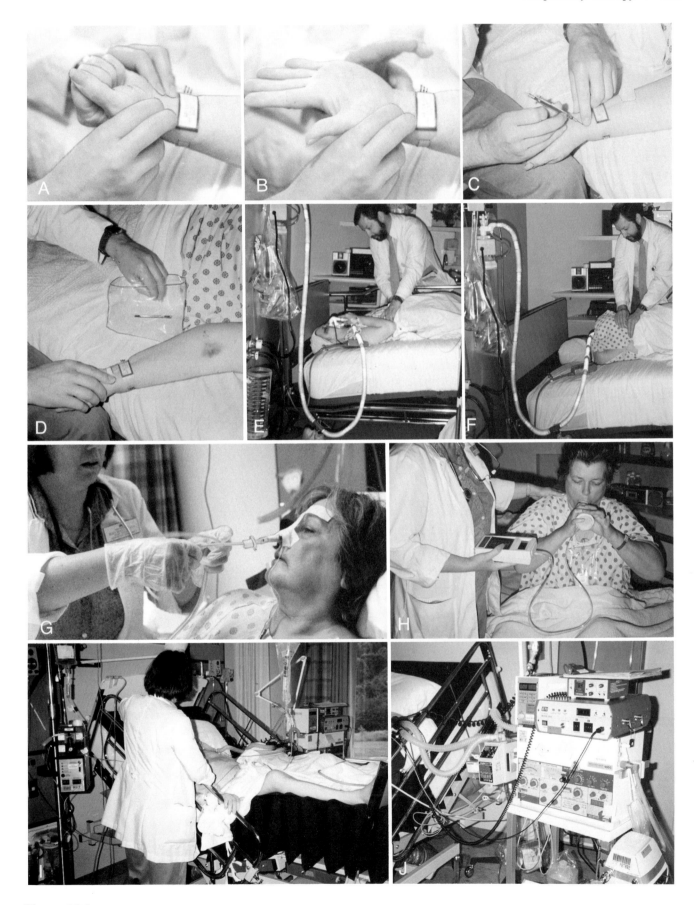

Figure 18.1.

19

Sexuality in Trauma

William H. Winkler, Ph.D.

Physical trauma often results in both psychological and organic sequelae, which frequently affect an individual's libido and sexual functioning in adverse ways. Successful sexual adjustment to traumatic conditions seems to be mediated by psychosocial adjustments. Specific issues of adjustment vary somewhat, according to the patient's sex, age, marital status, social support network, severity and type of disability, and premorbid level of psychological adjustment. Nevertheless, most sexual and psychological adjustments to traumatic injuries are quite difficult and painful and are tremendously anxiety-provoking.

Rather than present the disabled as different from the nondisabled, it is more helpful to view the variable to sexual adjustment as a continuous variable. Many nondisabled individuals have opportunities for gratifying sexuality. Individuals who were poorly adjusted prior to their injuries generally have the most difficulty with sexual adjustment after trauma. More important, and perhaps prognostic of adjustment, however, are positive views of sexuality, flexibility to change, potential for sexual and emotional creativity, and capacity for intimacy.

Following traumatic injuries (e.g., spinal cord injury, amputation, or head trauma), a set of total body reactions often affects the brain and sexual arousal mechanisms. The rehabilitation practitioner is apt to encounter an individual who is passive, depressed, and suffering from an ego-identity crisis. Self-esteem and sex role conflict are usually present as is considerable anxiety concerning openness to intimacy and physical touching. A general sense of helplessness prevails. Body image distortions are often present. In rehabilitation settings, the first approach is to provide a supportive environment. This is accomplished more easily by promoting not only the maximization of physical abilities but also the maximization of psychological and psychosocial strengths.

Opinions vary somewhat as to the appropriateness of introducing sex information early in the rehabilitation process. Perhaps the best approach is on a case-by-case basis. Providing an atmosphere of permission to explore sexual issues is of the utmost importance. Many patients often use ego defense mechanisms of denial and avoidance if the rehabilitation atmosphere and staff attitudes reflect repressive attitudes toward sexuality or exploration of sexual issues. Opportunities for privacy and sexual exploration following a period of medical stability

are also important to overcome the tendency of the patient to avoid or avert his or her self-image as a sensual and sexual being.

Some progressive rehabilitation centers provide a full complement of services, including physiatry, urology, gynecology, physical and occupational therapy, psychology, and sex therapy. Unfortunately however, the availability of one-to-one sex counseling is apt to be less than 50% of nation-wide spinal cord injury centers. The imbalance of services needed for delivery is even more alarming when considering a survey in the VA Hospital and Kaiser Hospital in Portland, Oregon of patients with spinal cord injury that showed that 85% of men and 50% of women would, if they could choose, return to normal sexual functioning rather than ambulation. This rather shocking statistic points out the need for a comprehensive shift in the focus of rehabilitation centers toward meeting the patient's need for information, education, and treatment in the sexual area.

Sex therapy should be provided by individuals who are knowledgable in psychology or sex therapy as well as in the anatomy and physiology of sex and disability. Prior to initiating any treatment, an adequate sexual history needs to be obtained. Sexual history combined with realistic goal setting are the foundation upon which the therapeutic endeavor is built. The therapeutic team in sex therapy also includes medical and allied medical staff to deal with such issues as contraception, bowel and bladder difficulties, and sexual positions. Every individual's level of sexual responsiveness will vary according to the type and level of injury. Regardless of whether an individual can procreate, achieve and maintain erection, ejaculate, or have orgasm, the goal in sex therapy should be to provide a sense of comfort, self-esteem, and sensual enjoyment. Therefore, there should be a shift in orientation away from the focus of erection-penetration-orgasm and toward enjoying the total experience of intimacy, which is more likely to occur in a nondemand sexual environment. Because the patient's level of injury may preclude any typical avenues of sexual arousal and performance, reorientation and relearning usually are necessary. The individual can be taught to appreciate the use of sexual fantasy, sexual apparatus, sexual talking, and sensate focus. In this context, a multitude of pleasurable stimuli encompasssing verbal, tactile, auditory, olfactory, and visual modalities can be used as expressions of intimacy, caring, and love. In achieving this end, the practitioner may recommend educational classes, support groups of other injured patients, group therapy, and couples groups. Problems concerning arousal, avoidance and relationship conflicts as well as specific sexual problems should be referred to a certified sex therapist. The American Association of Sex Educators, Counselors, and Therapists (AASECT) publishes an international directory of certified sex therapists, and is an excellent resource for making specialized referrals.

20

Social Work: Vocational and Social Rehabilitation of Traumatized Patients

Daniel Pinter, M.S.W.

Rehabilitation is comprised of various medical measures as provided by traumatotherapy, vocational measures, and, as necessary, supplementary social measures, which are all directed at restoring the disabled person's health to a degree that will enable him or her to participate in vocational and economic activities and to hold an adequate social position (Social Insurance Law, 1977). [Legal definition of rehabilitation in Austrian law (Social Insurance Law, § 172/2, (Suppl. 32, 1977)]. In accordance with these legal provisions, social accident insurance provides not only for traumatotheraphy (i.e., medical rehabilitation), but also for vocational and social rehabilitation measures. Specially trained social workers and rehabilitation advisers carry out the regulations as provided by law.

There are three basic tasks of social work in rehabilitation: *(a) client-centered tasks, (b) team-centered tasks,* and *(c) environment-centered tasks.*

CLIENT'S CENTERED TASKS

Social work can only be effective in an atmosphere of confidence. Therefore, the most important initial task of the social worker is to win the patient's confidence. An openly displayed readiness of the social worker to place his or her knowledge and experience at the patient's disposal together with a demonstrated understanding of the patient's situation usually create the necessary basis of confidence. This basis is consolidated by emotional support, interest in the arising problems, and expressed confidence in the abilities of the patient undergoing rehabilitation. From this basis, the social worker can succeed in helping the patient to overcome his or her handicap. This help is especially required to overcome the anxieties aroused in most persons by an accident and a handicap resulting from it. These anxieties include fear of life, fear of being left alone, and fear of having to surrender.

The knowledge and experience of the social worker can contribute much to the reduction, as well as to the control, of anxieties. Information about the complicated system of social insurance, and the financial aid provided by it, can relieve the anxiety and fear regarding economic security during and after rehabilitation.

By discussing the possiblities of rehabilitation and by carefully explaining the rehabilitation aim, anxieties are further reduced. For a continuing diminution of anxieties,

the social worker needs profound expert knowledge; and for the determination of rehabilitation goals, the possibilities, wishes, and conceptions of the disabled person must be respected. As the patient overcomes anxieties, he or she undergoes a process of change. Previous concepts of vocational and private aspects of life have at the least become questionable, and in many cases must be changed completely (especially with severe injuries). The patient must form a new self-image in accordance with the consequences of his or her handicap. The task of social work in this respect is to reconcile the new role and the expectations with the real possibilities. For this purpose it is necessary to find out whether the traumatized patient is conscious of his or her disability at all. Although the doctor informs the patient about the kind and extent of the disability, it often is found that the full significance is not immediately realized due to the patient's unconscious denial of his or her injury or the performance of the injury. In the previously mentioned atmosphere of confidence, however, the social worker, together with other team members, can help the patient to "accept" the disability and to try to master the resulting consequences. To support these attempts, the social worker must not only provide adequate information and the necessary support throughout each phase of adjustment to the disability but also must continue in these roles after the disability has been accepted.

After the patient has accepted his or her new image and has regained psychological stability, the social worker should attempt to develop a rehabilitation plan together with the patient. The aim of this rehabilitation plan is to develop a strategy that will enable the patient to achieve as great an independence as possible with his or her remaining capacities.

TEAM-CENTERED TASKS

The social worker must fulfill a variety of tasks within the rehabilitation team. The most important among these is the establishment of a *social diagnosis,* This means not only a social anamnesis, but also includes, for example, consideration of the way a patient copes with the handicap, how he or she experiences the stay at the rehabilitation center, or anxieties about which he or she complains. Social diagnosis also includes information about the motivation of the patient, how much strain can be imposed on the family, and the impressions and experiences the social worker gains from the contact with the patient (see Fig. 20.1). The social worker also must take into consideration the relationship of the patient to his or her environment and his or her stage of development (i.e., adolescent or adult). As it frequently changes during rehabilitation, the social diagnosis rarely is written, but is instead mostly transmitted orally to the other team members.

The social worker, like all other team members, not only furnishes the team with information, but also receives information. Regular team conferences are necessary to enhance this interchange. Since it is often essential for the social worker to obtain certain information without delay, he or she should arrange team conferences to gather additional information when necessary.

Finally, the social worker, provided he or she is familiar with group dynamics, should try to solve any problems arising in the teamwork together with the psychologist during the conferences.

ENVIRONMENT-CENTERED TASKS

Although the work and the close personal contact with the patient and other team members are the first priority tasks of the social worker, his or her efforts will not be successful in the long run if he or she does not also incorporate the environment of the patient (i.e., family and public) in his or her work. Members of the patient's family, especially, should be important partners for the social worker. They should be contacted as early as possible. As mentioned earlier, social work is only possible in an atmosphere of confidence. The social worker must, therefore, also win the confidence of the patient's family. The family's anxieties, which often are similar to those of the patient, must be relieved, and expectations must be revised. But they must also be made conscious of their special responsibility to the patient. The social worker must quite often overcome problems with communication (differences in the command of the language according to educational background are notable) by taking over the role of a mediator. In addition, the social worker should encourage the patient and the family to improve their ability to communicate (e.g., to express wishes, and to verbalize feelings, needs, and wants).

To support this work with the patient and the family, the social worker should never miss a chance to be an advocate for the understanding of the disabled in public. Of course there is no need to travel throughout the country like a soapbox orator, but talks with colleagues and employers about traumatized patients as well as lectures in schools and at institutions for adult education can very well help to improve the public's knowledge about disability, the possibilities of rehabilitation, and how the disabled population can be integrated into society.

Social work presents many vocational as well as social possibilities.

VOCATIONAL POSSIBILITIES OF ASSIMILATION

Legal accident insurance, such as workmen's compensation, starts from the principle that vocational rehabilitation activities shall enable the tramatized patient to practice his or her former, or if this is not possible a new, vocational goal. The measures provided to achieve this goal include:

1. Vocational training for recuperation or improvement of the ability to obtain employment
2. Granting of insurance and medical benefits
3. Assistance with obtaining suitable employment

How these measures will be carried out depends on the severity of the traumatic lesions; the intelligence, character, and age of the handicapped person; and the available opportunity in the labor market in relation to current economic trends. Therefore, working closely with vocational counselors and social workers in rehabilitation is necessary.

In drafting the rehabilitation plan, the patient's abilities (e.g., remaining efficiency, qualifications, preferences, and possiblities for the compensation of his or her handicap) as well as the possibilities provided by the service list of the legal accident insurance (which can be obtained by vocational rehabilitation professionals) must be taken into consideration. The rehabilitation plan should not consist of rigid obligatory directions concerning the measures that must be taken, but should instead be a flexible definition of rehabilitation goals. After the rehabilitation plan has been worked out together with the patient, the social worker must implement the particular measures and must make preparations for them.

Certain measures concerning the continuation of the patient's former employment usually can be implemented by the social worker. For instance, the social worker can contact the patient's former employer while the patient is out of work due to his or her handicap, and can try to find him or her another job in the same firm. In all those cases where financial aid from the legal accident insurance is necessary to regain the patient's working ability (e.g., expenses for training, tuition, transportation, and cost of living), the social worker can take all necessary preparatory steps by making a few phone calls on behalf of the patient.

After the authorization of the rehabilitation plan by a rehabilitation committee of the accident insurer, the realization of the plan is incumbent on the rehabilitation advisers of the insurer. If necessary, the rehabilitation advisers are also responsible for the accompanying care of the patient during vocational training. A close cooperation of the social workers (employed by hospitals for accident cases or rehabilitation centers) with the rehabilitation advisers is absolutely necessary to attain the rehabilitation aim.

SOCIAL POSSIBILITIES FOR THE ATTAINMENT OF THE REHABILITATION AIM

The social possibilities of rehabilitation comprise services, besides medical treatment and vocational measures of rehabilitation, that are designed to contribute to the attainment of the rehabilitation goal as defined in the introduction of this chapter. With regard to the economic situation of the disabled, three main measures come into question:

1. Income or loans that make possible or facilitate the adaptation of apartments or separate homes for use by the handicapped
2. Contribution to the expenses of acquiring a driver's license
3. Income or loans for the purchase or adaptation of a motor vehicle

Further measures of social rehabilitation include:

1. Promotion of athletics for the disabled
2. Promotion of rehabilitation workshops and institutions of occupational therapy

The increasing number of very severely disabled during the past few years has made the adaptation of housing to accommodate the disabled more and more important. Especially for paraplegic patients, adaptations are essential in most cases (Fig. 20.2). The social worker should obtain a complete description of housing conditions early enough to be able to advise the patient and his or her family. As options for adaptive housing are becoming more and more complicated and costly, it is advisable to seek early the assistance of experts (e.g., architects, technicians, or craftspersons). As an adaptation always entails considerable expenses that must be recovered from the insurer, the social worker should correlate these activities with the insurer's rehabilitation adviser responsible for following the care of the patient. An acceptable compromise must be achieved between the wishes of the disabled and the financial responsiblities of the insurer. In this situation, the social worker usually takes the role of an advocate of the patient, as he or she knows about the sources of the insurer to help his or her client. The economic aspects from the insurer's point of view is presented to the patient by the representatives of the authorities.

In order to compensate for the impairment of mobility, legal accident insurance gives handicapped persons the chance to acquire a driver's license, to adapt an already available car (see Figs. 20.3 and 20.4), or to buy a new motor vehicle with the financial aid of the accident insurance. The social worker, with the help of a driving school, has the task of informing the patient about prerequisites for acquiring or reacquiring a driver's license. The social worker should advise the patient on the purchase or adaptation of a motor vehicle and help him or her with purchasing it.

Legal accident insurers also contribute much to social rehabilitation by promoting and sponsoring athletics for the disabled. This particular insurance scheme, which owns and administers the trauma hospitals as well as rehabilitation centers, provides for all of the elaborate facilities and personnel to allow for physical education and reeducation and pays for competitive sport events and participation of the patients. The social worker should therefore try to motivate patients toward the participation in sports. This helps patients establish personal contacts, improve their self-respect, and participate in a physical exercise program.

Also, the promotion of the establishment of rehabilitation workshops and institutions for occupational therapy enables the social worker to give hope of an occupaton to those very severely disabled who strongly desire to resume an activity but who cannot be employed in the general labor market (see Fig. 20.5).

Figure 20.1.

A. The social worker conducts a conference at bedside
B. During progressive care and treatment, and
C. Along with orientation, prior to social training.
D–I. The social worker carries out social training.

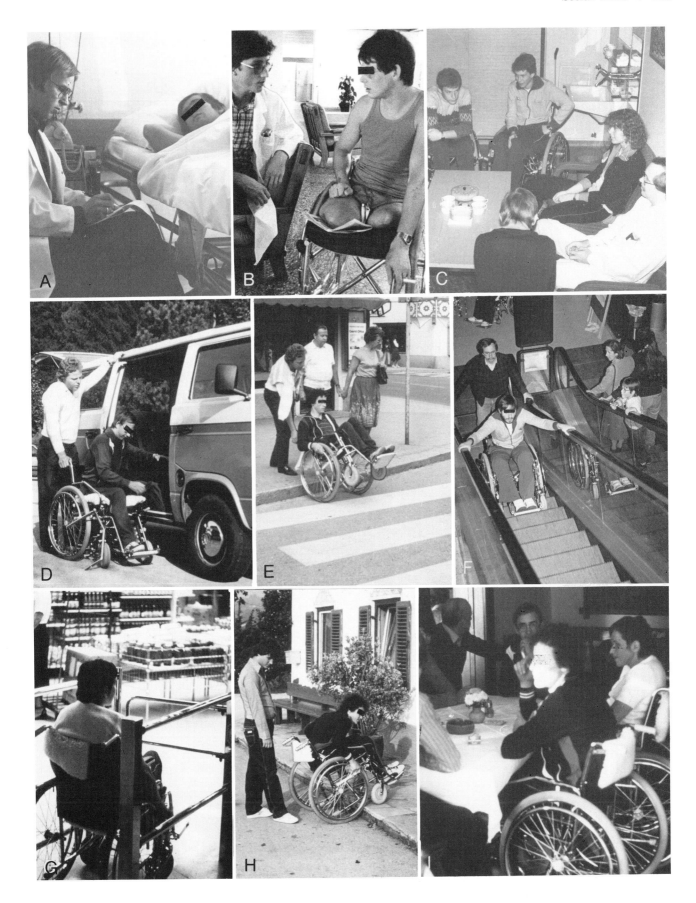

Figure 20.1.

Figure 20.2. Social training in the home involves

A–C. Bathroom modifications
D–F. Living room modifications
 G–I. Stair lifts
   J. An outside lift, and
K–L. A stair climber.

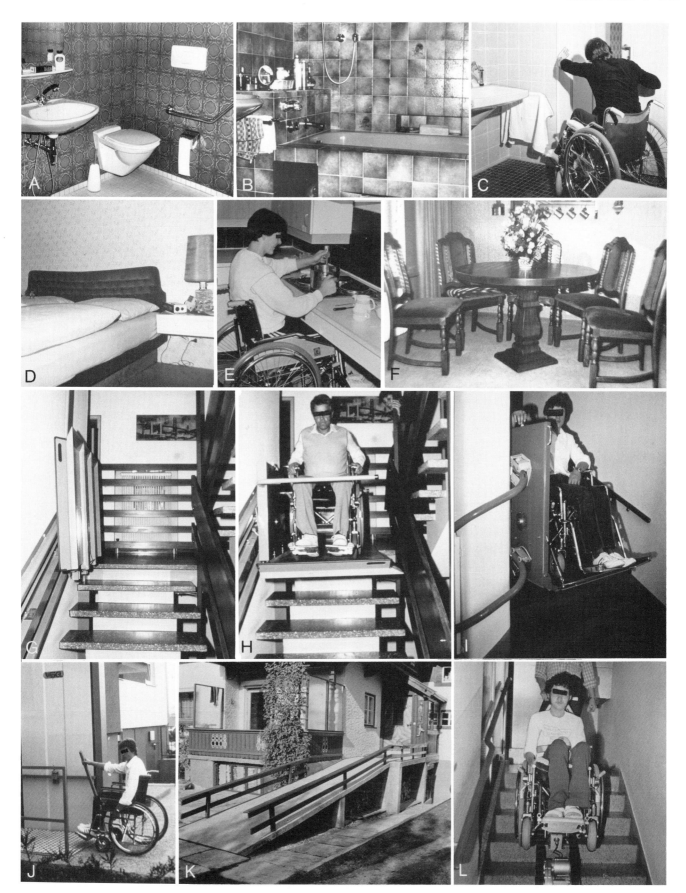

Figure 20.2.

Figure 20.3.

    A. Manual controls are used in driver training, along with

  B–I. Independent transfer of a paraplegic patient and his wheelchair into a car.

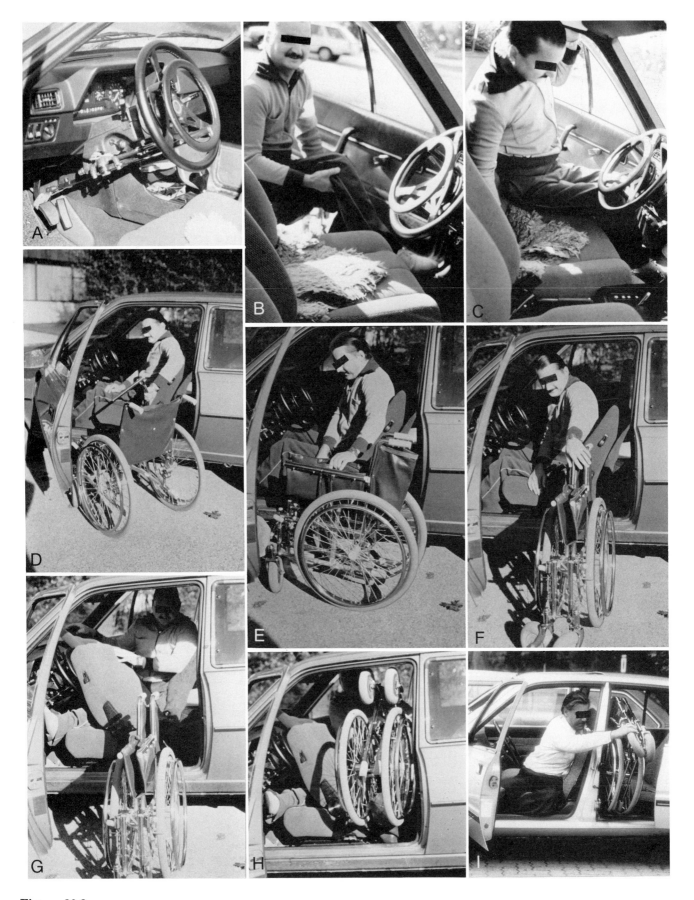

Figure 20.3.

Figure 20.4.

A–D. Outside lift for wheelchair patient transfer on back of van.

E–F. Side lift for wheelchair patient transfer into van.

   G. Outside key-switch to operate sliding door and side lift.

H–J. Special foot controls to drive car by patients with nonfunctioning upper extremities (Courtesy Prof. Marquardt, Orthopedic Dept. University of Heidelberg-Germany).

   K. Simple modification of a two-wheel scooter for operation by a paraplegic patient (two lateral wheels are attached).

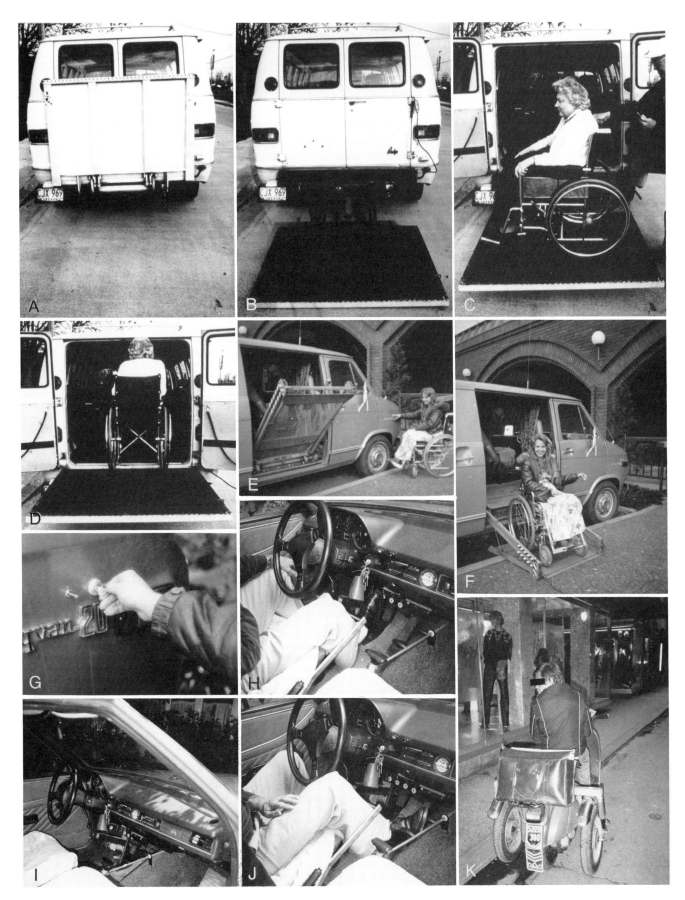

Figure 20.4.

Figure 20.5.

A–H. Work possibilities in a sheltered workshop are numerous.

    I. Self-employment possibilities include setting up a federal franchise stand (to sell stamps, magazines, pipes, etc.).

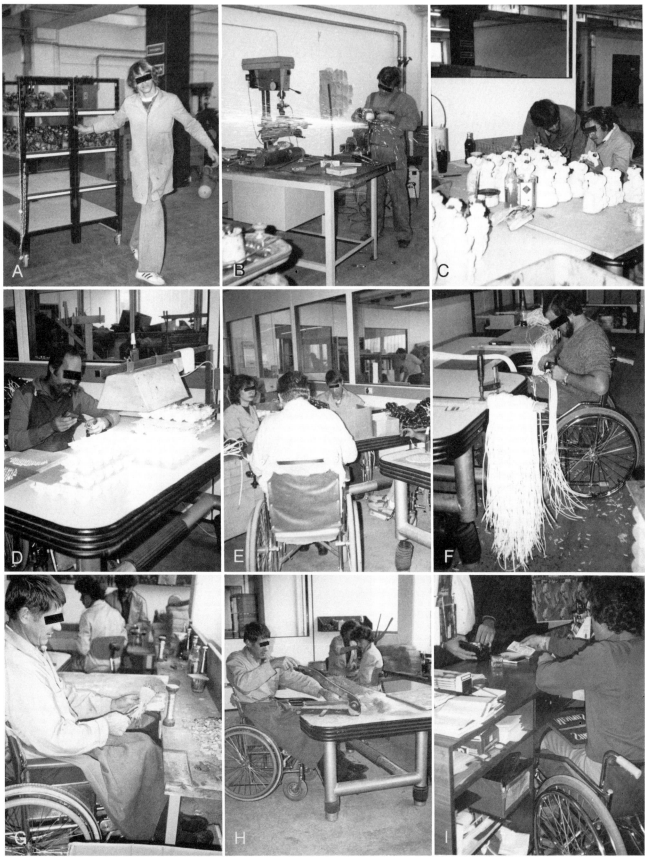

Figure 20.5.

21

Speech and Language Pathology: Treatment of Trauma Patients with Communication and Swallowing Disorders

Lance Tsugawa, M.S., C.C.C.

Traditionally, speech pathology services have focused primarily on the treatment of articulation (sound production) and voice disorders. Patients who have sustained a traumatic injury often present a complicated profile of medical, physical, emotional, cognitive, and communicative disabilities. As a member of an interdisciplinary trauma team, the speech-language pathologist has expanded his or her traditional activity to include a variety of associated disorders. Together with the management of speech disorders, treatment for deficits in language, cognitive ability, and swallowing have become part of the speech-language pathologist's concern. Management of these deficit areas is performed in close cooperation with other members of the trauma team.

LANGUAGE DISORDERS (APHASIA)

Deficits in language ability, or *aphasia*, commonly are seen in patients with traumatic injuries to the left cerebral cortex. Language is a symbolic process in which verbal, graphic, and gestural symbols stand for referents in the world, i.e., objects, actions, ideas, and feelings. Disorders of language are therefore deficits in the use of linguistic symbols. Patients with aphasia may have difficulty with comprehension of the written or spoken language. They may be unable to name objects or verbally describe their activities in a well-formulated manner.

The speech-language pathologist on the trauma team diagnoses and treats these disorders in an effort to aid language recovery. The trauma patient with aphasia may be confused and overwhelmed with his or her sudden lack of communication. The speech-language pathologist attempts to organize and structure the recovery process for the patient to mitigate the effects of this sudden isolation. Stimulation tasks should be presented in a manner that will challenge and facilitate the patient's residual abilities.

Speech directed to the aphasic patient may be received as a chaotic influx of incomprehensible jargon. The clinician's task should be to organize this input so that the patient can learn gradually and systematically to decode the language stimuli around him or her. Treatment designed to stimulate and facilitate the patient's verbal ability should be provided. Patients may be taught strategies for remembering words or formulating their ideas into coherent sentences.

A high percentage of traumaticallly brain-injured patients demonstrate language problems that are secondary manifestations of underlying cognitive disorganization. They may show deficits in attention, concentration, and organization of internal mental processes. The speech-language pathologist, in cooperation with the neuropsychologist, should structure treatment to aid the patient in the reorganization of these cognitively mediated language functions. Structured activities to improve alertness, memory, discrimination, and information processing will serve as a foundation for improvements in activities of daily living, communication, and job-related skills.

SPEECH DISORDERS (DYSARTHRIA)

Trauma patients may demonstrate a slurred and distorted quality of speech due to weakness and incoordination of the oral musculature. This disorder, known as *dysarthria*, is a common seqeulae of traumatic injury due either to head injury or to damage to the oral or neck areas.

Management efforts should focus on retraining the vocal mechanism in the areas of articulation, voice, respiration, intensity, and rate. In extreme cases where patients have lost the ability to speak, the speech-language pathologist may train the patient to use an augmentative communication system (see Fig. 21.1). These efforts may be as fundamental as using an alphabet board or picture system to communicate basic needs. More sophisticated systems have been developed to utilize portable, miniature typewriters and computer-based and electronically scanned communication boards, activated by tread switches or "joysticks."

SWALLOWING DISORDERS (DYSPHAGIA)

Dysphagia, or disorders of swallowing, have presented a particularly troublesome management problem for professionals dealing with the trauma patient. Damage to the brain or oral/neck areas may make feeding a laborious, and often dangerous, process. In severe cases, deficits in swallowing may allow food or liquid to be aspirated into the patient's lungs, posing a high risk of aspiration pneumonia.

The speech-language pathologist will often be the team member to determine whether the patient can be fed safely by mouth or must be fed by an alternate, nonoral means (Fig. 21.2). If oral feeding is indicated, a determination should be made of appropriate positioning, feeding techniques, and diet texture to be used with the patient. Team management is essential in these cases. Physical and occupational therapists may designate proper positioning of the patient, self-feeding techniques, and utilization of assistive devices. Consultation with a nurse and a clinical dietitian is important in planning appropriate diet textures and insuring adequate nutritional intake.

In summary, speech-language pathologists assist in the management of trauma patients with deficits in speech, language, cognitive functioning, and swallowing. An interdisciplinary approach to rehabilitation of these patients is vital. Successful management hinges on communication among team members as well as a coordination of therapeutic tasks to facilitate patient recovery in a logical and functional manner.

Figure 21.1.

A. The examiner begins an oral examination as a basis to assess swallowing.

B. Palpation of the larynx is used to assess the extent and strength of laryngeal excursion.

C. The patient's swallowing ability for pureed foods is evaluated. Proper positioning for a safe swallow demands sitting at 90 degrees. However, this trauma patient has hip precautions, limiting elevation to 45 degrees only.

D. Small amounts of liquid (3 to 5 cc) are administered by a straw pipette.

E. Swallowing of thin liquid is assessed using a small amount of fruit juice (3 to 5 cc).

F. Family counseling and instruction is a necessary adjunct to therapy.

G. Techniques may be demonstrated to family members to be practiced during hospital visits and later at home.

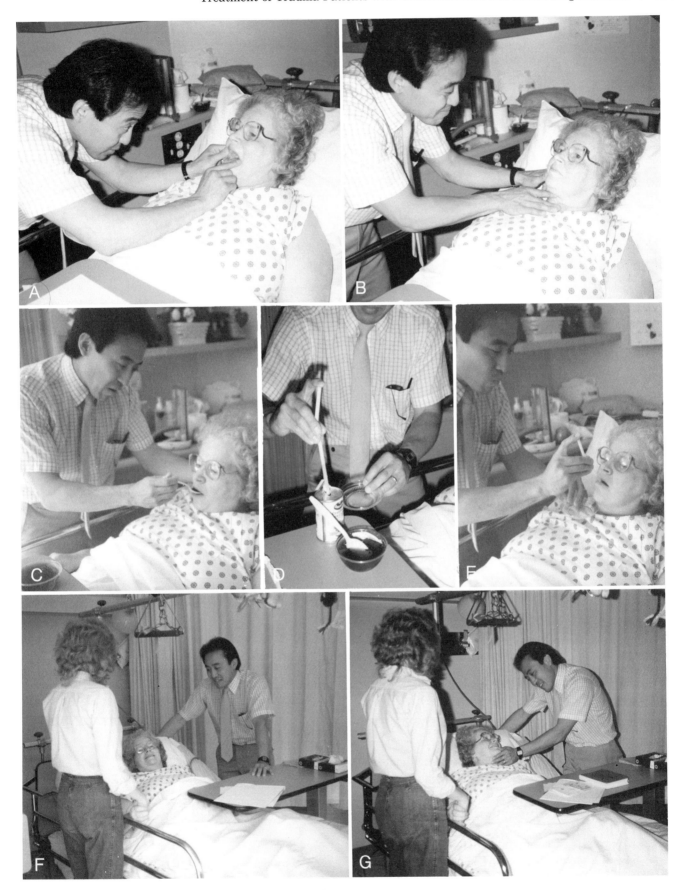

Figure 21.1.

Figure 21.2.

A. For articulation treatment for verbal apraxia, the clinician models a lip posture for the vowel /oo/.
B. The patient makes several attempts to approximate the sound.
C. The patient produces the correct lip movement for the sound.
D. The pathologist tests letter recognition.
E. Auditory comprehension may be tested by having the patient identify objects named by the examiner.
F. The clinician teaches word-retrieval strategies in a simple naming task.
G. A nonverbal patient learns to type messages with the Canon Communicator, a portable augmentative communications device.
H. Cognitive and perceptual retraining can be done with a standard personal computer system.
I. For this nonverbal patient, writing has become the primary means of communication.

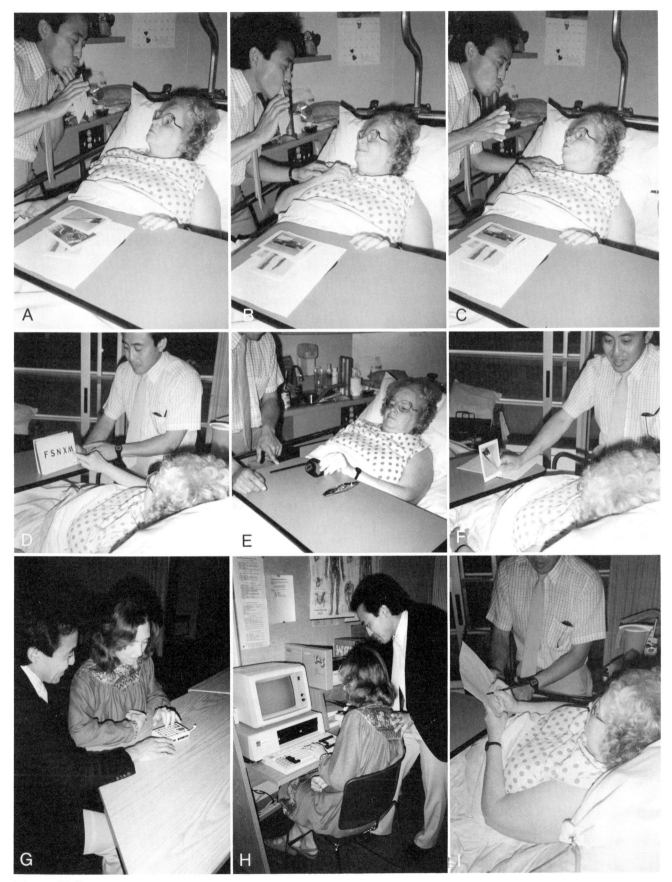

Figure 21.2.

22

Sports for the Disabled

Eckhart Reiner, M.D.

INTRODUCTION

Rehabilitation is a challenge not only for the patient, physician, psychologist, nurse, and therapist, but also for all unimpaired persons. For them, the challenge is to accept the disabled again as a full member of society. Sports constitute an ideal activity to serve as a bridge back to society, as they are an extremely important factor in social life, greatly influencing the thoughts and feelings of old and young persons throughout the world. Almost all aspects of human life can be influenced by sports activities.

DEVELOPMENT OF SPORTS FOR THE DISABLED

The development of sports for the disabled can be traced back to the beginning of the 20th century, although most of the growth and understanding of its therapeutic value has occurred since World War II. During that period, many persons disabled in war gathered to form sports groups. At that time, Sir Ludwig Gutmann initiated the development of wheelchair sports for paraplegics at the National Spinal Injured Center in Stoke Mandeville, England. Since 1948, international championships have taken place there every year. Over many years, rules and regulations for a number of individual kinds of sports were developed. Today, sports for spinal cord injured patients use the guidelines of the International Stoke Mandeville Games Federation (ISMGF) worldwide.

In addition to the ISMGF, which is responsible for paraplegics, two other organizations have been formed: the International Sports Association for the Disabled (ISOD) and the International Blind Sports Association (IBSA).

GOALS OF SPORTS FOR THE DISABLED

Treatment

Specific goals for sports in rehabilitation therapy vary with the kind of disability. For *amputees*; the emphasis is on strengthening stump muscles, exercises for balance, and training patients in the use of compensatory techniques for prosthetic replacements. For *paraplegics*; strengthening the muscles with preserved function and training balance and handling a wheelchair are the priorities. For *blind persons*, goals include training of orientation and compensatory senses to increase independence. Sports for the disabled constitute one of the most promising available therapeutic measures. The general aim of sports for all disabled persons is to activate available abilities, and to improve strength, endurance, and physical skills.

Integration

A goal of sports for the disabled is to promote positive development of the individual's personality structure by enhancing his or her self-image and self-confidence. Every success in sports, even those as small as mastering the correct pattern of a motion, creates the emotional experience of success. In addition, sports are of considerable sociological significance. Success in sports, small or big, may be associated with the approval of friends, which facilitates integration into society.

Preservation and Restoration of Physical Fitness

Sports are the best and most natural way for disabled persons to preserve or improve their physical ability through exercise. They present challenges for the disabled beyond those of daily life. Regular sports involvement preserves and improves general physical fitness.

Prevention

The following quote represents the feeling of many disabled patients:

I wish that all rehabilitation centers would make available to the patient the benefits of regular training and sport activities. Every disabled person should know, at the completion of his clinical treatment, that he can regain the full joy and happiness of his life only if he can prevent secondary effects of disability, especially the effects of immobility. My long experience in sports for the disabled made me convinced that active sports is the best prevention of secondary disabilities, along with medical measures and vocational rehabilitation (H. Hornof, personal communication).

KINDS OF SPORTS FOR THE DISABLED

Rehabilitation Sports

During rehabilitation therapy, the disabled person learns, perhaps for the first time, that sports can be adapted for his or her condition. He or she becomes familiar with the great variety of opportunities that exist for a disabled person to become engaged actively in sports. The therapist should evaluate and promote the interests and abilities of the individual to create a basis for further activity after discharge from the rehabilitation center.

Recreational and Fitness Sports

These include sports with regular teams or groups and the preparation for smaller competitions mainly of a social nature. The author's survey on the motivation for participation in sports for the disabled have indicated that the majority of the persons list "fellowship, team spirit, or being together with friends" as the principal reasons for their membership in a sports group.

Competitive Sports

To be effective in modern major sports competition requires knowledge of the entire field of present-day athletic training theory. Participation in international championships with disabled sportspersons from all over the world necessitates prolonged and intensive training (Fig. 22.1). Disabled sportspersons are competing for the honor of their nation in the Olympic Games as well as world and European championships.

CLASSIFICATION OF DISABILITIES

Disabled sportspersons do not want to be persons who "might have been." A matching or adjusting for disabilities must be possible. Therefore, various degrees of disabilities are classified in standardized groups.

Classifications for Blind Persons

B1 Completely blind
B2 Residual vision up to 3/60 (after best possible correction)

Classifications for Amputees

A1 Bilateral above-knee amputees
       Above-knee amputee on one side, below-knee on the other
A2 Unilateral above-knee amputees
A3 Bilateral below-knee amputees
A4 Unilateral below-knee amputees
A5 Bilateral above-elbow amputees
A6 Unilateral above-elbow amputees
A7 Bilateral below-elbow amputees
A8 Unilateral below-elbow amputees
A9 Combined upper/lower extremity amputees

Classifications for Paraplegics

There are six classifications of sports for paraplegics. They are listed according to the level of spinal cord injury.

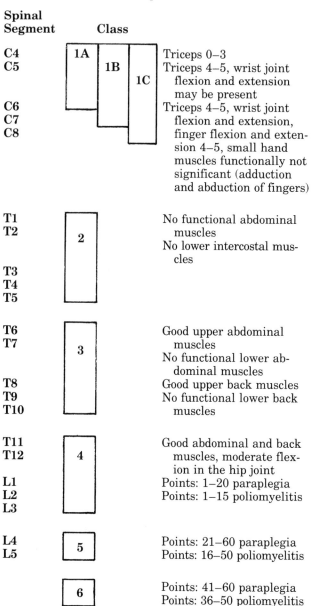

Spinal Segment	Class	
C4	1A	Triceps 0–3
C5	1B	Triceps 4–5, wrist joint flexion and extension may be present
	1C	
C6		Triceps 4–5, wrist joint flexion and extension, finger flexion and extension 4–5, small hand muscles functionally not significant (adduction and abduction of fingers)
C7		
C8		
T1	2	No functional abdominal muscles
T2		No lower intercostal muscles
T3		
T4		
T5		
T6	3	Good upper abdominal muscles
T7		No functional lower abdominal muscles
T8		Good upper back muscles
T9		No functional lower back muscles
T10		
T11	4	Good abdominal and back muscles, moderate flexion in the hip joint
T12		Points: 1–20 paraplegia
L1		Points: 1–15 poliomyelitis
L2		
L3		
L4	5	Points: 21–60 paraplegia
L5		Points: 16–50 poliomyelitis
	6	Points: 41–60 paraplegia
		Points: 36–50 poliomyelitis

BRANCHES OF SPORTS

Winter Sports

Winter sports for paraplegics include:

Cross-country skiing in the cross-country toboggan 2.5, 5, and 10 k
Ice-spiking: 100 , 500, 1000, and 1500 m

For amputees, winter sports are:

Cross-country skiing: 5, 10, and 15 k
Alpine skiing: slalom, giant slalom, and downhill racing (see Fig. 22.2)

Blind persons can participate in:

Cross-country skiing: 5, 10, and 20 k
Alpine skiing: slalom, giant slalom, and downhill racing

Summer Sports

Paraplegics participate in:

Track and field: discus, club, javelin, shot put
Wheelchair racing: 100, 200, 400, 800, 1500, and 5000 m
Wheelchair slalom, pentathalon
Archery: short metric round (30 and 50 m), advanced metric round (30, 50 and 70 m) and Fita-round (30, 50, 70 and 90 m)
Lawn-bowling: singles and doubles (similar to "boccia," with bowling balls having an eccentric center of gravity)

Amputees can enjoy:

Track and field: discus, javelin, shot put, high jump, long jump (standing start), long jump (running start) (see Fig. 22.3)
Running: 100, 400, and 1,500 m; race walking; 100 and 400 m (Class **A1**); wheelchair racing: 100 and 400 m (Class **A1**); Pentathalon
Archery: fita-round (Fig. 22.4)
Lawn-bowling: singles and doubles

Blind persons can participate in:

Track and field: discus, shot put, javelin, high jump (running start), high jump (standing start), long jump, triple jump (hop-step and jump)
Race walking: 3000 and 5000 m
Lawn-bowling: singles and doubles

Indoor Sports

For paraplegics, indoor sports include:

Shooting: Air rifle and air pistol
Fencing: Foil (single and team); épée (single and team); saber (single and team) (see Fig. 22.5)
Swimming: 25, 50, 75, 100, 200, and 400 m as well as 4 × 25 m and 4 × 50 m individual medleys in four strokes—breaststroke, backstroke, freestyle and butterfly (see Fig. 22.6)
Weightlifting: Bench press in various weight categories

Amputees participate in:

Shooting: air pistol
Swimming: same strokes and distances as paraplegics
Weightlifting: in various weight categories

Blind persons may enjoy:

Swimming: distances from 100 m and up as in the other classes of disabilities

Games

Paraplegics can participate in

Basketball
"Rebounding" ballgames (e.g., prellball)
Table tennis (singles and doubles team)

Amputees might enjoy:

"Sitting" ballgames (e.g., sitzball)
Volleyball (sitting and standing)
Table tennis (Fig. 22.7)

Blind persons can participate in:

Goal ballgames (e.g., torball)

ORGANIZATION OF SPORTS FOR THE DISABLED IN AUSTRIA

The organization of Sports for the Disabled in Austria is an example for combining all kinds of disabilities in one sports association. The following scheme of this organization (see Table 22.1) is worthy of use in other sports associations, as it coordinates all types of disabilities and all varieties of sports:

BOARD OF DIRECTORS OF THE AUSTRIAN ASSOCIATION FOR DISABLED SPORTS (ÖVSV)
Directorate of the Association of Spinal Cord Injured in Austria
Austrian Skiing Association Department for Disabled Sports

SPORTS COMMISSION OF THE ÖVSV (Federal)
Chief coach and managers for each of the following types of sports:
Track and field
Swimming
Skiing
Ballgames
Sports for the blind
Sports for the paralyzed

STATE ASSOCIATIONS OF THE ÖVSV
Exercise groups, sports clubs, sections, suboffices of the Association of the Spinal Cord Injured of Austria (VdQuÖ), game partnerships.

Figure 22.1.

A–B. Wheelchair skill riding training is done in the gymnasium and
C–D. On the track (for practice and training).
E–F. Wheelchair racing is popular in competitive sports.

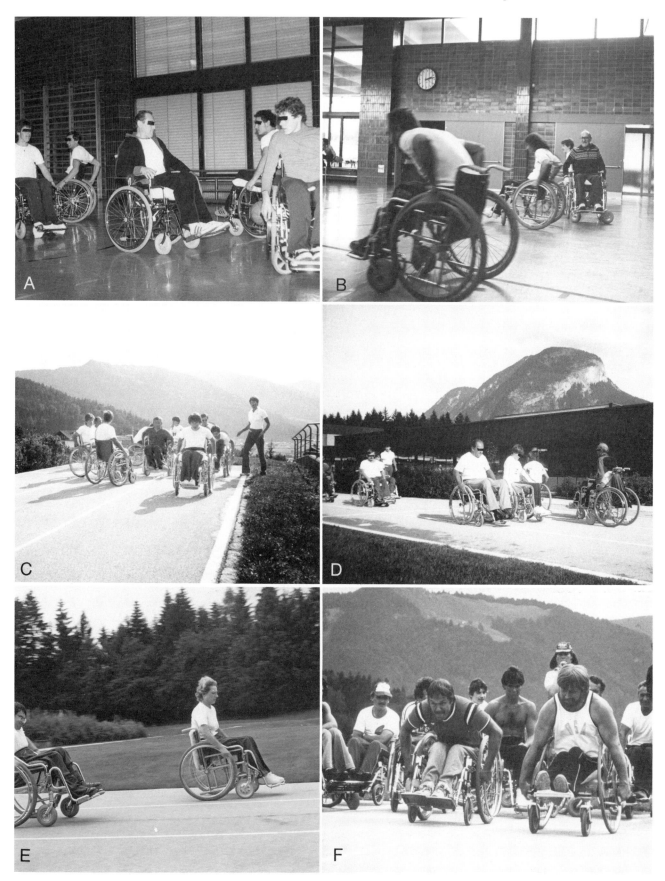

Figure 22.1.

Figure 22.2.

A–C. Amputees compete in ski gymnastics (after dry training).

D–E. Below-knee amputees compete in Alpine free skiing, and

F. Above-knee amputees in downhill ski racing.

G. Special sports equipment is necessary for ice spiking, and

H–I. An Alpine toboggan for paraplegics.

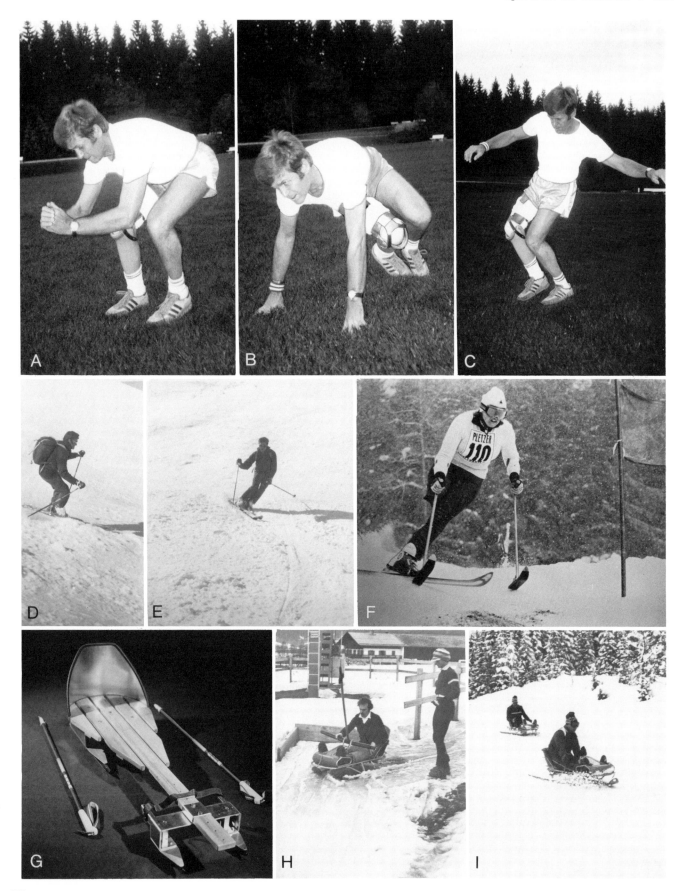

Figure 22.2.

Figure 22.3.

    A. Amputees compete in discus throwing.
    B. Race walking
    C. Running
D–E. Long jump (with a standing start),
    F. High jump, and
G–H. Shot putting.

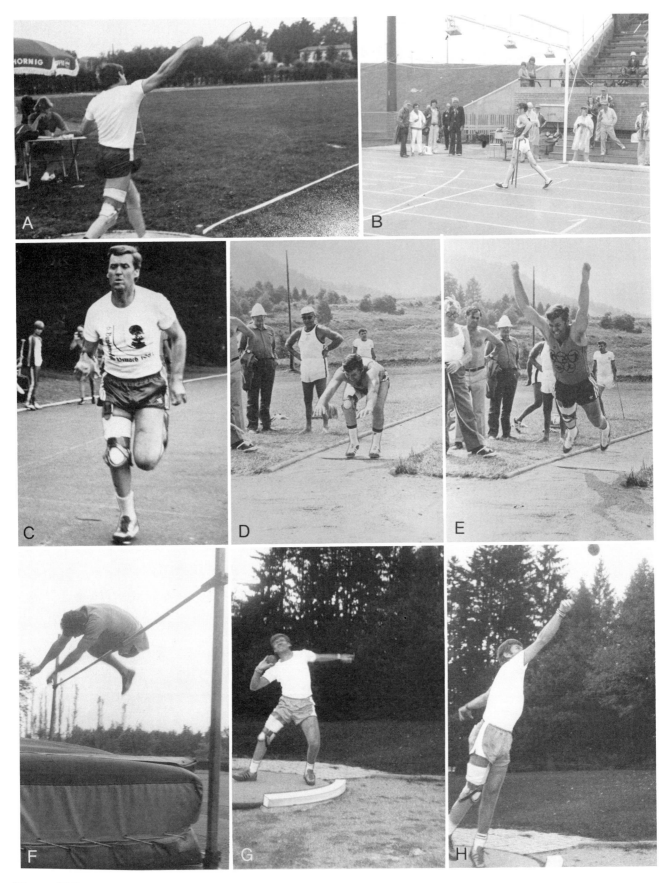

Figure 22.3.

Figure 22.4.

A–B. Archery: tetraplegic patient in action is shown.

C–E. Assistive devices in archery for both hands of a tetraplegic patient are shown.

F. Pronation of the hand trips the holding mechanism, and the arrow is released.

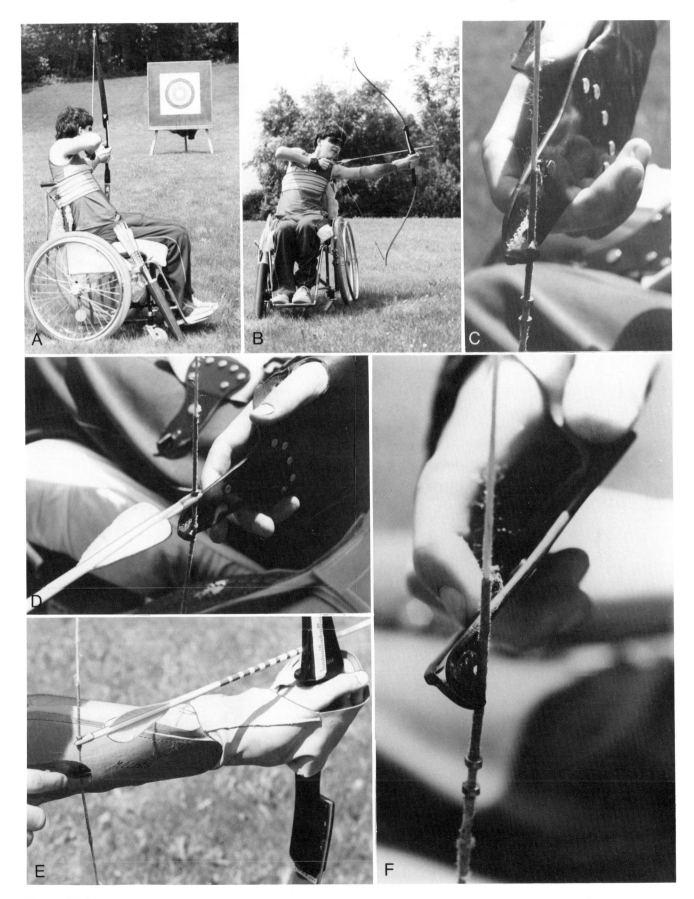

Figure 22.4.

Figure 22.5.

A–B. Club throwing is done by tetraplegics, and

C–D. Javelin throwing of paraplegics.

E–F. Paraplegics also participate in discus throwing

G–H. Shot putting, and

    I. Fencing.

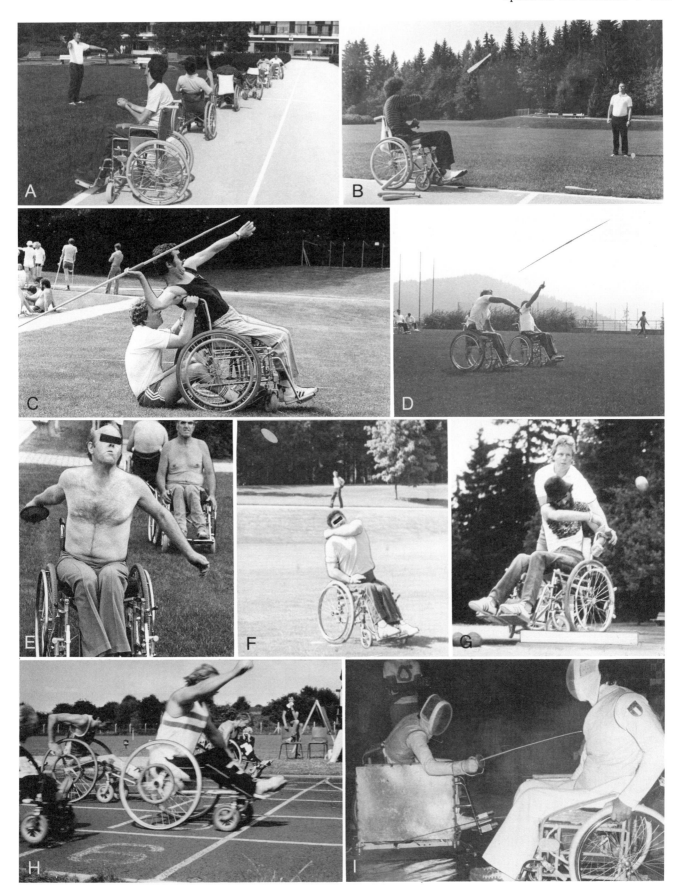

Figure 22.5.

Figure 22.6.

A–C. Paraplegics compete in swimming.
D–J. Amputees compete in swimming.

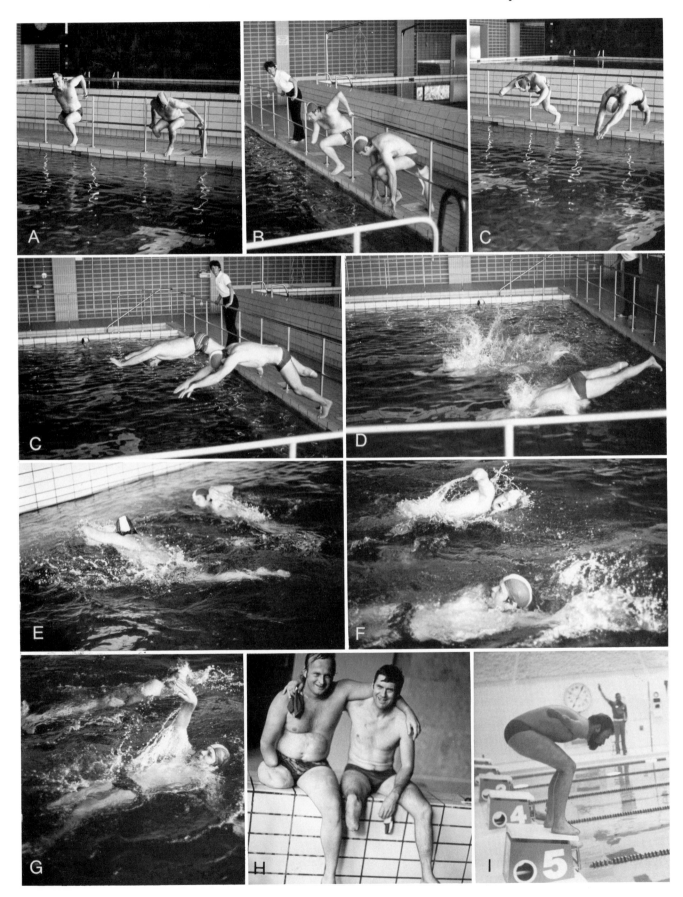

Figure 22.6.

Figure 22.7.

A–B. Volleyball of arm amputees is done using a light-weight beachball.
   C. Amputees also participate in basketball.
D–E. Sitzball, and
F–H. Tennis.

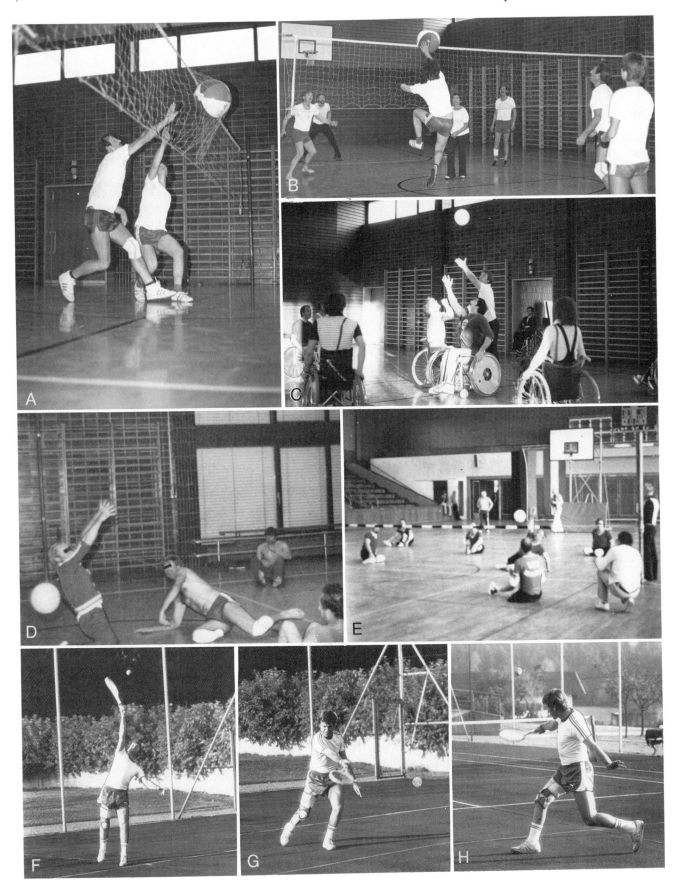

Figure 22.7.

23

Sports Prosthetics

Joseph Zettl, C.P.O.

Many sports activities can be performed without the aid of a prosthesis. Examples of these sports are swimming, scuba diving, snorkeling, kayaking, snow skiing, skydiving, and parachuting. Some exceptional adolescents with high-level amputations, such as short above-knee and hip disarticulations, are effectively participating in ping-pong, badminton, racquetball, tennis, baseball, basketball, football, and horseback riding without a prosthesis. An amputee soccer team in Seattle, Washington, plays regularly without their prostheses, just using crutches.

However, most amputees prefer to perform in these sports with their prostheses if at all possible and can extend their activities to include hiking, jogging, sprinting, hunting, golfing, cycling, mountain climbing, rope jumping, and snow skiing (Fig. 23.1).

The more advanced sport enthusiasts, or those seeking the ultimate in performance and achievement, seek the aid of specialized prostheses. Specially fitted and aligned prostheses have been designed for such activities as ice skating, snow skiing, water-skiing, running, and jumping sports.

To enhance these high performance prostheses and to achieve exceptional performances, the Seattle foot was developed (Fig. 23.2). The principal advantage of the Seattle foot over conventional types is that it stores gravitational energy in midstance, which is released in the toe-off phase of gait. This action aids in running and jumping activities and improves the performance level of the amputee, including the comfort level of the residual limb. Other specialized limbs are waterproofed and are fabricated for taking showers, swimming, launching a boat, or fishing—activities that require submerging the prosthesis for prolonged periods in water. Some peglegs or rockerbottom pylon prostheses are preferred by hunters or hikers who encounter muddy terrain and who prefer this prosthetic adaptation over conventional prostheses.

Figure 23.1.

A. A below-knee amputee runs the 100-yard dash.

B. A hiker has below-knee endoskeletal prosthesis.

C. A jogger is a below-knee amputee.

D. A golfer is an above-knee amputee.

E. A racquetball player is a below-knee amputee with an endoskeletal prosthesis.

F. A skydiver amputee wears a stump protector.

G. A downhill skier is an above-knee amputee and wears a stump protector.

H. Snorkeling is done by a person with a hip disarticulation.

I. A cyclist is a below-knee amputee.

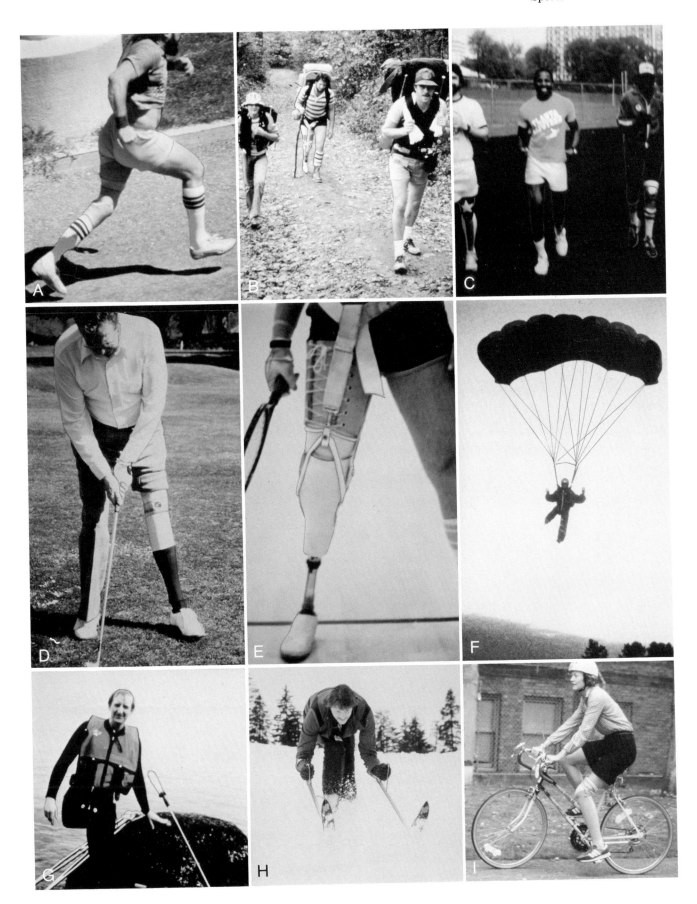

Figure 23.1.

Figure 23.2.

A–B. A below-knee amputee swims, wearing a patellar tendon-bearing (PTB) sports prosthesis.

    C. An above-knee amputee swims, wearing a prosthesis.

    D. This Seattle foot is an improved model.

    E. This 1984 Seattle foot model has a cosmetic finish.

    F. An above-knee amputee uses another type of swim prosthesis.

    G. An above-knee amputee uses a prosthesis for sports, hunting, and farming.

    H. A rockerbottom below-knee prosthesis is used for taking a shower.

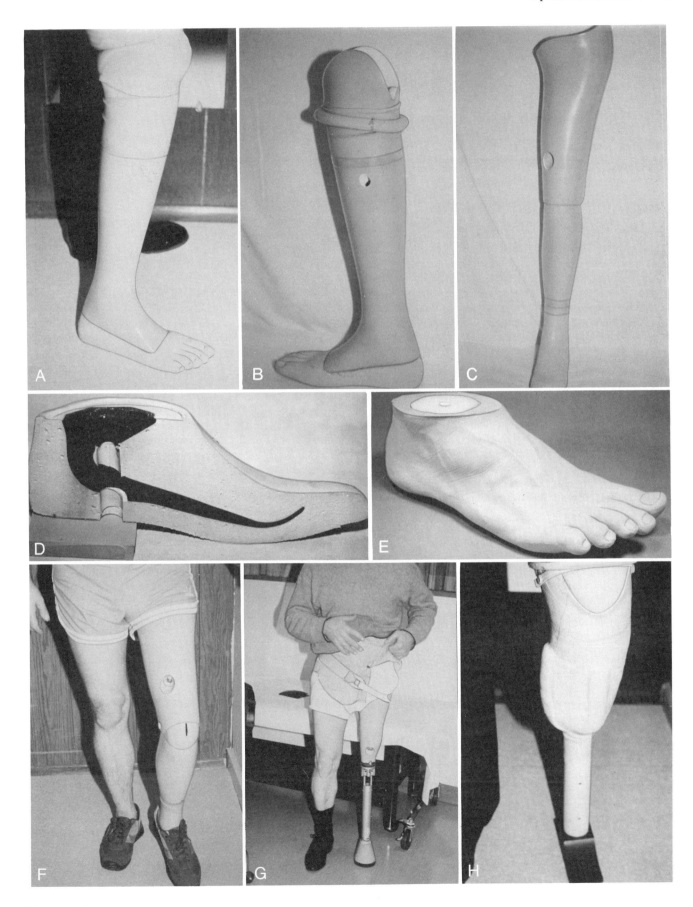

Figure 23.2

24

Vocational Rehabilitation

Philip S. King, M.D.

For the disabled individual who is younger than the accepted retirement age, vocational rehabilitation considerations must be assigned a very high priority. For some, remunerative employment will be an economic necessity to supply basic needs for himself or herself and dependents; but for almost all, it can be of tremendous psychological and social value, enhancing self-esteem and satisfaction with life; providing important experiences, contacts, and activities; and establishing a generally more satisfactory status in society.

The vocational rehabilitation counselor is of great importance in helping the patient achieve optimal goals in this area and should play an active part in the team process from an early phase of the management. The counselor's evaluation requires detailed knowledge of: the patient's prior education, skills, work experience, and avocations; the effect of the functional impairment on ability to perform previous or related types of work; other types of employment that are compatible with existing qualifications and limitations; the client's interest; and attitudes toward future training and employment. This must include very detailed information in such areas as sitting and standing tolerance, ambulation and/or transfer abilities; ability to lift, reach and manipulate objects; and any special environmental needs. Extensive formal psychometric, neuropsychological, interest, aptitude, personality, and skill testing are often important. The counselor then must correlate these data for the client with a deep professional background of knowledge in such areas as qualifications for specific jobs, current availability of job openings, utilization of services from available government agencies and organizations, accessibility and facilities in various employment and training sites, and many similar fields.

From this complex base of information, the counselor should work with the client in the development of a plan designed to lead toward optimal employment. For some, the plan can be as simple as improving accessibility to the previous workplace, or of devising adaptive techniques or equipment for the old job. Frequently, however, more complex plans are necessary. Sometimes the counselor's role must include facilitating changes in attitude and expectations of employer, client, and others. The employer may regard the impairment as a greater handicap, the prognosis worse, or the client's needs more demanding than is actually the case. The patient may need to accept undesired limitations or changes in employment. Often, evaluation is required while actually performing tasks in the work environment. Sometimes a period of formal training is required, either in an academic or vocational setting; and, in the case of younger clients, a relatively longer educational program may be well justified. For some patients, a sheltered workshop or similar supportive environment is necessary, at least initially. Final achievement of the vocational goal occurs with actual job placement and adequate follow-up to ensure mutual satisfaction of client and employer.

25

Wheelchairs

Richard Altenberger, P.T.

The problem of selecting and prescribing a wheelchair is well expressed in a remark made by a wheelchair patient: "A wheelchair must be adapted to a handicap in a way which does not add to the handicap."

The prescription for the wheelchair, which is usually made at about the midpoint of the initial rehabilitation hospitalization, must be accomplished by experienced members of the team. Various types of wheelchairs are available and must be utilized according to the disability and specific needs of the individual patient.

The progressive popularity of athletics for the disabled has produced great advances in the wheelchair industry. Various modifications of operation and seat positions were first used by handicapped athletes before they were implemented by the wheelchair industry.

There are six components of a wheelchair: (*a*) driving wheels, (*b*) swiveled casters, (*c*) seat, (*d*) back support, (*e*) legrests, and (*f*) armrests. All of these components must be combined in the most effective way to compensate for the physical handicap.

CHOOSING THE RIGHT WHEELCHAIR

The choice of the right wheelchair depends on the patient's handicap. Various indications for wheelchairs may be identified. For example, an amputee needs a different wheelchair from a paraplegic. Another consideration should be the physical requirements of a handicapped person. These requirements must be taken into account on an individual basis. One paralyzed patient is not like all other paralyzed patients. The size of the patient, extent of his or her lesions, and the patient's life-style are all variable and must be considered in selecting features for the wheelchair.

For Amputees

Amputee wheelchairs are available from various manufacturers. Amputees usually do not use the wheelchair the entire day but only periodically. The shift of the patient's center of gravity toward the back of the chair requires shift of the axle for stability on hills and ramps.

For Paraplegics

Most paraplegic patients rely on the wheelchair as their only means of locomotion. Therefore, the paraplegic's wheelchair must be adapted to the person's disability.

Driving Wheels

The type of wheel chosen should allow the patient to advance as quickly and as easily as possible. Driving wheels are available with or without hand rim projections. Wheels with projections usually are employed only with very high cervical lesions (above C6) or in other conditions with marked impairment of grasp.

Steering Casters

The casters give the wheelchair its maneuverability and allow change of direction, which is transmitted from the propulsion of the wheels. The choice of casters is limited.

Seat

The seat must be large enough so that no part of the body is cramped. However, a wide seat necessitates a broad wheelchair. Wheelchairs should be no wider than necessary, to facilitate passage through narrow doors, between pieces of furniture, etc.

Back Height

The height of the back must provide adequate trunk support yet permit all possible mobility of the upper extremities. The average appropriate height of the back is 36 cm, but should be varied with patient size and trunk stability.

Legrests/Foot Supports

These are available in various different forms. They must be adjustable to the patient's leg length, and any cushions that are added must be properly aligned to distribute pressures optimally and to provide comfort. Elevating legrests are also available and are prescribed for patients with dependent edema or other conditions requiring elevation of lower extremities.

Armrests

The armrests serve as lateral support to prevent slipping from the seat, but they must not impede arm motion during propulsion.

TYPES OF WHEELCHAIRS

Electric Wheelchair

The electric wheelchair should only be prescribed if a valid indication exists as in, for example, severe functional loss of the upper extremities. In any case, care must be taken to prevent weakening or loss of function by the use of an electric wheelchair.

In the prescription of an electric wheelchair, residual function must be taken into consideration for control. The wheelchair can be adapted for control by hand, head, or other movement (Fig. 25.1).

Manual Wheelchair

This is the type of wheelchair most frequently prescribed. There are two types of manual wheelchairs: (a) the "active" wheelchair, and (b) the universal wheelchair. The active wheelchair is especially suitable as a first wheelchair, as it is easy to handle and can be used for sport and everyday activities by both amputees and spinal cord injured patients; it meets all requirements of a good, all-purpose wheelchair.

Universal wheelchairs (Fig. 25.2) include the light-weight wheelchair, and they also are used frequently. For this type of wheelchair, a great variety of exchangeable components is available that allows individual adaptation to the patient's requirements.

Shower and Toilet Wheelchairs

If a wheelchair is necessary for these special activities of everyday life, it is sensible to prescribe such a wheelchair (Fig. 25.3). Yet, if possible, the patient should not depend on such aids, but learn to use usual installations.

Figure 25.1.

    A. Truss pads for trunk correction.

B–E. There are various types of electric wheelchairs.

    F. A stairlift may be necessary.

G–I. The universal amputee wheelchair is operated manually.

J–L. The active wheelchair has different axle settings.

M–N. Universal wheelchairs can also be used by children.

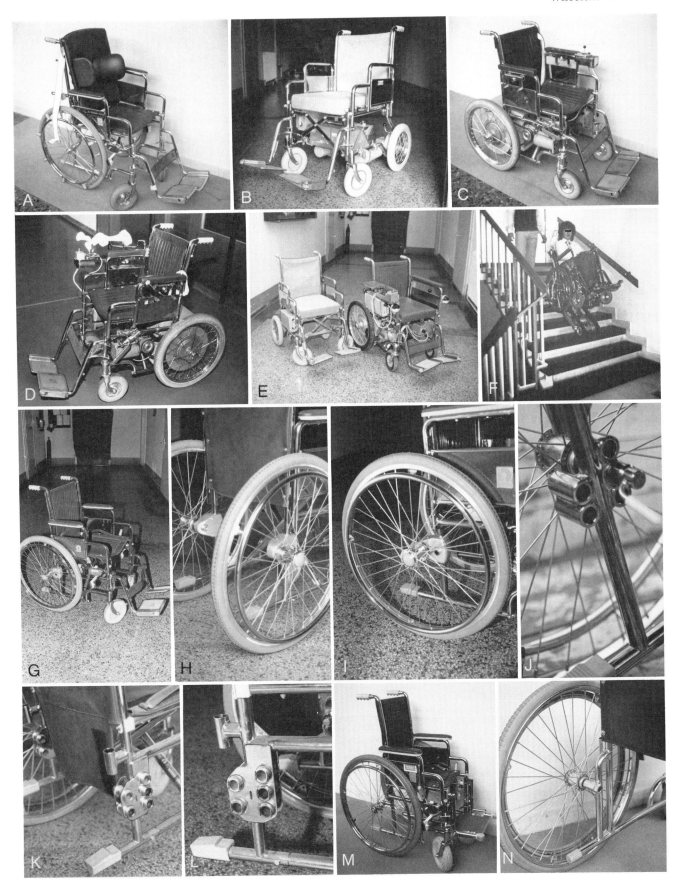

Figure 25.1.

Figure 25.2.

    A. The universal wheelchair has adjustable legrests.

B–E. Wheelchairs can be constructed for one-hand operation.

    F. Types of wheelchairs include lift-up,

G–K. Active, and

    L. Racing wheelchairs.

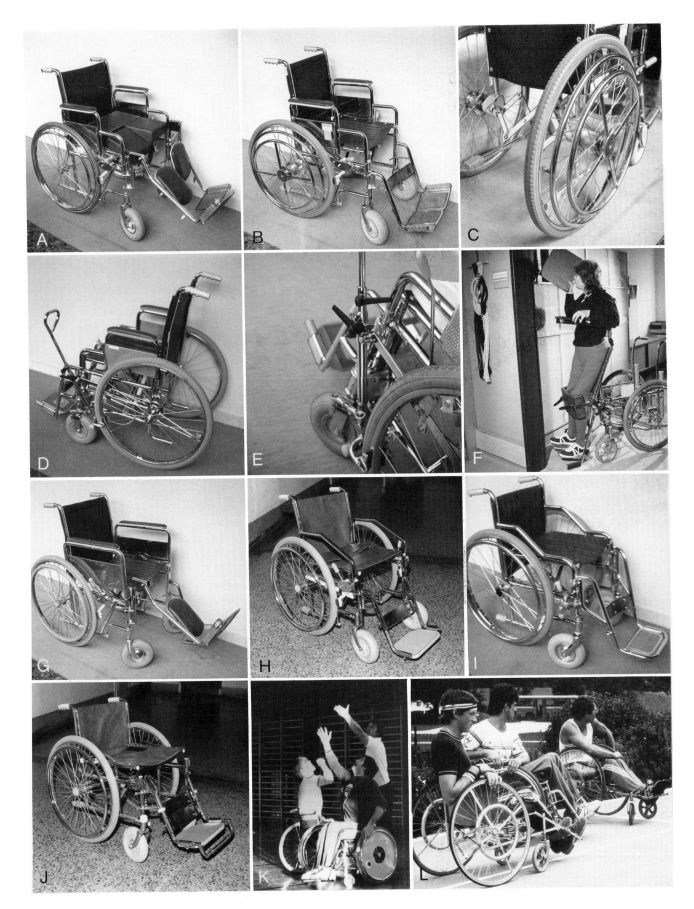

Figure 25.2.

Figure 25.3.

A–B. The shower wheelchair is one type of manual wheelchair.

C–F. Special shower or toilet seat which can be lifted with the patient with a lift from a wheelchair frame and placed on a caster frame. The caster frame can be pushed into a shower or over a toilet bowl.

G. Universal wheelchair with pneumatic wheels and casters.

H. Universal wheelchair with rubber wheels and rim projections.

I. Universal wheelchair with pneumatic wheels, rim projections, and a reclining extended backrest.

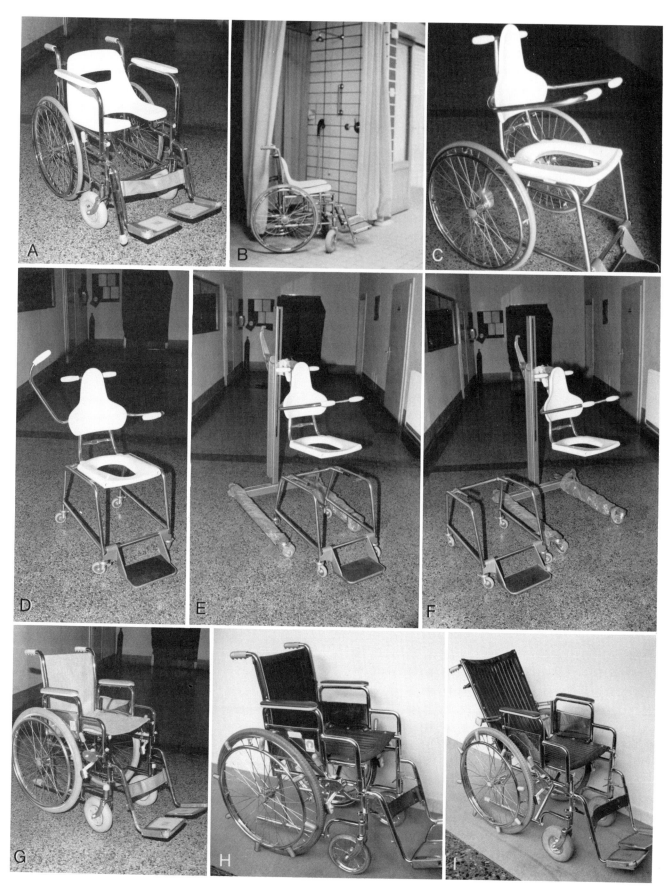

Figure 25.3.

SECTION
4

REHABILITATION OF SPECIFIC DISEASES

26

Amputations

Bernd Schwaiger, M.D., and John J. Gerhardt, M.D.

INTRODUCTION

Amputation of an extremity produces substantial losses for the patient in not only motor function, which results in the impairment of balance, and sensory feedback, the extent of which varies with the level of amputation (complicating the ability to acquire skills necessary to use functional substitutes, i.e., prosthetic training), but also cosmetic impairment. This chapter discusses various amputation levels as they relate to five topics: (a) surgery, (b) physical and occupational therapy, (c) prosthetic fittings, (d) social work, and (e) special considerations in children.

GENERAL DISCUSSION OF THE FIVE TOPICS

Regardless of the indication for the amputation, the operative shaping of the stump, or *surgery*, should always be performed under the supervision of an experienced surgeon. Knowledge and experience in the area of prostheses and their fitting are also important for optimal results.

In traumatology, amputation techniques and levels are largely determined by the condition of the soft tissues, particularly with regard to circulatory capabilities. Generalized procedures for amputation are obsolete, and each case must be individualized. Optimal functional length of the residual limb should be preserved in adults. The prospect of good prosthetic and overall function and cosmesis, rather than only maximum length of the residual limb, must be considered.

Physical therapy should include, as early as possible, postoperative breathing exercises, general flexibility and strengthening exercises, and exercises for the residual limb. Mobilization of the patient and gait training follow, utilizing any ambulation aids that are necessary. *Occupational therapy* activities for the amputee should include upper extremity prosthetic training, functional exercises after finger amputations, training in activities of daily living and homemaking, and prevocational evaluation and vocational retraining as indicated.

For *prosthetic fittings*, the prescription usually is prepared by a prosthetic team, including an orthopaedist, physiatrist, physical or occupational therapist, and prosthetist.

Preliminary planning for all necessary *social work* measures should start early. These include socioeco-nomic assessment; evaluation of the home, family status, and resources; and vocational planning. A team approach is important. Vocational guidance, including testing and consultation by a psychologist, is often necessary. Assistance is given in any necessary modification of home or workplace, in obtaining self-help or adaptive devices, and in automobile modification (e.g., hand controls and lifts).

Special considerations in children are necessary because only 10 to 15% of all amputations in the adult population are traumatic, whereas 75 to 80% of all amputations in children are caused by trauma. The psychological and physical problems after amputations can be overcome relatively rapidly by children when instruction and guidance of the parents and a good home environment are provided.

In general, children learn the use of prostheses easily. Wound healing complications are rare. Basic problems after amputations in children arise from disturbances of bone growth, i.e., differences in the growth potentials of proximal and distal epiphysis of the long bones. Another problem arises from the bony overgrowth of diaphyseal amputations with tapered distal ends.

There are five general maxims to follow when dealing with amputations in children:

1. Preserve the maximum possible length of residual limb in primary operation.
2. Preserve the epiphysis whenever possible, with consideration of disarticulation, if no fragment distal to the joint can be preserved.
3. Apply immediate postsurgical prosthetic fitting whenever possible.
4. Provide meticulous follow-up (with frequent checks of residual limb and prosthetic fitting).
5. Instruct and counsel parents.

Figure 26.1 shows the remaining growth in the normal distal femoral and proximal tibial epiphyses as a function of bone age in (a) girls and (b) boys (Anderson, Green, Messner: *J. Bone Jt. Surg.* 45-A). Relative contributions of osseous epiphyses to total limb growth are shown.

LOWER EXTREMITY AMPUTATIONS

Amputations of Toes

Surgery: Plantar flap: Disarticulation of the metatarsophalangeal joint except for the great toe, where proximal phalanx stump should remain. No resection of subchondral bone should be done to avoid hematoma formation, and no shaping of articular cartilage is necessary.

Physical and Occupational Theapy: Use general postoperative measures.

Prosthetic Fitting: An arch support with filler should be used.

Amputations of Metatarsal Region

Surgery: In amputations of the first through fifth rays, preservation of the general foot configuration should be tried. In transverse transmetatarsal amputations, plantar convex rounding of metatarsals is necessary (Fig. 26.2). No significant functional imbalance is to be expected.

Physical Therapy: Prophylaxis against equinus position. General measures should be taken.

Prosthetic Fitting: Shoes with long steel shank, molded supports and filler are necessary.

Special Considerations in Children: Tapering of distal ends of amputated metatarsals during growth leads to pressure problems, including "mal perforant du pied." Therefore, in children, the primary amputation is done at the diaphyseal-metaphyseal junction (transmetatarsal amputation by the technique of Sharp-Jäger-Bona).

Lisfranc's Amputations

Surgery: Muscular imbalance occurs with this amputation mainly because of the loss of the tendon insertions at the bases of metatarsals I–V. With suitable local conditions, transosseous reinsertion or suturing to the plantar fascia is recommended. Appropriate surgical technique and postoperative treatment usually produce a well-balanced functional stump with good active flexibility of the ankle joint.

Physical and Occupational Therapy: Passive and active prophylaxis should be used against equinus position along with general measures.

Prosthetic Fitting: For good functional stumps, only a high top shoe with insert and filler is needed.

Chopart's Amputations

Surgery: Without appropriate preventive measures, the muscular imbalance created by this amputation leads inevitably to equinovarus deformity. If the local situation is appropriate, functional stumps without defective position can be achieved by Marquardt's tenomyoplasty. In the case of major problems at the end of the stump due to imbalance of trophic disturbances (Fig. 26.3), secondary operations are often necessary. These operations include Pirogow-modifications of Spitzy or Günther (talus resection, tibiocalcaneal arthrodesis with horizontal (calcaneal angle 0 degrees), according to Günther, and physiologic calcaneal angle of 25 degrees, according to Spitzy.)

Physical and Occupational Therapy: The rare cases of a balanced Chopart's stump can be fitted with shoes. In the case of deformities or problems with the end of the stump, prosthesis with patellar tendon weightbearing can be used. The same is true for other amputations in this area.

Social Work: In all amputations in the foot region, only patients engaged in certain occupations require special measures, such as vocational retraining.

Special Considerations in Children: Arthrodesis of tarsal bones is only indicated if this can avoid higher amputations.

Syme's Amputation

Surgery: This is the lowest possible below-knee amputation, immediately above the distal articular surface of the tibia with resection of the malleoli (Fig. 26.4). A good functional stump can be obtained if there is good skin coverage. Good hemostasis and satisfactory drainage to avoid hematoma are necessary. Cosmesis is only fair, and this may be objectionable in the female patient. Caution: injury to the tibial artery is a possibility.

Special Considerations in Children: A good functional level is possible if epiphyses are preserved.

Diaphyseal Below-Knee Amputation

Surgery: In the extremely distal-diaphyseal region, frequent problems are encountered with soft tissue coverage and skin breakdown. Further proximally, myoplastic amputation (see Figs. 26.5 and 26.6) is possible and preferable. One advantage of the long below-knee stump is that there is a large area for the distribution of weight bearing pressure and good lever arm. A good range of motion with full-knee extension is necessary, however. For amputations proximal to the distal third of the tibia, Dederich's (von Ertl's) techniques are recommended; for amputations through the proximal half of the shaft, myoplastic surgery (Weiss, Burgess, Dederich, and others) is recommended.

In short stumps, abduction of the fibula may be a problem. In the case where this results in pressure problems, stump revision with resection of the entire fibula should be considered.

The highest possible below-knee amputation level with a functional stump can be obtained by preservation of the tibial tubercle and, if necessary, reinsertion and fixation of the ischiocrural flexor muscles (hamstrings).

Even with a short below-knee stump, a knee joint with active motion is a functional advantage to the patient. All possible attempts to preserve the knee joint, therefore, are absolutely justified; in the case of skin problems, secondary full thickness skin graft is possible (e.g., with neurovascular pedicle flaps). Even if failure should occur and secondary reamputation at the knee level becomes necessary, the functional result is as good as with a primary higher amputation.

Physical and Occupational Therapy: Following all conventional below-knee amputations, bandaging of stumps, for shaping and shrinking, is necessary along with exercises for the knee joint and for flexibility and strengthening of the thigh and arm muscles (especially triceps and shoulder depressors for crutch walking and limiting weight bearing on the stump). Immediate postoperative rigid dressing and prosthetic fitting is preferable to any other method (see Gerhardt et al., 1982).

Prosthetic Fitting: Below-knee prostheses, including ankle-foot components, are chosen according to level of amputation, shape and condition of stump as well as functional considerations. They are described in Chapter 13.

Social Work: If knee function is preserved, the below-knee amputee does not need special controls to operate a motor vehicle. However, it should be reported to the local division of motor vehicles. Other social work measures depend on the individual case.

Special Considerations in Children: As with upper arm amputations, there is a danger of skin perforation due to bone overgrowth and distal spike formation. Revisions may become necessary, and parents should be informed early of this possibility. For long and medium below-knee stumps, Dederich's bridging technique may be used.

In higher level below-knee amputations, caution is indicated in regard to stump revisions, as each produces at least 1.5 to 2 cm of additional bone shortening.

A secondary bridging, by Dederich's method, can be attempted, even after further bone overgrowth. Creation of a myoplastic stump should always be attempted.

Knee Disarticulation

Surgery: This is a good amputation level, and in certain cases better than above-knee amputation (see Fig. 26.7), especially in the geriatric amputee with fair general condition. Knee disarticulation allows quick and least traumatic surgery and wound healing.

Other advantages include: full endbearing capacity without ischial seat, good muscular control through preservation of the muscular insertions, no opening of subchrondral bone, and therefore diminished danger of hematoma formation and good wound healing. The patella is positioned at the level of the corresponding articular surface of the femur. Kirschner wire fixation of the patella at the distal end of the femur is not recommended. Optimal position of the postsurgical scar is achieved by placement somewhat posteriorly between the femoral condyles, but atypical flaps are also acceptable to avoid above-knee amputation.

Physical and Occupational Therapy: Hip and joint mobility should be achieved by following the same general measures as in below-knee amputees.

Prosthetic Fitting: Apart from minor cosmetic considerations, there are no special problems. The mechanical knee joint is usually a four-bar linkage joint, with the pivot center outside the construction. The thigh is slightly longer and the leg is slightly shorter than the remaining limb, which is most apparent in the sitting position.

Special Considerations in Children: As in adults, knee disarticulation is preferable to any higher amputation. In spite of the preservation of epiphyses, there usually is moderate impairment of growth, which can be advantageous as it allows better accommodation of the mechanical knee joint later.

Callander Amputation

Surgery: Metaphyseal amputations through the femur have become obsolete. Knee disarticulations and diaphyseal amputations are used.

Diaphyseal Above-Knee Amputation

Surgery: With higher amputation levels, increasing muscular imbalance favoring the iliopsoas muscle is present. Hip flexors and gluteus medius and minimus muscles (abductors) cause additional imbalance deformity. Muscle stabilization by myoplasty and myodesis or myopexy of at least one muscle group (using the methods of Dederich, Burgess, or Murdoch) is absolutely necessary to prevent migration of the femur and complications. Rigid dressing with new simplified suspension, using the method of Zettl, and immediate prosthetic fitting are always desirable.

Physical and Occupational Therapy: Correct bandaging of the stump, stump exercises, correct positioning, general conditioning, and gait training are necessary.

Prosthetic Fitting: Quadrilateral socket with an ischial seat is often used. Recently newer socket designs evolved, such as the ISNY (Islandic-New York) and CAT-CAM (Contoured Adducted Trochanteric-Controlled Alignment Method). The type of suspension, knee joint, and foot components are determined by consideration of age, general condition, vocation, climate, and family home environment of the patient.

Special Considerations in Children: Like all diaphyseal stumps in children, early overgrowth with spiking tendency is present, but usually there is no danger of perforation. There is impaired growth of the bony stump relative to the soft tissues. Surgical revisions are common. Immediate postsurgical prosthetic fitting should be applied.

Hip Disarticulations

Surgery: These rarely are performed in trauma patients. In such cases, the femoral head is often left in the acetabulum.

Prosthetic Fitting: Hip disarticulation prosthesis is used.

UPPER EXTREMITY AMPUTATIONS

Amputations of Fingers

Surgery: Extensive description of the primary surgical technique and surgical reconstruction can be found in the literature of traumatology and hand surgery. Measures for prevention of Sudeck's dystrophy should be observed. Predisposing factors often include inadequate primary care, faulty cast (too tight, too loose), insufficient fixation, and lack of motion of uninvolved joints and muscles.

Physical and Occupational Therapy: Range of motion exercises, grasping, prehension exercises, and stump conditioning are all necessary.

Prosthetic Fitting: Occasionally, a cosmetic glove is used.

Amputations in the Metacarpal and Carpal Region

Surgery: If the wrist joint function and the soft tissue coverage are good, the primary operation produces functional stumps (Fig. 26.8). After transverse amputation in the distal metacarpal region, the secondary formation of an active cleft hand is possible.

Prosthetic Fitting: A cosmetic glove is used and, at times, an open-end work prosthesis is attached by a quick disconnect mechanism.

Physical and Occupational Therapy: Therapy should start as early as possible according to the instructions of the hand surgeon.

Social Work: Early socioeconomic assessment and follow-up should be made according to individual needs.

Wrist Joint Disarticulations

Surgery: Amputation level is good; adequate soft tissue coverage can be achieved by partial resection of the styloid process. Pronation and supination remain largely unaffected (Fig. 26.8). This procedure is not recommended if myoelectric prosthesis is being considered because it results in excessive length of the forearm/hand.

Physical and Occupational Therapy: Range of motion exercises of elbows and shoulders should be done. Forearm pronation and supination can also be done as soon as permitted.

Prosthetic Fitting: Fitting with almost any kind of prosthesis is possible. Moderate lengthening of the extremity as compared to the remaining extremity may occur because of needed space for prosthetic components.

Special Considerations in Children: This is a favorable amputation level because the epiphyses are preserved. Moderate growth impairment on the amputated side helps to compensate later for the necessary excessive prosthetic length (similar to elbow and knee disarticulations). An immediate postoperative prosthetic fitting should be applied to prevent rejection of prosthetic devices by the child.

Diaphyseal Below-Elbow Amputations

Surgery: With a progressively proximal level of amputation, the active ability for pronation and supination is reduced, but soft tissue coverage is more easily obtained.

The shortest possible *functional* below-elbow stump requires preservation of the insertion of the biceps tendon on the radius (see Fig. 26.8). However, a shorter residual forearm with the elbow fused in moderate to 90 degree flexion can lead to a functional result if soft tissue coverage is adequate. (Suspension of the prosthesis is the same as with angulation osteotomy and provides good control.)

Krukenberg's operation surgically separates the two forearm bones. Active motion of the two segments is provided by separation of the forearm musculature, which produces an excellent functional organ, but cosmesis is objectionable to some. Those who have this procedure like it very much because of good function and *preserved sensation.* A prosthesis with a cosmetic hand can also be worn. The ideal indication is blindness in a person without hands or one hand. In bilateral amputees, this type of surgery is usually done on one side.

Physical and Occupational Therapy: Therapy should be started as soon as possible, at first with passive, and later with active, forearm rotation and elbow exercises and also shoulder ranging. After the Krukenberg's operation, therapy should be given according to the specific instructions of the surgeon.

Prosthetic Fitting: Only with extremely long below-elbow stumps can an elbow unit be omitted, similar to the prosthetic fitting of the wrist joint disarticulations.

Social Work: As with all previously mentioned amputations, such measures are taken as indicated by the individual case. Early estimation of the functional result is possible, so adequate steps for necessary interventions or assistance can be commenced at once.

Special Considerations in Children: There is no perforation tendency by distal overgrowth and spike formation. There is a marked impairment of longitudinal growth. (Only about 25% of the growth potential is preserved, so that distal diaphyseal amputations in children lead to a relatively short stump in the adult.) Whenever possible, wrist joint disarticulation should be performed. Of utmost importance is the application of the immediate postoperative prosthetic fitting principles and techniques to prevent the rejection of prosthetic devices often encountered when fitting is delayed.

Elbow Disarticulation

Surgery: If soft tissue coverage is adequate in an elbow disarticulation, a good stump can be created for prosthetic suspension and control.

Physical and Occupational Therapy: Shoulder flexibility should be the goal of therapy.

Special Considerations in Children: If a functional below-elbow stump cannot be secured, the primary elbow disarticulation operation is preferable to every metaphyseal or diaphyseal above-elbow amputation as it preserves the epiphyses. Immediate postsurgical prosthetic fitting should be applied.

Diaphyseal Above-Elbow Amputation

Surgery: There is no problem as to the amputation technique. Usually, the longer the above-elbow stump, the better the active flexibility of the shoulder joint is, provided that postoperative treatment is adequate.

Good range of motion of the shoulder can theoretically be preserved up to an amputation level immediately below the attachment of the deltoid muscle and the shoulder girdle musculature (Fig. 26.9). Experience shows, however, that the shoulder socket of the prosthesis, which is necessary for stumps shorter than half of the humeral shaft, considerably reduces the range of motion of the shoulder joint. Prosthetic control provided by the shoulder girdle is sufficient. Marquardt's angulation osteotomy is indicated in individual cases. Operative anterior angulation of the bony end of the stump facilitates prosthetic suspension without a shoulder socket and provides good rotatory control.

Physical and Occupational Therapy: Range of motion of the shoulder joint should be the goal of therapy. Postoperative treatment includes intensive specific exercises to avoid functional scoliosis, which develops secondary to muscle imbalance between the affected and unimpaired side of the trunk.

Special Considerations in Children: There is a perforation tendency of the bony end of stump, especially after early amputations, because of the prevailing growth potential of the proximal humeral epiphysis.

Countermeasures include Marquardt's angulation osteotomy for long- and medium-length above-elbow stumps in children. Osteoplastic stump coverage (Stumpfkuppenplastik) after Marquardt's for short above-elbow stumps is recommended if there is a perforation tendency. Both operations are done as secondary procedures. Immediate postoperative prosthetic fitting applies.

Shoulder Joint Disarticulation

Surgery: If possible, the humeral head (even if it is nonfunctional) should be left in the joint for cosmetic preservation of the shoulder contour. The forequarter amputation (interthoracoscapular ablatio), which includes amputation of the entire upper extremity and the scapula, is usually performed for orthopaedic reasons (e.g., tumor surgery). Trauma cases requiring this type of amputation are extremely rare.

Physical and Occupational Therapy: Long-term treatment is necessary to avoid functional scoliosis.

Prosthetic Fitting: Prosthetic fitting is usually rejected by patients, with the rate increasing with higher levels of the above-elbow amputations and the time elapsed between the amputation and the prosthetic fitting. Only in cases of bilateral impairment is prosthetic use relatively frequent. Immediate postsurgical prosthetic fitting is therefore also extremely important in the upper extremity amputee, especially in children.

THE IMPORTANCE OF THE IMMEDIATE AND EARLY POSTSURGICAL PROSTHETIC FITTING IN THE LOWER EXTREMITY AMPUTEE

In conventional methods of prosthetic fittings, the patient's stump is treated postsurgically like any other part of the body is treated: with dressing changes, drain removal, etc. The stump must be bandaged for shaping and shrinking over many weeks, and a temporary prosthesis must be used before a definitive prosthesis can be applied successfully. There is considerable morbidity, time loss, and expense. The disadvantages of this method also include delayed healing because of unfavorable moisture, temperature, and sterility in the conventional dressing, poor pressure gradient, often proximal constriction, and poor protection against the damage from postsurgical edema.

Wilson (1922) reported that early prosthetic fitting and ambulation produced physiological, psychological, and economical advantages for lower extremity amputees.

It is now largely accepted that immediate prosthetic fittings minimize postsurgical edema, reduce pain considerably, promote healing and maturation of the stump, and produce profound psychological benefits. Most studies (Wilson, 1922; Burgess et al., 1967; Malone, 1984) including the author's own experiences indicate that it also will reduce hospitalization and disability time. For the lower extremity amputee, early ambulation as part of the procedure can reduce the many complications of inactivity. In general, there are fewer problems with contractures and muscle conditioning than with conventional techniques (Figs. 26.10 and 26.11). With proper application of early postsurgical prosthetic fittings, many above-knee amputees could have been amputated successfully below the knee, which would have had an extraordinary impact on the patient's rehabilitation process and outcome. This is especially important in traumatic amputations in patients with preexisting vascular disease (e.g., diabetes and arteriosclerosis).

Meticulous attention to details is the key to success in immediate and early postsurgical prosthetic fittings. Surgeons should become familiar with the technique; it is worth the effort because the benefit for the patient and society are truly great. (For an extensive discussion of the advantages of this technique and its application, see Burgess et al., 1967, Gerhardt et al., 1982, 1986.)

In spite of excellent results in special centers, this method has not gained general use because of the necessary commitment. This is most unfortunate. A team (the prerequisite for success) can be well trained in a rather short time. The authors trained cast room technicians to apply rigid dressings and experienced no problems as long as the program was closely supervised and only specially trained personnel were used. The plaster socket must be changed whenever it becomes loose. Suspension must be maintained at all times.

There is much confusion as to the use of the term "early postsurgical prosthetic fitting." If delayed ambulation seems necessary, most practitioners disregard also the immediate application of the rigid dressing in the operating room. The crucial factor in immediate as well as in early postsurgical prosthetic fitting, however, is the application of the rigid dressing *immediately after surgery in the operating room* to prevent edema, which damages the already embarrassed circulation and the developing collateral vessels; to reduce pain; and to provide the best wound healing environment. The attachment of the prosthetic pylon and foot can either be done immediately or can be delayed for individual reasons (such as when the patient is unable to apply limited

weightbearing; when there is infection or borderline circulation; or when the patient's general physical or mental condition dictates one or the other). The early fitting without the immediate rigid dressing, on the other hand, deprives the patient of all the benefits of the technique and is just what it says: an early fitting of an amputee after conventional amputation. The exception of an acceptable early definitive prosthetic fitting is the method of Pierre Botta (CPO), director of the Orthopedic Technology Institute in Biels (Bienne) Switzerland (see Fig. 26.12). After initial treatment in the Controlled Environment Treatment dressing bag (CET), special pressure pads over specific soft tissue areas of the stump are applied, and the edema is squeezed out and prevented from reappearing by constriction of a soft insert (which must be split to permit donning and doffing). The outside of the insert is built up to fit into a plastic prosthetic socket. If there is further shrinkage of the stump, only the insert rather than the entire socket is changed. Frequent changes usually are not necessary. To be successful, however, this method requires exquisite knowledge of anatomy, physiology of circulation and wound healing, and kinesiology, along with profound prosthetic skills.

At Bad Häring Rehabilitation Center, cast-resin sockets are used routinely for the early prosthetic fitting. For outpatients, plaster of Paris or temporary Resur sockets are sometimes applied. During this time, measures for stump shaping and shrinking as well as gait training are started. After adequate preparation of the stump, patients are supplied with a definitive prosthesis.

In the following example, management of a severe injury with fracture of the lower extremity and preservation of the all important knee joint is shown.

A 17-year-old patient was injured in a motor vehicle accident. The right leg below the knee was pulseless, cold, and anesthetic, and showed no motor function. There was a compound displaced fracture of the proximal tibia and severe crushing injury to the leg with skin loss and wounds extending to midthigh. Arteriogram on the operating table showed that branches to the upper leg were intact. Patient was febrile, mildly toxic, and edema developed rapidly. Four-compartment fasciotomy was done for decompression. Because of small vessel damage a below-knee amputation was done initially 13 cm below the knee 2 days after admission and the fracture was stabilized with steel pins. The stump was left open until 19 days postinjury, when it was closed using rotational flaps and split thickness grafts. Two subsequent surgical revisions were necessary to obtain skin/soft tissue coverage, and the final length of the below-knee residual limb was 5 cm. Rigid dressing was applied. On the 26th day (7 days post skin closure and grafting), the dressing was changed and a pylon with SCAP-I set for 15 lbs weightbearing applied. Limited weightbearing ambulation was started 4 days later (4 weeks after admission), and the patient was sent home.

He had no difficulty in being independent at his trailer house, ambulating with SCAP-I. Casts were changed as soon as they started to get loose, and after 4 more weeks, the stump healed and the grafts took completely in spite of, or as the author believes, *because of* the limited early weightbearing. Patient is now gainfully employed wearing a PTB prosthesis (courtesy of Dr. David Long, Kaiser-Permanente Health Care System, Portland).

THE IMPORTANCE OF THE IMMEDIATE POSTSURGICAL PROSTHETIC FITTING IN THE UPPER EXTREMITY AMPUTEE

The immediate postsurgical prosthetic philosophy is equally important for the upper extremity amputee—in certain ways, it is even more important. As the upper extremity is not weightbearing, fewer precautions are necessary. Patients can learn to use terminal devices of the prosthesis effectively before they become accustomed to function with one hand only (see Figs. 26.13 and 26.14). For this reason, the frequent rejection of the functional prosthesis, especially by women and children, is minimized. The early use of the residual limb prevents secondary disabilities, such as contractures, disuse atrophy, weakness, and pain. In a short time, the patient is ready for a definitive prosthetic fitting. Prolonged training is not necessary, as patients learn the technique of operating the terminal device while wearing the rigid dressing.

Indications and Contraindications

As far as the lower extremity amputee is concerned, the only two prerequisities for use of this method of management are (a) the potential ability of the patient to stand and walk with assistance after surgery, and (b) the absence of flagrant infection at the amputation site. The first consideration obviously necessitates careful evaluation of the patient's physical ability, mental capabilties, and attitudes. In general, the patient who has been able to stand and walk, with or without ambulation aids, shortly prior to surgery will be a satisfactory candidate. Others must be given individual consideration as to their defects, and some of these will develop the necessary ability with suitable therapy. The process will be less demanding for below-knee amputees. Even for those who will not be able to walk with a prosthesis, the use of the rigid, total contact dressings may be beneficial because of the advantages of healing.

Contraindications to the complete program include: severe debilitation, marked senility (particularly with cerebral arteriosclerosis), severe cardiac disability, severe neurological disability, known inadequate life expectancy (as with metastatic neoplasm), severe mental illness, and intractable unwillingness to cooperate. It may be difficult to interpret apparent lack of cooperation or motivation; it is possible to be misled by reversible conditions, such as situational depression or toxic mental changes. Another contraindication is flagrant, uncontrolled infection. Localized controllable infection does not interfere with the procedure. Unless a suitability trained team of physicians, prosthetists (or other persons skilled in application of rigid dressings), therapists, nurses, and other attendants is available continuously during the entire period of the procedure, the method cannot be used effectively, and disappointment in results will be inevitable.

The best possible prosthetic fitting and training is provided in special rehabilitation centers with well-trained staff, including instructors who are amputees themselves.

Even in the outpatient, close supervision of the rehabilitation program and prosthetic fitting, as well as checking out the definite prosthesis for workmanship, function, and safety are mandatory. This supervision should be done only by physicians who are specially trained and knowledgable in the kinesiological aspects of the amputee as well as in prosthetics and orthotics.

Appendix

Advice to My Fellow Amputees

Lt. Col. Helmut Hornof

Utilize the time in the rehabilitation center to the utmost. The entire team wants the best for you, so work actively with them as a team member. It is ultimately for your benefit.

Cooperate with your prosthetist and guide him in the corrections which are always necessary during the period of healing and stump maturation.

Follow the instruction of your therapist and practice, practice—but don't overdo, to gradually harden your residual leg.

Observe your stump and take meticulous care of it to prevent infection and pressure. Wash your stump thoroughly with tepid or cold water and soap and after drying, apply thinly elk suet or a special cream for amputees. (I am using the French product "Akilortho.")

Keep your stump socks clean, and change them every day. Rinse them after washing repeatedly in lukewarm water to remove all remnants of soap or detergent which could cause skin irritation. Use the recently available stump socks with a terrycloth type inside layer, which is more absorbent and softer.

Do not wear your prosthesis even if only superficial skin infections have developed, and use crutches until the lesions have healed.

Exercise your residual limb muscles regularly several times a day. You can do it while wearing your prosthesis by applying 6-second isometric contractions and relaxations in addition to regular stump exercises without the prosthesis morning and evening.

Choose a standard shoe model with low rubber cushion heel right at the outset and never change the heel height. Don't pay attention to changing fashions or styles.

Choose a prosthesist with whom you can work and who has a good reputation. Try to get a second socket for your temporary prosthesis to have a spare and use it after work at home or at leisure time. Have also two soft inserts so you can change the soft socket if you work up a sweat such as during heavy work or sports. It can prevent stump breakdown in times of prolonged activity.

Talk to your employer and discuss prosthetic problems with him so he understands your special needs or occasional absenteeism.

Keep in touch with your physician and the rehabilitation center and report any problems without delay.

Phantom pain can be very annoying or outright bothersome. The best treatment I found was accupuncture on the remaining leg applied in five-day intervals for 20 minutes. Five to six treatments are sufficient to keep me free of pain for 6 to 12 months.

Make sure that the prosthetic suspension is functioning to prevent pumping.

Keep your weight constant, as weight fluctuations alter the size of your stump and produce it an ill-fitting prosthesis. Observe nutritional measures for good health.

Engage in sports. You will find congenial, understanding handicapped friends and fellowship. In sports clubs for the handicapped, you can increase your general fitness under the guidance of expert teachers and experienced athletes with handicaps. The best sports for amputees are swimming, bicycling, and cross-country skiing.

Swimming: Water provides best massage and exercises for your stump. Freestyle and backstroke are best.

Bicycling: Obtain a lightweight race bike (not over 10 kg [20 lbs.]). Try to bike 40–50 km a week on side roads with not much traffic.

Cross-country skiing: Equipment is relatively inexpensive. Courses for handicapped are usually offered, and you should attend one if you are not experienced. For the below-knee amputee, I'm recommending the "Scootertechnik" to lessen the strain. Keep the prosthetic leg stationary on the ski, and propel forward with the remaining leg and both ski poles. The only time you need the diagonal step technique is on the uphill slope. For Alpine skiing, use short skis initially. Use only a low, 2 cm (¾ inch) wedges under the prosthetic heel. The previously used 6 cm (2¼ inch) wedge is considered outdated.

Hiking and touring: I recommend use of lightweight adjustable crutches which can be carried in a backpack if not needed, such as during climbing, and used when walking downhill or on rocks. During longer hikes, always take the second soft socket as well as additional stump socks. Change socks/socket as soon as sweating is noted and air dry the used one.

If you like sauna, use plastic swim prosthesis rather than crutches. They are hazardous on wet cement floors.

Lower back pain: Muscle imbalance and uneven weightbearing in the amputee can lead to painful ligamentous sprains and scoliosis. Have your therapist teach you suitable preventive exercises. In standing, try to distribute weight evenly between the prosthesis and remaining leg.

Mobilize all your energy. Leave your past problems behind and turn to the present and immediate future. You can do more than you think you can. Learn from the handicapped who have been successfully rehabilitated and establish a personal mental and physical training program to fit your needs and goals.

As you become successful, joy and sunshine will return into your life and you will feel handicapped no longer in spite of recurring problems, ailments and pain. If you also accept as your mission the assistance of weaker and more suffering neighbors, and help provide them with a living example for their attitude and (perhaps) emulation, then you have been privileged to perceive the true meaning of your life.

Figure 26.1.

A. Growth remaining in normal distal femur and proximal tibia following consecutive skeletal age levels (means and standard deviations derived from longitudinal series 50 girls and 50 boys). This growth chart which may be used as a guide in estimating the amounts of growth which may be inhibited in the distal end of the normal femur or the proximal end of the normal tibia by epiphyseal arrest at the skeletal ages indicated on the base line.

B. Relative contributions of osseus epiphyses to total limb growth are shown.

From Anderson, Green, Messner: *J. Bone Jt. Surg. 45-A.*

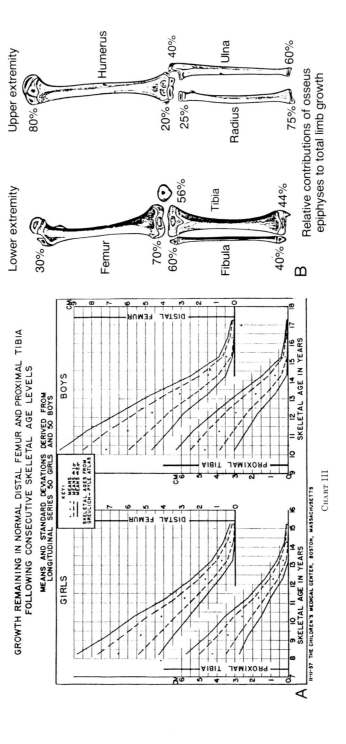

Figure 26.1.

Figure 26.2.

   A. X-ray view of toe amputation 1–5 shows the stump of proximal phalanx of digit 1 (big toe) and disarticulation in the metatarsophalangeal joint 2–5.

   B. X-ray view of transmetatarsal amputation and

   C. X-ray view of proximal transmetatarsal amputation according to Sharp-Jäger-Bona (1961) are shown.

D–E. Transmetatarsal amputation (*right*) and Lisfranc's amputation (*left*) are shown.

   F. X-ray view of Lisfranc's amputation is shown.

G–H. These functional photographs are of a Lisfranc's stump.

 I–J. Clinical photographs and X-ray views show the Chopart's amputation in malposition.

   K. Resection-fusion of the posterior foot according to Spitzy (1914).

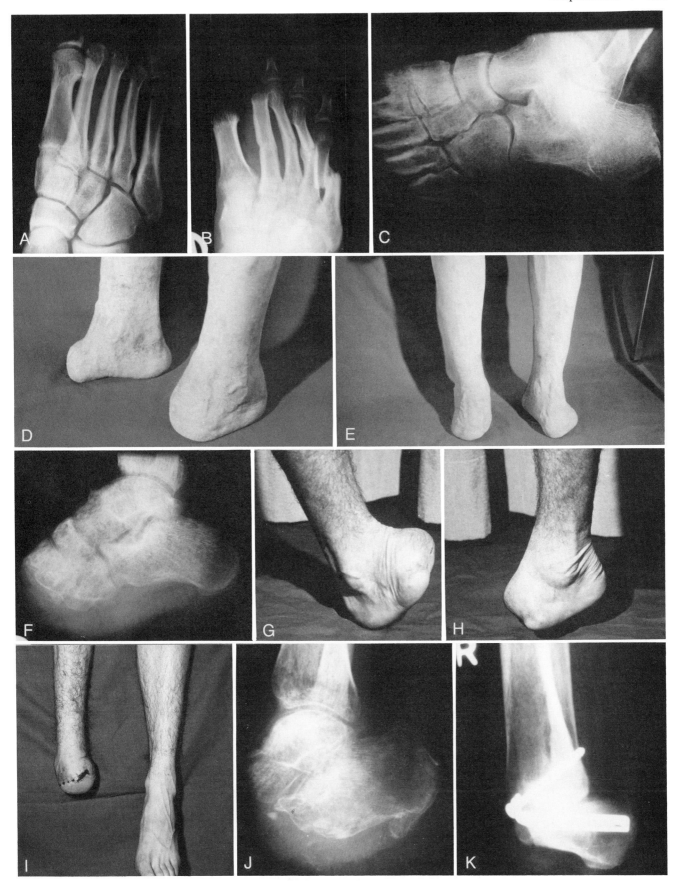

Figure 26.2.

Figure 26.3.

A. Ventral and dorsal incision for hip disarticulation.

B. Boyd's approach for hip disarticulation.

C. Approaches for various levels of above-knee amputations and knee disarticulation are shown.

D. An alternate approach to knee disarticulation is to create a medial and lateral flap instead of the conventional AP flaps.

E. Equal length AP flaps in below-knee amputaton in cases with normal, unimpaired circulation include typical flaps for Syme's amputation.

F. Long posterior flap is done in amputations for vascular reasons. Optimal amputation level is at about one-third tibial length but may be at one-quarter tibial length, or shorter if necessary. Even the shortest possible below-knee stump is functionally better than a knee disarticulation or above-knee amputation. The length of posterior flap is about one-third of tibial length. On rare occasions, where there is uncertainty as to the blood supply to the posterior muscles (such as in traumatic cases), a guillotine amputation is done further distally. Then the muscles are explored via medial and lateral incisions and, according to the blood supply, a longer anterior or posterior flap is created. With modern prosthetics, it is completely irrelevant where stump scars are located.

G–H. Approaches for various levels of upper extremity amputations and disarticulations.

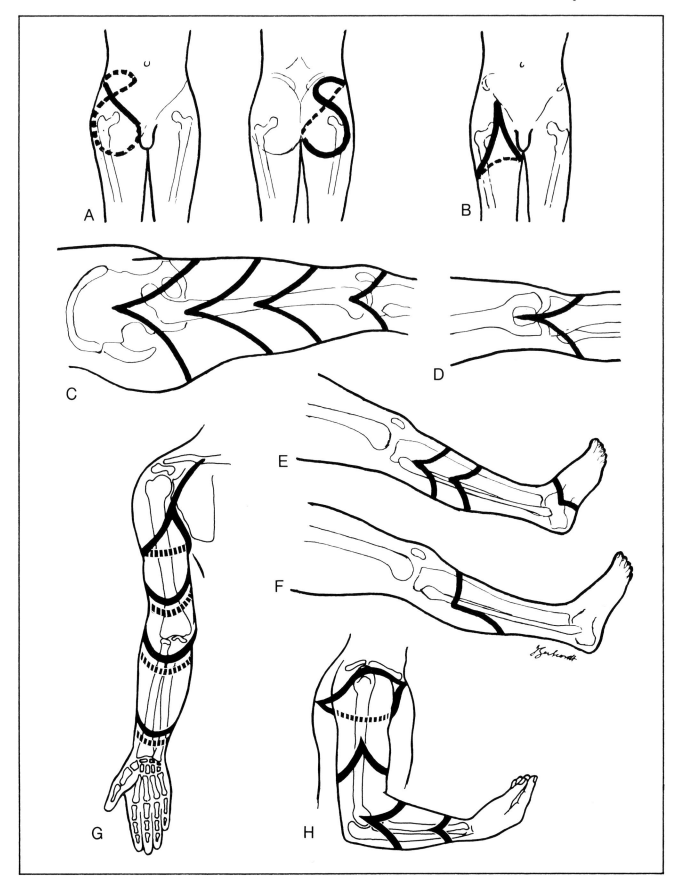

Figure 26.3.

Figure 26.4.

A. X-ray views of Syme's amputation,

B. Of below-knee amputation through the distal diaphysis of the tibia, and

C. Of below-knee amputation at midlength are shown.

D. A shorter below-knee amputation with fibula in abducted malposition is shown.

E. Below-knee amputation with spontaneous bony bridging between tibia and fibula is shown.

F. X-ray view of below-knee amputation shows an intended bone bridging of tibia and fibula according to Dederich (von Ertl).

G. This X-ray view is of a very short below-knee amputation with capitulum fibulae in situ.

H. In this X-ray view, a very short below-knee amputation is shown with fibula head removed.

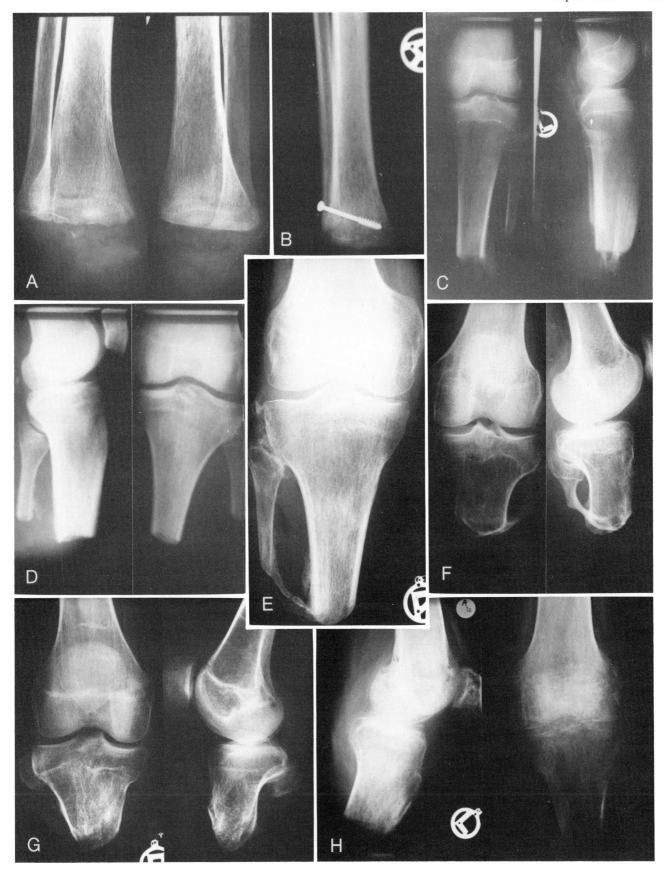

Figure 26.4.

Figure 26.5.

  A,C. A 29-year-old male with a very short (3.8 cm or 1½ inch below knee stump shows good extension and flexion of the knee.

E,B,D. X-rays of the knee with residual limb are of same patient; AP view and lateral views in extension and flexion are shown.

  F–G. The same patient ambulates with a Prosthese Tibiale Supracondylienne (PTS prosthesis), showing excellent gait and using no assistive devices. He is fully employed.

    H. This patient is able to elevate and hold the prosthetic limb elevated in spite of the very short stump. He has better than antigravity extension and flexion against resistance of the knee with the PTS same prosthesis.

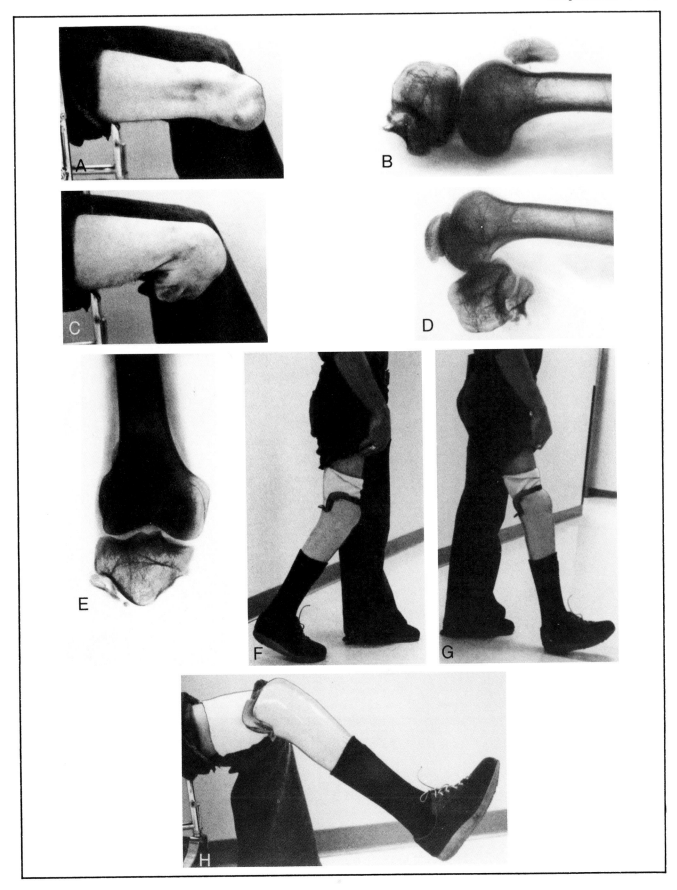

Figure 26.5.

Figure 26.6. Technique of application of rigid dressing in a below-knee amputee using first two elastic plaster of Paris bandages, which allow better control of tension and pressure gradient. Thereafter, regular plaster of Paris is used for added rigidity and stability. Patient in supine position.

A. The first turn is circular, lateral to medial with little tension to anchor the felt relief pads.

B. The second turn is from posterolateral to anteromedial in order to avoid displacement of gastrocnemius. Considerable tension is applied.

C. The third turn is placed similar to the second turn, but further medially. The tension should be the same in order to avoid pulling the bandage between the felt pads (*arrow b*). This turn is then reversed, taking extreme care not to overstretch the large arc (*arrow a*) and to avoid formation of deep ridges at the chord of the arc. Also avoid sharp turns to prevent wrinkling and sharp margins.

D. The fourth turn applies tension over the distal and medial aspect of the stump.

E. The fifth turn is similar to the fourth, but further medially.

F. From now on the turns are rolled on with evenly diminishing tension toward the knee in order to promote and facilitate blood flow. Extreme care is used to avoid proximal constriction.

G. Turns of first elastic plaster bandage completed.

H. The second elastic plaster bandage is rolled on with diminishing pressure gradient, and over and above the knee it is merely layed on in even overlapping turns.

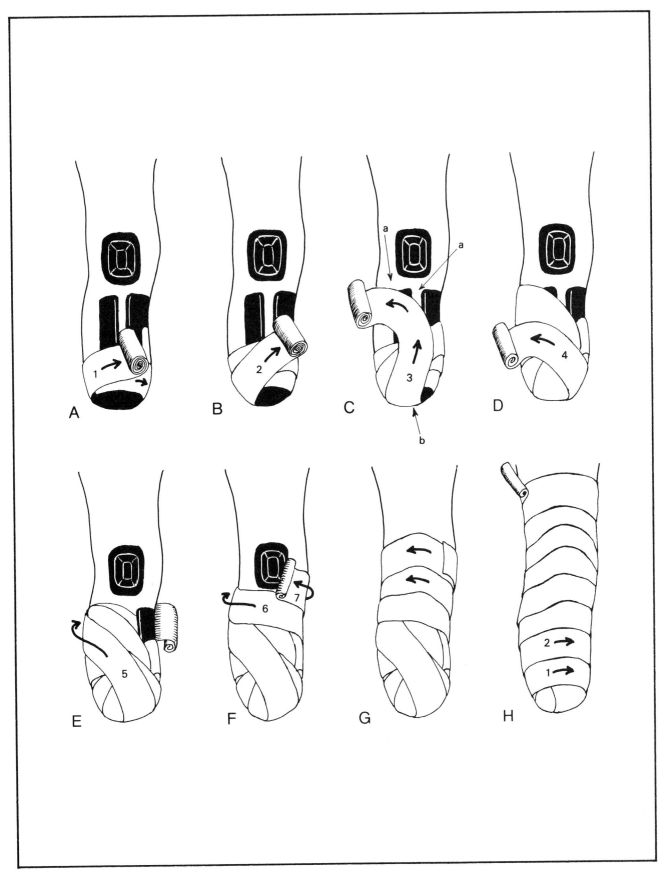

Figure 26.6.

Figure 26.7.

   A. A knee disarticulation stump is shown.

B–C. This trial is to preserve a residual limb at the knee disarticulation level. Note femoral fracture stabilized with intramedullary rodding on the amputated side.

D–E. In this diaphyseal above-knee amputation, note a "dog ear" (Polsterzipfel) on the lateral aspect of the stump. Minimum 4 inches of space above the knee joint is needed to accommodate a mechanical prosthetic knee.

   F. This above-knee amputation was done in childhood. X-ray views show bony overgrowth with spiking.

   G. Very short above-knee and below-elbow amputations.

   H. X-ray of the very short above-knee residual limb, AP and lateral, is shown. Note bony spike formation not removed from periostal shreds.

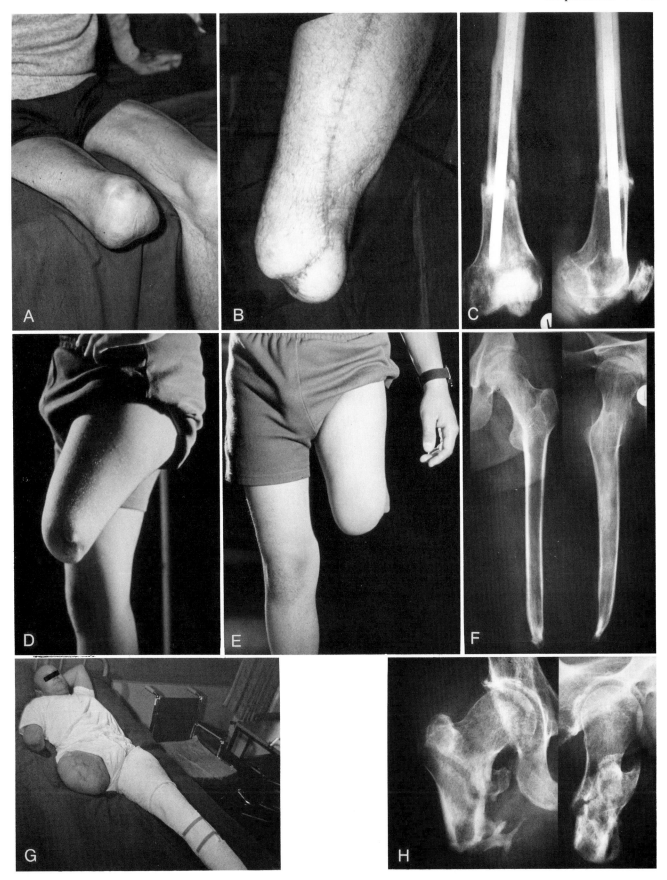

Figure 26.7.

Figure 26.8.

   A. This X-ray view shows amputation of the thumb. The patient has also combined median and ulnar nerve paresis.
   B. X-ray views of the thumb and index finger amputation.
   C–D. Wrist amputation of the hand at the carpal level.
   E. Wrist disarticulation stump.
   F–G. Below-elbow amputation. Osteosynthesis of fractured radius and ulna was attempted to preserve length of the residual limb and the rotation of the forearm.
   H–I. Satisfactory amputation level for consideration of Krukenberg's operation, fitting with conventional prosthesis, or with a myoelectric prosthesis.
   J–K. Short below-elbow residual limb which can be fitted with a Münster socket or step-up double socket prosthetic elbow unit.

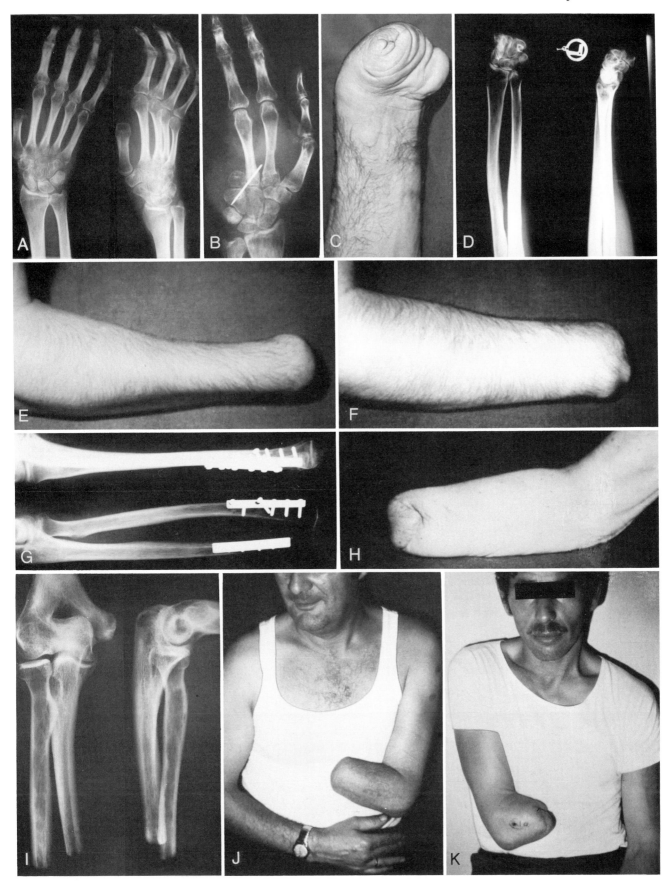

Figure 26.8.

Figure 26.9.

A–C. Different levels of very short above-elbow amputation are shown.

D. Short, above-elbow stump with fibrous ankylosis is shown.

E–F. X-ray views of shoulder disarticulation show very short, soft tissue stump.

G. X-ray view of a short above-elbow stump is shown in the proximal one-third of the humerus.

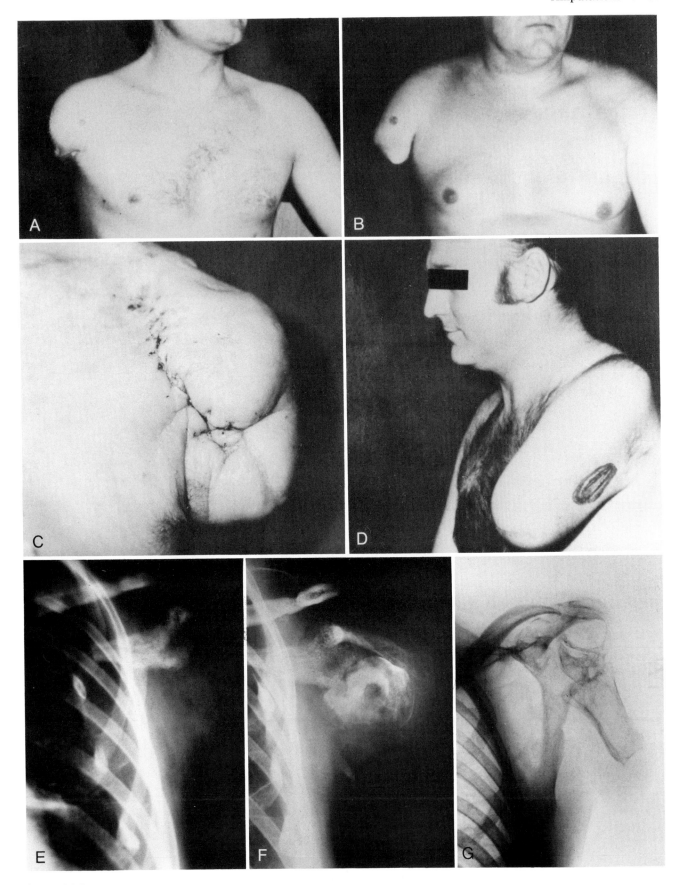

Figure 26.9.

Figure 26.10.

A–B. X-rays of residual limb below knee in rigid dressing with prosthetic unit attached are shown. Note Steinman pin for fracture fixation to preserve the all important knee.

C–D. X-rays of residual limb show a final length of 5 cm (2½ inches) after revision and removal of pin because of irritation of skin by posterior spike and difficulties with definitive prosthesis. There were no further complications.

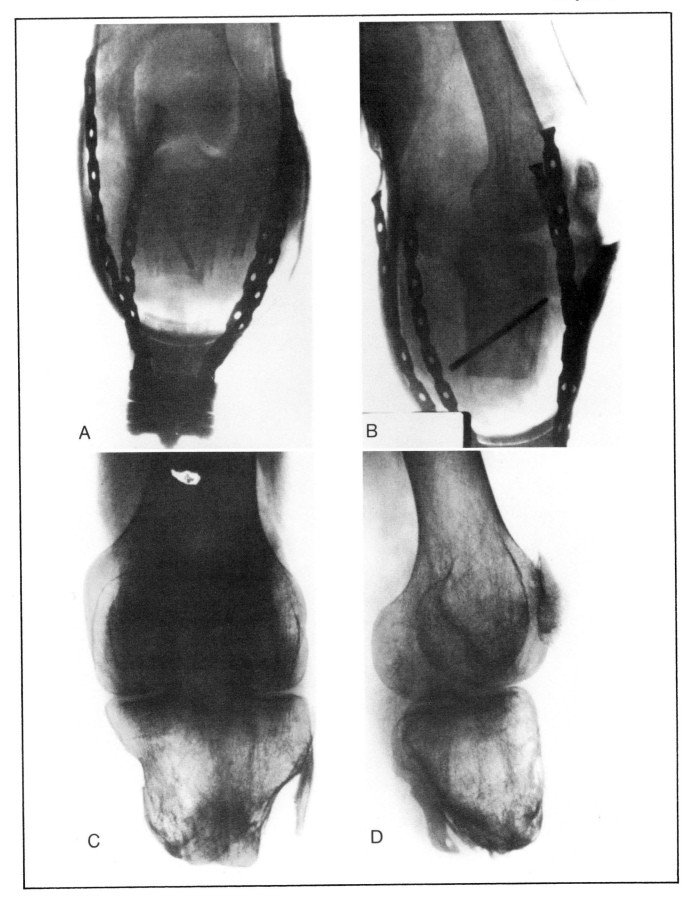

Figure 26.10.

Figure 26.11.

A. Residual below-knee limb has a final length of 5 cm (about 2½ inches).

B. Pylon with pressure warning device (SCAP I), attachment device, SACH foot and patient's shoe are shown.

C. A patient attaches pylon to the rigid dressing before leaving home.

D. The same patient ambulates with limited weightbearing, monitored by SCAP I on the sidewalk in front of his home.

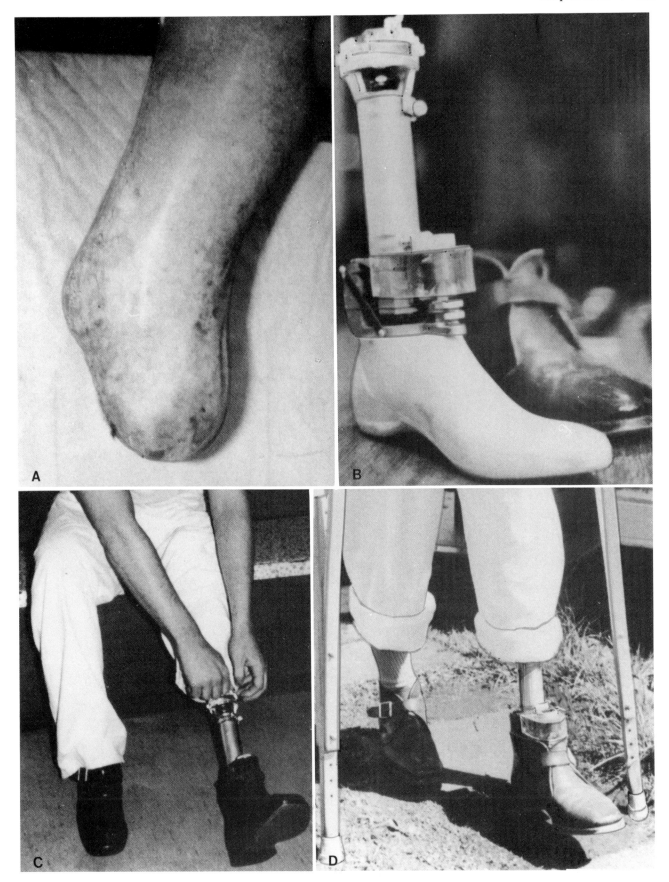

Figure 26.11.

Figure 26.12.

Steps in preparation of an early definitive below-knee prosthesis:
A. Especially cut plaster of Paris splints and tubigrip are sewn at the distal end.
B. Splints are applied over tubigrip with molding and pressure over soft tissue. The positive mold is modified over the soft tissue areas (made about 3-ply sock thickness smaller).
C. This finished plaster mold has the shape of the residual limb.
D. A soft socket is built up on the outside over the depressed areas to provide smooth outer surface for the hard socket, and then split laterally to allow application under tension.
E. A hard-laminated PTS socket is applied over the soft socket.
F. A hard socket is shown in place.
G. A socket is mounted on an adjustment rig and pylon for alignment and initial gait evaluation. One thin nylon sock is worn under the soft socket.
H. SACH foot is carved for better cosmesis and reduction of weight.
I. In the final fit of prosthesis with cosmetic cover, the total weight is about 1 kg (about 2 lbs). It can be worn 10 to 12 months with fitting provided by application of additional stump socks (courtesy of Pierre Botta, CH - 2500 Biel, Neuhausstrasse 24, Switzerland).

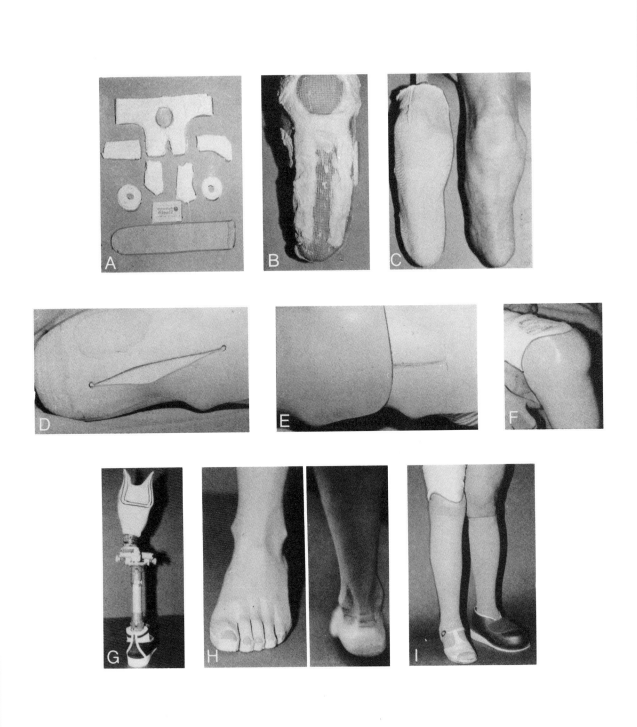

Figure 26.12.

Figure 26.13.

A–B. A 35-year-old patient had a forearm amputation following an accident with a meat grinder.

C. The below-elbow stump is shown immediately after surgery.

D. Immediate postsurgical prosthetic fitting (IPPF) with below-elbow rigid dressing and terminal device attached to the cast are shown.

E. The same case is shown 28 days and

F. 37 days postinjury.

G. Definitive below-elbow prosthesis with Münster socket is shown 40 days after surgery.

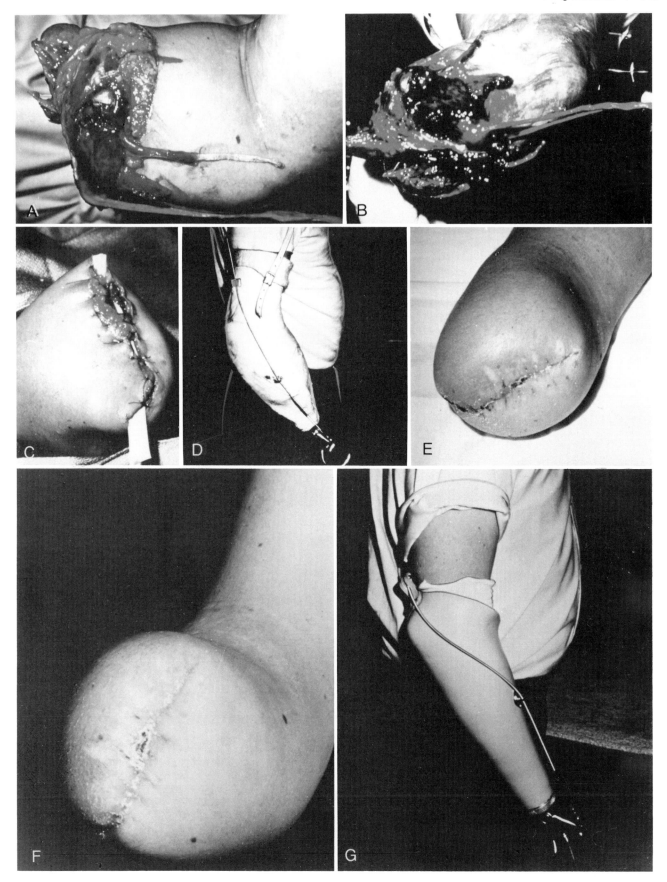

Figure 26.13.

Figure 26.14.

> **A.** Traumatic wrist disarticulation is treated with an immediate postsurgical prosthetic fitting. A terminal device is attached to the rigid dressing.
>
> **B.** The stump is shown at 22 days.
>
> **C.** And 36 days postsurgery.
>
> **D–E.** Definitive prosthesis is shown 45 days post amputation.

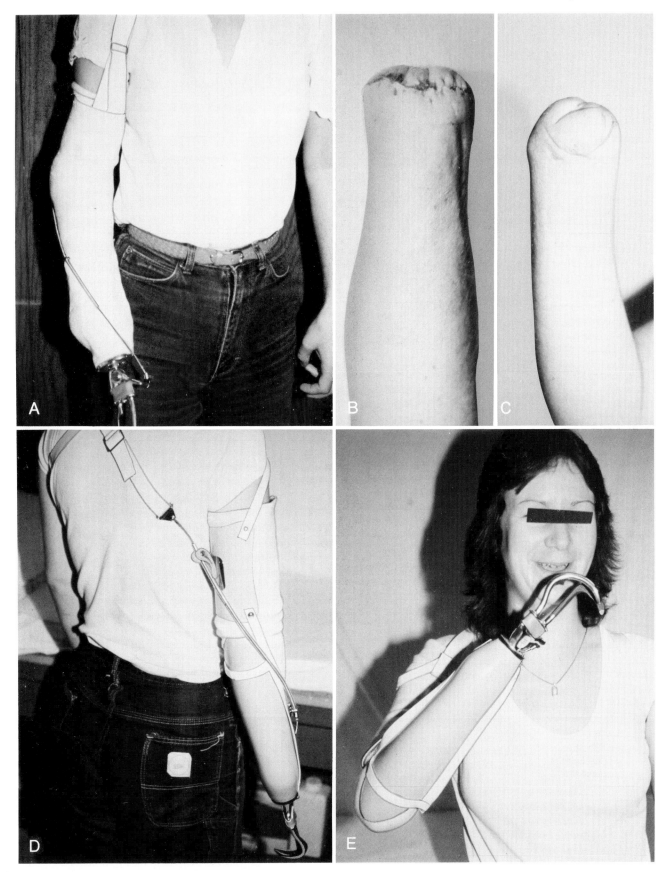

Figure 26.14.

27

Burns

Jolene Heitmann, O.T.R. and Philip Parshley, M.D.

Burn injury is one of the most serious and devastating forms of trauma. Those hospitalized require specialized care. With the multiple aspects of care required, comprehensive quality management requires the knowledge and skills of a multidisciplinary team.

Rehabilitation begins at the time of admission because all that is done for the patient during hospitalization directly contributes to his or her return to society. Complete rehabilitation requires attention to functional usefulness, cosmesis, psychological adjustment, and vocational rehabilitation. Only some of these aspects are represented in this chapter.

POSITIONING AND SPLINTING

Therapeutic positioning (see Fig. 27.1) is implemented to reduce edema by elevation and extension of extremities and to preserve function by proper body alignment and use of anticontracture positions. Specific injury site positioning is designed to counteract the forces and patterns of wound contraction and scarring. For example, patients with axillary burns are positioned with the shoulder at 90 degrees abduction and slight flexion, with supination of forearm and extension of the elbow. Critically ill and other patients who are immobile require frequent monitoring and repositioning.

Splinting is a component of the positioning program. It is indicated when the patient is unable to maintain proper positions voluntarily, when voluntary positioning is ineffective, or when the patient must be immobilized for extended periods, i.e. post grafting.

Immediate attention is placed on hand burns and their splinting needs. With dorsal or circumferential burns, often the support of the wrist is the key to the positioning of the whole hand. With early excision, wound closure, and motion, full hand splints are not always required.

Duration of wear is determined by the specific problem requiring intervention and the patient's ability actively to use the involved part. Low temperature thermoplastic materials are used in the fabrication of splints in the acute phase. Because of their molding characteristics, it is easy to revise the splint's contour. Measurements and application of splints are done after a thin layer of dressings has been applied to the burn area. They may be secured by gauze wrap, ace bandages, or Velcro straps. Frequent assessment on a daily basis by the occupational therapist is the key to effective splinting, thus ensuring proper fit and function.

Splints may be used with nearly every type of burn wound treatment, including grafts and other biological dressings. Traction, sling suspension, and dynamic splinting may also be used to assist in positioning, and with exposed joints, internal fixation may be required. In the event of existing deformity serial or progressive splinting is used for nonsurgical correction of contracture. They are designed to apply pressure and stretch to the scar. As the contracture is resolved, the splint is altered progressively until full motion is obtained.

EXERCISE

A major complication of severe thermal injury is serious loss of joint function. To avoid this, each patient should be evaluated and an exercise program established according to his or her individual needs (see Fig. 27.2). The overall goals of an activity program are to decrease edema and to maintain a normal range of motion and functional strength. Early excision and wound closure have facilitated a dynamic rehabilitation program resulting, in faster recovery and fewer functional disabilities.

Prolonged immobility should be avoided and early motion encouraged following skin grafting, usually within 3 to 5 days or when the graft is secure. Slow sustained stretching of burned areas is preferable to multiple, vigorous, and repetitive stretching because of extremely strong contractile tendencies of burn scars. The patient should be encouraged to achieve his or her optimal active range of motion by the therapist assisting in the increase of that range. Because of pain, apprehension is often a major deterrent to successful exercise programs. If this is a major problem, the contract-relax method is valuable in gaining motion without increasing pain. Lubrication and paraffin to healed areas will assist in softening the skin and assist in stretching. Precautions in exercise include taking special care to exposed tendons and extremities in dependent positions. With exposed extensor tendons of the hand, a patient should be instructed not to make a fist but to flex the metacarpophalangeal (MP) joints actively with the interphalangeal (IP) joints extended. IP flexion is accomplished with MP joints in a neutral position. Extremities in dependent positions should be wrapped with elastic bandages for additional vascular support. Coordination exercises are often needed and may involve both gross and fine motor reeducation. Tactile reeducation and early pressure to the hand is used for skin hypersensitivity.

Neuromuscular complications of thermally injured patients require special attention as do electrical injuries and their associated problems.

AMBULATION

Mobilization should begin as soon as the patient is medically stable, to prevent respiratory congestion, pulmonary emboli, general loss of muscle tone, and stiff joints. With prolonged bedrest following grafting, a tilt table may be used by physical therapists to progress the patient to an upright postion. Brief but frequent ambulation is emphasized rather than prolonged standing. When sitting, legs should be elevated to encourage adequate venous return. Assistive ambulatory devices are discouraged except for specific reasons in weightbearing status as specified by the physician.

STRENGTHENING

Active resistive modes of exercise are more beneficial. These include cuff and ankle weights and dumbbells. When the patient is allowed off the burn unit, a more aggressive strengthening program is to be used including resistive weight equipment, for example, Cybex, Nautilus and Ariel, to promote full-body reconditioning and strengthening.

FUNCTIONAL ACTIVITY

Transfer of exercise techniques into meaningful activity is accomplished through activities of daily living. Setting realistic goals with the patient, allowing additional time to perform tasks, and actively reinforcing desired behavior assist in gaining independence and preserving motor skills and endurance.

Every effort should be made to facilitate participation in self-care. When possible, dressings over joints should be loose and have minimal thickness to avoid limiting joint motion. Fingers should be wrapped individually to allow the use of hands for feeding and other light activities. Assistive devices or compensatory techniques should be used if necessary to increase feasibility of performance. Play is commonly the means with which infants and small children are involved in exercising groups of joints and overall motion patterns. With a progressive program, the patient is functioning, prior to discharge, as near to his or her maximal level as possible. This is followed by a home program and/or outpatient visits. Instruction and training is given the family or others assisting in the home care.

PSYCHOSOCIAL CARE

All team members deal with the psychosocial needs of the burn patient daily as they implement programs to meet physical and functional goals. Professional help for the patient and family is available through the burn team psychologist. Peer counseling through the burn support group is most helpful. As with any patient population, burn patients are encouraged to be self-initiating in all aspects of daily living, including vocational planning, socialization, and dealing with the public.

HYDROTHERAPY

Nonambulatory patients can be cleansed, debrided, and exercised during immersion or, in some cases, rinsed only over the hubbard tank.

BURN SCAR COMPRESSION

As burn wound closure is accomplished and the healing process progresses, scar tissue formation becomes a primary concern. Third degree burns require more attention for closure; however, second degree burns often require more urgency for scar control. The resultant scar overgrowth may inhibit function markedly and is often associated with severe disfigurement.

Larson and associates (*J. Burn Care Rehabil.*, J.B.C. Publ. Co., 1975, pp. 119–127) reported reduction of hypertrophic scar formation following application of conforming isoprene splints and/or elastic dressings during the convalescent period. By exerting continuous pressure on the hypertrophic scar (Fig. 27.3), reduction in local interstitial edema and improved alignment of collagen fibrils are accomplished.

To be effective in scar control, pressure garments should be worn continuously 24 hr a day, with the exception of periods of skin care and, possibly, exercise. Although blisters may occur at any time, pressure garments are not to be discontinued unless major skin breakdown occurs. Foam pads applied beneath the garment may aid in controlling blistering and breakdown. Conforming splints (used to contour areas of the face and neck), and finger-webs, of silicone, high-density foams, and isoprene are often used with the pressure garment (Fig. 27.4) Measurements for pressure garments are taken when remaining wounds are less than 2.5 cm in diameter, when swelling of the affected parts has been minimized, and when general weight loss is less than 10 pounds. Prior to receiving garments, lightweight pressure may be initiated with an elastic bandage wrap or tubular elastic bandages. Use of pressure garments should continue until the scar tissue matures, that is, until it is no longer red and firm to palpation, often between 8 and 18 months. Two garments are required over the 24-hr-per-day period. Patients are instructed to contact their physician or therapist when garments are worn out or outgrown during the period of required wear or when weight change exceeds 10 to 15 pounds.

Figure 27.1. Positioning and splinting involves the use of:

A. A wrist cock-up splint is applied. Note finger position with metacarpophalangeal joints in mid flexion and proximal and distal interphalangeal joints extended; thumb is in opposition (intrinsic plus position).

B. A conforming axillary splint and

C. A prefabricated foot splint with foam inserts.

D. An acute burn patient is positioned.

E. A sling is used to position a shoulder in abduction.

F. Axillary and elbow contractures require positioning and splinting.

G. A patient is positioned postreconstructive surgery.

H. Axillary foam wedge allows a hand free.

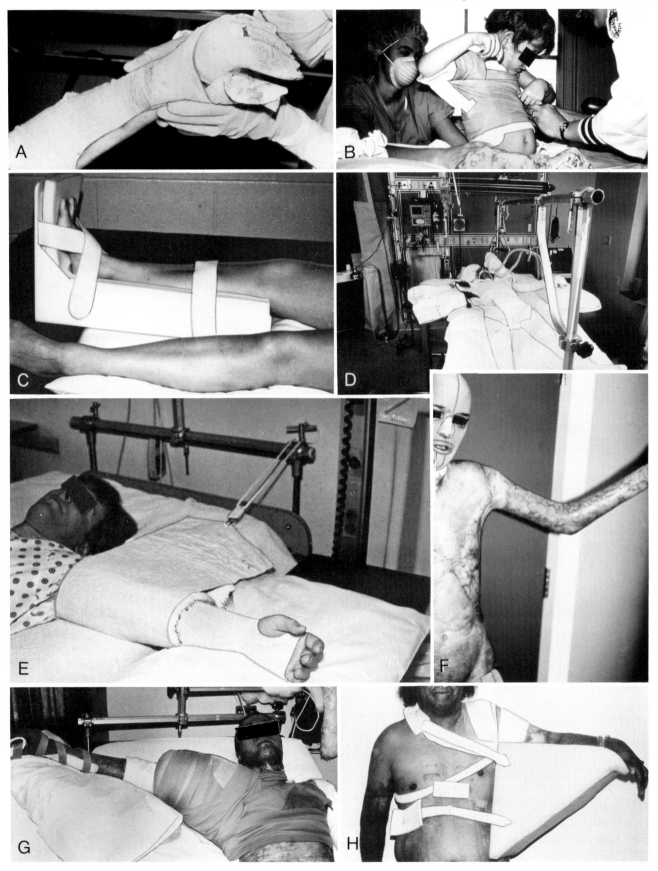

Figure 27.1.

Figure 27.2. Exercise and activities include:

A. Therapy putty for strengthening and
B. Coordination activities using pressure gloves.
C. Adaptive devices are used for eating.
D. Occupational performance is crucial in home, work, and school skills.
E. Exercises are done on isokinetic apparatus.
F. A patient ambulates off a tilt table between parallel bars.
G. Swimming and
H. Gross motor activities used in
I. Play/leisure skills involve coordination, dexterity, and socialization.

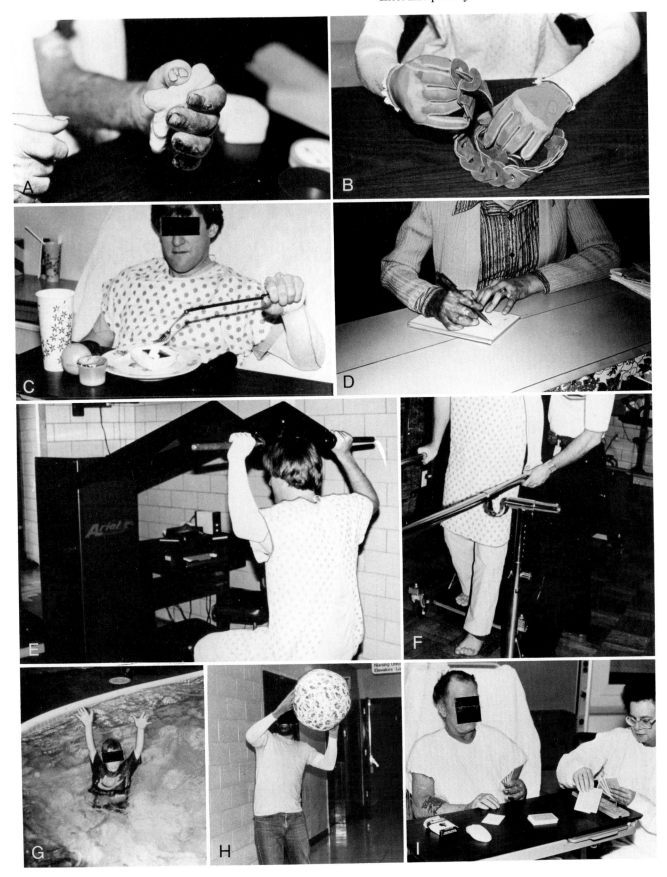

Figure 27.2.

Figure 27.3.

   A. Materials and utensils needed to construct or modify prefabricated splints and conformers.

   B. Thermoplastic material is molded into a conforming forearm splint.

   C. Patient with extensive hypertrophic scars is shown.

D–E. Neck-chin collar and compression garment are shown in the AP and lateral view.

   F. Microstomia prevention appliance (MPA) to prevent scar of the commissures of the mouth and full face mask are shown.

   G. Full face mask with conformers and head and neck compression garment with collar are shown.

   H. Cock-up wrist splint made out of perforated, low temperature thermoplastic material is molded over the forearm which is covered with a thin compression material.

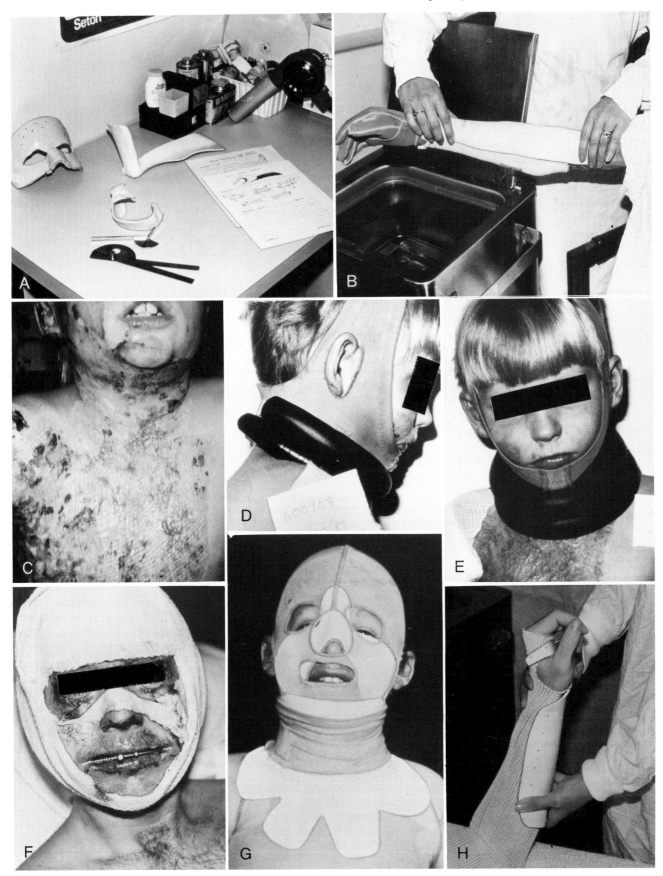

Figure 27.3.

Figure 27.4. Compression.

A. Various pressure materials and garments are used.

B. Special burn pressure garments are used for the patient's chin, torso, arms, and legs.

C. A pressure vest has conformers beneath it.

D. A temporary pressure support is used before a sleeve is custom fit.

E. Burn scars require pressure.

F. Temporary pressure wraps decrease swelling before measurement.

G. Finger-web inserts are worn beneath a pressure glove.

H. An Ace bandage is used to wrap toes to the upper thigh when the patient is in a dependent position.

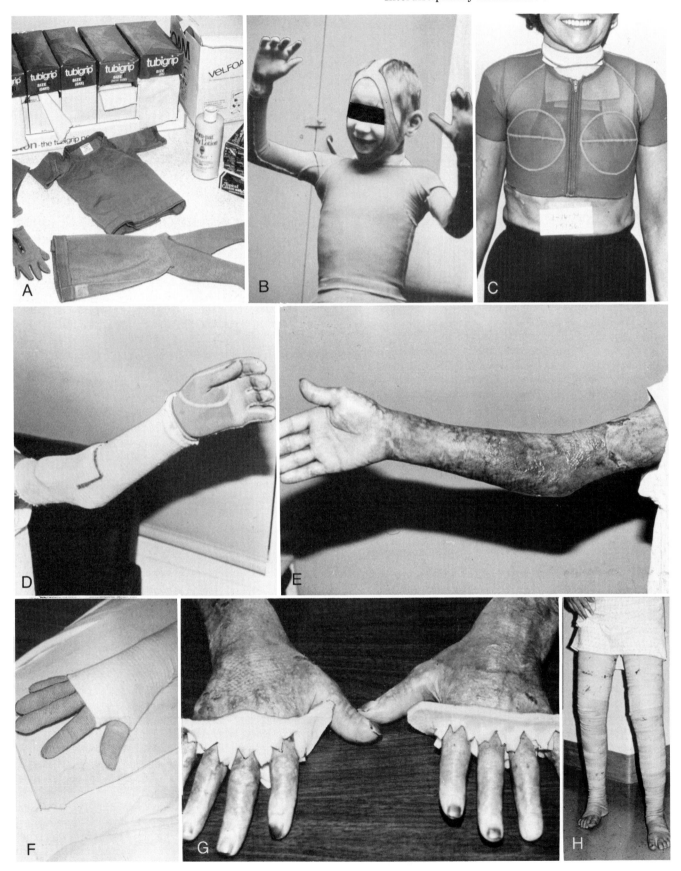

Figure 27.4.

28

Rehabilitation of Cardiopulmonary Injuries

William B. Long, M.D., and Victoria Azavedo, M.D.

REHABILITATION OF THE PATIENT WITH CHEST TRAUMA
William B. Long, M.D.

Rehabilitation of the trauma victim should begin at the time of resuscitation. Diagnostic and therapeutic decisions made at that time determine to a large extent the length of time the patient will stay in the intensive care unit (ICU), the acute care hospital, and the rehabilitation center. Decisions for single organ injury can be straightforward and there are algorithms in the literature detailing diagnostic and therapeutic approaches with expected outcomes (Moore, 1984a, 1984b). Complex trauma involving two or more organ systems invites a logarithmic increase in diagnostic and therapeutic choices that are not chronicled easily. Some authors have tried to reduce the complex to the simple with protocols and/or linear algorithms involving only one decision maker and one course of action (Gill and Long, 1979; Cowley and Dunham, 1981).)

This chapter involves three different types of chest trauma, illustrated by patient examples and how decisions during the critical phase of their illness affect the rehabilitation and overall outcome. Due to limitation in space, all types of chest trauma are not described and discussed.

Flail Chest with Pulmonary Contusion

The American College of Surgeons Advanced Trauma Life Support Manual (Committee on Trauma, 1984) lists flail chest as one of the immediate life-threatening chest injuries, and pulmonary contusion as one of urgent major chest injuries that should be identified in the secondary survey. Not every patient with flail chest has pulmonary contusion, and the converse is also true.

The degree of respiratory insufficiency caused by flail chest is in proportion to the amount of pain the patient suffers from rib fractures, compromise of normal lung mechanics, and the severity of preexisting lung disease. Thus, a frail elderly lady with moderate chronic obstructive lung disease and flail chest from three fractured ribs can develop more respiratory difficulties than a young man with flail chest involving eight fractured ribs. (The magnitude of trauma may not correlate with the degree of respiratory embarrassment. There may be a delicate balance between adequate respiratory function and chronic obstructive pulmonary disease [COPD] and the three fractured ribs may be enough to upset that balance.) Similarly, a full-term pregnant female with flail chest develops respiratory failure because the dia-

phragm cannot compensate for the loss in chest wall mechanical forces. (The gravid uterus limits diaphragmatic excursion and chest wall pain causes splinting.)

The initial management of these patients could dictate when rehabilitation takes place. The frail elderly lady who has only three fractured ribs on chest X-ray and "normal" blood gases, if consigned to a hospital room and treated with oral or parenteral analgesics and "respiratory therapy," probably will become too sedated, splint her respirations excessively, and then develop atelectasis and secondary pneumonia. These complications will necessitate a trip to the ICU, where she will be intubated, placed on a ventilator, and given intravenous antibiotics and frequent suctioning with or without bronchoscopies. If she survives the ICU, she is usually so weak from these complications and the treatment thereof, that rehabilitation with walking, deep breathing exercises, and stretching exercises usually is put off for weeks.

The same frail elderly lady, if admitted directly to the ICU and given local pain relief with epidural injections of morphine, will not "splint" her respirations as much, and she will be able to cough effectively and clear retained secretions. In addition, frequent monitoring of patient tidal volumes, inspiratory volumes and pressures and FEV_1, as well as close nursing observations, can detect impending respiratory difficulties long before serious pulmonary complications develop. The frail elderly lady managed in this way is usually out of the ICU in several days, is walking and is taking nourishment.

Physical therapy on the acute care floors is much more effective if the patient's pain has been controlled from the time of admission. The pain-free or pain-reduced patient is usually willing and able to get out of bed, ambulate, and take deep breaths. The rest of the physical therapy program during rehabilitation is designed to keep the patient as active as possible.

The following example demonstrates chest wall trauma complicated by management that delayed rehabilitation:

Figure 28.1 shows a patient was 20 years old when the motorcycle he was riding collided head on with a car. The patient was thrown from the vehicle and suffered a right flail chest (rib fractures 1–8), a right upper lobe pulmonary contusion, and a right hemopneumothorax. He was taken to the nearest hospital, where a right tube thoracostomy was inserted, and was transferred to a trauma center. On admission, the patient was in marked respiratory distress and he was intubated with a nasotracheal tube. He was placed on a ventilator in the ICU, where his right upper lobe pulmonary contusion became worse and blood, coming from his right upper lobe bronchus, caused infiltrates in his remaining lung fields (Fig. 28.1A–C). No bronchoscopy was performed initially to rule out tracheobronchial injury or to suction out retained secretions and blood not removed by endotracheal suctioning. He developed a staphylococcal maxillary sinusitis secondary to the nasotracheal tube and his right upper lobe pulmonary contusion became infected. Forty-eight hours after admission, he developed a right lung staph pneumonia (Fig. 28.1D), and despite antibiotics, his right lung condition deteriorated to a right pleural empyema, (Fig. 28.1D) which went unrecognized. He progressed to a bilateral staphylococcal pneumonia (Fig. 28.1E).

A thoracic surgical consult was then obtained, and after frequent fiberoptic bronchoscopies, his left lung infiltrates disappeared and his pulmonary function improved to the point where a right thoracotomy, empyemectomy, decortication, and tracheostomy could be done. He required two additional weeks of parenteral nutrition and ventilatory support in the ICU before he was weaned from the respirator and before rehabilitation was initiated (Fig. 28.1F). Before that, he was too sick and too weak to tolerate active and passive range of motion (ROM) physical therapy and breathing exercises.

His total hospitalization was 6 weeks. He required another 6 months of physical therapy before he could resume athletics. The therapy consisted of torso stretching and twisting exercises twice a day and rapid nonstop walking at least 3 miles per day. Two years later, he is now a track star with normal pulmonary function at a local community college (Fig. 28.1G).

Management of his pulmonary contusion affected the course of his acute hospital stay. Active bleeding from the right upper lobe bronchus collected in his airways and pain from his rib fractures prevented him from coughing effectively, despite endotracheal suctioning.

The placement of an epidural catheter with frequent injections of morphine to control pain would have improved his tracheobronchial toilet and might have avoided the use of the respirator. Frequent suctioning with a fiberoptic bronchoscope could have kept his airways clear and avoided infiltrates in the other lung fields. Frequent alternation of a nasotracheal tube with an oral tracheal tube, or the placement of a tracheostomy could have avoided the staph pneumonia, and subsequent development of an empyema.

Pain control, good tracheobronchial toilet, and avoidance of infection of the contused lung are hallmarks of management of flail chest and pulmonary contusion (Trinkle & Glover, 1980; Korban et al, 1984).

In the absence of avoidable complications, the patient's rehabilitation program could have been initiated in the ICU, his length of hospital stay halved, and disability for 6 months reduced to 2 months. Immobilization of the patient on a ventilator for long periods weakens not only respiratory muscles, but extremity and back muscles as well and delays effective patient progression from lying down, to sitting, to walking, to exercising.

Vascular Trauma in the Thorax

Thoracic vascular trauma from blunt injury usually is fatal at the scene of the accident. Parmley's (8) studies of motor vehicle accidents show that 90% of victims die from rupture from the heart and/or great vessels within 1 hr of impact. Of those that reach the hospital alive, 50% of the remainder will die each day the underlying disease goes undetected and is treated inappropriately (Parmley et al, 1958).

The diagnosis and treatment of these injuries is almost always angiography followed by surgery. Rehabilitation begins in the ICU following surgery and is directed at gradually increasing the patient's activities until the patient is ambulatory and ready for discharge.

Certain incisions for vascular access may inhibit this process. Median sternotomies for access to arch vessels are relatively pain-free incisions, provided that the sternum is wired together tightly. This tight union of a surgically divided sternum can be difficult if the patient has associated sternal fractures. Imbalance or unequal force applied to the upper extremities tends to cause a distraction of the sternum and may actually make the wires work loose and lead to nonunion. Patients who have "mushy" sternum from trauma or from osteoporosis and who have had a median sternotomy are not candidates for walking with the aid of crutches or with any other appliance causing unequal force applied to the sternum. Activities such as carrying objects greater than 20 pounds in one hand also tend to distract the healing sternum.

Lateral thoracotomy wounds can be extremely painful in the postoperative period. The use of intercostal nerve blocks for three rib interspaces above and below the incision or freezing the intercostal nerves with a cryoprobe are helpful techniques for relieving postoperative pain. The most effective pain reliever is the epidural catheter with intermittent injections of epidural morphine. Usually, if the pain can be controlled well for the first 3 to 4 days, the patient is able to cough more effectively and can get out of bed more easily. This in turn improves his or her pulmonary function and gives the patient confidence that he or she can recover and do things without incurring too much discomfort.

Surgical technique in closing the large muscles of the lateral thoracic wall also is important in reducing postoperative pain and disability. Anterior and posterior fascial closures for the serratus anterior and the latissimus dorsi muscles provide not only a strong closure, but also a smooth surface over which the patient's muscles can slide as the patient begins range of motion (ROM) exercises and other activities. Full ROM exercises for both shoulder girdles following thoracotomy is usually possible by the fifth through the seventh postoperative day.

Common to both incisions is the limitation of activities that might produce sudden and violent movements, causing pain and tearing of suture lines. For those reasons, thoracotomy and sternotomy patients are advised not to drive a car for at least 6 weeks following surgery in order to avoid situations where they might have to make a sudden swerving motion to avoid a collision but might be unable to do so because of pain and discomfort. Similar recommendations are given to younger patients who wish to resume swimming or riding a bicycle. Should the unexpected occur, they might not have the physical capabilities to cope with the situation.

Figure 28.2 shows a patient with blunt chest trauma, rupture of the innominate artery, and thrombosis of left vertebral artery. This female patient was 20 years old when she lost control of her automobile and rolled it over an embankment. Her body was unrestrained by seat belts and her chest was compressed between the roof of the car and the car door. There was momentary loss of consciousness at the scene of the accident. She was taken to a local hospital, where she was resuscitated. A chest X-ray showed a widened mediastinum. She was transferred to a trauma center, where a repeat chest X-ray showed bilateral hemathoraces, bilateral pulmonary contusions involving both upper lobes, and a widened mediastinum. The hemothoraces were relieved with tube thoracotomy, where an aortagram (see Fig. 28.2B) showed rupture of the innominate artery and thrombosis of the left vertebral artery. CT scans of the lower neck and upper thoracic vertebrae showed no evidence of any fracture dislocations, and she was taken to surgery for repair of her right innominate artery.

In surgery, she had hemopericardium and transection of the origin of her innominate artery—only adventitia held the artery together. The origin of the innominate artery was closed, and a gortex graft was placed in the proximal ascending aorta and sutured end to end to the innominate artery just proximal to its bifurcation. The left innominate vein was divided for purposes of exposure and reanastomosed following completion of the surgery. Fiberoptic broncoscopy showed no intrinsic tracheobronchial injury or disease.

She made an uneventful recovery in the ICU and was extubated the following day. Forty-eight hours postsurgery, she was transferred to the acute care floor, where she was placed on a progressive diet, and her chest tubes were removed. By the third postoperative day, she was ambulating without assistance in the hall. She developed some swelling of her left arm, probably secondary to compromised flow through her left innominate vein. The swelling disappeared after the patient took Coumadin for anticoagulation, and she wore an elastic sleevelet to decrease the left arm edema.

She was placed on progressive activity on her return home and was encouraged to walk at least 1 mile per day without stopping. By 3 weeks post injury, the patient had an almost normal chest X-ray (see Fig. 28.2D), and by 6 weeks post injury, she had returned to college and had resumed swimming. After 12 weeks of torso stretching and twisting, and upper extremity progressive weight exercises, she resumed snow skiing.

Young patients with vascular trauma within the thorax can make dramatic recoveries, despite life-threatening injuries, and can be ready to go home within a week after corrective surgery. Rehabilitation can be started early and the patient's family can help provide psychological support that promotes rapid recovery.

Combination of Severe Chest Wall Injuries and Thoracic Vascular Injuries

Combinations of vascular and chest wall injuries increase the complexity of decision making. Sometimes the operations can be done all at once; other times, the operations have to be staged. Figure 28.3 is an example where a combination of very serious injuries were perhaps appropriately dealt with during the acute phase, but not optimally managed in the recovery phase when rehabilitation should be taking place: An automobile accident victim had blunt chest trauma, right flail chest, right upper lobe pulmonary contusion, torn right main stem bronchus, fractured sternum, avulsion of the right subclavian artery and vein, and neuropraxia of the right phrenic nerve.

This female driver was 32 years of age when her pickup truck collided head-on with a car, which traveled over the top of the truck cab where she was seated. The patient sustained severe blunt chest trauma and was taken to the nearest community hospital, where she was intubated and resuscitated. A chest X-ray showed a right hemopneumothorax and a widened mediastinum. She received two tube thoracotomies and was transferred to the trauma center.

On arrival, she was in marked respiratory distress with hypoxemia. A repeat chest X-ray showed severe right pulmonary contusion, obvious right flail chest, and a widened mediastinum with right pleural capping. An emergency arch aortagram revealed thrombosis of the right subclavian artery 2 cm distal to its origin.

The patient was taken immediately to surgery, where a median sternotomy was performed and a transverse fracture of the manubrium was noted. Exposure of the right subclavian artery necessitated that the midline incision be extended out along the superior border of the clavicle and the medial half of the right clavicle be resected. The right subclavian vein was shredded by the fragments from the first and second rib fractures. The right phrenic nerve was markedly contused and stretched out over the avulsed and thrombosed right subclavian artery. The right subclavian vein was sutured and an interposition greater saphenous vein graft was placed between the innominate artery at the bifurcation and the distal right subclavian artery. The median sternotomy incision was closed after the fractured halves of the sternum were stabilized. The patient also had extensive upper and lower alveolar fractures, which were stabilized by the maxillofacial surgeon.

Her immediate postoperative course was characterized by high cardiac outputs, high concentrations of inspired oxygen to maintain normal arterial oxygen tensions, and blood-tinged aspirate from the tracheobronchial tree. She did not have a significant air leak from her right chest tube.

The first postoperative chest X-ray suggested a tooth might be in the right main stem bronchus and be contributing to her large shunt (Fig. 28.3B). Fiberoptic bronchoscopy revealed a heretofore unsuspected, almost complete, transsection of the right main stem bronchus and blood coming from her right upper lobe pulmonary contusion. There was no evidence of any foreign body in the tracheobronchial tree.

Because she was so sick, repair of the right main stem bronchus was delayed for another 96 hr. During that time, she had no increase in mediastinal air, nor did she develop any appreciable leak from her right chest tubes. When her condition improved, a right posterior lateral thoracotomy was performed, and her right main stem bronchus was repaired. During closure of the chest wall, several of her flail segments were immobilized with wire sutures.

Her postoperative chest X-ray 1 week following repair of the right main stem bronchus (Fig. 28.3C) showed good resolution of the good upper lobe pulmonary contusion and an elevated right hemidiaphragm. She was unable to be weaned from the ventilator for another 3 weeks because of neuropraxia of the right phrenic nerve, the right thoracotomy incision, and the right flail chest. Phrenic nerve stimulation revealed that diaphragmatic innervation was intact, and it would be a matter of time before she would regain sufficient movement of the right diaphragm to breath satisfactorily off the ventilator. A crycothyroidotomy simplified the tracheobronchial toilet.

The patient was in hospital for another 4 weeks before discharge home where she made a slow, but progressive recovery. A follow-up chest X-ray 1 year later revealed a relatively well-expanded right lung field. The patient was able to resume her duties as a housewife and participate in local aerobics classes.

Her residual disabilities are largely psychological, but she does have some physical limitations. She was left with a posttraumatic right maxillary sinusitis for which a local surgeon did a Caldwell-Luc procedure without symptomatic improvement. Because of right shoulder pain, she sought and obtained numerous consultations with orthopaedic surgeons and pain clinics without symptomatic relief.

She eventually returned for follow-up at the trauma center 1 year later and was referred to a psychiatrist and a pain clinic for blocking of intercostal nerve. She obtained symptomatic relief and psychological support from these consultations and declined offered surgery for related problems. She has plans to return to work.

Approximately 30% of patients with life-threatening trauma who are critically ill for weeks require psychological support during their rehabilitation phase. A careful assessment of the patient's psychological status during the critical care and acute recovery phase should detect which patients are not going to be able to cope with the magnitude of the injury and the intensive care experience. Many patients are troubled by the peri-accident amnesia so common to the majority of the severely injured patients. They develop feelings of guilt for possibly causing the accident and potential or actual loss of life, and some become concerned about underlying suicidal tendencies. Psychiatric consultations with both patient and family initiated during the critical care phase will do much to minimize posthospital discharge anxieties.

Approximately 50% of the patients who are involved in severe automobile accidents are intoxicated at the time of the accident. Close questioning of the patient, the family, and friends within 24 hr after admission when all are anxious about the outcome of the patient, will usually reveal that the patient has a problem with substance abuse. Appropriate consultation with substance counselors for both family and patient and friends, if appropriate, will do much to get the patient and his or her support system oriented toward a complete recovery for not only the physical injuries but also the behavior that leads to those types of injuries. Delaying counseling until the rehabilitative phase, when there is belief that the patient is going to recover and the "crisis" is over, frequently leads to noncompliance by both the patient and the support structure, and the patient reverts to old habits.

Postthoracotomy pain is a well-recognized entity and can be minimized with intercostal nerve blocks or epidural catheters with intermittent injections of epidural morphine, beginning immediately in the postoperative period. However, patients with multiple rib fractures and/or flail chest not infrequently develop chronic pain at the site of the rib fractures, especially if the rib fractures were located posteriorly and involve the upper four ribs. Usually, a skilled anesthesiologist with experience in peripheral nerve blocking can relieve patients of these symptoms. Some patients with first, second, or third rib fractures will go on to develop a thoracic outlet syndrome and will need to be evaluated by a neurologist.

The emphasis for all types of thoracic injuries should be stabilization of the patient's injuries with correction of those injuries that require surgery, control of pain, and early mobilization. Attention and sensitivity to the emotional aspects of major trauma (the behavior that caused the trauma or the psychological reaction to the traumatic episode) should decrease the chances that this will become a long-standing problem. Delays in considering rehabilitation during the acute care phase will only prolong the patient's recovery and may lead to more problems with subsequent patient management than necessary.

REHABILITATION OF CARDIOPULMONARY INJURIES
Victoria Azavedo, M.D.

Trauma is the third leading cause of death in the United States after cardiovascular disease and cancer. Cardiopulmonary problems in the trauma patient can be due to: (a) blunt chest trauma, (b) penetrating chest trauma, or (c) preexisting cardiovascular disease. Eighty percent of blunt chest trauma results from motor vehicle accidents. Seventy percent of automobile fatalities have chest injuries. Of patients with chest injury reaching the hospital, 3% die of their chest injuries. Blunt trauma to the lungs can produce a flail chest with severe respiratory distress, multiple rib fractures, fracture of the scapula (which is infrequent but, when present, indicates severe thoracic trauma), and tracheal and main bronchial injuries. Also, the diaphragm can be ruptured. Blunt trauma to the heart can produce myocardial contusion, rupture (rarely), injuries to the valves and their supporting structures, disruption, and thrombosis of coronary arteries, causing damage to the pericardium. Penetrating lung trauma is usually from low-velocity handguns and knives, producing pulmonary contusion, laceration, pneumothorax, hemothorax, and lung hematomas. Penetrating trauma can produce posttraumatic pericarditis or traumatic rupture of the thoracic aorta. The trauma patient may also have preexisting cardiovascular disease, such as angina, arrhythmias, or hypertension.

The rehabilitation of the cardiopulmonary trauma patient definitely should be a team effort among the primary physician, traumatologist, anesthesiologist, rehabilitation physician (physiatrist), respiratory therapist, physical therapist, occupational therapist, psychologist, dietician, and social worker. In cases of tracheostomies, a speech-language pathologist might also be needed. The patient may or may not have concomitant injuries, such as spinal cord or head injury, which requires special rehabilitation measures. The goals of cardiopulmonary trauma rehabilitation are:

1. To increase physical activity with a graded activity program, including teaching the principles of pacing and work efficiency
2. To return to work when applicable
3. To return the patient to as functional a life-style as possible; if the patient has preexisting cardiovascular disease, it is important to discuss diet, risk factors like hypertension, smoking, and obesity

Other important factors to be considered are:

1. Good patient communication
2. Education of the patient regarding his or her:
   Cardiopulmonary trauma
   Associated injuries, e.g., head injury, spinal cord injury, peripheral nerve injury, or fractures
   Diet
   Leisure skills
   Relaxation
3. Decrease in anxiety and depression
4. Pacing of activities
5. Family involvement
6. Coordinated interdisciplinary rehabilitation team approach, including discussions at least weekly of patient's progress and reassessment of his or her short- and long-term goals.

A program of physical exercise improves the efficiency of the heart by decreasing the heart rate and blood pressure response to a given level of activity. The cardiac output (volume of the blood pumped by the heart per minute) increases with physical conditioning. After cardiopulmonary trauma, the team should try to return the patient gradually to normal activity through a program of progressive exercise. The exercise prescribed should be individual and specific for each patient, based on the heart or lung trauma involved and patient evaluation. The heart beats per minute and the blood pressure are most likely the two best indicators of the work performed by the heart.

The practical approach to rehabilitation of cardiopulmonary trauma varies with the severity of the heart-lung trauma. It should be modified for concomitant injuries (e.g., head injuries, spinal injury, multiple injuries, or fractures) and consists of an *inpatient phase* of approximately 10 to 14 days. Exercise can begin as early as 2 to 4 days following cardiopulmonary trauma or 1 day after surgery if the patient is medically stable and off the respirator. In myocardial contusions, the exercise program is similar to that of myocardial infarction. (Metabolic equivalent table [MET] is the amount of energy the body uses per minute at rest—approximately 3.5 cc of oxygen per kilogram body weight per minute):

1 to 1.5 Metabolic equivalent table (METS) (lying)—Approximately 2 days
1.5 to 2.5 METS (sitting)—Approximately 3 to 6 days
2.5 to 4 METS (standing—Approximately 7 to 9 days
Low level exercise test—Approximately 10 to 14 days at the time of discharge

Outpatient Phase

The outpatient phase should begin immediately after discharge and last from 14 days to 2 to 3 months. The conditioning program should last 3 to 6 months before the patient's return to work.

After the patient's return to work, the program should continue as follows:

1 to 1.5 METS—Standing-walking 1 mile per hour
2 to 3 METS—Level walking 2 miles per hour or level bicycle 5 miles per hour
3 to 4 METS—Walking 3 miles per hour or bicycle 6 miles per hour.
4 to 5 METS—Walking 3½ miles per hour or bicycle 8 miles per hour.
5 to 6 METS—Walking 4 miles per hour or bicycle 10 miles per hour.
7 to 9 METS—Jogging 5 miles per hour.
Over 9 METS—Running over 6 miles per hour.

Inpatient Phase

The inpatient phase is designed for cases of uncomplicated myocardial contusion or cardiopulmonary trauma.

1 to 1.5 METS

Day 1

Range of motion (ROM)	(i)	*Passive* ROM to all four extremities four to five time qd or bid
Ankle	(ii)	Active foot circling q 1 to 2 hr while awake.
Breathing	(iii)	Deep breathing tid
Activities of Daily Living (ADL)	(iv)	Wash hands, face, brush teeth, feed self with arms supported in bed bid
Bathroom	(v)	Bedside commode
Bath	(vi)	Bed bath by R.N.
Mobility	(vii)	Dangle foot with support

Day 2

ROM	(i)	*Active assistive* ROM to all 4 extremities four to five times qd or bid
Ankle	(ii)	Active foot circling q 1 to 2 hr while awake.
Breathing	(iii)	Deep breathing tid
ADL	(iv)	Wash hands, face, brush teeth, feed self with arms supported in chair.
Bathroom	(v)	Bedside commode
Bath	(vi)	Bed bath with maximum assistance by R.N.
Mobility	(vii)	Up in chair 20 min two to three times a day with foot elevated

1.5 to 2.5 METS

Day 3

ROM	(i)	Active ROM to all four extremities four to five times qd or bid.
Ankle	(ii)	Active foot circling q 1 to 2 hr while awake.
Breathing	(iii)	Deep breathing tid

ADL	(iv)	Wash hands, face, brush teeth, feed self with arms supported in chair
Bathroom	(v)	Bathroom privileges with help
Bath	(vi)	Bed bath with moderate assistance by R.N.
Mobility	(vii)	Up in chair as desired with arms supported; up in chair for meals

Day 4

ROM	(i)	Active ROM to all four extremities four to five times qd or tid.
Ankle	(ii)	Active foot circling q 1 to 2 hr while awake
Breathing	(iii)	Deep breathing tid
ADL	(iv)	Wash hands, face, brush teeth, feed self with arms supported in chair
Bathroom	(v)	Bathroom privileges with help
Bath	(vi)	Bed bath with minimal assistance by R.N.
Mobility	(vii)	Up in chair as desired, walk in room two times a day for 30 to 60 min with assistance

Day 5

ROM	(i)	Active ROM to all four extremities sitting at the side of the bed tid; upper extremity exercise against resistance; flexion and extension of the knee against resistance
Ankle	(ii)	Active foot circling q 1 to 2 hr while awake
Breathing	(iii)	Deep breathing tid
ADL	(iv)	Wash hands, face, brush teeth at sink sitting down
Bathroom	(v)	Bathroom privileges with help
Bath	(vi)	Bed bath
Mobility	(vii)	Up in chair as desired, walk in room two times a day for 30 to 60 min with assistance

2.5 to 4 METS

Day 6

ROM	(i)	Active ROM to all four extremities sitting at the side of the bed tid; upper extremity exercise against resistance; flexion and extension of the knee against resistance
Ankle	(ii)	Active foot circling q 1 to 2 hr while awake
Breathing	(iii)	Deep breathing tid
ADL	(iv)	Wash hands, face, brush teeth at sink sitting down
Bathroom	(v)	Bathroom privileges with help
Bath	(vi)	Bathtub with help, especially getting in and out of the tub
Mobility	(vii)	Walk in room as desired, approximately 50 feet

Day 7

ROM	(i)	Active ROM to all four extremities four to five times tid standing
Ankle	(ii)	Active foot circling q 1 to 2 hr while awake
Breathing	(iii)	Deep breathing tid
ADL	(iv)	Wash hands, face, brush teeth at sink sitting down
Bathroom	(v)	Bathroom privileges with help
Bath	(vi)	Bathtub with help, especially getting in and out of the tub
Mobility	(vii)	Walk in the hallway, approximately 75 feet

Day 8

ROM	(i)	Active ROM to all four extremities four to five times tid standing, also warm-ups five times, three times a day
Ankle	(ii)	Active foot circling q 1 to 2 hr while awake
Breathing	(iii)	Deep breathing tid
ADL	(iv)	Wash hands, face, brush teeth, standing
Bathroom	(v)	Bathroom privileges with help
Bath	(vi)	Bathtub with help, especially getting in and out of the tub
Mobility	(vii)	Walk in the hallway, approximately 100 feet

Day 9

ROM	(i)	Active ROM to all four extremities 4 to 5 times tid standing, also warm-ups 10 times, three times a day
Ankle	(ii)	Active foot circling q 1 to 2 hr while awake
Breathing	(iii)	Deep breathing tid
ADL	(iv)	Wash hands, face, brush teeth, feed self standing
Bathroom	(v)	Bathroom privileges with help
Bath	(vi)	Bathtub with help, especially getting in and out of the tub
Mobility	(vii)	Walk in the hallway, approximately 150 feet

Day 10

ROM	(i)	Active ROM to all four extremities four to five times tid standing, also warm-ups 10 times, three times a day; may use 1-pound weights
Ankle	(ii)	Active foot circling q 1 to 2 hr while awake
Breathing	(iii)	Deep breathing tid
ADL	(iv)	Wash hands, face, brush teeth standing
Bathroom	(v)	Bathroom privileges with help
Bath	(vi)	Bathtub with help as desired
Mobility	(vii)	Walk 200 feet, walk down one flight of stairs, take elevator up

Day 11

ROM	(i)	Active ROM to all four extremities four to five times tid standing, also warm-ups 10 times, three times a day, active resistive exercise with 1-pound weights
Ankle	(ii)	Active foot circling q 1 to 2 hr while awake
Breathing	(iii)	Deep breathing tid
ADL	(iv)	Wash hands, face, brush teeth standing
Bathroom	(v)	Bathroom privileges
Bath	(vi)	Bathtub with help as desired
Mobility	(vii)	Walk as desired; walk down one flight of stairs; take elevator up

Day 12

ROM	(i)	Active ROM to all four extremities four to five times tid standing; also warm-ups 10 times, three times a day; active resistive exercise with 1-pound weights
Ankle	(ii)	Active foot circling q 1 to 2 hr while awake
Breathing	(iii)	Deep breathing tid
ADL	(iv)	Wash hands and face, brush teeth standing
Bathroom	(v)	Bathroom privileges
Bath	(vi)	Bathtub with help as desired
Mobility	(vii)	Walk as desired; walk down one flight of stairs; take elevator up

Day 13

ROM	(i)	Active ROM to all four extremities four to five times tid, warm-ups 10 times, three times a day; active resistive exercise with 2-pound weights
Ankle	(ii)	Active foot circling optional
Breathing	(iii)	Deep breathing tid
ADL	(iv)	Wash hands and face, brush teeth, dress independently
Bathroom	(v)	Bathroom privileges
Bath	(vi)	Tub bath without help
Mobility	(vii)	Can be up for half a day

Day 14

ROM	(i)	Active ROM to all four extremities four to five times tid, warm-ups 10 times three times a day; active resistive exercise with 2-pound weights
Ankle	(ii)	Active foot circling optional
Breathing	(iii)	Deep breathing tid
ADL	(iv)	Should be independent with dressing, grooming, hygiene, pacing activities
Bathroom	(v)	Should be independent
Bath	(vi)	Should be independent with tub bath
Mobility	(vii)	Walk up-, and downstairs; should be able to be up one full day pacing activities

Following discharge from the hospital to home, pace activities should be reinforced, and follow-up should be done by the primary care physician in 1 to 2 weeks and by the rehabilitation physician in 1 month. The patient should be involved in a conditioning and maintenance exercise program. Depending on age, work situation, severity of cardiopulmonary trauma and other associated injuries, the patient should either have a work evaluation to return to work, or if this is not necessary, then return to work for half a day, gradually progressing to a full day. It should be stressed that rehabilitation of the cardiopulmonary trauma patient is best achieved through a coordinated team approach after patient evaluation, monitoring day-to-day progress, having weekly patient care conferences, and setting goals. The ultimate goal is to return the patient to as normal a life-style as possible. Table 28.1 shows the approximate energy requirements of selected activities.

Table 28.1. Approximate Energy Requirements of Selected Activities

Category	Self-care or home	Occupational	Recreational[a]	Physical conditioning
Very light <3 METS <10 ml/kg/min <4 kcal	Washing, shaving, dressing Desk work, writing Washing dishes Driving auto	Sitting (clerical, assembling) Standing (store clerk, bartender) Driving truck[a] Crane operator[a]	Shuffleboard Horseshoes Bait casting Billiards Archery[a] Golf (cart)	Walking (level about 2 mph) Stationary bicycle (very low resistance) Very light calisthenics
Light 3–5 METS 11–18 ml/kg/min 4–6 kcal	Cleaning windows Raking leaves Weeding Power lawn mowing Waxing floors (slowly) Painting Carrying objects (15–30 pounds)	Stocking shelves (light objects)[b] Light welding Light carpentry[b] Machine assembly Auto repair Paperhanging[b]	Dancing (social and square) Golf (walking) Sailing Horseback riding Volleyball (six-man) Tennis (doubles)	Walking (3–4 mph) Level bicycling (6–8 mph) Light calisthenics
Moderate 5–7 METS 18–25 ml/kg/min 6–8 kcal	Easy digging in garden Level hand lawn mowing Climbing stairs (slowly) Carrying objects (30–60 pounds)[b]	Carpentry (exterior home building)[b] Shoveling dirt[b] Pneumatic tools[b]	Badminton (competitive) Tennis (singles) Snow-skiing (downhill) Light backpacking Basketball Football Skating (ice and roller) Horseback riding (gallop)	Walking (4.5–5 mph) Bicycling (9–10 mph) Swimming (breaststroke)
Heavy 7–9 METS 25–32 ml/kg/min 8–10 kcal	Sawing wood[b] Heavy shoveling[b] Climbing stairs (moderate speed) Carrying objects (60–90 pounds)[b]	Tending furnace[b] Digging ditches[b] Pick and shovel[b]	Canoeing[b] Mountain climbing[b] Fencing Paddleball Touch football	Jog (5 mph) Swim (crawl stroke) Rowing machine Heavy calisthenics Bicycling (12 mph)
Very heavy >9 METS >32 ml/kg/min >10 kcal	Carrying loads upstairs[b] Carrying objects (>90 pounds)[b] Climbing stairs (quickly) Shoveling heavy snow[b] Shoveling 10/min (16 pounds)	Lumberjack[b] Heavy laborer[b]	Handball Squash Ski touring over hills[b] Vigorous basketball	Running (≥6 mph) Bicycle (≥ 13 mph or up steep hill) Rope jumping

Taken from Wenger N, Kass H, & Hellerstein H. *Rehabilitation of the Coronary Patient* New York: Wiley, Ed.2, 1984.
[a]May cause added psychological stress that will increase work load on the heart.
[b]May produce disproportionate myocardial demands because of use of arms or isometric exercise.

Figure 28.1.

A. Flail chest with pulmonary contusion right upper lobe is shown on the admission film of a motorcycle accident victim.

B. The same patient is shown on a ventilator in the ICU, and

C. 24 hr post admission.

D. The same patient 48 hr post admission develops a staph infection of the right upper lobe.

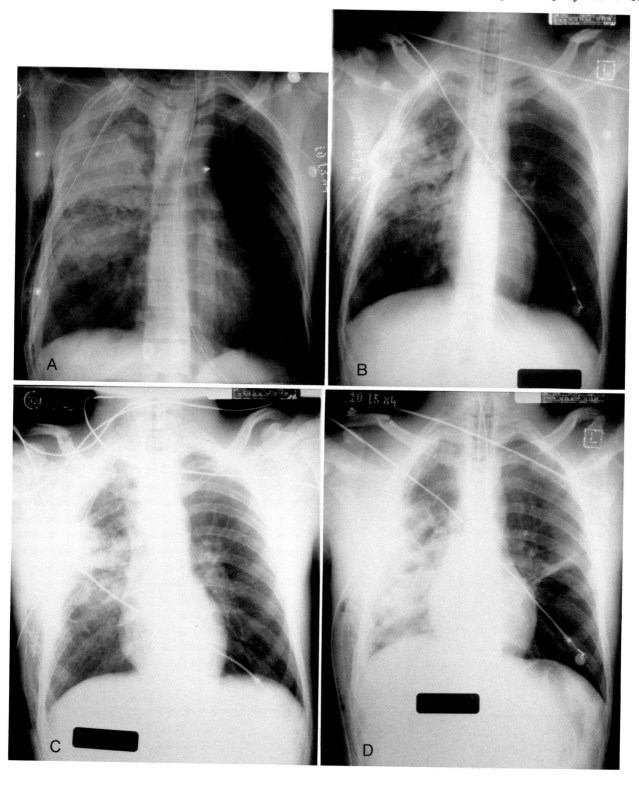

Figure 28.1.

Figure 28.1. (continued)

E. The same patient is seen 7 days post admission with empyema and staph pneumonia, and

F. Ten days post admission with bilateral staph pneumonia.

G. The same patient is shown 1 month post injury, 2 weeks post thoracotomy and decortication, and

H. One year post injury—field-and-track star at a local college.

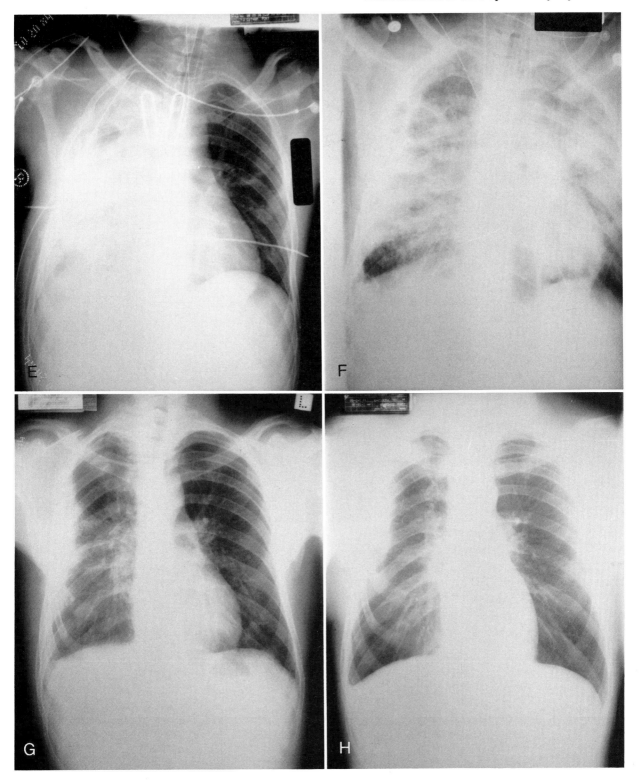

Figure 28.1. (continued)

Figure 28.1. (continued)

I. The patient is shown with a rupture of the innominate artery and thrombosed left vertebral artery; the aortogram was taken on the day of injury.

J. The same patient is shown 3 weeks post injury, exercising and as a student.

K. This patient has flail chest, pulmonary contusion, torn right main-stem bronchus, neuro-praxia right phrenic nerve, tears of right subclavian artery and vein, fractured sternum 4 weeks post injury, 1 week post repair of the right bronchus.

L. The same patient is shown 1 yr post injury, exercising, lifting weights, and as a housewife.

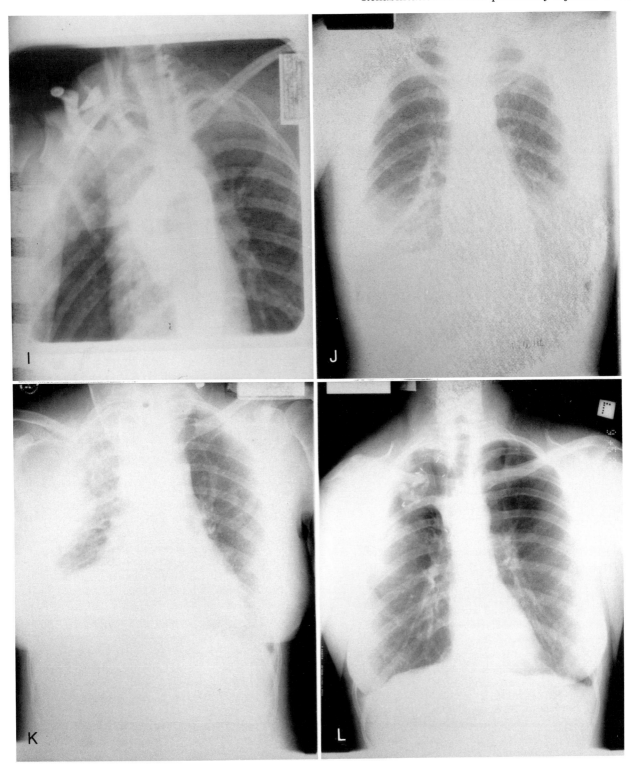

Figure 28.1. (continued)

Rehabilitation of Craniocerebral Injuries

Kiran Bhatt, M.D., and John J. Gerhardt, M.D.

There are eight basic types of head trauma:

1. *Scalp injuries.* May be simple lacerations or associated with linear or depressed skull fractures; any penetrating wound may be an avenue to spread of intracranial infection
2. *Cerebral concussion.* Transient posttraumatic brain dysfunction causing brief loss of consciousness and amnesia; no permanent organic brain damage
3. *Cerebral contusion.* Anatomical injury to brain, often occurring in conjunction with skull fracture and/or intracranial hematoma; *coup contusions*: directly beneath the impact; *contrecoup contusions*: on side of brain opposite site of external injury
4. *Acute extradural (epidural) hematoma.* Caused by low velocity injury and hemorrhage from middle meningeal vessels; associated with brief loss of consciousness and lucid interval followed by progressive neurological deficits; may progress to transtentorial herniation; posterior fossa hematomas mostly extradural
5. *Acute subdural hematoma.* Caused by high velocity impact; 20% are bilateral; often connected with contusion; is becoming more common than epidural
6. *Intracerebral hematoma.* Bleeding from intracerebral vessels causes large space occupying lesion; often associated with contusion of brain
7. *Chronic subdural hematoma.* Usually occurs in older age group with minor injury; patient complains of headache with decreased intellectual functioning and of mental alertness, which may gradually lead to loss of consciousness
8. *Subarachnoid hemorrhage.* May be spontaneous or associated with contusion as usual cause is bleeding from small cerebral vessels; hemorrhage from present ruptured aneurysm is spontaneous rather than trauma-related

Special techniques useful in the diagnosis of head trauma include CT scans, electrodiagnosis, diagnostic ultrasound, and angiography.

Contributors: Linda Allaway, R.R.T., Cheryl Kosta, R.P.T., Kathy Mitchell, M.S.W., Blaise Scollard, M.A., C.C.C., Nita Sharp, O.T.R., Anne Smith, and Nelson Stevland, M.D.

With the assistance of Professor E. Scherzer, Medical Director, Ilse Lebic, R.P.T., the staff of the Rehabilitation Center for Craniocerebral injuries, Vienna XII, Austria; R. Ehret, M.D., and E. Sattlegger, M.D., Neurological Clinic, Singen, West Germany; B. Brown, M.D., Radiology Department, Kaiser Sunnyside Medical Center, Clackamas, Oregon; W. Zinn, medical director, R. Hohmeister, M.D., V. Mutter, R.P.T., and the staff of the Medical Clinic Bad Ragaz and Rehabilitation Center. Valens, Switzerland

CT SCANS

The computerized axial tomography (CT) scan is one of the most important aids in diagnosing craniocerebral injuries. It utilizes specialized X-ray equipment to depict several cross-sectional cuts of the head (see Fig. 29.1). An X-ray tube and computer receptors rotate around the head while the computer reconstructs slices taken during different rotations (see Figs. 29.2 and 29.3). Contrast media may be used intravenously for enhancement.

ELECTRODIAGNOSIS

Evoked Potentials

Evoked potentials are electrical wave forms of biological origin that are elicited by, and temporally related to, stimuli delivered to sensory receptors or nerves. Three types of evoked potentials are often used (see Fig. 29.4):

1. *Visual evoked potentials* are elicited by light stimuli delivered to the eyes, thereby stimulating the optic nerve and recording over the cerebrum. P_1 is the most significant wave form recorded at latency of approximately 1000 msecs
2. *Brainstem auditory evoked potentials* are elicited by delivering sound stimuli to the ear, thereby stimulating the cochlear nerve (VIII) and recording early latency wave forms from the brainstem. Interwave latencies are measured wave I–III = 2.6 msecs; wave III–V = 2.4 msec; and wave I–V = 4.7 msecs
3. *Somatosensory evoked potentials* are electrical wave forms recorded from the head or trunk in response to electrical stimulation of peripheral sensory nerve fibers. P_{10} is derived from the brachial plexus; N_{19} from an early cortical wave; and P_{23} from the contralateral cerebral cortex

Electroencephalography (EEG)

No specific EEG pattern is associated with head injury. The most common EEG finding after head injury is diffuse slow wave abnormalities (see Fig. 29.5). With mild to moderate head trauma, slowing of the α-rhythm or diffuse theta may be present. After severe head injury, generalized delta slowing may be seen. Abnormalities are seen in about 90% of patients with subdural hematomas, with correct lateralization in about 75% of the patients. A normal EEG does not exclude the possibility of a subdural hematoma. Recovery from uncomplicated head injuries is usually associated with resolution of the slow wave abnormalities and a return to more normal background activity. The return of a normal EEG pattern does not exclude posttraumatic seizures or persistent neurological deficits as an outcome.

Diagnostic Ultrasound (Ultrasonic Echography)

Ultrasonic echography utilizes a crystal transducer, which acts both to transmit a brief pulse of ultrasonic energy and to receive echoes of the pulse as they are reflected from interfaces between internal structures of the body (brain) echo. The echoes are displayed on a time base line of the oscilloscope. Ultrasonic echography is used to determine the midline or shift of the midline in the intracranial diameter in brain injuries or diseases. In Figure 29.6, the test is demonstrated on a model. The method is rapid, consistent, painless, requires no participation of the patient, is noninvasive, and, therefore, is completely safe. It can be done anywhere and has been found quite accurate. In larger centers it has been replaced for studies of the brain by CT scans which provide more information.

Angiography

Angiography has a place in the diagnosis of head injuries when a CT scan is not available and also in the determination of fistulas. It is an invasive method requiring injection of a dye. With the introduction of water-soluble dyes, the risks have been reduced.

ACUTE PHASE TREATMENT OF HEAD TRAUMA PATIENTS

In treating head trauma patients in the acute phase, certain basic steps should be followed:

1. Maintain respiration
2. Position the patient. Remember: 10 to 15% of all head trauma patients have concomitant acute C-spine injuries
3. Control bleeding
4. Correct hypovolemia
5. Provide immediate surgical intervention in cases of depressed skull fracture, expanding intracranial hematoma, CSF leak, ruptured spleen or liver, and, if indicated, fracture of extremities
6. Provide medical adjunctive treatment, i.e., control of cerebral edema, fluid balance, osmotic diuretics, and steroids, administering of anticonvulsants as indicated by the neurologist or barbituate treatment; temperature control, administering of antibiotics for prevention, and observation for overt infection; and maintenance of adequate oxygenation
7. Provide late surgical treatment, i.e., evacuation of hematoma, closure of fistula in cerebrospinal (CSF) leak, evacuation of abscesses, shunting procedure, or cranioplasty

SPECIAL ASPECTS

Respiratory therapy intervention is primary to successful management of the craniocerebral-injured patient. These patients may present with immediate airway problems requiring intubation and/or tracheostomy.

Cerebral swelling may be reduced by hyperventilation and hyperoxygenation and may require utilization of a mechanical ventilator. Impingement upon the respiratory control center, as a result of the injury and alteration of respiratory patterns, may further complicate the course of these patients.

The nature of the insult and the invasive procedures utilized require precise monitoring of the pulmonary status of the patient. Aspiration and pneumonia are common and require extensive respiratory care techniques, such as postural drainage with percussion and vibration (Figure 29.7).

ASSESSMENT OF HEAD TRAUMA PATIENTS

Head trauma patients require a complete physiatric evaluation (Fig. 29.8) and the appropriate intervention. The evaluation would include, for example:

1. Body positioning
2. Nutritional status
3. Bladder incontinence
4. Bowel problems (e.g., constipation or incontinence
5. Psychosyndrome (state of consciousness, sensory deficit, speech, memory, and orientation disturbance) as assessed by a physiatrist, psychiatrist, and psychologist
6. Functional capabilities in mobility and activities of daily living (ADL)
7. Short- and long-term prognosis, assessment of i.e., rehabilitation potential as assessed by a physiatrist and psychologist
8. Social capabilities, as assessed by a physiatrist and medical social worker

The respective intervention procedures would be:

1. Instruction in positioning
2. Oroparenteral nutrition
3. Organization of neurogenic bladder program
4. Implementation of a neurogenic bowel program
5. Therapy by a psychiatrist, psychologist, and speech pathologist as indicated
6. Involvement in, and prescription of, physical therapy and occupational therapy
7. Establishment of a therapy plan and decision to transfer to special head trauma rehabilitation center
8. Counseling of patient and family, marital counseling, economic advice, and placement.

Rehabilitation Potential

The rehabilitation potential prognostic factors of each head trauma patient should also be assessed. These factors are:

1. Age
2. Duration of coma and posttraumatic amnesia (edema)
3. Premorbid personality
4. Anatomical location and extent of injury
5. Clinical severity, i.e., seizures, visual perceptual deficits, communication deficits, or neuropsychiatric sequelae
6. Other complications

Mental Outcome: Cognitive and Perceptual Functions

Until recently, a satisfactory and universally acceptable means of defining coma was lacking, chiefly because the hierarchy of physical signs, including the depth of coma and reflecting the severity of brain injury, had not been decided. As the patient recovers, the process of returning to awareness is continuous; during its course, a number of signs of specific neurological dysfunction of brain damage are apparent. To assess rehabilitation potential and outcome, various methods have been tried. These methods have included not only the routine neurological examination but also the evaluation of the physiological function of individual muscles or complex movements, such as gait analysis, using sophisticated equipment including videotapes, pressure plates, and specially designed computers. Serial multimodality evoked potentials (MEP), somatosensory cortical evoked responses (SER), visual cortical evoked response (VER), and brainstem auditory evoked response (AER) have been used extensively and represent the most accurate single prognosis indicant, with prognosis increased to 93%.

For everyday clinical use, however, simple functional scales with numerical values, e.g., length of amnesia or duration of coma, have proven very practical and useful. Russel (1971) correlated the severity of injury with the time it takes the patient from the injury to regaining continuous memory, and called it the period of Post-Traumatic Amnesia (PTA). The scale is known as the PTA Scale.

Teasdale and Jennett (1976) made the most significant contribution to modern understanding of the assessment of disordered consciousness in the immediate postinjury period. They constructed the Glasgow Coma Scale (GCS), which provides a high level of accuracy in predicting the early outcome of injury (Fig. 29.9). The GCS involves all disorders of neurological function, which are divided into three categories: eye opening (E), motor response (M), and verbal performance (V). These categories were considered to comprise the most sensitive measure of severity and predictors of outcome. In the GCS, responses are scored separately, giving a total derived from E + M + V, with a range of 3 to 15 points. Ninety percent of the patients with scores of 8 or less are in coma. These patients are regarded as having had a severe head injury, given that the low score is maintained for a minimum of 6 hr from onset. Patients with scores from 9 to 11 have injuries of moderate severity, and patients with scores more than 12 are regarded as having had minor injuries.

Neurological and Psychological Testing

The neurological evaluation of head trauma patients should include:

1. Mental state
2. Psychological testing (where indicated)
3. Evaluation of localized brain lesion
4. Cranial nerve examination
5. Cerebellar function testing
6. Posture and gait evaluation
7. Muscle testing
8. Testing of sensory function
9. Reflex testing, including pathological reflexes and signs

Evaluation of mental state, brain functions and brain areas (see Fig. 29.10) (Brodman) should include:

1. Level of consciousness, sensorium
2. General behavior
3. Mood, emotional status
4. Intelligence
5. Content, thought
6. Insight
7. Language, comprehension

As part of the total evaluation of the patient, a group of tests commonly are used by the trained psychologist for the assessment of: intellectual capabilities, personality traits, interests, evidence of organic brain disease, and related problems. These may be objective or projective in character, and are usually administered in a combination rather than as single tests. Among the more frequently used are the Wechsler-Bellevue Intelligence Test (for adult intelligence), the Stanford-Binet Intelligence Test (for children and adolescents), the Bender-Gestalt Test (for visual motor function), the Minnesota Multiphasic Personality Index (for personality profile), and the Rorschach Test (for projection of personality features, etc.).

MANAGEMENT OF HEAD TRAUMA PATIENTS IN THE REHABILITATION UNIT

Patients can be transferred to the rehabilitation unit when they are more stable medically, when they are able to follow simple instructions consistently, and when they have shown further rehabilitation potential.

A comprehensive assessment of the patient for his or her rehabilitation potential should be done by team members (physiatrist, rehabilitation nurse, physical therapist, occupational therapist, psychologist, speech therapist, dietician, recreational therapist, and social worker). A team conference should be held to set short- and long-term goals, to estimate the projected length of stay in the rehabilitation facility, and to outline treatment plans and strategies. The patient and his or her family should then meet with the team to discuss this as they are considered invaluable as team members.

Rehabilitation Nursing

Proper body positioning; nutrition maintenance; the prevention of decubiti, contractures, aspiration pneumonia; orientation training, regulation of the bowel and bladder; and the continuation of activities learned by patients in various therapies are all functions of the rehabilitation nurse (see Fig. 29.11). The nurse is also responsible for management of any complications that arise (see Table 29.1).

PHYSICAL THERAPY

Physical therapy deals with a variety of treatments for progressive mobilization, range of motion, stretching of tight muscles, development of muscle tone, bed mobility,

Table 29.1.
Management of Complications by Rehabilitation Nurses

Complications	Prevention/Treatment
Central	
Posttraumatic Epilepsy	Control EEG, antiseizure medication (e.g., Dilatin, Phenobarbital)
Hydrocephalus	Observe/shunt
Intracranial Hypertension	Observe/antihypertensives
Chronic Subdural Hematoma	Observe/surgical evaluation
Diabetes insipidus	Fluid restriction/pitressin
Intracranial abscess	Operative evacuation
CSF leakage	Fistula closure
Parkinsonism	Sinemet
Peripheral	
Aspiration Pneumonia	Positioning nasogastric (NG) tube or gastrostomy
Decubitus	Positioning/local dressing
Contractures	Physical Therapy: range of motion (ROM) stretching, splinting, surgical release
Fractures	Immobilization/internal or external fixation
Peripheral nerve injuries	Observe/operative repair
Shoulder/hand Syndrome	Physical therapy; ROM/ edema control; analgesics (sympathetic block by injection or electrical nerve block)
Periarticular Ossification Arthropathy (POA)	Gentle ROM/observe for maturation

sitting and standing balance, transfer training, and gait training with assistive devices, i.e., braces, crutches, and canes (Fig. 29.12). Modalities like cold or heat, ultrasound, and electricity are used as needed. Special techniques such as proprioceptive neuromuscular facilitation or Bobath inhibition of abnormal tone and movements are widely applied. Hydrotherapy and exercises in the swimming pool also prove very beneficial. Activities and games in groups are integrated into physical and occupational therapy programs.

PROPRIOCEPTIVE NEUROMUSCULAR FACILITATION

The normal healthy human body has neuromuscular mechanisms that enable it to respond to the everyday demands of life. The abnormal neuromuscular mechanism is not capable of these demands or normal responses. These abnormalities could be a result of a congenital problem, trauma, or disease. Manifestations of the above can be seen as weakness, incoordination, decreased range of motion, muscle spasm, or spasticity. Any one or a combination of these problems can be treated effectively with techniques of proprioceptive neuromuscular facilitation (PNF).

The techniques of PNF recognize potential in weakened areas of the body and utilize stronger body parts to strengthen the weakened ones. In treatment, exercise movement is purposeful and specific, directed toward functional goals and optimal development of strength, coordination, and endurance. Attention also is given to stimulate basic righting and equilibrium reactions. PNF techniques may be confined to increasing fine hand coordination or utilizing the gross motor ability and reflex integration of the developmental sequence (Fig. 29.13).

Credit for the development of the PNF approach to therapeutic exercise is given to Herman Kabat, who developed it over a 5-year period at the Kabat-Kaiser Institute in Washington, D.C. Dr. Kabat's work has been refined, published, and taught by Dorothy Voss and the late Margaret Knott.

Today, physical therapists throughout the world are utilizing techniques of PNF.

THE BOBATH TECHNIQUE

The Bobath technique of treatment is based on principles developed by Berta Bobath, a physical therapist, and Dr. Karel Bobath, a neurologist.

The basic concept is to treat the body as a whole by using techniques to facilitate movement on the paretic side and trying to gain symmetry of body and movement. Too often taught compensatory techniques have been utilized for the uninvolved side, and some of these techniques actually have contributed to the abnormal tone and posture on the involved side. The Bobath concept attempts to inhibit abnormal tone and movement so that normal patterns can begin to be facilitated until, through guidance and repetition, they become more automatic. The technique should begin in the acute hospital with correct positioning to encourage body symmetry and to decrease the development of abnormal tone.

From the beginning, the patient should be made aware of his or her paretic side by giving tactile input from the involved side. The patient should be told what is being done and why. The patient should be taught how to take care of his or her involved side as well as how to move in bed, come to a sitting position, transfer to a chair, and begin self-dressing (Fig. 29.14).

During the treatment sessions, it is important that abnormal tone is inhibited while the patient moves toward normal tone (see Fig. 29.15). The patient may need constant input from the therapist until he or she begins to feel this symmetrical posture in his head, neck, and trunk. As the patient is encouraged to bear weight through the affected side, the spasticity of the trunk, arms, and legs will be inhibited, making further treatment easier. This technique is most effective when applied by all members of the interdisciplinary team, not only physical and occupational therapists. Only a few physicians are familiar with the technique.

As Louise La Pitz, chief physical therapist in Bad Ragaz Switzerland (formerly, the Mayo Clinic) stated during the Congress of the International Rehabilitation Medicine Association (IRMA) in 1978:

Nurses are the people who are with the patients most of the time, not physical therapists and not occupational therapists—it's important that they are working with the team.

The Bobath technique to decrease spasticity should be taught to the entire team, including the patient and the patient's family, in order to secure its application to any activity the patient might be performing. In the brain-injured patient, as Dr. Wilhelm Zinn, Medical Director of the Clinic Valens in Switzerland, stated at the IRMA Congress in 1978 the greatest emphasis is placed on three-dimensional recognition and movement patterns. This is best achieved by communication between the patient and team members. Teaching and learning intertwine mutually and communication is by way of tactile/kinesthetic, rather than audiovisual channels. The Bobath technique provides just this.

HYDROTHERAPY

Water is an excellent medium for the mobilization of joints with restricted motion as well as for muscular re-education. It provides an environment for general and special handling of healthy as well as disabled persons.

Hydrotherapy has to be based on the mechanical and thermal capacities of water (hydrodynamics) and on the physics of the human body immersed in that medium. In this concept, the healthy or disabled human being is regarded as a mobile machine with levers, joints, contractile elements (McMillan) controlled by the central nervous system. On land it has to react against gravity at all times. In water, there is a second powerful force: buoyancy, and the human body has to develop new postural reactions to the combination of these two forces (Zinn, handout).

Some treatments can be applied in special tubs or tanks; others require a pool for the necessary buoyancy and space. Pool activities should be pleasurable, not perceived by the patient as "therapy." Water is not the natural environment of humans, therefore, therapists must rethink and relearn their approach in order to dispel fear that occurs in some persons, especially the handicapped.

There are four major rehabilitative approaches in the pool:

1. *Water-specific exercises*, which can be done in a proper tank using special techniques for orthopedic and neurological conditions (see Fig. 29.16).
2. *General exercises*, which can be performed in the pool for joint mobilization, training of weak muscles, improvement of posture, breathing, relaxation, and recreation.
3. *The McMillan-Halliwick method*
4. *Specific exercises with rings*, i.e., the Ragaz-Ring method, for mobilizing, strengthening, applying facilitation techniques, and getting the patient to become comfortably adjusted to the water environment in a nonthreatening way.

McMillan-Halliwick Method

The McMillan-Halliwick method of swimming instruction was introduced in 1950 at the Halliwick School for Handicapped Children in England. Initially, it was used for children with brain injuries. Later, the method was, and is still being, used successfully for all kinds of patients with impairment, disability, or handicaps. The method was developed by Dr. J. McMillan.

The principle of the McMillan-Halliwick method is to have fun and enjoyment in the water while learning. Introduction of the water environment as a place where the impaired patient can feel "able-bodied" and function without assistive devices in a pleasurable way makes him or her feel safe and secure. It minimizes the disability, maintains the health of the patient, and allows him or her to enjoy the newly discovered freedom of movements as well as improved function.

The program (see Fig. 29.17) is summarized in 10 points:

1. Mental adaptation to water environment
2. Disengagement from land situation and becoming independent in water
3. Learning vertical rotation—forward and backward, standing, and floating with assistance
4. Learning lateral rotation, rolling sideways
5. Learning combined rotation—vertical and lateral
6. Learning to feel for, and to utilize, buoyancy
7. Learning to balance and rest in water
8. Learning to float and glide in water
9. Learning elementary swimming movements
10. Applying first swimming style

The Halliwick method has proven that many musculo-skeletal- and neurologically impaired patients can be freed from the necessity of living with splints and assistive devices while in water. They need to learn to assume a "breathable" position in water and to return to such a position in any event and under any circumstances. Therapists need not be top athletes in order to teach this method, but they must be secure and comfortable in water and have special skills and understanding to guide the patient in working with buoyant forces and not against gravity, as on land. They need to see and assess the impairment of the handicapped person from the technical-mechanical, rather than medical, point of view and must apply the proper mechanics, which differ somewhat in every case. The body of the impaired patient may not be symmetrical any longer, as for example in a hemiplegic or hemiparetic patient after cerebral injury. Special corrective positions and movements must be taught to those patients to allow them to balance in water and to return to breathable positions.

Ragaz-Ring Method

The Ragaz-Ring method (Fig. 29.18) was developed for mobilization of joints with restricted motion, muscle re-education, and muscle strengthening. Using Bobath techniques, inhibition of abnormal tone and movements and facilitation of normal pattern can be enhanced.

The pelvis is supported with inflated rings (inner tubes) and the head, with a life-preserverlike inflated collar. This gives the patient a feeling of total security in water and allows him or her to perform the specific exercises without anxiety or fear. The therapist always should be with the patient in the pool.

OCCUPATIONAL THERAPY

Occupational therapists should be involved with head injury patients from the acute stage, through the recovery stage, and until the patient is back to resuming his or her maximum potential for all activities of daily living. Assessment of both cognitive and physical function is imperative at the acute stage so that the therapist can plan the treatment accordingly. The therapist needs to be aware of both cognitive and atypical stages of recovery and must be able to modify treatment procedures in order to maximize function. The therapist should consider also the premorbid social history, life-style, and family support available.

Mobility and techniques used to regain motor control should be based on the Bobath method of inhibiting abnormal tone or motor function prior to trying to strengthen motor control. The Bobath theory of not trying to superimpose normal tone on abnormal tone should be adopted. Thus, abnormal patterns and tone should first be inhibited. When the patient is able to feel normal pattern, he or she then can work with the therapist to regain and strengthen these patterns.

Other areas covered through occupational therapy are increasing activities of daily living, including feeding, dressing, grooming, personal hygiene, bathing, and training in these areas; increasing abilities to attend bimanual visual coordination tasks; increasing concentration and organization of multiple stimuli skills; decreasing distractibility; and increasing concreteness of thinking. As the patient progresses in cognitive retraining, advanced activities of daily living (ADL), such as planning meals, shopping, development of a budget for effective money management, and driver evaluation, should be addressed. Avocational and leisure-time skills may also be explored. Therapy that might be utilized in addressing these issues include training in the development of the ability to break tasks down into parts for problem solving, presenting the patient with increasingly complex cognitive testing drills, and possibly eventually focusing on the types of skills needed for employment. Rest and dynamic splints are applied as necessary. The occupational therapist finally performs prevocational assessment, assigns patients to manual arts therapy or industrial workshops, and designs a work hardening program (Fig. 29.19).

SPEECH LANGUAGE PATHOLOGY

Patients with closed head injury frequently progress through a series of stages in regaining cognitive and communication skills. Treatment programs must be designed to stimulate and facilitate the patient's abilities at each stage of the recovery process. For those patients functioning at a low level of consciousness, therapy should focus on stimulating the basic sensory modalities, i.e., auditory, tactile, olfactory, and gustatory. With the patient having severe dysphagia, oral motor stimulation to increase preswallowing skills should be utilized. Thereafter, special positioning and feeding techniques can be used to decrease risk of aspiration and to advance the patient through a series of dietary progressions, from pureed food with thickened fluids to a regular diet.

The receptive and expressive language disorders resulting from a closed head injury are directly influenced by the underlying cognitive deficits, i.e., attentional abilities, auditory and visual discrimination and comprehension, short- and long-term memory, and finally, abstract reasoning skills. For the nonverbal patient (unable to speak because of physical limitations resulting from trauma), augmentative communication systems, such as communication boards both mechanical and electronic, devices which print out words and stimulate speech and gestural systems, will be utilized to provide the patient with a means of communication.

As the patient's communication skills improve, greater emphasis should be placed on integrating the patient back to normal social interactions. This involves increasing pragmatic communication skills, for example, how to listen and make appropriate comments within the relevant context of a conversation. Therapy should also assist the patient in developing self-monitoring skills and in facilitating the patient's appropriate independent interpersonal communication (Fig. 29.20).

PSYCHOTHERAPY

Treatment of chronic posttraumatic psychosyndrome (specific therapy of psychological disturbances secondary to organic cause) should involve:

1. Reaction training
2. Memory training
3. Concentration training (see Fig. 29.21)
4. Behavior modification therapy
5. Counseling

Repetitive performance and problem solving exercises are preferred to actual psychotherapy.

SOCIAL WORK

Medical social workers provide the interdisciplinary team with an assessment of the hospitalized patient and his or her family from the standpoint of physical, psychological, and social health. At Kaiser Sunnyside Medical Center in Clackamas, Oregon, the medical social worker automatically provides an early assessment for all spinal cord-injured, brain-injured, and neurologically impaired patients, and notifies the rehabilitation team members.

Head injuries and strokes are traumatic events that constitute a life crisis. In particular, individuals and families often have difficulty coping with the variable effects and unpredictable outcome of these events. Furthermore, strokes in particular usually result in short acute care hospitalizations, which demand rapid mobilization and planning on the part of the family. Family and individual coping is also effected by previous experiences with neurological difficulties and individual or family history of other diseases or disabilities. Recent, and sometimes remote, experiences with bereavement are important, as is a history of substance abuse in assessing resources and predicting coping ability.

A social worker gathers information that will lead to an assessment of the individual and family's previous level of functioning and available coping mechanisms. Social supports and financial resources also should be assessed. An appropriate group of interventions and approaches, based on characteristics particular to each individual's situation, should be developed.

A brief, crisis-oriented model of treatment is appropriate for use in acute care hospitals. Treatment is aimed at helping the patient and his or her family maintain maximum control and independence. This model can be characterized by eight principles:

1. Immediate intervention
2. Action orientation
3. Limited goal
4. Realistic hope and expectations that clients can cope effectively
5. Support
6. Focused problem solving
7. Self-image protection and enhancement
8. Self-reliance

One aspect of social work treatment is the facilitation of appropriate discharge plans, such as placement in a skilled nursing facility (SNF) or rehabilitation hospital. When individuals are able to return home, various community resources may be used. These include home health agencies, for home therapy and nursing needs; the American Heart Association; stroke clubs; Loaves and Fishes; and mental health services. For individuals who require long-term custodial care, foster placement services and intermediate care facilities are available.

In working with neurologically impaired individuals, medical social work services intend to reduce, to the extent possible, the negative impact on the individual and family, by identifying and utilizing their assets and by mobilizing community resources to assist as needed.

Certain countries also have specially trained recreational therapists, who treat patients during recreational hours. They involve the patient in individual and group activities to improve orientation, socialization, and communication (see Fig. 29.22). Visual hand coordination and

problem solving skills are improved by games. They also develop programs of meaningful recreational activities, individualized for each patient on the bases of abilities, interests, and available resources, to improve the quality of leisure time after return to the community.

The medical social worker should provide weekly team conferences, discharge planning, and follow-up for the head trauma patient. Weekly team conferences monitor and guide the patient's progress, coordinate team effort toward common goals, and advise families of their involvement in patient care during various phases.

Discharge planning is initiated from the day of admission and should take into consideration the patient's need for adaptive equipment. Patient and family are advised as to the patient's activity level, precautions, and restrictions. The patient should be sent home overnight or for a weekend prior to his or her discharge. Assessment of long-term disability should be made.

As for follow-up, outpatient therapies should be continued. Referral to vocational rehabilitation is made. Clinical follow-up is done monthly at first to monitor medications (e.g., antispastic or anticonvulsant drugs), bowel and bladder program, gait, ADLs, driving, and return to work. Final outcome of head trauma disability usually takes longer than 1 year; hence, complete evaluation should be done every 3 to 6 months until progress is documented. The effort to rehabilitate head trauma patients is tedious; but, in the long run, dividends are paid.

SUPPORT GROUPS FOR FAMILY MEMBERS

Head injuries are called the "silent epidemic."

Long-term problems facing the brain-injured person and his or her family are many and complex (Fig. 29.23, also see Chapter 1). The family's need for support and acceptance is critical, from the time of initial hospitalization through discharge and the many months and often years following. Throughout the nation, there are support groups

Figure 29.1.

A. An enhanced CT scan of the head is prepared.

B. A CT scan of the head is taken (courtesy: University Hospital, Innsbruck, Austria).

C. A CT scan in a 6-month-old infant with craniocerebral injury is prepared. The mother is present to keep infant quiet and relaxed (Kaiser Sunnyside Medical Center).

D–E. A CT scan monitor (KSMC) and

E. X-ray evaluation are necessary in head injuries.

F. An X-ray of the skull of an injured child is taken upon admission in the shock room (courtesy: University of Innsbruck-Trauma Department).

G. a. The location of the middle meningeal artery is shown in the Krönlein's diagram, along with

b. An extradural hemorrhage and

c. A subdural hemorrhage (trephine holes are shown for each).

d. A subtemporal decompression is trephined after 1. A skin incision is made and position of burr holes are located. 2. A trephine and 3. Dahlgreen's forceps are used. 4. A spurting branch of the middle meningeal artery is ligated. The haematoma has been evacuated and is no longer visible. See the fracture line in the osteoplastic flap.

e. A depressed fracture of the cranial vault is elevated (from Russe, O: *An Atlas of Operation for Trauma*, Wien-Bonn, Wilhelm Maudrich).

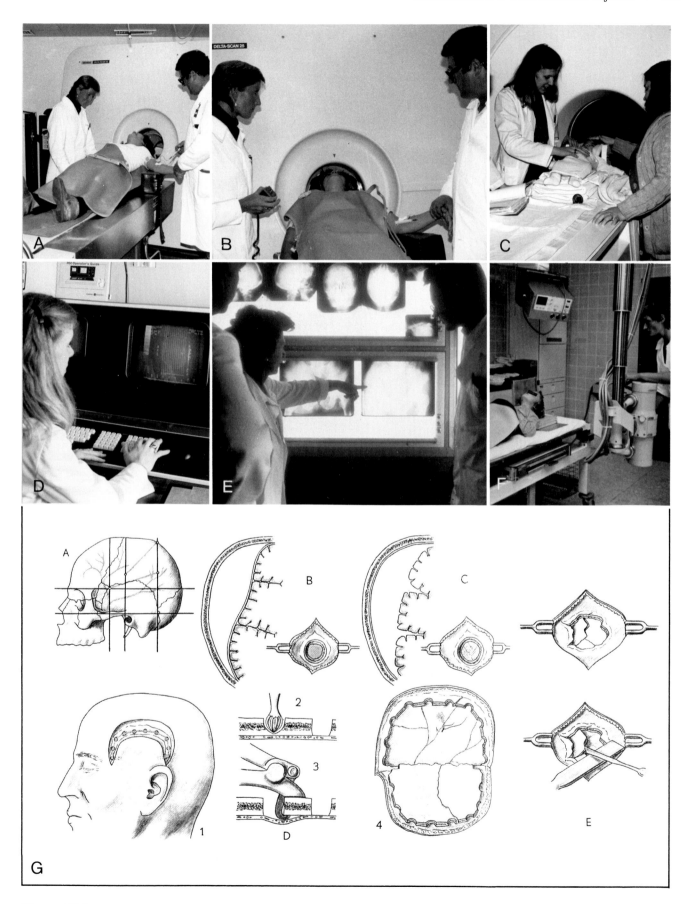

Figure 29.1.

for family members of the head-injured. These support groups offer families counseling, educational information, and a link with community resources. Support groups are comprised of both family members and professionals involved in the care and treatment of the head-injured. The primary caregiver often feels overwhelmed and isolated. A family support group offers acceptance, reassurance, and the more tangible help of respite care, activities for the head-injured, community service help, and the chance to share with others facing similar situations (Fig. 29.24).

The strength, social, and emotional support families derive from the support group is essential to their well-being and ability to continue as primary caregivers.

HIPPOTHERAPY

Hippotherapy is a relatively new approach in treatment of neurologically impaired patients. It has proven extremely beneficial in motor disorders with impaired balance and coordination secondary to craniocerebral injuries, cerebral palsy, and similar conditions (Fig. 29.25).

Figure 29.2. CT scans of various craniocerebral injuries.

A–C. Fronto basilar fracture (left), rhinorrhoea (*left*), facial paresis (*right*), and otorrhea (*right*) are shown. The patient is fully oriented and complains of headaches. The CT scan finds a clouding of the ethmoid sinus. Air is present in area of basal cisterns and subarachnoid space. Spotty changes are shown in the delineation of the brainstem and cerebral gyri, especially in the frontal and midline areas. Facial edematous contusion is shown in the left frontal and midline areas and facial edematous contusion in the left frontal and right parieto occipital areas. Air in ventricles is shown with the filling of the anterior horn.

D–F. An acute epidural temporobasal hematoma is shown on left. The hyperdense zone adjacent to the inner table of the middle cranial fossa is sharply delineated. Temporo basal fracture line, fracture of zygomatic arch, soft tissue swelling in upper eyelid, and discrete exophthalmos are shown. The sphenoid, ethmoid, and frontal sinuses are clouded. There is a suspicion of basal CSF fistula with equivocal air in region of basal cisternae. This was proven surgically.

G–H. In this fronto basal contusion, the intracerebral bleed on the right side is greater than on the left side. Facial edema and coagulated blood are shown in bilateral frontal and basal regions. There is a discrete shift of ventricles and an extrinsic compression of the right anterior horn. There is asymmetry in the area of the pars centralis and spontaneous resolution.

I. In this traumatic intracerebral hemorrhagic contusion, there is a midline shift with a flattening of spots in the low-density zone. Multiple spotty hyperdense foci are consistent with coagulated blood in the right superior parietal cortex.

Courtesy of R. Ehret, M.D., E. Sattlegger, M.D., Singen/West Germany. Review of the English version, Ben M. Brown, M.D., Dept. Radiology, Kaiser Sunnyside Medical Center, Clackamas, Oregon.

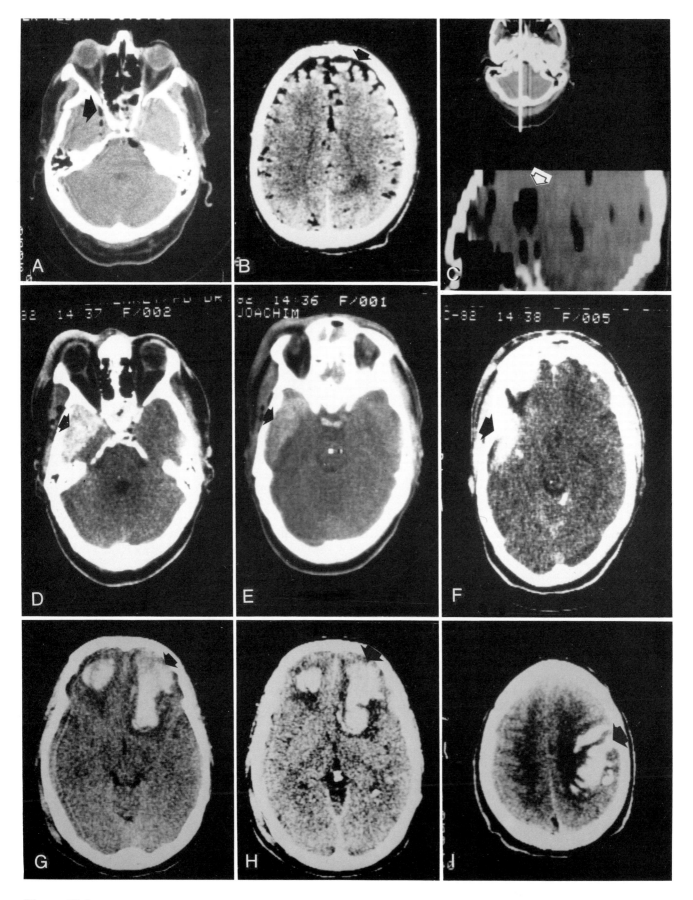

Figure 29.2.

Figure 29.3.

A–B. Isodense space occupies this subdural hematoma. The ventricle shift is from left to right and the pars centralis is compressed, the superior fronto-parietal and occipital gyri are flattened, and there is indirect evidence only of an isodense collection of fluid.

C. Subacute subdural hematoma on right. Mixed high- and low-density areas (7 only) consistent with blood, and CSF density with crescentric layering, displacement of brain, ventricular shift, and bilateral compression of gyri right greater than left.

D. In this chronic subdural hematoma in the left fronto parieto occipital region, the low-density, sharply marginated zone is consistent with edema, mixed with multiple areas of high density, consistent with blood overlying the right hemisphere and focal cavity formation. The gyri on left is flattened; the gyri on right, normal.

E. The status of this patient after severe craniocerebral injury is prolonged coma. Traumatic rupture of A-V fistula is suspected, and there is a high-density, streaky zone originating either at posterior cerebral artery or posterior communicating artery with drainage, confluence of the vein of Galen with the straight sinus.

F. Cerebrofrontal and cerebrobasal contusions are shown on the left. Low-density, sharply delineated zone of edema is shown in the anterior white matter in the left frontal area. Hyperdense focus is consistent with blood in the left frontal area.

G. The patient's status after a cerebral contusion is a shift of the right posterior horn with dilatation. The adjacent, sharply marginated cerebrospinal fluid (CSF) density focus is consistent with porencephaly.

H. The spontaneous subarachnoid hemorrhage is secondary to an aneurysm. High-density layering of blood is in basal perimesencephalic cisterns. Blood density covers over the gyri (isodense after a few days). Disturbance of CSF resorption and flow is seen with obstructive hydrocephalus.

I. In a minor cerebral injury in this patient on anticoagulant therapy, high-density space occupies a lesion with blood in the right frontal area. (Traumatic interacerebral hematoma is facilitated by anticoagulant therapy.)

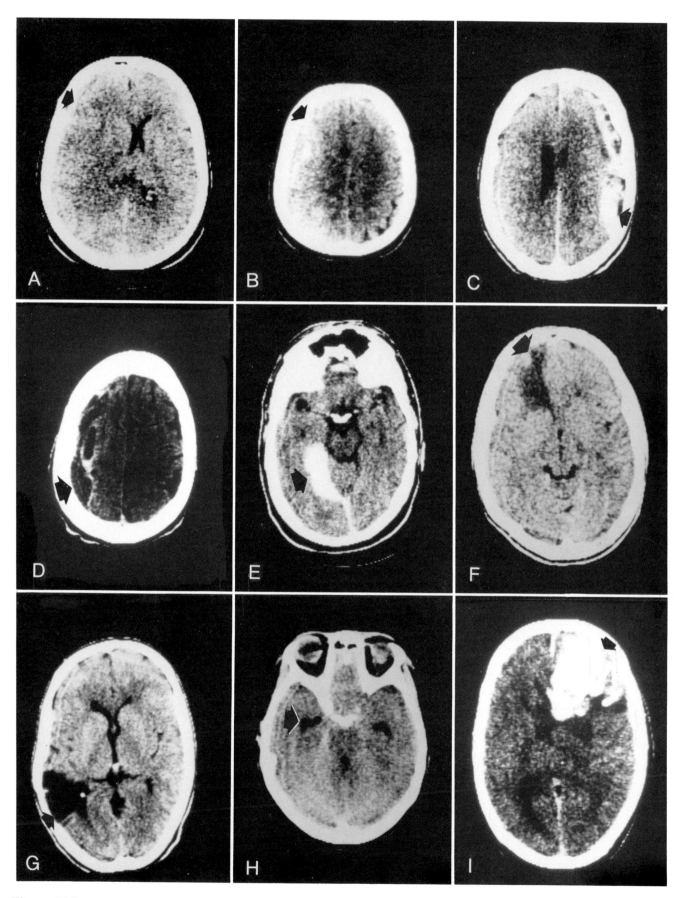

Figure 29.3.

Figure 29.4.

A. In this Visual Evoked Potential (VEP), left is normal; the right, absent. Diagnosis: Right intracerebral hemorrhage.

B. In this brainstem Evoked Potential (BSEP), Waves I and II are present; Wave III shows small amplitude, and Wave V is absent. This represents cerebral ischemia.

C. A normal BSEP is shown (courtesy of David R. Hampton, Ph.D., Director of Clinical Research; and Clarence Washington, M.D.; Cadwell Laboratories, Inc., Kennewick, WA 99336).

D. A normal Somatosensory Evoked Response is shown (courtesy of Neuro Diagnostics, Inc. Santa Ana, CA 92707).

E. Set-up for an auditory evoked potential study is shown.

F. Set-up for visual evoked potential study is shown.

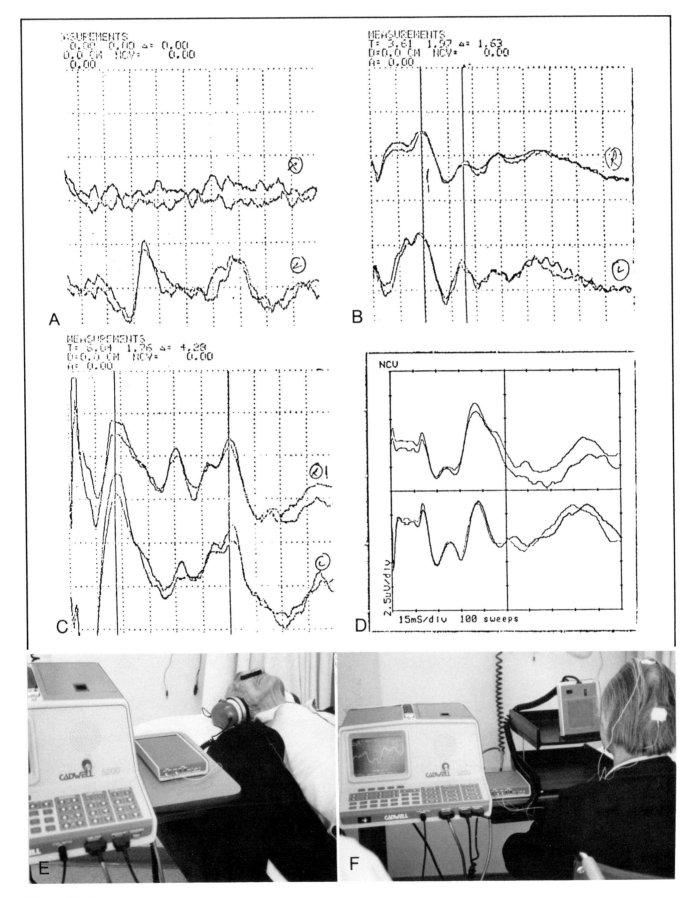

Figure 29.4.

Figure 29.5.

A. A normal EEG is shown in an alert adult.

B. An abnormal EEG demonstrates diffuse, bilateral slowing of EEG activity and attenuation of the faster frequency activity on the left and prominent left frontal focal slow activity. The findings suggest diffuse, bilateral cerebral dysfunction with greater dysfunction on the left plus focal cerebral dysfunction in the left frontal region. The EEG is from a 23-year-old man who sustained a head injury in a motorcycle accident, requiring the removal of an acute left frontoparietal subdural hematoma.

C. An EEG is recorded with the patient supine.

D. EEG equipment is shown.

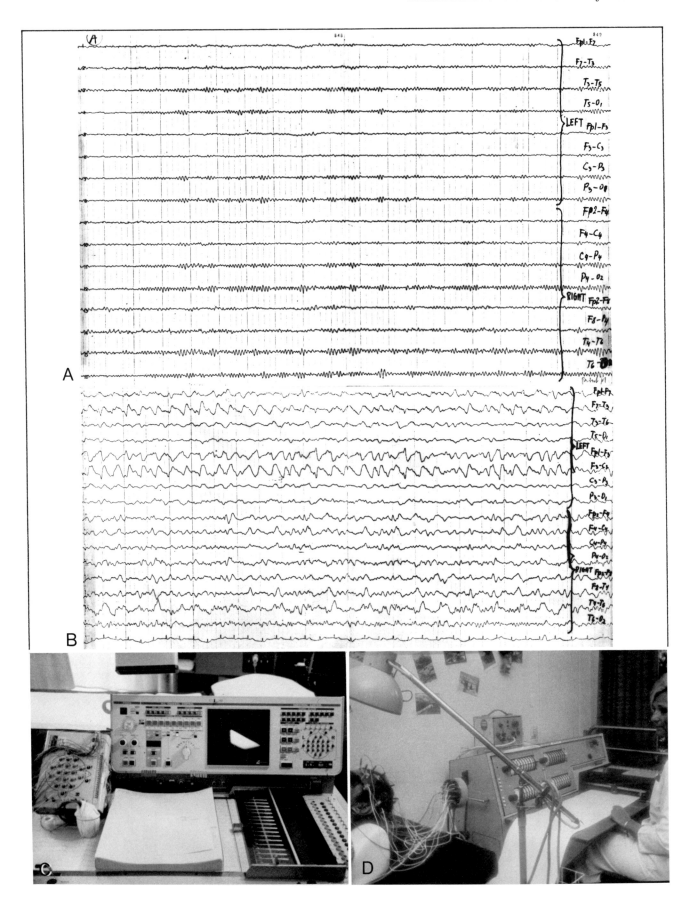

Figure 29.5.

Figure 29.6.

    A. An A-scan ultrasound and

    B. B-scan are shown.

    C. This normal ultrasonic echogram shows
        Nearside skin and face of transducer
        Nearside outer table of skull
        Nearside inner table of skull
        Normal midline echo
        Farside inner table of skull
        Farside outer table of skull, and
        Farside skin.

    D. This midline shift is away from the space occupying a supratentorial lesion (e.g., subdural hematoma).

    E. This angiography is in progress.

    F. The modern angiography unit has a monitor control table (Kaiser, Sunnyside Medical Center).

G–H. Cerebral angiogram, AP and lateral are shown.

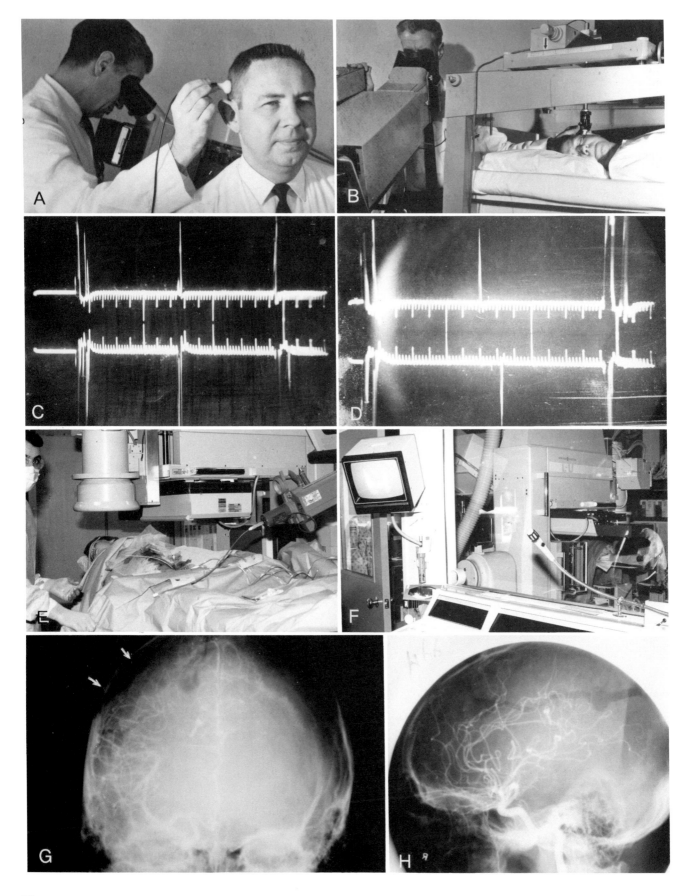

Figure 29.6.

Figure 29.7.

    A. Vibration massage is used to assist in loosening and removal of bronchial secretions. This is done for bronchial hygiene.

    B. Active breathing exercises are done with the use of a blow tube.

    C. A nasotracheal tube is suctioned.

    D. A nasotracheal tube is connected to an automatic respirator.

    E. A patient in intensive care who has a craniocerebral injury is positioned and a tracheostomy, hyperalimentation, respiration, and supervision of bowel and bladder evacuation are done

    F. This patient has polytrauma, including extremity fractures, and is in traction.

G–H. This patient with head trauma is in the regular ward of the acute hospital. Active range of motion (ROM) exercises are done with a protective net around the bed to prevent secondary injury because of transient confusion and disorientation. (Pictures A, B, and E–H courtesy Trauma Hospital Vienna XII) Director Professor Dr. Jahna

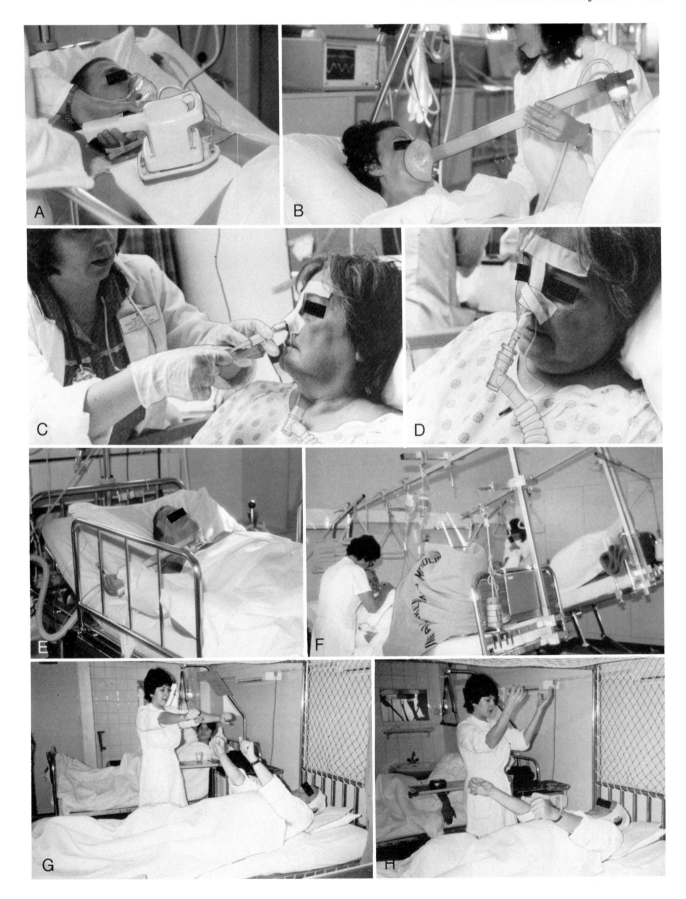

Figure 29.7.

Figure 29.8.

A. A neurological evaluation is conducted.

B. A visual field evaluation is conducted.

C. A fundoscopic evaluation is done.

D. Speech and level of consciousness are assessed by conversation.

E. Perceptual testing is done by an occupational therapist with figure ground cards.

F. Assessment of perceptual skills is done with spatial orientation sheets.

G. Testing and training visual recall are assessed using playing cards in general cognitive retraining.

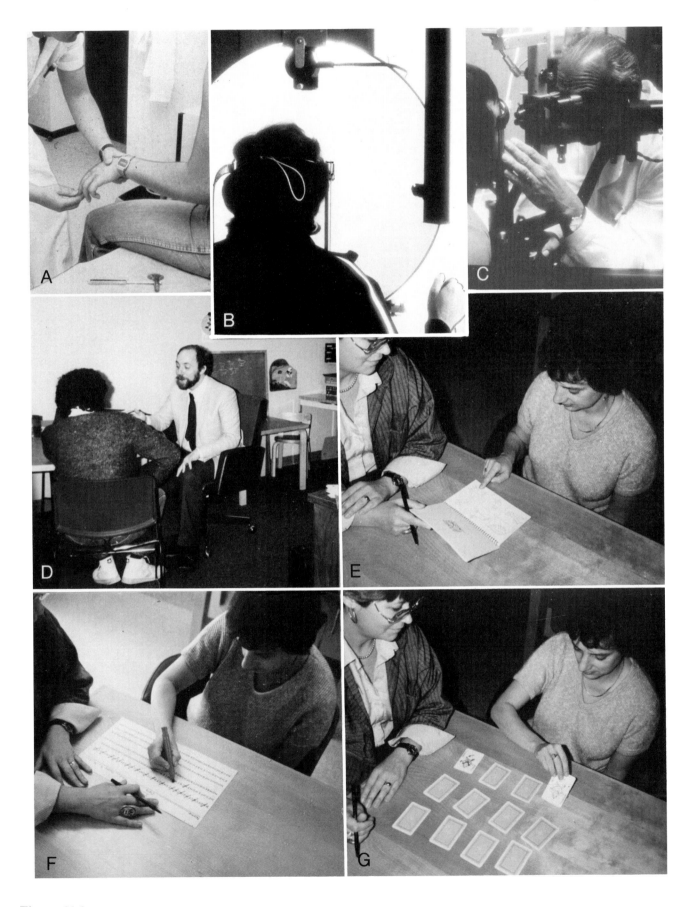

Figure 29.8.

Figure 29.9.

A. The Post Traumatic Amnesia (PTA) Scale is shown.

B. The Neurophysical Scale is shown. Its score is correlated with the PTA-Scale, the Social Scale etc.

C. In the Glasgow Coma Scale, scores of eye opening (E), best motor response (M) and verbal response (V) are added for a total ranging from 3 to 15. A score of 8 or less indicates severe brain injury if it is low for minimum 6 hr. A score from 9 to 11 indicates moderate severity and over 12, minor injury.

A

POST TRAUMATIC AMNESIA—PTA SCALE (Russel)

PTA: less than 10 minutes = very mild injury 1 hour to 1 day = moderate
    from 10 minutes to 1 hour = mild injury 1 day to 1 week = severe
                         longer than 1 week = very severe injury

B

NEUROPHYSICAL SCALE (Roberts)

Deficit	Score	Deficit	Score	Deficit	Score
Motor Deficit		*Speech*		*Cranial Nerves*	
Monoparesis	1	Partial aphasia	2	Each nerve	1
Monoplegia	2	Complete aphasia	4	Exception:	
Hemiparesis	3			Vision 1 eye	2
Hemiplegia	4	*Ataxia*		2 eyes	4
		Each limb		Hearing 1 ear	1
Sensory Deficits		Mild/moderate	1	2 ears	2
One arm/leg, partial	1	Severe	2		
One arm/leg, full	2	Dysarthria		*Physical Deficits*	
One arm/leg and part		Mild/moderate	1	Mild/moderate	1
trunk	3	Severe	2	Severe	2
Arm/leg and truck	4	Dysphagia			
		Mild/moderate	1		
		Severe	2		

C

GLASGOW COMA SCALE (Teasdale and Jennett)

Examiner's Test		Patient's Response	Score
Eye opening	Spontaneous	Opens eyes on own	E4
	Speech	Opens eyes when asked to in a loud voice	3
	Pain	Opens eyes when pinched	2
	Pain	Does not open eyes	1
Best motor response	Commands	Follows simple commands	M6
	Pain	Pulls examiner's hand away when pinched	5
	Pain	Pulls a part of body away when examiner pinches him	4
	Pain	Flexes body inappropriately to pain (decorticate posturing)	3
	Pain	Body becomes rigid in an extended position when examiner pinches victim (decerebrate posturing)	2
	Pain	Has no motor response to pinch	1
Verbal response (talking)	Speech	Carries on a conversation correctly and tells examiner where he is, who he is, and the month and year	V5
	Speech	Seems confused or disoriented	4
	Speech	Talks so examiner can understand victim but makes no sense	3
	Speech	Makes sounds that examiner can't understand	2
	Speech	Makes no noise	1
Coma Score (E + M + V) = 3 to 15			

Figure 29.9.

Figure 29.10.

Frontal Lobe
4 Principal motor area (Pre-Rolandic), lesion: paralyses, alexia
6 Premotor area (part of extrapyramidal tract circuit), lesion: forced grasping
8 Frontal eye movement and pupillary change area
9
10 Frontal association areas (higher intellectual and psychic function; lesion: changes of per-
11 sonality and character
12
44 Motor speech (Broca) area; lesion: motor asphasia, agraphia

Parietal Lobe
3
1 Postcentral principal sensory areas; lesion: paraesthesia, anaesthesia, anarthria
2
5
7 Sensory association areas; lesion: astereognosia
39
40 Association area; lesion: sensory and amnesic aphasia, ideomotor apraxia, alexia

Temporal Lobe
41 Primary auditory receptive area; lesion: auditory agnosia
42 Associative auditory cortex
38
40
20 Association areas
21
22

Occipital Lobe
17 Primary visual receptive cortex (striate); lesion: visual agnosia, visual field defects, visual
   hallucinations (macular blindness?)
18
19 Visual association areas; lesion: defective visual orientation (spatial)
23
24 Pronounced sensory and motor autonomic (sympathetic) effects; (muscle tone)
47 Anterior insula
   Autonomic effects (respiration, blood pressure)

(Reprinted with permission from Russe, Gerhardt, King, *An Atlas of Examination, Standard Measurements and Diagnosis in Orthopedics and Trauma*, Hans Huber, 1972).

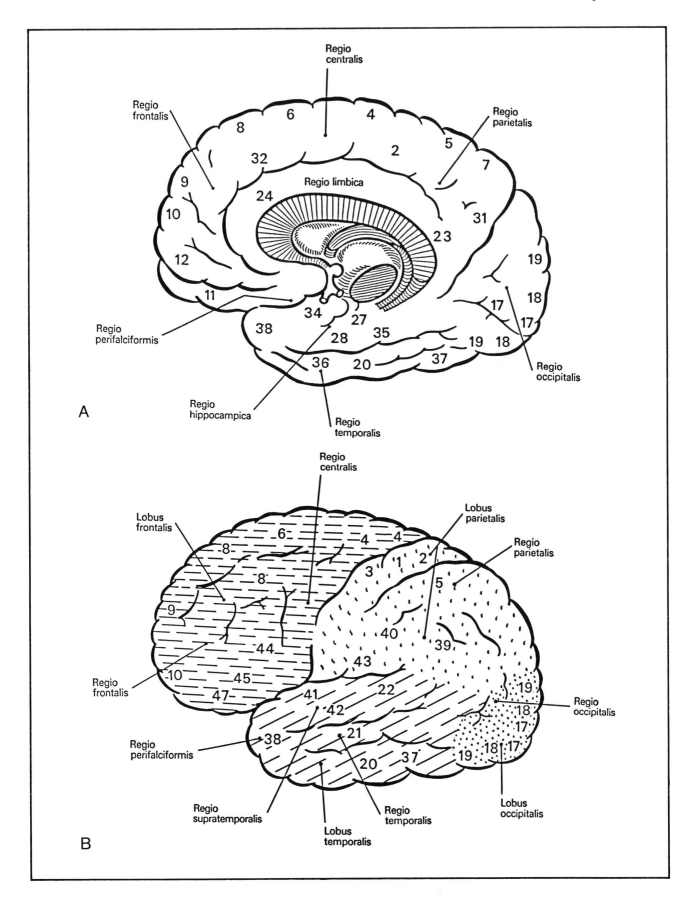

Figure 29.10.

Figure 29.11.

A. Positioning in bed.

B. In positioning in bed, areas of frequent decubitus sites are marked on the patient for teaching purposes.

C. An X-ray of a Periarticular Ossification Arthropathy (POA) is shown. This condition occurs in craniocerebral injuries frequently, also in joints of the upper extremity.

D. An X-ray of aspiration pneumonia is shown.

E. Harris/Bobath sling is shown.

F. A Schanz cervical collar is used in head and C-spine injuries.

G. A training belt is used for spasticity.

H. A closed circuit television system is useful for nursing supervision of patient rooms and hallways.

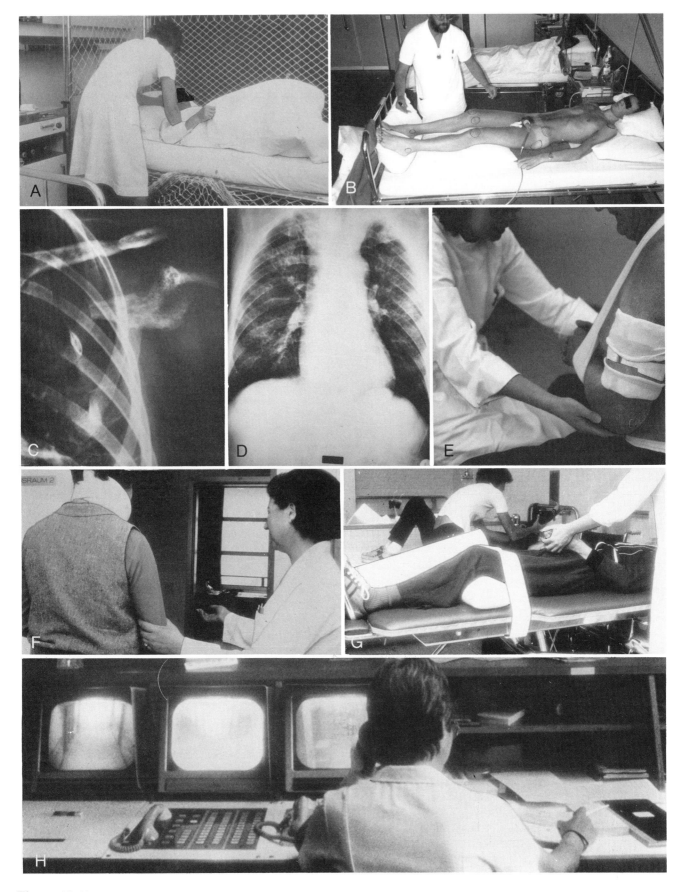

Figure 29.11.

Figure 29.12.

A. Upper and lower extremity ataxia after craniocerebral injury are shown. Build-up of muscle tone is done in a standing position. Previous preparation for gait training was done with the PNF technique.

B. Gait training in parallel bars after PNF training.

C. Severe spastic right hemiparesis. Lower extremity is in flexor synergy pattern. Paretic leg is splinted in extension to enable gait training. Lofstrand crutch provides additional ambulation aid.

D. Gait training using Bobath technique in a patient with right hemiparesis. Therapist controls pelvis. Upper extremity is in reflex inhibitory position.

E. Shoe and Perlstein Splint in order to restrain movement of foot into pathological pattern; namely, plantar flexion and inversion. An improvised peroneal strap was applied to support splint only during therapy.

F. Improvised peroneal strap using elastic bandage and tongue blade. Dorsiflexion and eversion of foot can be effectively secured. This is used only in mild hemiparesis.

G. Severe left spastic hemiparesis with upper extremity predominance. Gait training with three-point cane. Therapist applies hip and knee control.

H. Severe left spastic hemiparesis. Therapist applies knee and heel control during gait training.

(Fig. 29.12–29.16 courtesy of Special Rehabilitation Center for Cranio Cerebral Injuries, Vienna XII).

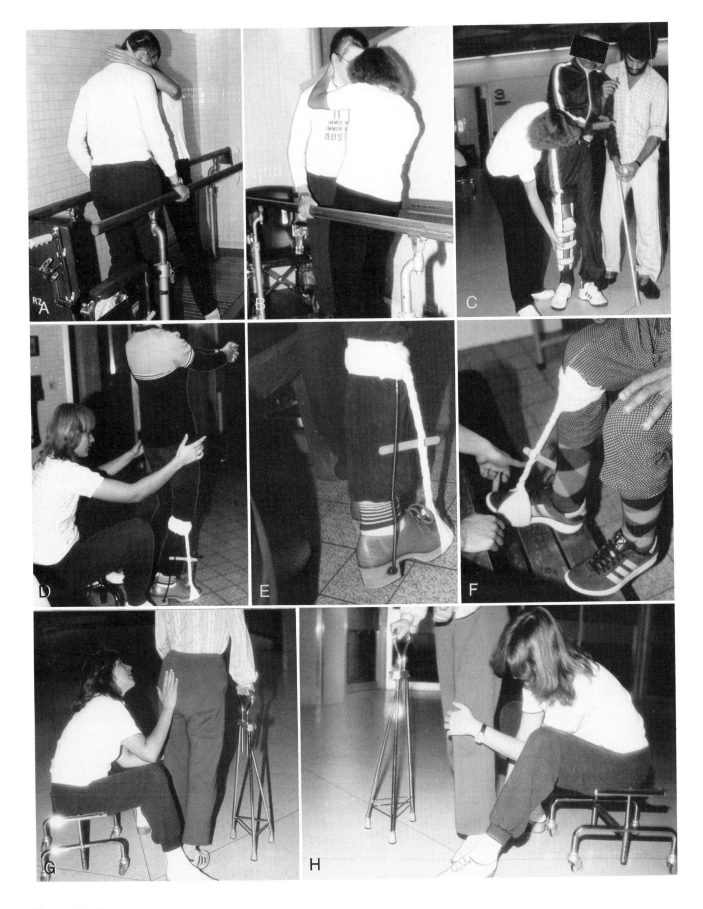

Rehabilitation of Craniocerebral Injuries / 373

Figure 29.12.

Figure 29.13.

    A. Severe cerebellar ataxia: muscle tone building exercises are done with distal resistance in a diagonal pattern. A patient is prepared for wheelchair-to-mat transfer.

    B. In the wheelchair-to-mat transfer, the therapist provides pelvic control while agonist and antagonist muscles are contracted. (The therapist pushes patient in the desired direction, with patient resisting the movement.)

    C. Stabilization in quadruped position should be done in all directions, including diagonal. Head control is important.

D,E,F. In PNF, body rolling is done while therapist applies resistance to the patient's head; then the patient holds position.

    G. In PNF, body rolling is done with resistance on the lower extremity and

    H. On the upper extremity.

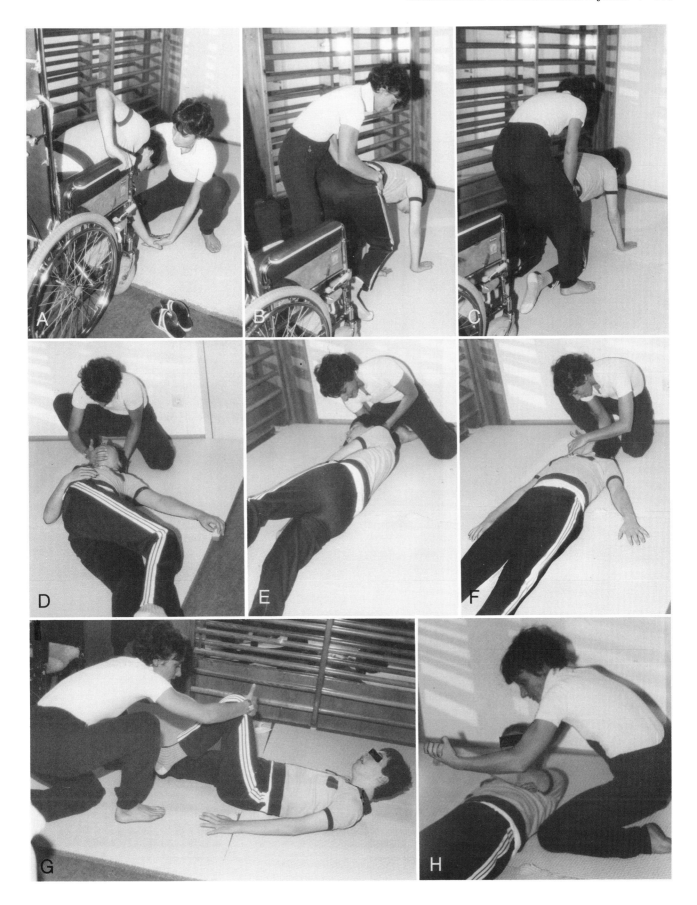

Figure 29.13.

Figure 29.14.

A. In a left spastic hemiparesis, facilitation of activity in shoulder and elbow is done functionally as the patient holds an air-filled balloon in both hands.

B. The patient is prepared for controlled sitting up from the supine position over the affected side.

C–D. A certain sequence is followed in sitting up from the supine position over the affected side.

E. The patient is prepared for transfer from bed to wheelchair.

F. Transfer from bed to wheelchair is done with the assistance of the therapist.

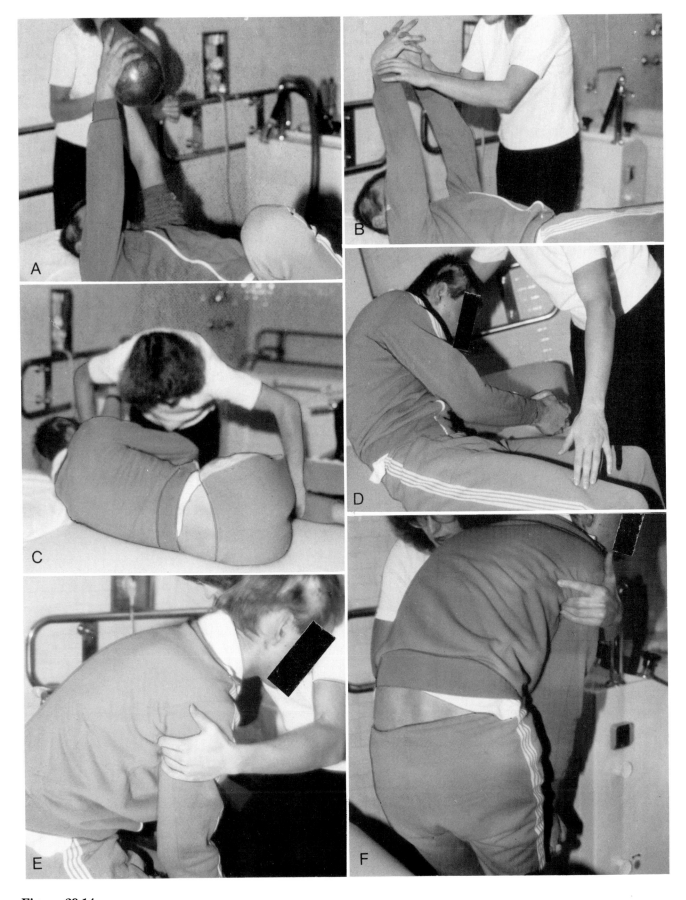

Figure 29.14.

Figure 29.15.

A. In left spastic hemiparesis, balance exercises are done on a bolster. Controlled sitting and rotation lower muscle tone.

B. Weight shifting, lengthening of left side, and rotation to reduce muscle tone also are helpful. Fingers are interlocked to inhibit hand motion (left spastic hand is to the right of midline).

C. In pushing up on the bolster, the patient's weight is shifted forward on both arms to reduce muscle tone.

D. To achieve a sitting position, the patient shifts his or her weight forward to his or her arm; then raises the pelvis and shifts the body weight onto lower extremities to reduce muscle tone.

E. Weight shifting to the left side and weight bearing on the left reduces muscle tone.

F. In this quadriparetic child, post craniocerebral injury, muscle tone-reducing exercises are done on a Bobath ball.

G. Patients with spastic quadriparesis also do balance exercises on the ball.

H. Balance exercises on a Pezziball are done in a sitting position. The patient raises to standing position with upper extremity facilitation.

I. Spastic quadriparesis exercises for full weight bearing and hip and knee control are done on a rocking board.

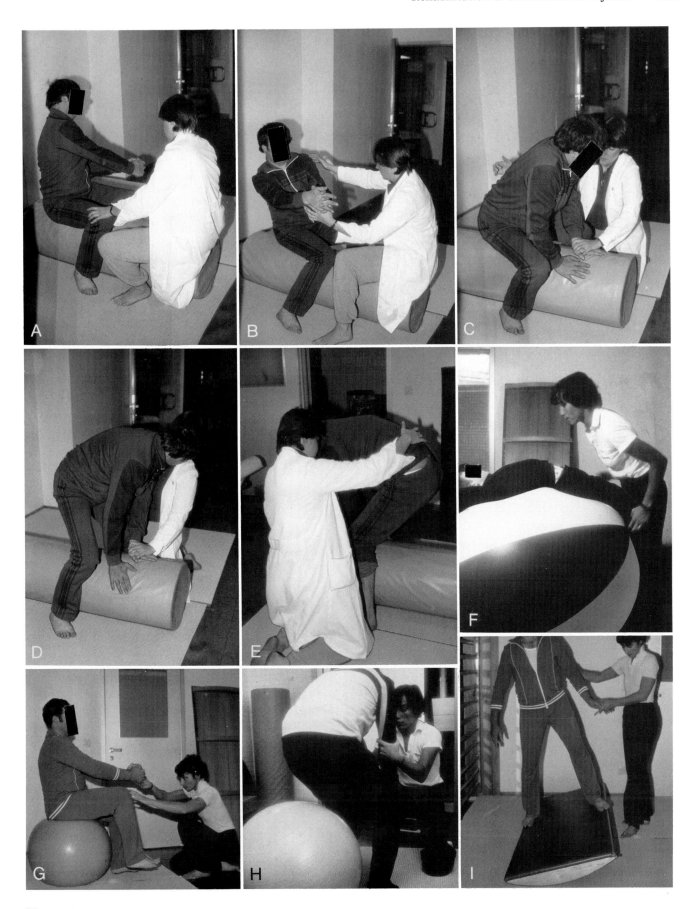

Figure 29.15.

Figure 29.16.

A–B. Hydrotherapeutic techniques include treatment in the Hubbard tank,
    C. the Stanger bath, and
    D. Underwater massage with water pressure, directed by the hydrotherapist.
    E. A wading pool is used.
    F. Exercises in a pool are beneficial.
    G. Group treatment in pool can involve the McMillan-Halliwick method.

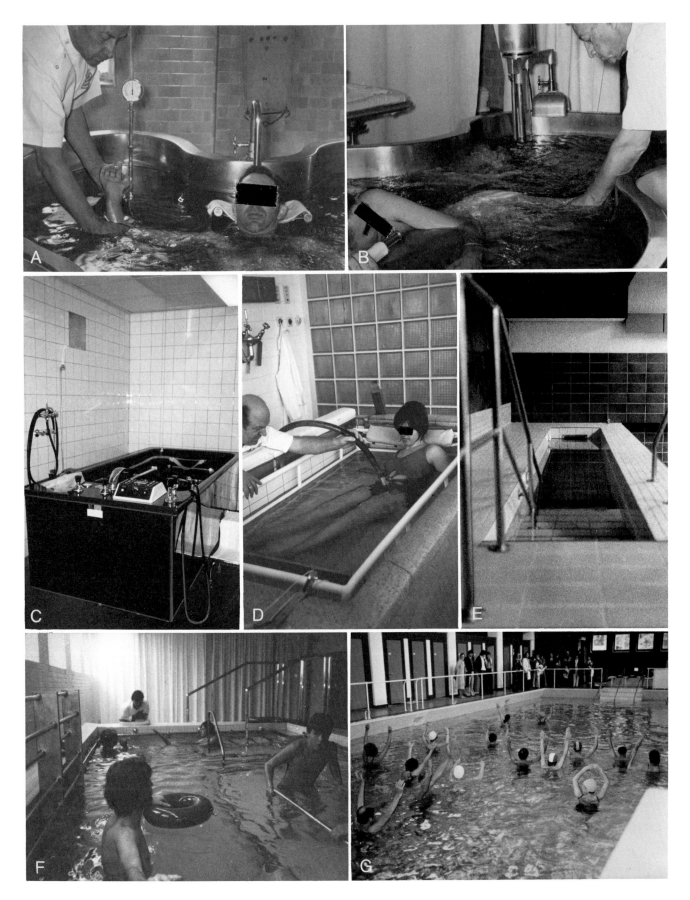

Figure 29.16.

Figure 29.17.

A. In sitting balance exercises, the starting position (ASTE) is with the long axis of the body stabilized. The goal is to accomplish balance through control of vertical and lateral rotation. This ASTE is beneficial for bilateral arm activities, scapular protraction, and in hemiplegia for inhibition.

B. Sitting balance can use a smaller support surface. More control of vertical rotation is required. In balance reaction, head and trunk are important for "balance stillness."

C. In horizontal floatation, the ASTE is supine floating and the goal to control very unstable lateral rotation by balance reaction of head, trunk, and extremities.

D. A smaller supporting area can be the approximate size of the supporting hands of the therapist. The weight of the patient's hands is exposed to gravity. The effect is the uplift of the caudal part of body (which prevents sinking of caudal parts). This is used when vertical rotation is not well controlled.

E. In swimming, the ASTE is horizontal floatation and the goal, head position reaction, trunk symmetry, control of pelvis, and breath control.

F. When the ASTE is horizontal with lateral rotation (i.e., toward the hemiparetic side), the goal is movements over the hemiparetic side. Other goals are: breath control and strong balance reaction of the trunk through lengthening of the hemiparetic side (similar to good inhibition of trunk spasticity), (courtesy of Veronika Mutter RPT, Clinic Valens, Switzerland).

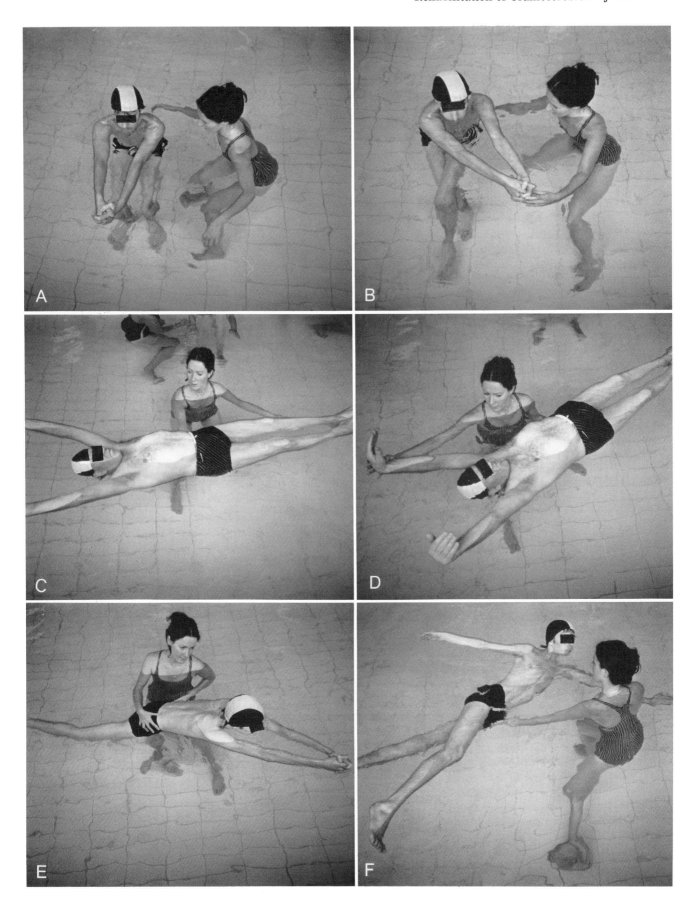

Figure 29.17.

Figure 29.18.

A. An apprehensive brain-injured patient is introduced to pool therapy. The therapist takes a shower with the patient to reduce tension.

B. The therapist should be with the patient at all times. The therapist should face the patient and in a friendly manner encourage him or her to relax while the patient's pelvis is supported by an inflated ring and the head by a life preserver-type collar.

C. As the patient gains confidence, coordination exercises are started. To improve trunk stability, the therapist places the patient's arm over her own shoulder.

D–E. Various inhibition as well as facilitation techniques, like Bobath and PNF, also are used in water.

F–G. The therapist works on the lower extremities while patient is supported by ring and collar.

H–I. In patients with ataxia, water is used as assistance in order to facilitate movements. Better coordination is accomplished. Additional resistance is given by the therapist. Arm abduction and adduction against resistance reduce ataxia.

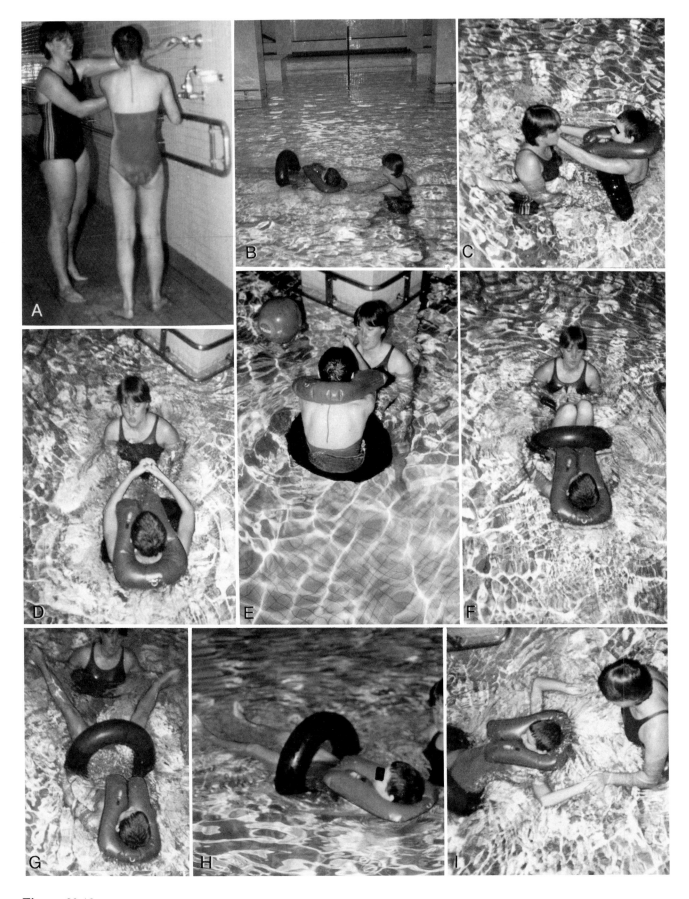

Figure 29.18.

Figure 29.19.

A–B. The involved extremity is retrained using Bobath technique of inhibition of abnormal tone.
  C. Memory (sequencing by memory) and coordination training is conducted.
  D. Coordination exercises are done on drums in the music room.
  E. Sequencing and judgment training is conducted.
  F. Memory and concentration activities are useful.
  G. Advanced Activities of Daily Living.
  H. An occupational therapy room has various work set-ups.
   I. A brain-injured patient practices on the computer.

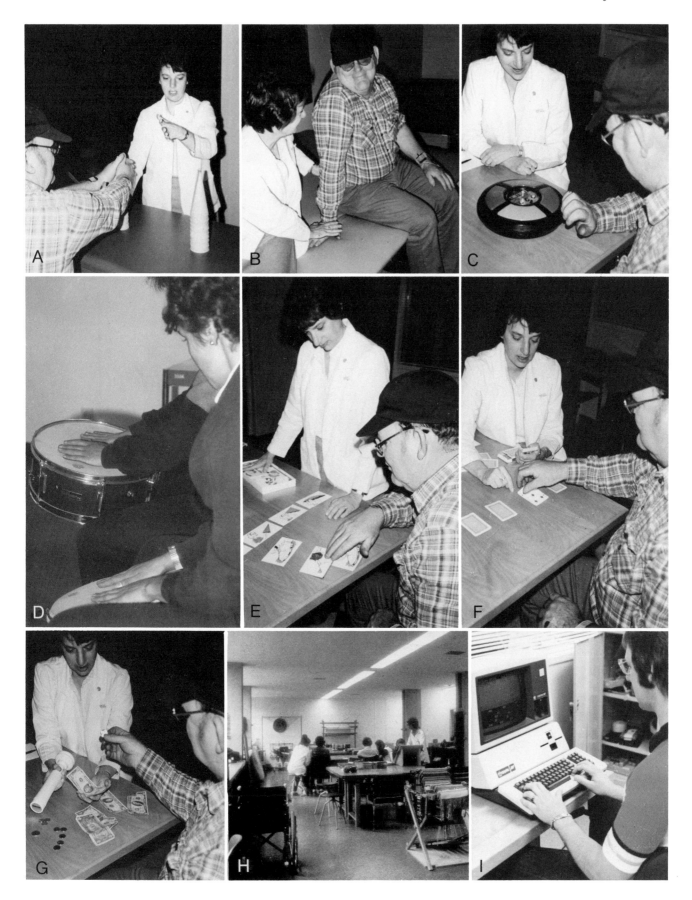

Figure 29.19.

Figure 29.20.

A. A beginning feeding program for patient with dysphagia is applied by the speech pathologist. The patient was unable to be fed at the normal upright sitting position due to physical limitation.

B. A cutaway cup is utilized to keep head posture tilted slightly to prevent aspiration with the dysphagic patient.

C. A patient is instructed in the use of a nonverbal communication device (Zygo board).

D. Word finding skills of a closed head injury patient are evaluated.

E. Therapy increases the use of correct grammatical forms with the aphasic patient.

F. Reading skills are evaluated at the simple phrase level.

G. Picture recognition and naming exercises are done.

H. Syntax building is done using pictures. This is the patient's first attempt to build simple sentences with a pictorial aid.

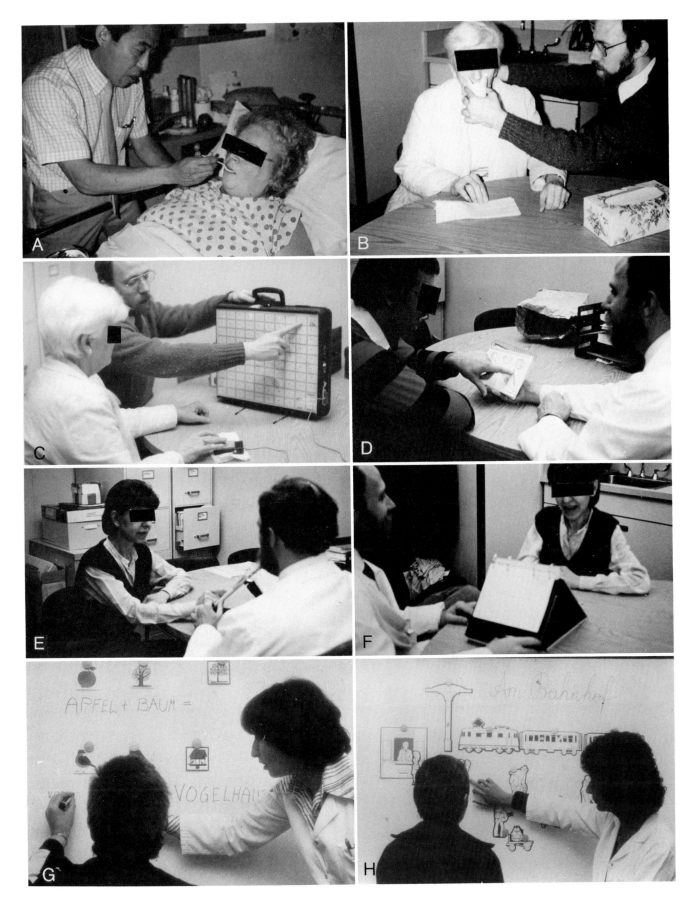

Figure 29.20.

Figure 29.21.

A. Interview and counseling is done by a medical social worker. Information also is given to the family.
B. Family conference takes place.
C. In psychology, concentration training is useful.
D. A psychological test determines visual flicker frequency response.
E. Psychology reflex-reaction response training is conducted.
F. Electroencephalogram measures bioelectrical potentials.

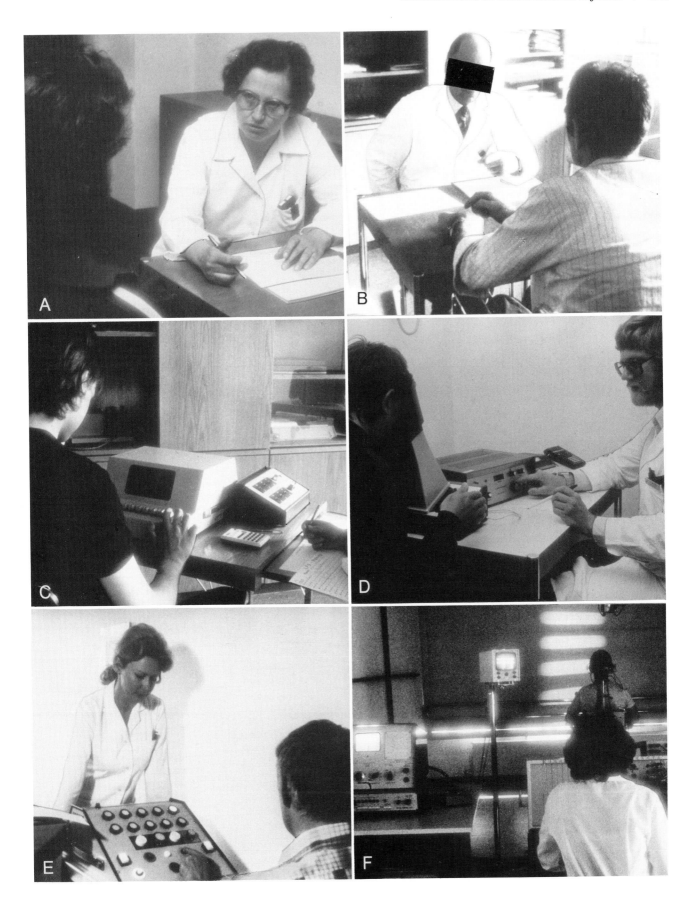

Figure 29.21.

Figure 29.22.

A. Psychological group therapy is helpful to head-injured patients.
B. A weekly rehabilitation learning conference should be held.
C. Outdoor group physical therapy is also beneficial.
D. Reflex inhibition is done through positioning.
E. Patients do unilateral trunk stretching exercises.
F. Manual arts therapy takes place in a metal workshop.

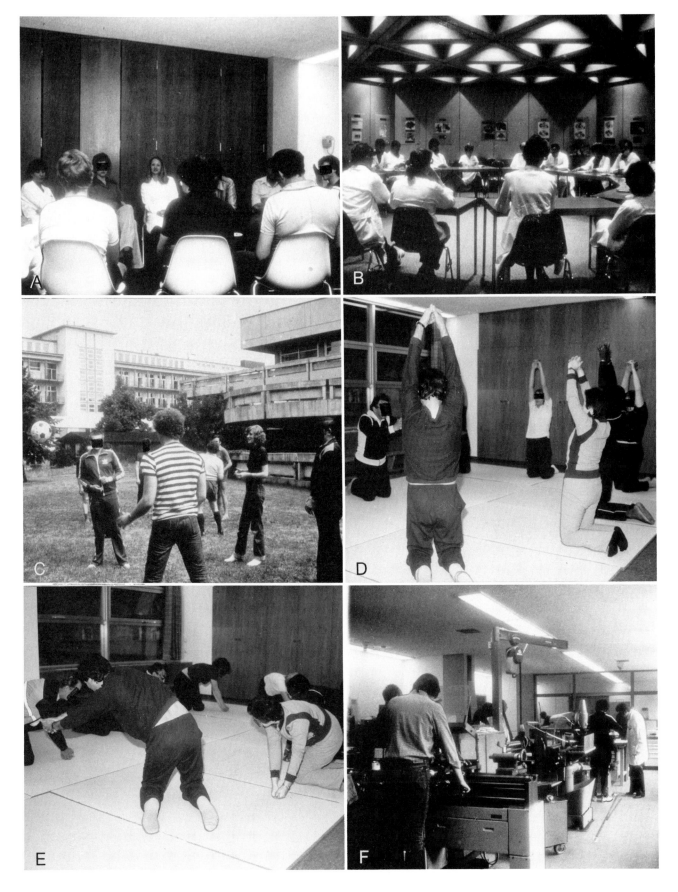

Figure 29.22.

Figure 29.23.

    A. A patient learns to turn on an electric stove.
    B. Stir contents of a pan.
    C. Make coffee.
    D. Get a bowl.
    E. Transfer hot food from pan to bowl.
    F. Get a cup from the cupboard.
G–H. Drink from a cup and glass in a coffee shop.
    I. Rinse and wash dishes.

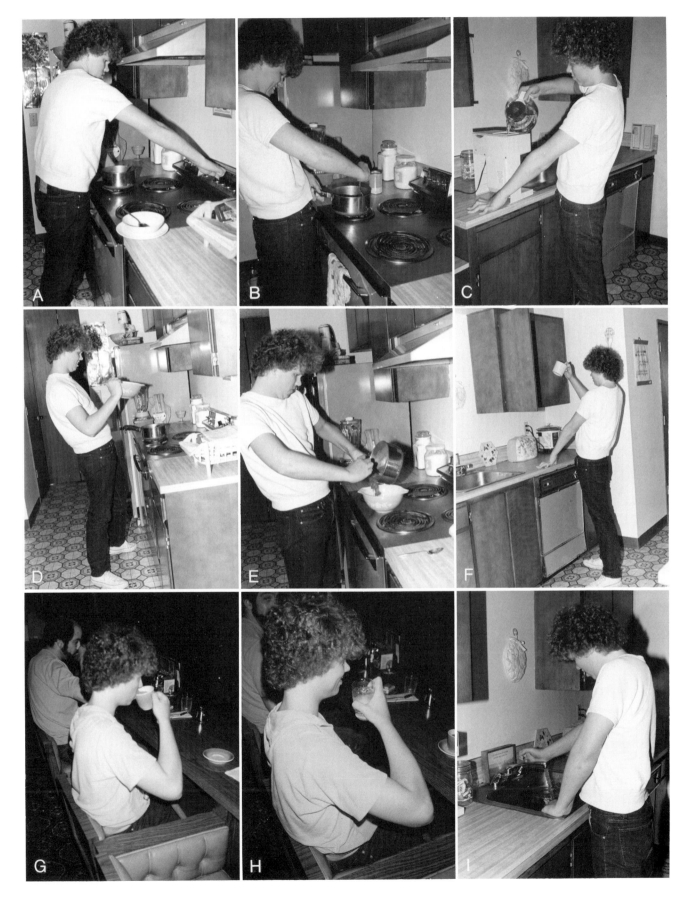

Figure 29.23.

Figure 29.24. Sheltered workshops include

    A. A metal workshop.

    B. A special loom is used.

    C. Woodworking is also helpful.

    D. A weaving room makes a good workshop.

    E. Team conferences are important.

F–G. Goodwill Industries (courtesy of Goodwill Industries, Portland, Oregon, 1985) is an important source of support.

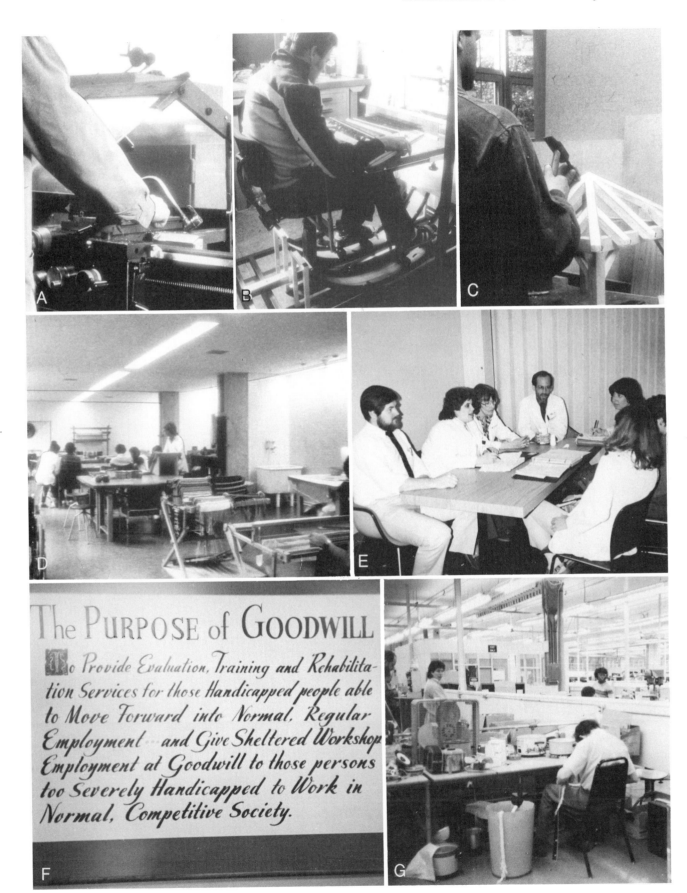

The PURPOSE of GOODWILL

Ko Provide Evaluation, Training and Rehabilitation Services for those Handicapped people able to Move Forward into Normal, Regular Employment...and Give Sheltered Workshop Employment at Goodwill to those persons too Severely Handicapped to Work in Normal, Competitive Society.

Figure 29.24.

Figure 29.25.

A. In hippotherapy, a patient with craniocerebral injury and paraparesis is lifted up to the horse and

B. Arranges the reins.

C. The patient assumes free sitting balance on the horse with arms apart.

D. Sitting balance on a moving horse is accomplished with two persons' standby assistance; a third person guides horse. The rhythmic motion facilitates responses.

E. The patient prepares for dismounting. The assistant supports the patient's right shoulder and pelvis.

F. Independent horseback riding can be achieved.

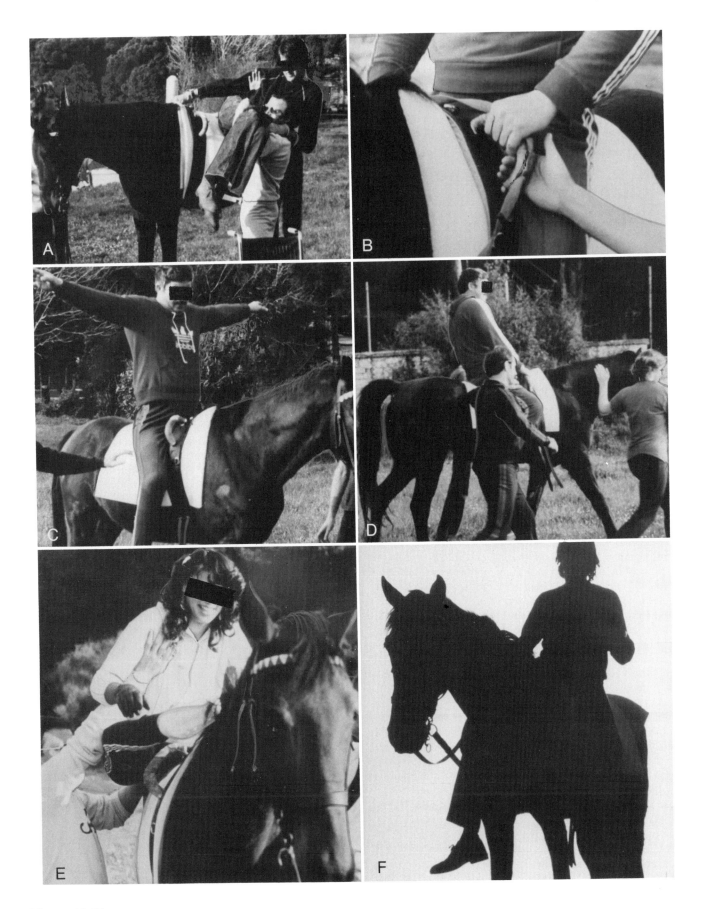

Figure 29.25.

30

Rehabilitation of Hand Injuries: A Case History in Team Approach

Kenneth D. Meadows, R.P.T., Peter A. Nathan, M.D., and Martha F. Rushing, O.T.R.

REHABILITATION OF THE PATIENT WITH HAND INJURIES
Kenneth D. Meadows, R.P.T.

The human hand is essential for its ability to perform functional activities, and it is through the hand that creativity is often expressed. The hand also has an added dimension in interpersonal relationships because it is through reaching out, touching, or gesturing that many social roles are fulfilled. Injury and the resulting disability of the hand can be an intensely devastating experience because of the hand's varied and important functions, and rehabilitation of the hand therefore becomes a vitally important task.

To assure optimal recovery from hand injuries, it is more effective to carry out the rehabilitation process in a *team approach* than in a fragmented, multidisciplinary fashion. The patient and the patient's family are essential members of the rehabilitation team and should be given every opportunity to contribute to the rehabilitation process. The professional disciplines involved in the team will vary depending upon the needs of the patient, but a typical rehabilitation team may consist of a physician, surgeon, physical therapist, occupational therapist, mental health professional, and vocational counselor.

Unfortunately the patient and the patient's family are all too frequently given passive roles by the professional members of the rehabilitation team. The success of the rehabilitation process greatly depends upon the patient and family having an understanding of the realistic treatment goals and committing themselves to achieving those goals. A motivated, cooperative, and well-informed patient-family unit can mean the difference between a rehabilitation program that is successful and one that fails. It is important that the patient and family view the members of the rehabilitation team as a single unit with a common goal and not as separate disciplines functioning autonomously and isolated from the rest.

In the small clinical setting, it is often necessary for the treating physician to bring other team members in from the outside. This may be time consuming and inconvenient, but it is essential in order to maintain the team concept. The enhanced outcome of the rehabilitation effort is sufficient reward to justify the additional scheduling and logistical problems involved in bringing a group together from unrelated settings.

Once the members of the rehabilitation team have been identified by the treating physician, it is important that these persons interact frequently. Team input should not be limited to treatment modalities but ought to be considered in the evaluation process as well. All team members should participate in carefully assessing the patient's vocational, avocational, and social needs and in establishing a set of treatment goals based on these needs. Once the goals have been established, it can be determined if surgery is indicated to alter or restore the involved anatomy to the point that physical rehabilitation will be feasible. If surgery is required, the surgeon's role must not be limited to simply performing the mechanical aspects of the surgery. The surgeon's involvement with the rehabilitation team should begin with consideration of surgery and extend throughout the entire rehabilitation process.

As rehabilitation proceeds, the team needs to meet frequently to assess the patient's progress and revise the treatment protocol as necessary. The composition of the rehabilitation team may need to be modified as the patient's needs are met in a particular phase or as new problems are encountered. The primary treating physician or surgeon will continue to facilitate and coordinate the efforts of the team as a whole and must assume the ultimate responsibility for the patient's recovery.

To illustrate the importance of the team approach the following case history focuses on a patient who began treatment without benefit of an interdisciplinary rehabilitation team: The patient was an 11-year-old boy who 15 months earlier sustained an accidental gunshot wound to the left arm with multiple sites of pellet penetration and with lesion of the left ulnar nerve. The patient underwent surgery for forearm pedicle skin flap and ulnar nerve repair with sural graft. Following surgery, he became involved in a rehabilitation program that did not use a team approach. When the patient was released from care, he had extremely limited functional use of his left upper extremity.

At the time of the initial evaluation by the rehabilitation team, the patient demonstrates contractures of the left elbow and wrist and severe claw deformity of the hand. There was a positive Tinel's sign found in the forearm in the area of the pedicle graft. The patient's stated goal was "I would like to have my whole arm better." He stated he was able to play baseball with his right arm only. He admitted that he felt like crying at times because of his significant deformity.

After several sessions of mutual evaluation and goal setting involving the patient and his family, the surgeon, a physical therapist, and an occupational therapist, it was determined that realistic physical rehabilitation goals would include providing functional range of motion (ROM) and strength to the elbow, restoring the wrist motion to at least a neutral position and restoring a functional grasp. The global objective for this patient was to provide enough return of function to bolster his level of self-confidence and help him to view his injured extremity as a potentially functional part of his anatomy rather than as a disfigured, useless appendage that needed to be hidden.

The treatment process involved four surgeries and a staged program of physical and occupational therapy that spanned many months. Physical and occupational therapy was administered both prior to and after surgery. The patient and his family were critically important members of the team since they lived 85 miles from the treatment center and much of the physical and occupational therapy had to be accomplished through a home program.

Although this patient's initial treatment was of good quality, it was delivered in a fragmented manner without a set of goals first having been determined for the rehabilitation process. In the absence of specific goals and without a team structure to facilitate communication, the initial surgery and the postoperative rehabilitation program fell short of expectations and resulted in frustration for all concerned. The patient viewed his impaired physical state as being permanent, and became depressed and angry at having been deprived of the ability to enjoy his normal, active life-style.

The patient and his family questioned whether another attempt at rehabilitation would be beneficial, and they were reluctant to again invest the time and energy needed for the rehabilitation program. Once exposed to the team rehabilitation approach and strongly encouraged to be an active part of the treatment team, however, they became enthusiastic and the rehabilitation process proceeded in a positive direction.

Because of the severity of this patient's injury, rehabilitation could not overcome all of his physical limitations, but through a team effort it was possible to maximize his functional strengths and minimize his weaknesses. The positive result is an individual who is independent, physically active, and once again able to participate in vigorous activities, such as camping, fishing, and in varsity wrestling on his high school team.

The success of any rehabilitation team is dependent upon full participation by *every* member, each contributing as much as possible within his or her area of expertise. Individual contributions should be made in such a manner that the efforts of the other team members will be enhanced rather than discouraged. Although it is important that each team have a designated leader, it is essential that the leader not overshadow the participation of the other individuals on the team. The leader's primary responsibilities are to elicit the best performance from each discipline represented on the team and to orchestrate the team in such a way that the set goals are achieved in concert with the patient and the family.

REHABILITATION OF HAND INJURIES
Martha Rushing, O.T.R.

The hand is a marvelous and complex tool. When the hand is injured, the best efforts of a well-trained treatment team are essential in order to realize its goal, which is the return of maximal function of the hand. The treatment team is guided by the physician and consists of an occupational therapist, a physical therapist, and often, a social worker. Each has a specific role in the recovery and rehabilitation of the patient. Comprehensive treatment of the hand-injured patient is a very complex issue, as evidenced by the volumes of literature on the subject. This chapter provides an overview of care for the hand-injured patient. Many excellent texts are dedicated to a more detailed analysis of care of the hand-injured patient.

In the most basic sense, hand therapy can be thought of as occurring in three realms: evaluation, treatment, and splinting. When evaluating the patient, the therapist's own hands are among the best tools available. The therapist should observe the patient functioning spontaneously, and then palpate the tissues of the injured hand. The experienced therapist can identify problem areas by palpation. Figure 30.2A shows the therapist examining a hand that has very dense scar tissue, with significant limitation of mobility in the carpus.

The therapist also should evaluate the patient's sensibility. Watching the patient function spontaneously gives the therapist clues to the degree of sensibility experienced by that patient. In addition, the therapist should conduct an objective measurement of sensation by looking at a variety of parameters.

After vibratory stimuli are assessed and recorded, moving touch, constant touch, and 2-point discrimination should be measured (Fig. 30.2B). Range of motion (ROM) can be measured and recorded in a variety of planes.

Figures 30.2C and D show the available active ROM of a patient in flexion and in extension. Distal edema is often a problem with the patient who has sustained an injury to the hand. Patients can be instructed in a variety of methods to control edema. A volumeter provides an objective measure of edema, using the principle of water displacement (see Fig. 30.2E–G). Results of measurement should be recorded for comparative purposes.

A variety of evaluation tools are used to gather objective data, which are recorded and provide a base from which a set of goals and treatment plan can be devised (see Fig. 30.2H). The data base should be updated constantly, and the treatment should reflect the patient's current status with current goals. Useful instruments include a Jamar dynamometer, which measures grip strength; a 2-point discrimination gauge; a paintbrush, used to desensitize very sensitive tissue; a Jamar pinch gauge; tuning forks to assess vibratory stimuli; and a variety of goniometers used to measure ROM.

Graded treatment tools are shown in the center horizontal row with a variety of sponge balls of different sizes and density (see Fig. 30.2I). These usually are used with persons who have very little grip strength. The top horizontal row of these tools offers more resistance, and the bottom row consists of more difficult media.

All treatment programs must be such that they can be carried out easily at home. The patient should always be in a home program to augment visits to the clinic for therapy. Often, the injury has resulted in severely diminished earning power for the individual. If the patient is to be expected to work on his or her own therapy at home, simple media readily available in the person's environment must be devised.

Figure 30.3A shows the forearm and hand of a 71-year-old male who arrived in the authors' clinic 3 months post-injury with a circular saw. In addition to dense scar tissue and limited ROM, the patient experienced significant pain. His treatment program must address all of the areas of concern discussed in this chapter. The application of cold packs is helpful to reduce inflamation, edema, and often pain (see Fig. 30.3B). The therapist can use massage to treat very dense scar tissue (see Fig. 30.3C). Often, patients are not able to do their own massage at home between clinic visits. Usually there is a family member who is very pleased to help the patient by doing massage at home, once the therapist has taught him or her the procedure.

Often, a very limited web space can develop as a result of an injury (see Fig. 30.3D). Massage, stretching, and often splinting may help increase the patient's web space. Transcutaneous electrical nerve stimulation (TENS) can be very helpful in reducing pain symptoms (see Fig. 30.3E).

Vibration is a form of mechanical stimulation to the tissues that often helps reduce pain as well as scar tissue (see Fig. 30.3F).

Evaluation and treatment plans must be designed individually (see Fig. 30.3G). However, a group treatment setting is very effective. A "skateboard" can be a means for providing active assistive ROM and can easily be duplicated at home (see Fig. 30.3H).

Splints are an integral part of the therapy program as well. Splints are categorized as either *static* (stationery) or *dynamic* (allowing for movement). Splints must be designed and fitted well or the result may be more harmful than helpful.

Figure 30.4A shows the hand immobilized in a splint in the functional position: metacarpophalangeal joints in flexion, proximal and distal interphalangeal joints in extension.

The finished splint is made of plaster of paris (Fig. 30.4B).

Figure 30.4C is a static splint used to hold the thumb stable while a tendon repair heals.

Figure 30.4D is an example of a dynamic splint. The purpose of the splint is to extend the PIP joint of the index finger while allowing for active flexion of the digit.

The glove splint shown in Figure 30.4E is a simple, inexpensive, dynamic splint which is very effective in gaining flexion in some types of injuries.

Figure 30.4F shows the use of the paraffin bath which is a heat modality effective in softening tissue prior to ROM exercises and is often very soothing to the painful hand. The patient shown had all four digits amputated. The surgeon was able to replant the long ring and small, however, the index finger could not be saved.

Figure 30.4G shows a patient exercising while in a full cast. It is very important to retain whatever ROM one can to prevent unnecessary joint stiffness.

Figure 30.4H demonstrates that a patient can work on maintaining ROM and strength while some other joints are supported by a static splint.

A group therapy setting is the focus of Figures 30.4I and J. Once the baseline data is gathered and a set of goals is established, the treatment plan is put into practice both in the clinic and at home. The therapist reassesses the treatment plan regularly as a result of changes that take place in the baseline data. The information is communicated to the referring physician on a regular basis.

Group settings can be very helpful to the patient, as he or she will encounter people with injuries similar to his own who are making progress. This will motivate the patient to work for his or her own progress. Patients see injuries that are perceived as more severe than their own when a group situation occurs. There is open dialogue around these issues and a positive healing climate is generated which speeds the patient's recovery.

Hand therapy, when carried out by experienced therapists, under the guidance of a trained physician, can be very successful for the patient and a rewarding experience for the treatment team.

Figure 30.1.

A. Maximum extension: elbow, wrist and fingers, at time of presentation for evaluation by Rehabilitation Team.

B. Prehension with functional extension at elbow and wrist following surgeries and treatment by rehabilitation team is demonstrated.

C. A patient grasps with extended reach provided by wrist and elbow extension following conclusion of treatment by the rehabilitation team.

D. A patient participates on the school wrestling team.

E. Active grasp is demonstrated.

F. Active extension of wrist and digits is shown.

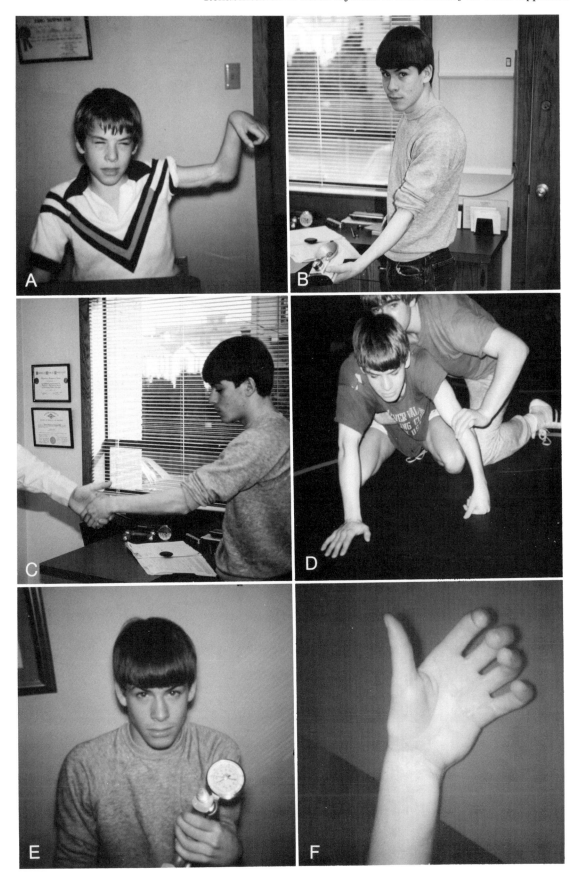

Figure 30.1.

Figure 30.2.

    A. A therapist examines a hand with very dense scar tissues.

    B. Vibratory stimuli are assessed and recorded.

C–D. The available active ROM of a patient in flexion and in extension is shown.

E–F. A volumeter measures edema.

    G. Useful instruments include (from *left* to *right): Jamar dynamometer, 2-point discrimination gauge, paintbrush, Jamar pinch gauge, tuning forks, and a variety of goniometers.*

    H. Graded treatment tools include a variety of sponge balls.

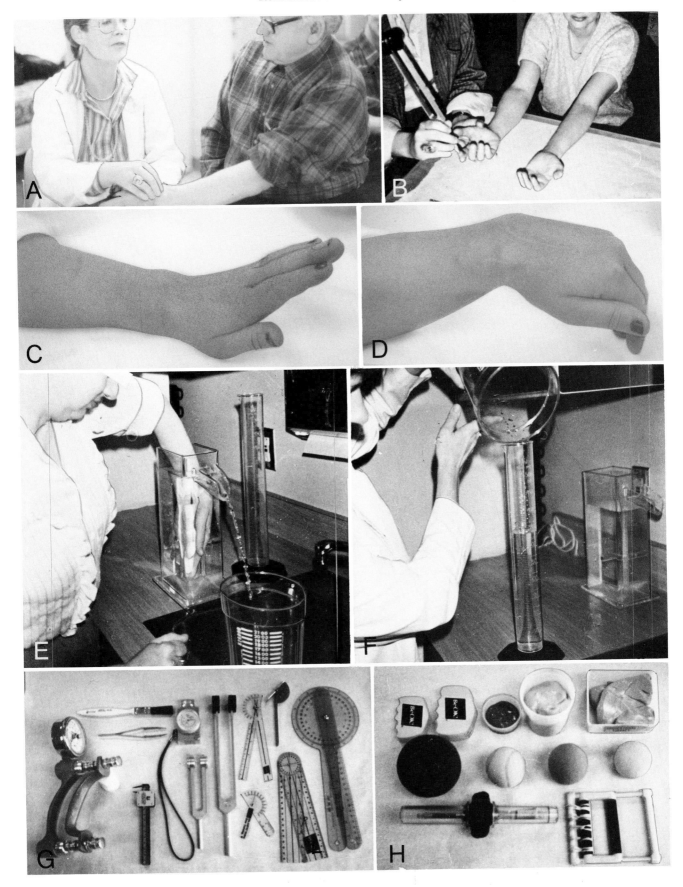

Figure 30.2.

Figure 30.3.

A. The forearm and hand of this patient shows dense scar tissue and limited ROM.
B. Cold packs are applied.
C. Limited web space resulted from the injury.
D. Massage is used to treat scar tissue.
E. A TENS unit is applied to a patient.
F. Vibration is used to reduce pain and scar tissue.
G. Two patients engage in therapy on an individual basis.
H. This patient who had sustained a brachial plexus injury, works on a skateboard.

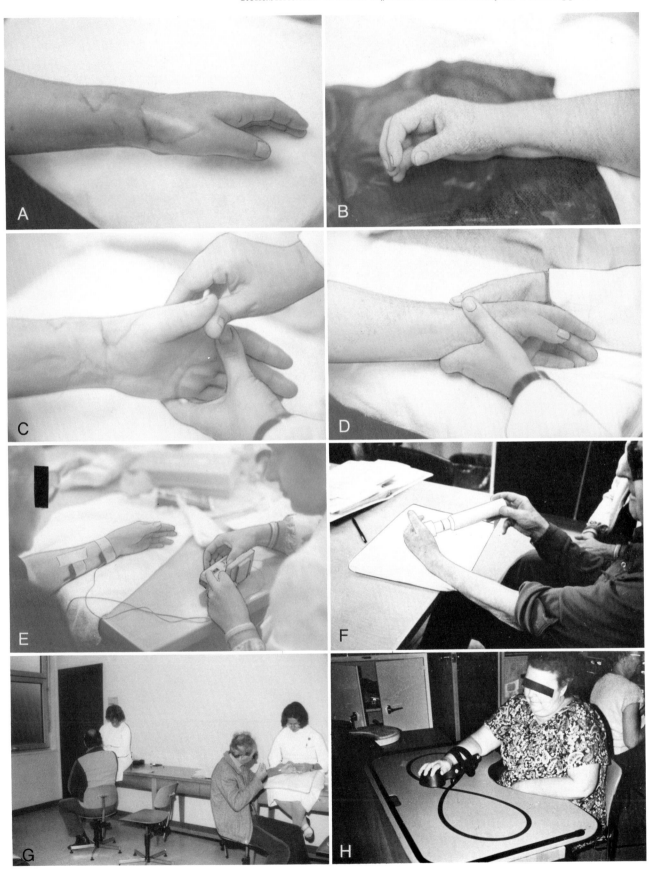

Figure 30.3.

Figure 30.4.

    A. This hand is immobilized in a functional position.

    B. A plaster of Paris splint is shown.

    C. A static splint is shown.

    D. The dynamic splint extends the PIP joint.

    E. The glove splint is shown.

    F. A paraffin bath is used.

    G. A patient in a full cast exercises.

    H. A patient wearing a static splint works on maintaining ROM and strength.

I–J. A treatment plan is put into practice.

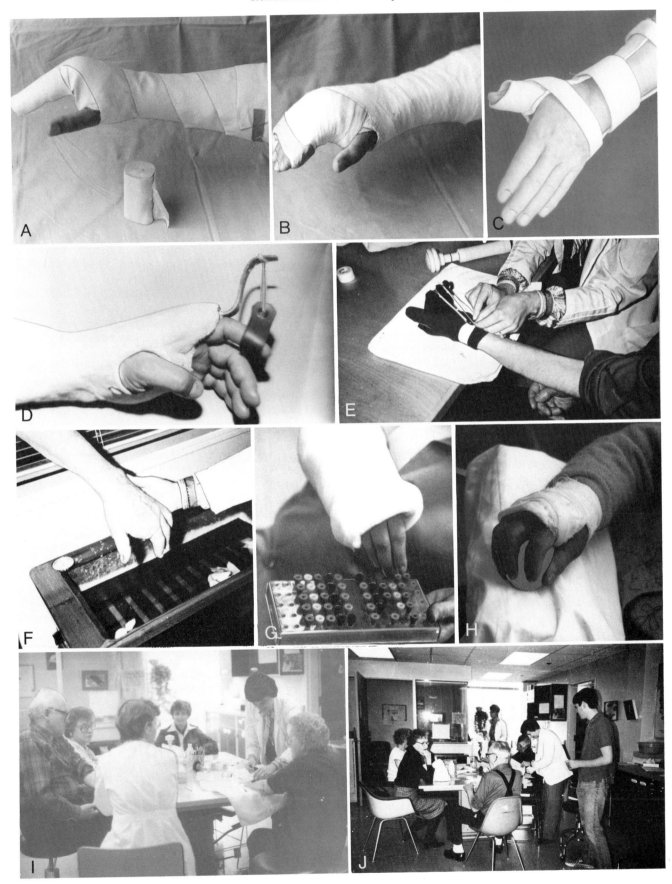

Figure 30.4.

31

Rehabilitation of Spinal Cord Injuries

Stephan Spanudakis, M.D.

REMOVAL

Management at Site of Trauma

The rehabilitation of patients with spinal cord injuries begins at the site of the accident. Meticulous management is essential to avoid further damage. The number of persons required for the transfer of the patient depends on the level of the lesion. Injuries at the cervical level, for instance, require four persons—one to keep the patient's head in constant traction while the others lift the patient and transfer him or her onto a hard stretcher.

The transfer of a patient with a thoracic cord injury can be accomplished by three persons as no traction of the head is required. The patient should be positioned on a hard stretcher, with the physiological curves of the spine supported by cushions or folded clothes and the region of the suspected fracture hyperextended. Edged and sharp objects must be removed from the patient's pockets to avoid pressure sores. Transport by helicopter is preferred because it is the fastest means and puts the least strain on the patient. Patients suffering from injuries with spinal cord involvement suffer a period of so-called spinal shock (see Fig. 31.1), which may last days, weeks, or rarely, up to several months.

Neurological Aspects

With spinal injuries accompanied by neurological damage, accurate, early neurological examination is crucial for the assessment of the extent of the injury. The observation of motor or sensory deficits will reveal the level and completeness of the lesion (see Fig. 31.2). Continuous checks and observations during the first hours after the injury will show whether the paralysis has remained stable or has become better or worse. The evaluations, together with additional examinations, like X-ray, myelography, and computerized tomography (C.T.) scans, constitute the basis for decisions regarding further treatment measures (whether conservative or surgical).

Figure 31.3 shows the functional abilities of a patient with complete motor loss. They include:

1. *Tetraplegia C5.* Restricted tidal volume; complete dependence; wheelchair dependent for mobility
2. *Tetraplegia C7.* Restricted tidal volume; functionally independent or nearly so; wheelchair dependent for mobility; aids for forearm and hands; and controls on automobile for driving
3. *Paraplegia C8.* Restricted tidal volume; functionally independent (minimal personal needs can be satisfied); wheelchair-dependent for mobility; standing between parallel bars with knee-ankle-foot orthoses (KAFOs) possible; driving a car is possible with hand controls.
4. *Paraplegia T1–T2.* Restricted tidal volume; functionally independent; wheelchair-dependent for mobility; with two KAFOs long braces, swing through gait between parallel bars possible (although not functional for ambulation otherwise); driving a car possible with hand controls.
5. *Paraplegia T3–T9.* Complete independence; wheelchair-dependent for mobility; swing through gait with long leg braces and forearm crutches possible (although usually not practical because of high energy demands); car driving with hand controls
7. *Paraplegia from L4 downward.* Functionally independent at home and outdoors; independent ambulator with two ankle foot orthoses and two forearm crutches or two canes; car driving with hand controls

CONSERVATIVE TREATMENT OF SPINAL FRACTURES WITHOUT SPINAL CORD DAMAGE

Following closed reduction and appropriate padding, fractures or dislocations of the cervical spine can be immobilized successfully in a Minerva jacket. Regular radiological follow-up examinations are necessary to control fracture healing.

Fractures of the lower thoracic or the upper lumbar part of the spine are immobilized in a Böhler plaster corset. The reduction is usually accomplished in suspended position after appropriate padding. When applying the plaster cast, the epigastric region is not enclosed. The heavy plaster corset may eventually be replaced by synthetic material (Neofract). The advantages of the Neofract corset are that it is lightweight and can be removed for hydrotherapy and when the patient is resting in bed (after the sixth week). The principle of fabrication is the same as for the plaster cast.

CONSERVATIVE TREATMENT OF SPINAL FRACTURES IN PARA-/TETRAPLEGICS

For the treatment of complete transverse lesions in the thoracic and lumbar regions after reduction, hyperextension at the fracture site by appropriate positioning in bed is sufficient (Fig. 31.4). This position of hyperextension must be maintained when the patient is turned. For fractures of the cervical spine, continuous traction with Crutchfield clamps or halo traction can be used. Initially, a traction of 6 kg or more must be applied until reduction is achieved; thereafter 2 to 3 kg continuous traction will be sufficient. Regular radiological checkups are essential. Both methods require hyperextension of the cervical spine, which is achieved by appropriate padding between neck and shoulders. Frequent evaluations and care of the insertion points are necessary.

SURGICAL METHODS

Stabilizing surgery is the method of choice for the treatment of spine fractures. Laminectomy, to release spinal cord compression without stabilization, was formerly a frequent procedure, but now has been abandoned. Surgical treatment at the cervical level is possible by Cloward's bone plug blocking. In this method, the bone fragments and parts of the intervertebral discs are removed and replaced by bone graft. A method similar to this is the spondylodesis, in which the addition of a simple or H-plate is used for better stabilization.

Other methods of surgical stabilization in the region of the thoracolumbar junction and the lumbar spine are those of Roy-Camille and Harrington.

TYPES OF BEDS FOR THE POSITIONING OF PARA-/TETRAPLEGICS

For the positioning of paraplegics and tetraplegics, different types of beds are available, ranging from the common bed to the mechanically operable bed. Positioning and turning paralyzed patients are still best and most accurately accomplished by hand, although this method is certainly also the most expensive one because it requires a large number of nursing personnel. The patients can be mechanically turned in a Stryker frame (see Fig. 31.5). The disadvantages of this frame are that only prone or supine positions can be utilized, and the patient's circulation may be stressed if the frame is not rotated slowly enough.

The Egerton-Stoke-Mandeville bed can be operated more easily and with less strain on the patient. The patient can be adjusted to three different positions (two lateral and one supine). A rubber sheet is required for hygienic reasons. Natural fleece, synthetic fur (easy to maintain), gel cushions, and various pillows are used for the positioning of the patient to avoid pressure sores.

Special beds are also available for the positioning of paraplegics with decubitus ulcers. These are an air bed (Mediscus) or a sand bed (Clinitron). Both types of bed are based on the same principle of pressure relief, and the patient can be positioned on his or her ulcer without any further tissue damage. The temperature of the beds can be regulated as desired. Even following plastic surgery, patients can be placed in one of these two types of beds without any interference with wound healing.

POSITIONING OF PARA-/TETRAPLEGICS

Due to the paralysis, the patient cannot, like the non-injured person, relieve skin pressure by movement. In addition to this, circulation of the tissue is reduced by the absence of vascular regulation and the loss of sensibility. The patient is in danger of developing a decubitus ulcer. The areas at risk are especially those where the bone is immediately below the skin (see Fig. 31.6). From the time of the injury, the patient must be turned regularly every 2 hrs, and if the skin is very delicate, even more often. The patient can be positioned prone, lateral, or supine.

Supine Position

The patient is placed on fleece and pillows. Both shoulder joints are progressively abducted from slightly to 90 degrees at regular time intervals. In the same progressive pattern, the elbow joints are flexed and extended and the forearms pronated and supinated. The hand and finger joints are brought into functional position (foam rubber padding in the palm and fist bandage). This kind of positioning is used with tetraplegics. Positioning of the lower extremities is the same for both tetraplegics and paraplegics. The legs are slightly abducted at the hip, hyperextension of the knee joints must be avoided, and the feet must be in a neutral position.

Lateral Position

The back is placed in a position so that the frontal plane is vertical, and supported by pillows and fleece. With tetraplegics, the shoulder joints are abducted up to 90 degrees by padding. The legs are abducted and supported by pillows and fleece.

Prone Position

The patient is brought into the so-called bridging position by cushions and fleece with the fracture site in hyperextension. Other precautions are the same as for the supine position, but with additional care taken to avoid complications with the genitals.

INDIVIDUALIZED EXERCISE

Incorrect positioning, immobilization of the patient in bed, and insufficient passive motion may lead to contractures of the paralyzed joints. Application of motion is often overlooked during the period of spinal shock.

The individualized therapy to maintain full joint mobility of tetraplegics must include measures to compensate for the physiological countertraction of various muscles and groups of muscles in order to avoid contractures (see Fig. 31.7). Neglect of physiotherapeutic measures in tetraplegics with a lesion at the level of C6, for instance, may lead to a flexion contracture of the elbow caused by full biceps function in the presence of severe triceps weakness. In paraplegics, the same measures are necessary in the lower limbs to prevent contractures. The time that individualized therapy is started is determined by the patient's condition. Movement should be started as soon as possible.

For the passive movement of the lower limbs, the stability of a vertebral fracture must be considered to provide undisturbed healing. Complete passive mobilization of the lower limbs is possible with fractures down to the level of about the 7th thoracic vertebra. With fractures below this level, more precautions must be observed in mobilization of the hip joint. For example, with fractures at the 9th thoracic vertebra, hip joint flexion may be permitted up to 90 degrees; at the 11th thoracic vertebra hip joint flexion up to about 45 degrees. In such cases knee and foot joints can only be mobilized adequately if the hip joint is abducted.

PREVENTION OF COMPLICATIONS OF THE RESPIRATORY SYSTEM

In patients with damage of the cervical and upper thoracic part of the spinal cord, complications of the respiratory system are frequent. The respiration of such patients is maintained by the phrenic nerve (diaphragm) and the cervical muscles. Coughing is partly impaired in high paraplegics and extremely impaired in tetraplegics, due to loss of intercostal muscle function. Physiotherapeutic measures must therefore be started immediately (Fig. 31.8). The patient needs to learn how to breathe in and out correctly and how to cough by compressing the lower margin of the thorax and the abdomen. Compression is only possible in cases where no secondary injuries to the rib cage and abdomen contraindicate, such as in rib fractures and injuries in the abdominal region. Initially, a high tetraplegic (who has lost the ability for expectoration by the loss of function of thoracic and abdominal muscles) must be enabled to clear pulmonary secretions by the compression of the thorax, which requires the help of one or two auxiliary persons. In the course of rehabilitation, the patient should be taught how to compress the abdominal region by using his or her hands.

The bronchial lavage of tetraplegics is accomplished by aspiration; in some cases, it will not be possible to avoid a tracheotomy, which considerably facilitates the bronchial lavage. The aspiration and the regular change of cannula must be accomplished (under sterile technique). As an additional therapy circulatory support, inhalation, and antibiotics will be required.

PREVENTION OF THROMBOSES AND DIFFERENTIAL DIAGNOSIS OF PERIARTICULAR OSTEOARTHROPATHY (POA)

In the presence of lower extremity paralysis, the venous blood flow in the affected areas, especially the deep pelvic veins and veins of the lower limbs, is impaired. In these areas, thromboses frequently are caused by the venous stasis. Treatment must therefore be started immediately after the accident. At first the use of heparin is necessary to reduce the danger of venous thrombosis. About 1 week later, anticoagulative therapy might be given orally. The natural muscle-vein pump is replaced by passive movements (applied by the therapist or assistant). If a thrombosis already exists, a thrombosis bandage is required in addition to drug therapy (see Fig. 31.9). This bandage consists of 5 mm foam rubber and an elastic bandage. The leg must be bandaged from the toes up to the proximal end of the thigh. Swelling of the thigh is not always the result of thrombosis. Sometimes a differential diagnosis between thrombosis and heterotopic new bone formation is neces-

sary. The increase in alkaline phosphates in the blood, X-ray, and the scintigram can help to establish the diagnosis.

Heterotopic new bone formation develops in the soft tissues adjacent to the joints, but the joint cavity is spared. The cause of this is unknown.

The most frequently involved joints are the hip and knee joints. Involvement of shoulder and elbow joints is rare. The disease occurs both symmetrically and unilaterally and is found in about 10% of all para-/tetraplegics. An effective therapy does not exist. Treatment with steroids, calcium, or irradiation has sometimes been given, although without success. Didrinal has been tried.

If heterotopic ossification is suspected or diagnosed, physical therapy must be reduced but not completely abandoned. After the process has stopped, the ossification can be removed surgically in the rare cases where significant reduction of joint motion results, but success is not always guaranteed as recurrences of bone formation are possible.

CARE OF THE INTESTINES

Spinal cord injuries usually are associated with constipation and permanent sphincter dysfunction. These concomitant problems initially should be treated with drugs (e.g., stool softeners, bulk laxatives), diet, colon massage, and motion therapy (Fig. 31.10). Serious cases are treated with drugs promoting the peristaltic motion (e.g., prostigmin injections), or else with oral laxatives, suppositories, or enemas.

The diet should include a large amount of bulk foods and should avoid substances that produce flatulence, including aerated drinks. A daily colon massage also should be administered. The massage should follow the course of the large intestine, from right to left. In cases of significant flatulence, a flatus tube also should be inserted. Motion therapy increases the intraabdominal pressure and so facilitates the passage of feces and gas through the bowels.

INITIAL MOBILIZATION

After the fusion of the vertebral fracture, which is accomplished after about 6 to 8 weeks, mobilization should be commenced, with sitting on the edge of the bed as the first activity. The circulation of the patient is impaired, both by posttraumatic neurogenic factors in cases of high lesions, and also by the long period of recumbancy. When the patient sits up in bed, the blood pools in the abdomen and in the paralyzed lower limbs due to the loss of the muscle vein pump and the vascular regulation. Apart from cardiovascular agents, management of these circulatory complications includes elastic bandaging of the lower extremities or support stockings and an abdominal binder or bandage. Mobilization can be accomplished with regular monitoring of pulse and blood pressure.

WHEELCHAIR MOBILIZATION

When the circulation is stable, mobilization in a wheelchair is possible. The following must be considered for this: The paralyzed lower extremities tend to rotate externally, which may lead to pressure sores on the legs caused by the wheelchair edge. Those tetraplegics who lack the upper extremity strength required to bring the legs into the proper position are particularly at risk. To avoid pressure areas, the thighs should be kept in position by a belt with Velcro closure. This belt must not be excessively tightened to avoid pressure to the medial surface of the knee.

SPASTICITY

When spinal shock has resolved, spasticity will occur in most of the cervical and thoracic injuries as well as those involving the conus medullaris. Excessive spasticity can be controlled by several therapeutic measures. Diazepam (Valium), derivatives of butyric acid (Lioresal), dantrolene sodium (Dantrium), or combinations of these preparations can be administered.

In the past, spasticity was managed by the intrathecal application of alcohol. This method was soon abandoned because of various side effects, including skin lesions and loss of bladder reflexes. The operative treatment of spasticity may include the transection of tendons, muscles, nerves, and nerve roots. Physical therapy can prevent contractures and influence spasticity by appropriate mobilization therapy and adequate positioning in splints (see Fig. 31.11). Ice treatment of individual joints and the ice bath will reduce spasticity for some time. Also, swimming in warm water, at a temperature of about 32°C, occasionally gives relief. The variety of therapeutic measures employed reflects the difficulty in managing spasticity.

Spasticity also produces other problems. A spastic patient may be at risk of falling out of his wheelchair, so he or she should be secured to the chair by two belts, one around the trunk and another one around the lower legs. Spasms of the adductors may lead to pressure areas at the medial aspects of the knee joints. This can be avoided by a foam rubber wedge between the legs or by a padded spreader. Spasticity may also produce problems in the care of the patient. Correct positioning of the patient is essential. In unusually severe cases of spasticity, the patient can be brought into good hyperextended position by the use of padding with fleece or synthetic fur. The legs are tied to the bed with a sheet in order to avoid a change of position by spastic movements. This also prevents the patient from falling out of the bed during severe spasms. For very intense spasms, another sheet should be tied around the pelvis of the patient.

DECUBITUS ULCERS

Conservative Treatment

In the first stage of decubitus ulcers, due to loss of sensation, the para-/tetraplegic may suffer skin damage without realizing it because of pressure-produced ischemia. Even slightly excessive time of pressure on the skin leads to prolonged erythema and later to superficial skin damage by blistering. The next stage is necrosis followed by the formation of ulcers. The last stage is osteomyelitis; or infection of the underlying bone.

For mere reddening associated with minimal tissue damage, it is sufficient to relieve the skin for several hours and to rub it with heparin or similar ointments. The reddening will soon fade away. Blistering indicates superficial damage of the skin. The blister should be removed under sterile precautions and dressed with a sterile sponge.

The lesion will soon be dry. After that, a protective dressing and some days of avoiding any further pressure will be sufficient.

If necrotic areas already exist, they should be removed surgically, the skin can then be treated with hydrotherapy, e.g., baths with chamomile decoction or Kamillosan and ointment dressings (Fig. 31.12). In cases where the necrotic material cannot be removed, e.g., in patients with defective coagulation, debridement with enzyme ointments can be utilized. Decubital ulcers can be treated conservatively as long as they are small. Larger ones, however, must be treated by surgical removal and closure. Decubitus ulcers that also involve the bone can *not* be treated by conservative means. The osteomyelitis will produce recurring fistulae drainage through the superficially healed skin. Surgery is therefore required. Before any surgical closure, conservative pretreatment for the cleansing of the wound is necessary.

Surgical Treatment

Various different operative procedures are used. Very small ulcers may be grafted by Reverdin's skin transplant method. The patient can be mobilized after about 2 weeks.

Small, and sometimes medium-size decubitus ulcers over the sacrococcyx have been covered by Thiersch's graft or plastic mesh, but results have not been satisfactory. For larger decubital ulcers, the use of rotation flaps (see Fig. 31.13) is the method of choice. The decubitus ulcer is excised, the affected bone is removed, and the defect covered by full thickness skin graft. In case the defect is very large, a double rotation flap must be used to avoid tension in the suture area. In each case, one or two Hemovac drains are required to guarantee the free drainage of blood from the wound area, as blood is a good culture medium for bacteria, increasing the danger of wound infection.

For decubitus ulcers in the ischial region, Guttman's pseudotumor technique is applied. This technique involves three steps:

1. Packing the ulcer cavity with gauze
2. Removing the "pseudotumor" (bulging soft tissue)
3. Resecting the ischium and finally closing the wound in layers

One or two Hemovac drains should be inserted and progressively withdrawn during the following days until they are removed completely (after 10 days, at the latest).

On the twelfth day, the sutures are removed, and after 3 weeks, the limited resumption of pressure over the wound can be started and gradually increased. These surgical methods of treatment can mobilize the patient within about 3 weeks.

DYSREFLEXIA OF THE URINARY BLADDER

Injuries of the cervical and upper thoracic part of the spinal cord (down to T6) are frequently accompanied by a dyssynergia between the sphincters and the detrusor of the bladder. Voiding of the bladder is therefore impeded. A full bladder results in stimulation of the sympathetic nervous system, which may lead to autonomic dysreflexia. Dysreflexia in turn produces hypertension (paraxysmal hypertension 200 mm Hg and above), tachycardia, and headache. Tachycardia might not be present when the vagus nerve is intact. If the dysreflexia is not treated, it may lead to the rupture of a cerebral vessel, with subsequent hemiplegia or other neurological deficits.

As an emergency measure, the urine should be withdrawn by catheterization; bladder distention is the most common cause of other infections. If this is not sufficient, an indwelling catheter is required until the signs disappear. Frequent recurrences of dysreflexia from bladder distention are an indication for sphincterotomy. Drug treatment consists of the administration of spasmolytics (e.g., Buscopan), antispasmodics (e.g., diazepam), and α-receptor-blockers. In case of dysreflexia, emptying the bladder is essential; every patient should therefore learn self-catheterization. This is easy to learn for the paraplegic, but only a few tetraplegics can do it adequately with the use of orthoses or special aids (Fig. 31.14).

Should an indwelling catheter be necessary for reasons mentioned above, the following rules should be observed:

The lumen of the permanent catheter should not exceed 12 to 14 Charrière in order to avoid pressure areas on the mucosal lining of the urethra.

The penis must be held upward over the abdomen to avoid the development of pressure areas with ulceration at the penoscrotal junction.

To minimize the chance of bacterial invasion of the bladder the care of the meatus must not be neglected.

The indwelling catheter should be attached to a closed system to ensure sterility.

Incrustation can be minimized by using a Silastic catheter; the formation of calculi in the bladder can be prevented by irrigation with mandelic acid.

BLADDER TRAINING AND SELF-CATHETERIZATION

After spinal shock with neurogenic bladder, various different voiding patterns can develop. With injuries above the sacral vesical center, a reflex bladder (automatic bladder) usually develops; with injuries in the sacral center and below, an autonomous bladder (vesical autonomy) develops. This is common, but also mixed forms are observed.

Following spinal shock in the higher lesions, the detrusor becomes active, which is manifest as the spontaneous passing of urine. This is the time when bladder training should be started. Contractions of the detrusor can be caused by tapping over the suprapubic region. The same effect can be achieved by slight strokes (Guttmann's trigger method) or by light skin stimulation over the thighs (Fig. 31.15). These stimuli lead to several contractions of the detrusor at short intervals and therewith to short passings of urine. By repeated application of the above-mentioned procedure, emptying of the bladder can be achieved. (This often takes about 15 min.) With lesions of the vesical center and below, the detrusor cannot be activated (areflexia). For these, emptying of the bladder is accomplished passively by increasing the intraabdominal pressure (valsalva-abdominal press) or by pressing against the vesical region with one or both hands (Credé). Frequently, both abdominal press and Credé are required.

If the bladder does not compensate and the patient does not consent to sphincterotomy, the patient should be taught self-catheterization. This must be carried out under sterile or "clean" technique. Scissors, compresses, lubricant, sterile catheter (12 or 14 Charrière), and an antiseptic area are required. Preliminary measures for self-catheterization include cutting off the tip of the catheter case, soaking the compresses with antiseptic, and opening the lubricant. The male patient should then clean the glans penis with the compress and disinfectant, always from the top downward to wipe the bacteria away from the meatus. The lubricant should then be instilled into the urethra, the catheter inserted, and the urine withdrawn. The female patient cleans the vulva after spreading the labia in similar fashion, lubricates the tip of the female-type catheter, inserts it into the urethra, and withdraws the urine.

Figure 31.1.

A–B. A spinal cord-injured victim is removed.
  C. Objects must be removed from the spinal cord-injured patient's pockets. (Anesthesia can rapidly lead to pressure sores.)
  D. A spinal cord-injured victim is transported by helicopter.

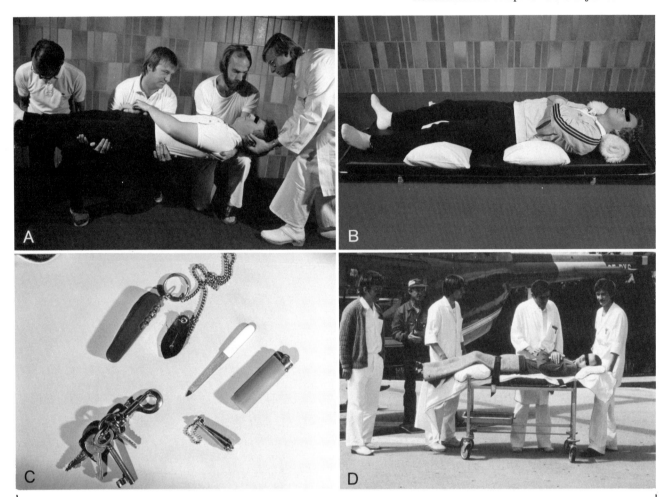

Figure 31.1.

Table 31.1. Spinal Shock: Symptoms that Appear Below the Level of Injury (Duration: 1 Day to 4 Weeks, Occasionally Several Months)

Complete paralysis of the muscles
Absence of deep reflexes
Absence of vascular control and heat regulation
Detrusor areflexia, urinary bladder paralysis and possibility of overdistention
Impairment of kidney function, oliguric and polyuric phase
Change in electrolyte balance
Complete paralysis of the bowels, initially subileus

Figure 31.2. Neurological aspects of transverse cord lesion are shown, including:

A. Segmental dermatome distribution anterior view

B. Dermatomes posterior view, and

C. Residual function in relation to level of lesion.

Figure 31.2 Spinal Cord Injury Functional Assessment (Translation of C)

Quadriplegia C5
Respiratory volume diminished. Complete dependency. Wheelchair indispensable.

Quadriplegia C7
Respiratory volume diminished. Almost complete dependency. Wheelchair indispensable. Support and assistive devices for forearms and hands.

Paraplegia C8 T1
Respiratory volume diminished. Partial dependency; minimal for personal needs (ADLs). Wheelchair indispensable. "Swing to" gait possible; Bilateral lower extremity corset, hip locks; two Canadian forearm crutches or two standard crutches. Driving car possible with hand controls and automatic transmission.

Paraplegia T1–T2
Respiratory volume diminished. Complete independence. Wheelchair indispensable. Swing through gait possible. Two orthoses for lower extremity with or without corset, two Lofstrand crutches. Driving car possible with hand controls, with or without automatic transmission.

Paraplegia T7
Complete independence. Wheelchair indispensable. Swing through or 4-point gait. Bilateral orthoses for lower extremities with or without corset, two Lofstrand crutches. Driving car possible with hand controls, with or without automatic transmission.

Paraplegia T12 L1
Complete independence. Wheelchair indispensable. 4-point gait or swing through; bilateral orthoses for lower extremities, two Lofstrand crutches. Driving car possible, with hand controls.

Paraplegia L4
Complete independence at home and outside. Wheelchair dispensable. Normal gait with foot dorsiflexion assist and two Lofstrand crutches. Eventual orthoses for knee stabilization. Driving car possible, with hand controls.

MUSCLES

Diaphragm—(C2), C3, C4

Biceps brachii—C5–C6

Triceps brachii—(C6), C7, C8

Latissimus dorsi—C6, C7, C8

Hand Muscles—C6, C7, C8, T1

Intercostals—T1–T11

Abdominals—(T6), T7, T12, L1

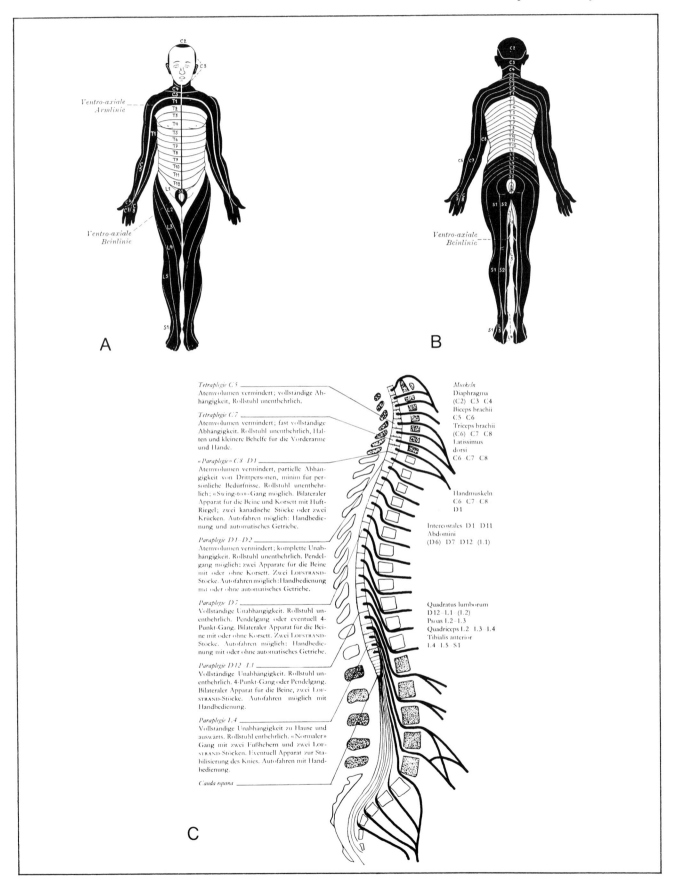

Figure 31.2.

Figure 31.3. Conservative management is provided for a spinal injury without cord lesion

A–C. A Minerva jacket, anterior and lateral view, is used in a cervical spine injury with instability

    D. A vertebral fracture in dorsal suspension is reduced (hyperextension).

E–F. A plaster of Paris corset is used.

G–H. A Neofract (thermoplastic) corset is fitted.

     I. A Neofract corset is shown on a standing patient.

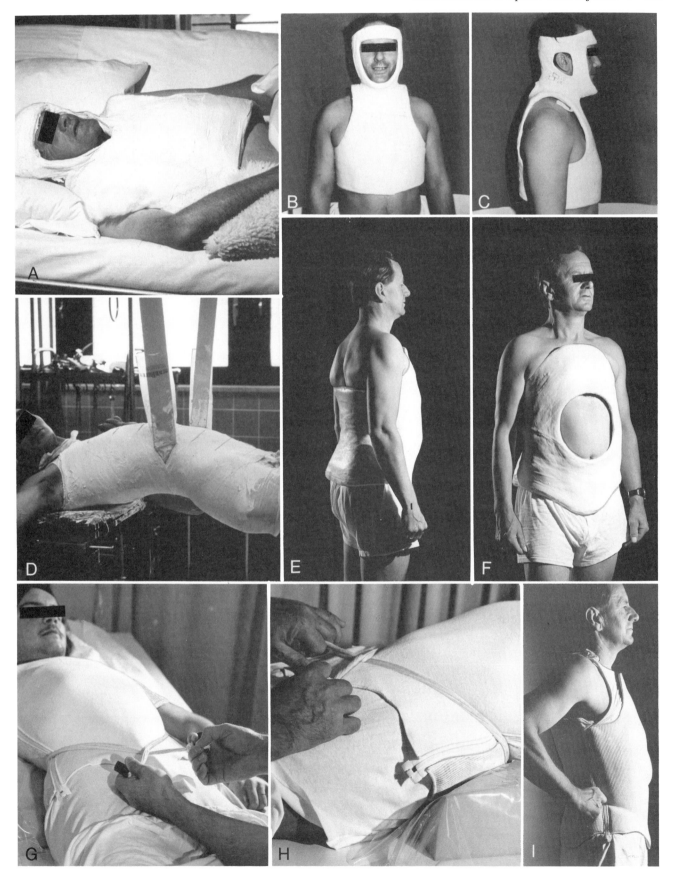

Figure 31.3.

Figure 31.4. Conservative treatment in transverse cord lesion includes:

    A. Positioning of patient in bed in thoracolumbar hyperextension
    B. Crutchfield tong traction
C–D. Traction in a halo, surgical treatment
    E. Stabilization with bone graft (block)
    F. Stabilization with an H-plate
    G. Stabilization with a Roy-Camille plate, and
    H. Stabilization with Harrington rods.

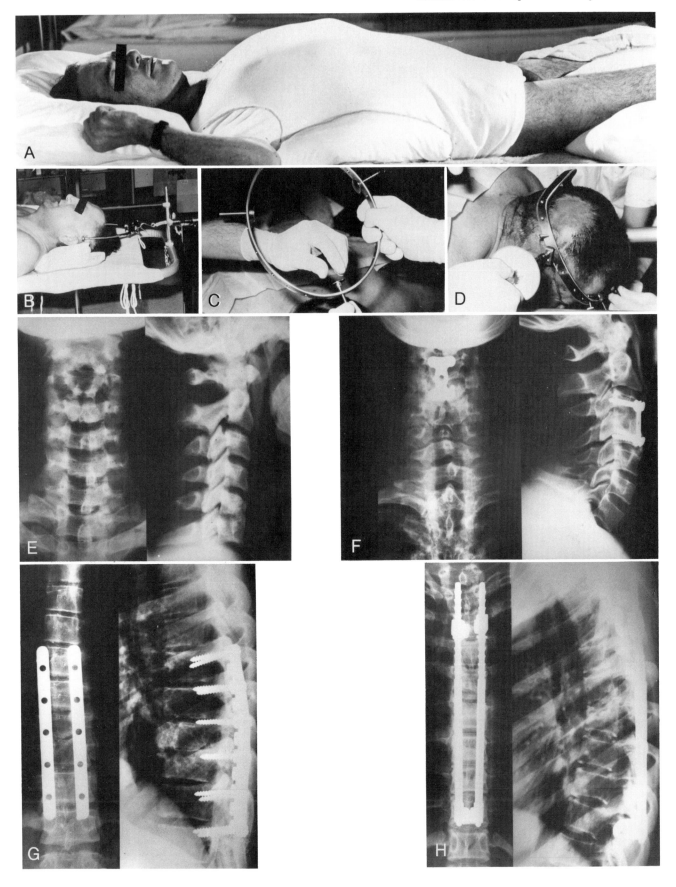

Figure 31.4.

Figure 31.5. Bed types include

    A. The Stryker bed

B–C. The Guttmann bed (Egerton-Stoke-Mandeville)

D–F. The standard hospital bed with pads and support

    G. The Mediscus bed, and

    H. The Clinitron bed

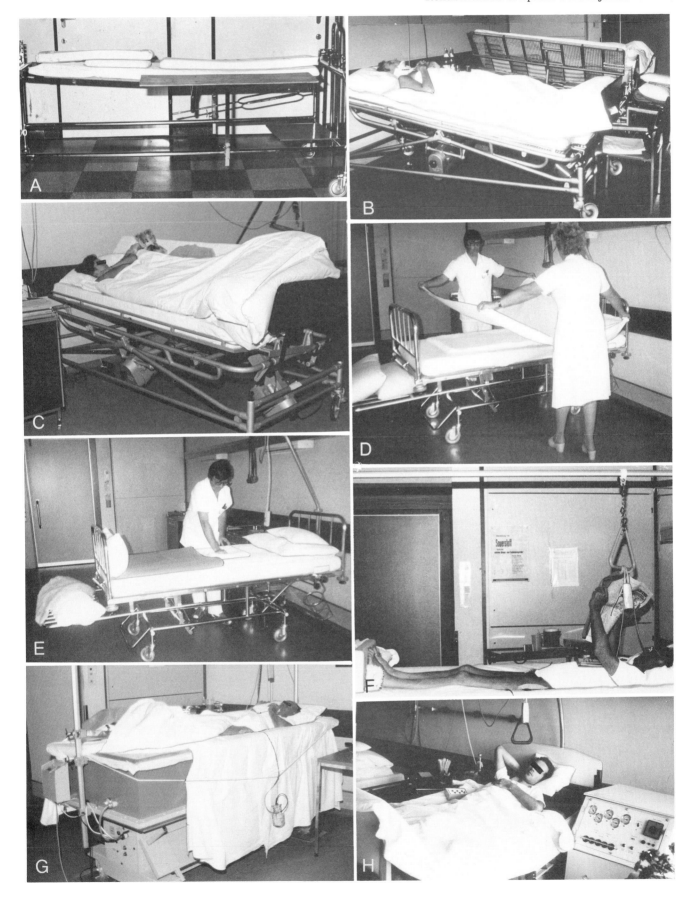

Figure 31.5.

Figure 31.6. Positioning

A–B. Areas at risk for decubitus ulcers are marked on the anterior and posterior side.
   C. The patient is shown in the supine position.
D–E. Positioning of upper extremity is done in pronation and supination.
   F. Side lying position is also used.
   G. Hand bandaging is in the fist position in tetraplegics.
   H. The prone position is shown.
    I. The feet are positioned.

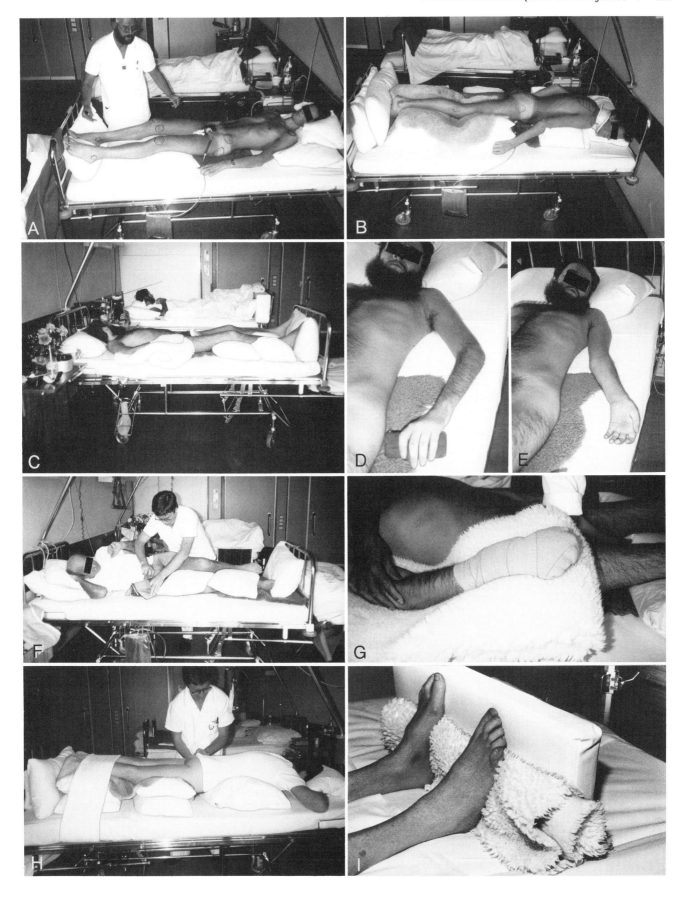

Figure 31.6.

Figure 31.7. Individual exercises are done in bed prior to patient being permitted up.

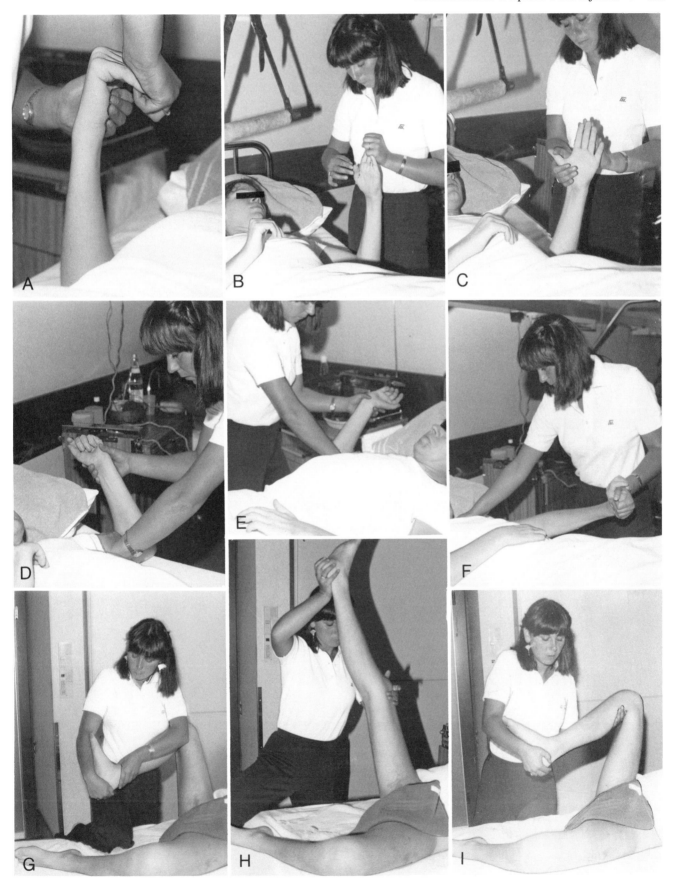

Figure 31.7.

Figure 31.8.

A–C. Breathing exercises are done.
D–F. Cough assistance is used.
G–I. Bronchial hygiene includes respiratory care, suction, and change of the tracheostomy tube (cannula)

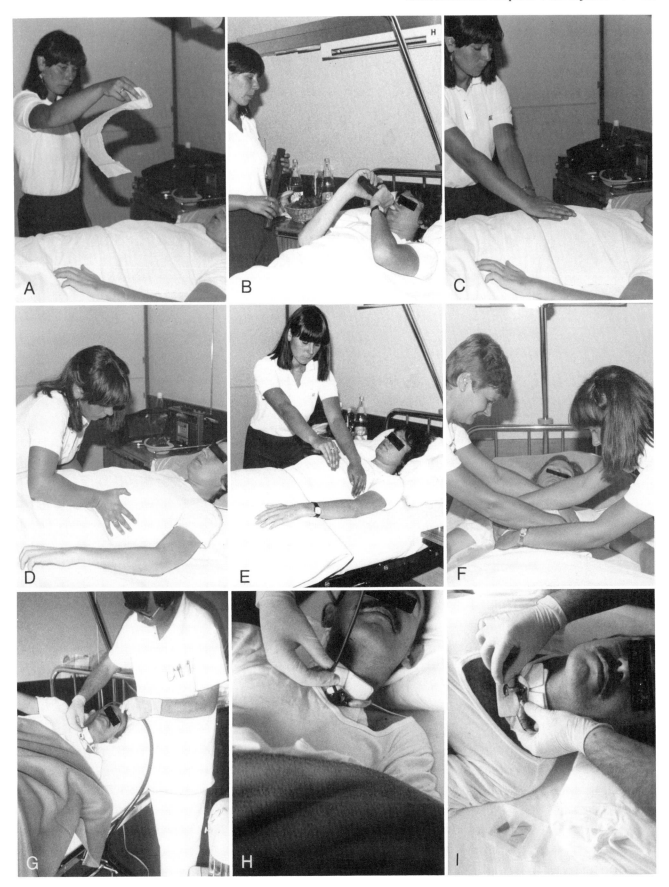

Figure 31.8.

Figure 31.9.

   A. Phlebo-thrombosis is shown in the left leg of a patient.

B–C. Bandaging is done on a leg with thrombosis, using a foam-elastic bandage.

D–E. Periarticular ossification arthropathy (POA) is shown in both hips of a patient. The early and final phases of the ossification process are represented.

F–H. A unilateral POA is shown in the early, intermediate, and late phases of the process.

   I. POA in both hips is shown (final phase).

J–L. POA involving the hip, ilium, and femur is shown in progression.

   M. POA of the knee is shown.

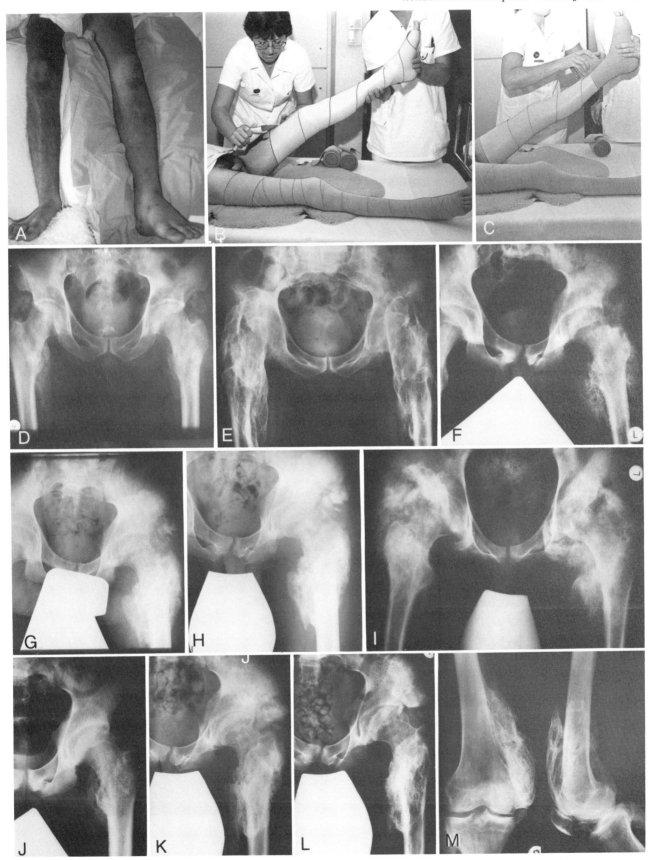

Figure 31.9.

Figure 31.10. Bowel care is important.

    A. Peristalsis is stimulated by abdominal massage.

    B. Bowel function is increased by exercises.

    C. Bandaging of legs is done with elastic bandages.

D–E. An abdominal binder is applied for support while the patient dangling.

F–H. For patients who sit in a wheelchair, there are rules for prevention of pressure sores, e.g., apply belt to keep hips from pressing against sides of chair.

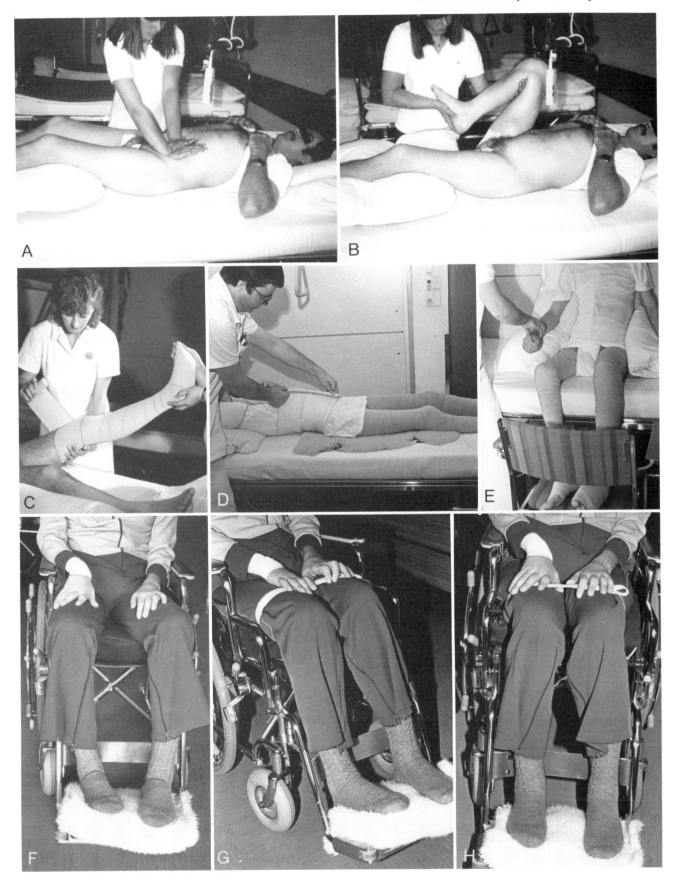

Figure 31.10.

Figure 31.11. Spasticity necessitates special considerations.

A. In the spastic hand, there is a risk of contractures;
B. These can be prevented by daily ROM exercises and
C. Splinting.
D. Extensor spasms in the wheelchair may injure feet and cause falls by propelling the patient out of the wheelchair.
E. Extension spasm of the legs can be prevented by application of a belt; adduction spasm can be prevented by insertion of foam wedges between the patient's knees.
F. Spreading of thighs using spreader bar in a patient with adductor spasticity.
G–I. The legs are stabilized during recumbency by using a folded bed sheet to tie them down.
J. Other measures that are helpful include an ice bath
K. Ice pack and
L. Swimming.

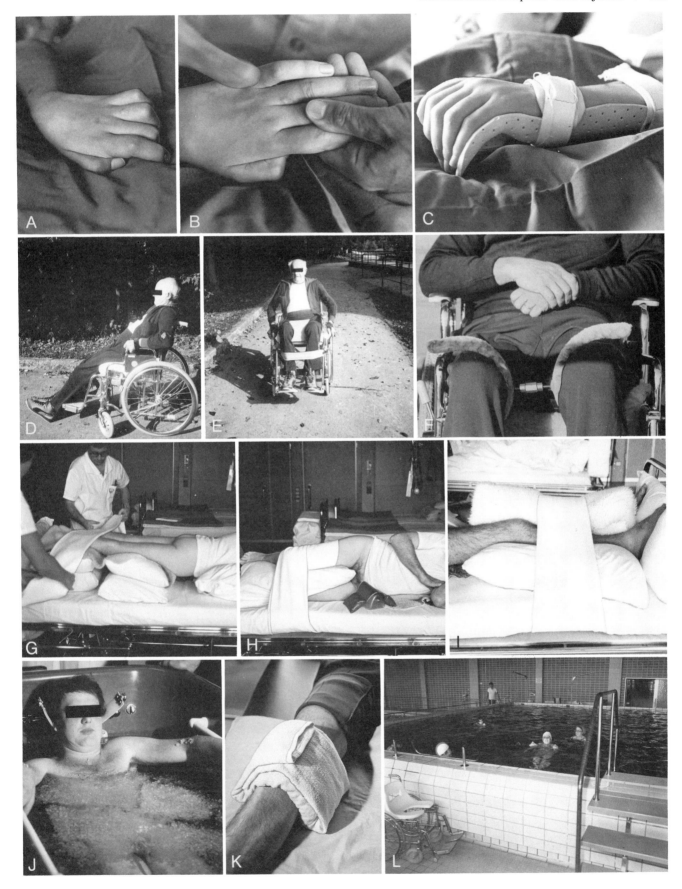

Figure 31.11.

Figure 31.12. Decubitus ulcers are treated conservatively by

  A. Bathing.

  B. Debridement of necrotic tissue, and

  C. Dressing.

  D. A patient with multiple ulcers is shown prior to conservative treatment.

  E. The same patient is shown after completion of conservative treatment.

  F. Decubitus on lateral aspect of foot is shown.

  G. Decubitus over the left trochanter is shown.

  H. Decubiti over anterior superior iliac spine and crest.

  I. Decubitus in complete spinal cord transsection from plaster of paris corset is shown.

J–K. Decubitus on the heel prior to and after completion of conservative treatment is shown.

  L. Decubitus over the coccygeal area is shown.

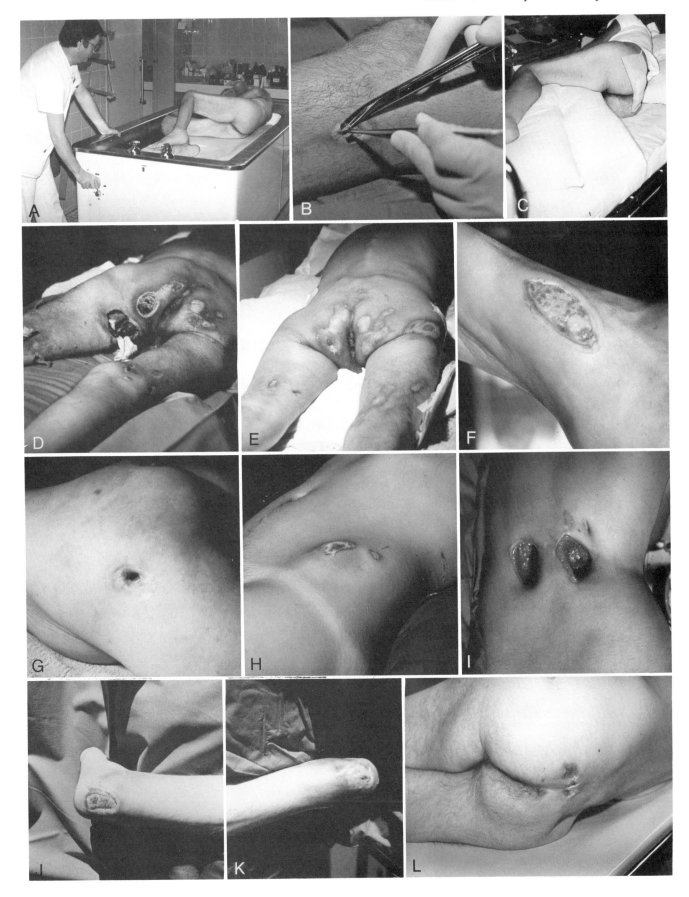

Figure 31.12.

Figure 31.13. Decubitus ulcers are treated surgically by

A–F. Double rotation flap, and

G–K. Resection of tuber ossis ischii and plastic closure

L. Plastic surgery about the trochanter.

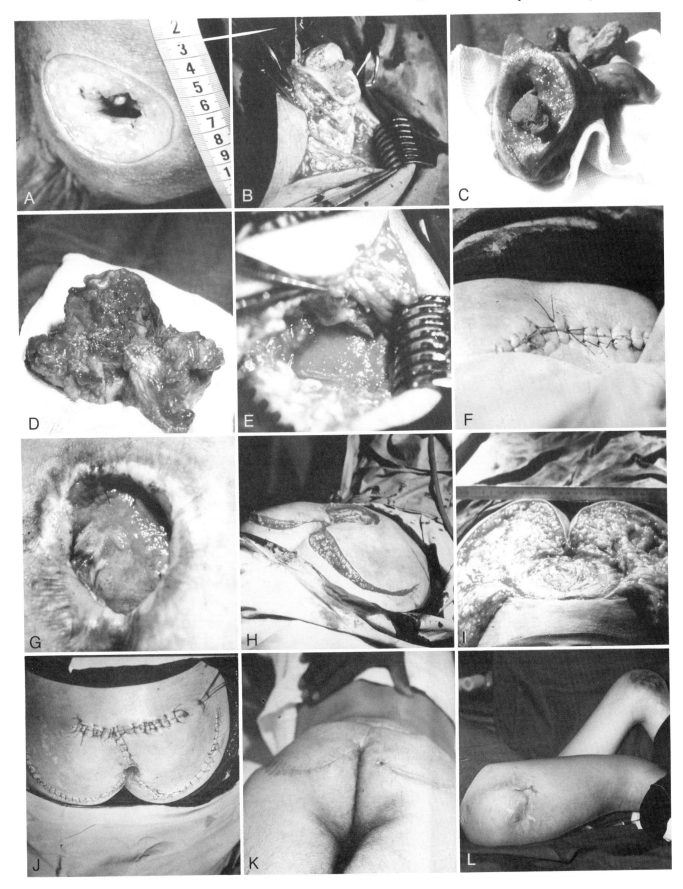

Figure 31.13.

Figure 31.14. In autonomic dysreflexia,

A. An indwelling catheter is used.

B–C. Self-catheterization is done by a tetraplegic using an orthotic device.

D–I. Procedure of self-catheterization in a high-level tetraplegic is shown. Note opening and closing of the zipper with a hook.

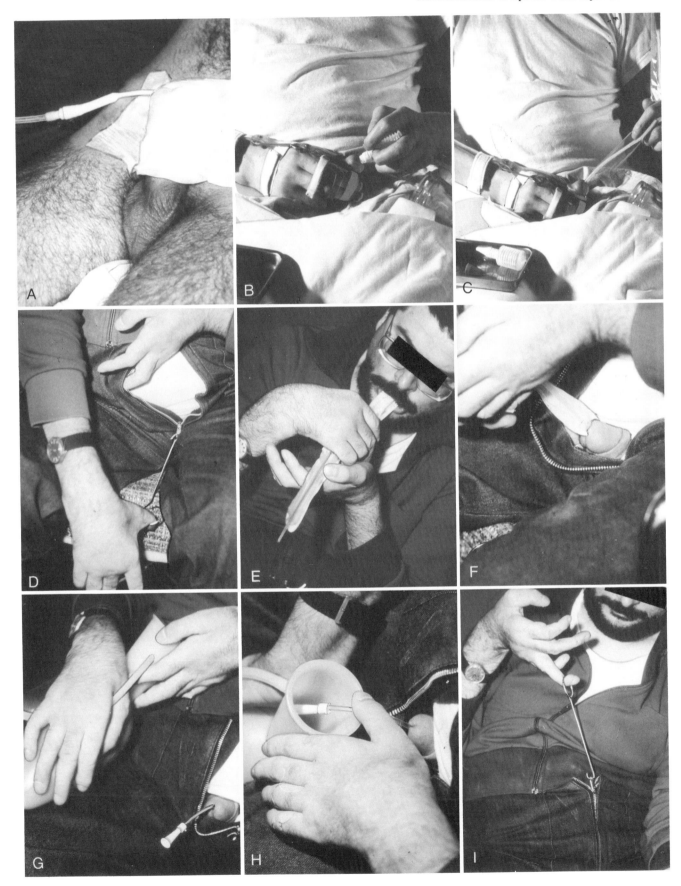

Figure 31.14.

Figure 31.15. Bladder training and self-catheterization are used in paraplegia.

A. Percussion of lower abdomen is shown over the bladder area.

B. Triggering, after Guttman is shown.

C. Credè is used here with one hand.

D. Credè is used here with both hands.

E–L. These utensils and procedures are necessary for self-catheterization

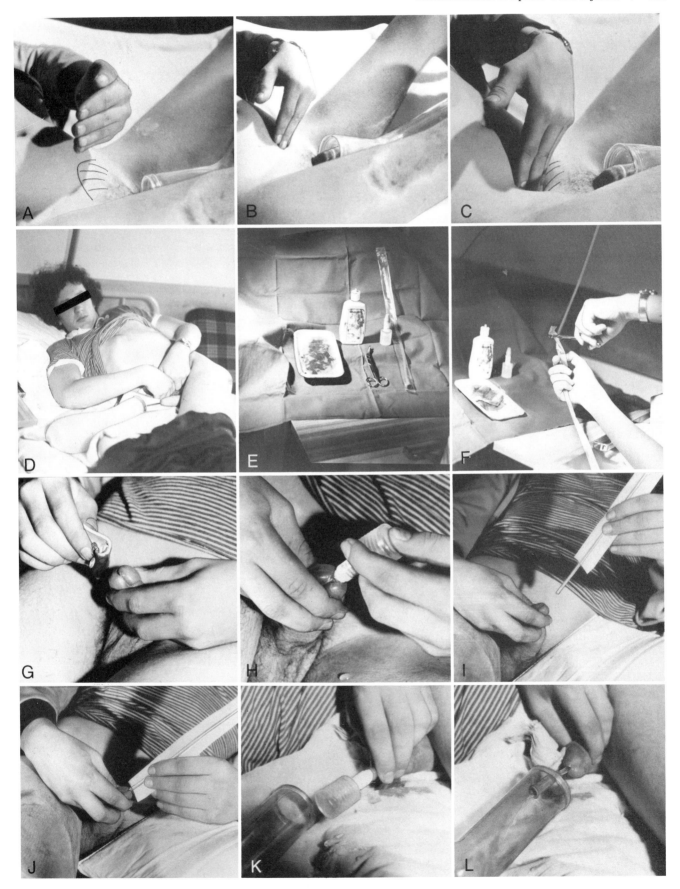

Figure 31.15.

32

Urological Management of Spinal Cord Injured Patients: Diagnostic and Therapeutic Aspects

Helmut Madersbacher, M.D.

Spinal cord injuries usually cause disturbances of the genitourinary system and micturition, which if not adequately managed, frequently lead to kidney failure. Therefore, the life expectancy of the spinal cord injured patient depends to a great extent upon his or her urological management. The principles of rehabilitation medicine are to preserve what function is left, to use it judiciously, and to substitute for lost function to the greatest possible extent. This applies also to the urological treatment, especially in regard to the emptying of the bladder. Understanding the underlying pathophysiology is absolutely necessary for appropriate management of the patient with a neurogenic bladder.

PHYSIOLOGY AND PATHOPHYSIOLOGY

The urinary bladder and its sphincter are one functional unit. In the normal situation, when the detrusor contracts, the sphincter opens; at the same time, the bladder neck changes its shape, forming a funnel. This is hydrodynamically favorable as it keeps voiding resistance at the lowest possible level.

Interplay between detrusor and sphincter is only possible when the pathways carrying nerve impulses from the bladder to the spinal cord, brainstem, and cortical centers are intact. Efferent pathways from the brain to the spinal cord nuclei and peripheral nerves to the bladder must also function to provide adequate emptying. The sacral portion of the spinal cord (S2–S4) contains the center controlling micturition. This center contains cells through which inhibitory and facilitatory impulses reach the bladder.

Contraction of the bladder is only possible when the parasympathetic sensory stretch receptors are intact. Sympathetic cells located between T10 and L3 also influence bladder contraction by relaying touch, temperature, and pain sensations. Normally, emptying of the bladder is under voluntary control with no residual urine present.

TYPES OF NEUROGENIC BLADDER

Reflex Bladder

Interruption of the pathway between the sacral spinal cord (S2) and brain leads to development of a reflex bladder after spinal shock subsides (see Fig. 32.1). Emptying of the bladder is regulated by the spinal reflex mechanism. However, in the absence of a central regulatory mechanism, there is a deficiency of interaction between the bladder and sphincter. During bladder contraction, there is spasm of the external sphincter. This is called the detrusor-sphincter dyssynergia. It causes increased outflow resistance, prevents coordinated voiding, and increases residual urine volume. Voluntary control is lost, and there is no sensation of urgency or voiding.

Autonomous Bladder

If the sacral spinal cord and peripheral nerves innervating the bladder and bladder neck are damaged, the bladder is physiologically cut off from the central nervous system (CNS). The reflex mechanism at the spinal cord is lost and the bladder becomes autonomous. If the cauda equina is completely destroyed, the bladder and pelvic floor muscles become paralyzed and flaccid. Clinically, there is a combination of detrusor arreflexia and pelvic floor muscle paresis.

Other Neurogenic Bladder Types

The type and severity of bladder and sphincter problems vary according to the pattern of primary lesion. An exact and detailed understanding and knowledge of these patterns is a prerequisite to proper and adequate management of incomplete neurogenic bladder.

DIAGNOSTIC CONSIDERATIONS IN VOIDING DISTURBANCES OF NEUROGENIC BLADDERS

The history and clinical-urological evaluation are the most important tools in the understanding of neurogenic voiding disturbances. History should include not only the voiding habits, but also sexual and bowel habits, because neurogenic pathways for these three activities are either shared or in proximity.

The neurological evaluation should include checking the tone of the anal sphincter, its active contraction, the anal or wink reflex, bulbocavernosus reflex, and sensation of touch and pain in the sacral (S2–S4) segments.

Radiological Urodynamic Evaluation

Intravenous Pyelogram (IVP)

This is still the basic examination of the function of the urinary tract. It gives information regarding the mor-

444

phology and shape of kidney, ureters, and bladder and also provides clues to kidney function. Voiding and postvoiding views give additional information about the lower urinary tract and efficiency of the bladder-emptying mechanism (Fig. 32.2).

Urethrogram

This is done by injection of contrast media into the urethra. With this method, the contour and pathological changes (e.g., strictures of the urethra can be recognized.

Cystogram and Voiding Cystourethrogram

The bladder is filled with contrast media until it's fullness or urgency is felt. Filling and bladder emptying are observed in a supine, sitting, or standing position, according to patient's voiding preferences (time and habits). It is done easily using an image intensifier with a television display. The changes of shape of the bladder and bladder neck allow identification of the type of the neurogenic bladder. Other severe voiding disturbances, such as vesicle-ureteral reflux also can be recognized clearly.

Uroflowmetry

This test shows peak flow rate, mean flow rate, and often the more important flow rate curve (voiding in a time-related curve).

Cystometrogram

The numerous methods used to measure intravesicular pressure can be divided into two main categories: (a) devices that use fluids for bladder filling (Fig. 32.3), and (b) devices that use gas, usually CO_2.

Construction of these devices allows continuous and exact graphic display of the intravesical pressure. In fluid manometry, a two-channel catheter is used. One channel allows continuous bladder filling, while the second channel is attached to measuring system and graph recording the pressure. In gas cystomanometry, there is only a single-channel catheter using variable speed of gas flow, and bladder resistance is measured and recorded. Simultaneous measurement of intravesical and intrarectal pressure is done by insertion of a rectal probe (see Fig. 32.4). Extravesical pressure increase can thus be measured and recorded during coughing, laughing, talking, and straining in order to differentiate other pressure from detrusor contraction. Bladder tone is important in the assessment of cystometrograms because its status during the filling period relates primarily to the elastic properties of the bladder wall.

Questions that should be asked are: "Is there presence of detrusor contraction?" and, if so, "Can it be influenced by voluntary action or can involuntary detrusor contraction be produced by coughing, position change, etc.?"

A cystometrogram also provides information about bladder sensation. Even simple measurements of the intravesical pressure give much more information than merely the pressure if a skilled interpreter observes the procedure.

Characteristic curve patterns are at times more important than measurable absolute values. From this point of view, the cystomanometry becomes an indispensable screening test for the evaluation of functional bladder disturbances.

Simultaneous Pressure, Flow, Electromyography, and Radiography

Recording relevant parameters for continence and micturition during bladder filling and emptying can be determined exactly by sequential recording with the aid of modern instrumentation. Bladder filling and intravesical pressure can be measured either by thin suprapubic or transurethral catheters, intrarectal pressure by rectal probe, electromyogram (EMG) activity of the pelvic floor muscles or the sphincter ani and external urethral sphincter by wire or needle electrodes, and the urinary flow by means of the uroflow meter. Filling and emptying phases are observed radiologically with the image intensifier on a television screen and permanently recorded on videotape. With this method, it is possible to make an exact analysis of the detrusor as well as the sphincter mechanism, especially the external sphincter.

Endoscopic Diagnosis (Cystourethroscopy)

Changes in the bladder and urethra, which can be seen during an endoscopic examination, develop secondary to disturbances in the emptying mechanism of the neurogenic bladder and increase with the duration of the illness.

Dislocation and deformation of the ostia and formation of trabeculation and diverticuli are not seen in early lesions; likewise, pathological chances in the urethra, such as caverns and stones of the prostate (the so-called trigone sclerom, diverticuli, and fistulas) are not seen until later in the disease process. In order to recognize catheter incrustations, cystoscopy is indispensable (see Fig. 32.5).

Urinary Drainage in Patients with Acute Spinal Cord Injuries

Care should be taken to provide adequate bladder emptying during the so-called spinal shock phase, in which the micturition reflex is absent.

There are three options for bladder emptying:

1. Indwelling urethral catheter
2. Suprapubic catheter
3. Intermittent catheterization

The indwelling catheter treatment, which superficially appears as a simple and nonproblematic method, actually carries major risks, mainly that irritation of the urethral mucosa causes abacterial urethritis. Bacteriuria results, followed by urinary tract infection, with attendant complications, such as epidydimitis, stone formation, contracted bladder, and urethral reflux. Permanent catheter pressure leads to ureteral ulceration with periurethritis and urethral diverticuli. The most endangered location is the penoscrotal junction.

For the above reasons, indwelling urethral catheter drainage in acute spinal cord injured patients should be restricted to the following indications: when exact monitoring of fluid intake and output is necessary (e.g., in multiple trauma), during parenteral feeding, and in severe febrile urinary tract infections.

To prevent urethral erosion at the penoscrotal junction, the catheter should be lifted up and loosely taped to the lower abdomen. A small, well-tolerated catheter should be used (12 to 16F silastic) in a closed drainage system.

With suprapubic cystostomy the traumatization of the urethra is eliminated, but there is still a foreign body in the bladder. For this reason, infections and incrustation cannot always be prevented.

With intermittent catheterization, the patient is catheterized several times a day, and sterile precautions must be observed. With careful techniques, the infection rate is extremely low, and paraurethral abscesses and epididymitis almost always can be avoided. The only danger of the intermittent catheterization is overdistention of the bladder by insufficient frequency of catheterization of increased diuresis. This can be prevented by strict fluid balance and adequate catheterization intervals. The apparent increase of time and material used in this method can be easily justified because urinary tract complications in the early phase of spinal cord lesions can be reduced to a minimum.

BLADDER TRAINING

Technique of the Noninstrumental Emptying of the Bladder in the Spinal Cord Injured Patient

The bladder, even the neurogenic bladder, can be emptied by various methods according to the type.

The Reflex Bladder

Emptying can be induced by reflex triggering of the detrusor contraction. The customary trigger mechanisms leading to detrusor contraction are: tapping of the suprapubic area (Fig. 32.6); rhythmic compressions of the suprapubic area; stimulation of the skin over the lower abdomen, external genitalia, or the inside of the thighs; deep breathing, coughing, and sneezing; or rectal stimulation.

Prerequisites for successful "triggering" are: (a) the sacral reflex arc must be intact and functional, and (b) the bladder should be full but not overdistended. The optimal stimulus for a reflex contraction of the bladder should be determined empirically; "triggering" requires patience, time, and endurance. Only regularly scheduled bladder emptying with measured fluid intake leads to dryness between emptyings. Instruction and inspection by the physicians and nursing personnel, as well as experimentation, in close cooperation with the patient are prerequisites for success.

Autonomous Bladder

If the spinal reflex arc is absent, "triggering" is meaningless. However, emptying of the bladder can be achieved by the Credé maneuver or abdominal strain, provided that the pelvic floor muscles are also paralyzed and flaccid. The intravesical pressure necessary for this type of emptying, however, must be much greater than the physiological micturition pressure. The reason is that in this form of emptying, the bladder and posterior urethra are being pushed downward; the urethra is squeezed against the muscles, even if the pelvic floor muscles are paralyzed and flaccid. A functional stenosis of the urethra results during micturition. It is possible that additional pathological sympathetic reflex mechanisms play a role as well. The harder the patient presses or strains, the more squeeze is exerted upon the urethra and the more difficult bladder emptying becomes. Through experience, some patients have learned that bladder emptying can be substantially facilitated by manual counterpressure against the perineum (while applying the Credé maneuver). Triggering and passive emptying of the bladder are only compensatory mechanisms with many disadvantages. Even in seemingly excellent emptying of the bladder, with either of the above ways, regular, life-long urological reevaluations are necessary for early recognition and correction of problems and prevention of harmful secondary changes.

Management of Incontinence in Patients with Neurogenic Bladder

Even in patients who have been trained optimally in management of their neurogenic bladder, there are times that uncontrollable incontinence is experienced: in the reflex bladder, secondary to spasms, and in the autonomic bladder, (with flaccid paresis of the pelvic floor muscles) because a of sudden increase of the intraabdominal pressure.

At home, patients often get by without the use of a collecting device. Outside of the home, however, these patients should be provided with a well-fitted condom or other external collecting devices for hygienic and social reasons. The condom is affixed to the penis either by a medical adhesive or a double-faced adhesive tape strip, which is wrapped around the penis and then connected to a drainage system (Fig. 32.7). It is especially suitable for nonambulatory wheelchair persons. The condom should be changed daily.

Unfortunately, at present, there is no suitable collecting system for women. Only a strict regimen of fluid intake and emptying of the bladder may reduce the urinary incontinence to a socially acceptable level. If residual urine is the main cause of a reflex or overflow incontinence, intermittent self-catheterization becomes the method of choice.

The treatment or continuous long-term drainage with an indwelling catheter seems only justified after all other therapeutic measures have failed.

The surgical alternative in the treatment of incontinence seems to be the insertion of a hydraulic sphincter, which was developed by Scott. The implantation is, however, recommended only in a bladder with arreflexia or hypocontractility of the detrusor and with no residual urine after emptying of the bladder. Any existing reflux must be corrected beforehand. Generally, several preparatory operations, such as sphincterotomy, notching, or sacral rhizotomy, are necessary. Technical problems with the implanted sphincter system require at times "reparatory" surgical procedures. Therefore, indications for implantation of Scott's hydraulic sphincter in spinal cord injured patients with neurogenic urinary incontinence is limited.

Intermittent (Self-) Catheterization

Intermittent catheterization (Fig. 32.8) can be taught to, and practiced by, the patient or performed by relatives and caretakers. It is a useful alternative for patients in whom adequate emptying of the bladder cannot be achieved by conservative methods (e.g., trigger mechanism, abdominal straining, or Credé). The patient, however, according to the type of the lesion, is continent and one in whom (in all probability) a surgical procedure would lead to incontinence.

This method is also of great value to female patients in whom adequate bladder emptying cannot be achieved and in whom high residual urine results in reflux or overflow incontinence.

The ground rules for intermittent catheterization apply also to self-catheterization. Overdistension of the bladder must be prevented because it increases the risk of infection and prevents recovery of the detrusor. Emptying of the bladder must be complete to avoid rapid increase of infection rate.

The method of choice is the intermittent catheterization using disposable catheters under as clean conditions as possible, (e.g., "out of the envelope" method).

Thirty-year follow-up evaluations have shown that intermittent self-catheterization is a reliable method for managing patients with low-pressure arreflexia bladder.

Operative Measures for Improvement of Bladder Emptying

Present surgical procedures are limited basically to the transurethral procedures at the bladder neck. The procedures are technically simple. They require, however, very good knowledge of pathophysiology of the neurogenic disturbances and bladder emptying as well as of exact urodynamic assessment.

Basically, the indication for a transurethral procedure is imbalance between the detrusor force and the bladder outlet resistance, that cannot be corrected by conservative measures. This leads to unsatisfactory bladder emptying. The doctor must consider carefully, case by case, after discussions with the patient and his or her relatives or caretakers, whether to consider bladder emptying by intermittent catheterization in the presence of an arreflectic detrusor and spasm of the pelvic floor and, thus, preserve continence; or, whether satisfactory emptying of the bladder should be accomplished by a transurethral procedure at the price of incontinence.

Choices for reduction of the increased outflow resistance secondary to detrusor-external sphincter dyssynergia are the transurethral sphincterotomy, with or without incision of the bladder neck, and resection of a chronically inflamed and enlarged prostate.

Figure 32.1.

A. Brainstem reflex for micturition is similar to other vital function reflexes. It utilizes long spinal tracts via the brainstem.

B. Bladder neck assumes the shape of a funnel during normal bladder emptying, when there is normal coordination between the bladder and sphincters.

C. In the reflex bladder, micturition is controlled by spinal reflex only, which has many disadvantages.

D. In the reflex bladder, there is often simultaneous contracture of the bladder and the external sphincter called detrusor-external sphincter dyssynergy. This is caused by loss of central control.

E. In the autonomous bladder, the sacral cord is damaged, and the bladder as well as bladder outlet are separated from the central nervous system; there is arreflexia of the detrusor with flaccid paresis of the pelvic floor muscles.

F. In incomplete neurogenic bladders, the detrusor and sphincter can be damaged to various degrees and the following types can be identified:
1. Spastic detrusor with spastic pelvic floor
2. "Spastic" detrusor with flaccid pelvic floor
3. "Weak" detrusor with spastic sphincter
4. "Weak" detrusor with flaccid sphincter

Translations to Figure 32.1: A, Brainstem with pons; C, Cord transsection above S_2, Mass reflex!; E, Brainstem; F, types of neurogenic bladders.

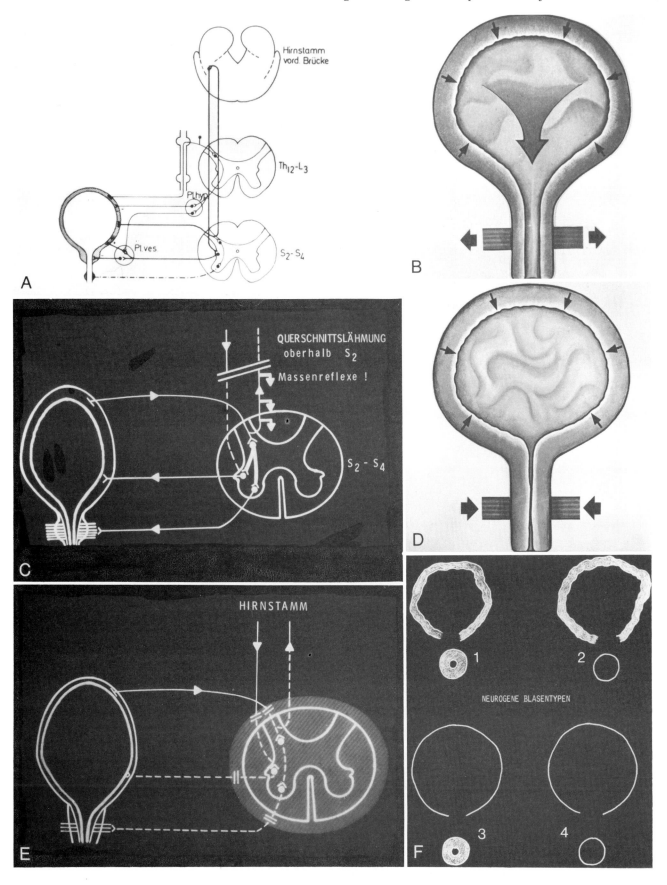

Figure 32.1.

Figure 32.2.

A. Intravenous pyelogram shows a normal renal pelvis, calyces, and ureters.

B. Massive dilatation of the renal pelvis, calyces and ureters secondary to detrusor-external sphincter dyssynergy in reflex bladder is shown.

C. In this urethrogram; leakage of contrast media at the penoscrotal junction in paraurethral abscess is secondary to continuous use of a Foley catheter during the spinal shock phase. (Taping of the penis and catheter to the abdominal wall may prevent fistula).

D. This voiding cystourethrogram shows the sequela of paraurethral abscess after prolonged use of a Foley catheter—a large urethral diverticulum developed. It acts as a reservoir for sludge and bacteria leading to recurrent urinary tract infections and poor urinary flow.

E. This voiding cystourethrogram shows vesicoureteral reflux, which endangers the kidney. Contrast media initially introduced into the bladder is seen in the ureter and the kidney.

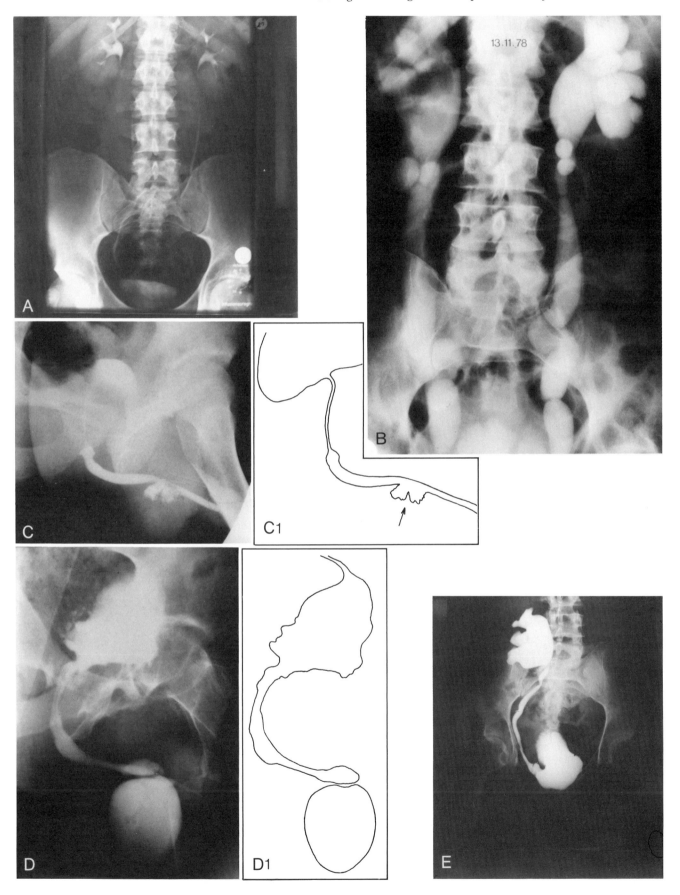

Figure 32.2.

Figure 32.3.

A. Already in 1882, Mosso and Pellicani had evaluated the influence of the psyche on bladder pressure with this cystometer.

B. This diagram shows fluid cystometry using dual channel transurethral catheter.

C. This graph of intravesical pressure changes during bladder filling shows the normal range for adults would be seen within the shaded area.

D. Dual-channel CO_2 cystomanometer for simultaneous intravesical and intrarectal pressure recording is shown. Through a transurethral catheter, the bladder is inflated with CO_2, and its resistance is measured by a transducer incorporated in the cystometer. Transrectal catheter allows recording of the intrarectal pressure, substituting for the intraabdominal pressure.

E. The so-called "reflex bladder"-single channel CO_2 cystomanometry is shown. At about 200 mm of CO_2 filling, there is detrusor contraction which can be recognized by the increase in the intravesical pressure; the patient, however, is only aware of some sensation of dysesthesia in the back.

Translations to Figure 32.3: B, H_2O or contrast media, recorder, monitor pressure (transducer); E, spinal cord lesion, heat sensation in back, CO_2 cystomanometry, micturition.

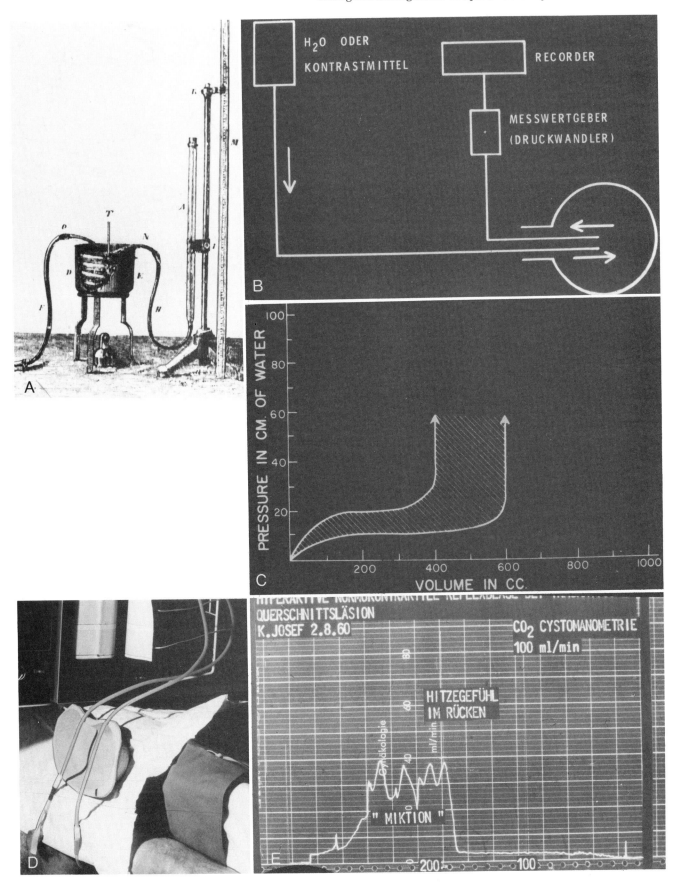

Figure 32.3.

Figure 32.4.

A. Layout of combined urodynamic evaluation with simultaneous measurements of the intravesical pressure, intrarectal pressure. EMG of the pelvic floor or the external anal and urethral sphincters is shown. The urinary flow and the voiding volume is measured with the uroflowmeter. When filling the bladder with contrast media one can also observe the radiological picture of the bladder and the trigone during filling and emptying phases in addition to the urodynamic parameters.

B. This layout and instrumentation for combined urodynamic and radiological evaluation at the rehabilitation center in Bad Häring shows the 8-channel printer for recording pertinent parameters. In the middle is the X-ray table with television monitor and, beside it, the image intensifier. A tape recorder is in the background. The examination is shown with the patient in the supine position but the same parameters can be obtained in sitting position.

C. Urodynamic study of bladder emptying in a patient with benign prostatic hypertrophy without suspected additional disturbances is shown. From *bottom* to *top*: intravesical pressure, EMG of pelvic floor, intrarectal pressure, voiding volume, and urinary flow. With onset of detrusor contraction, seen as a rise of intravesical pressure, bladder emptying follows whereby, the pelvic floor muscles totally relax. The intrarectal pressure remains constant as a sign that the increase of the intravesical pressure was accomplished by detrusor contraction alone.

D. Urodynamic study of the so called reflex bladder with detrusor-external sphincter dyssynergy is shown. With onset of detrusor contraction, there is spasm of the pelvic floor muscles which can be recognized as an increase in EMG activity. A final brief emptying of the bladder can be seen after the detrusor contraction and EMG activity have subsided.

E. Urodynamic study of bladder emptying by Credé maneuver in the so-called autonomous bladder, with arreflexia of the detrusor and flaccid paresis of the pelvic floor muscles is shown. *Bottom* to *top*: intravesical pressure, intrarectal pressure, EMG of pelvic floor, differential pressure between bladder and rectum, and urinary flow and voiding volume. By using the Credé maneuver, there is simultaneous increase of pressure in the bladder and the rectum. The EMG shows only motion artifacts. The differential pressure shows only minimal oscillations because of synchronous increase in both bladder and rectal pressure. In spite of high intravesical pressure values, the urinary flow is weak and bladder emptying is only possible in stages.

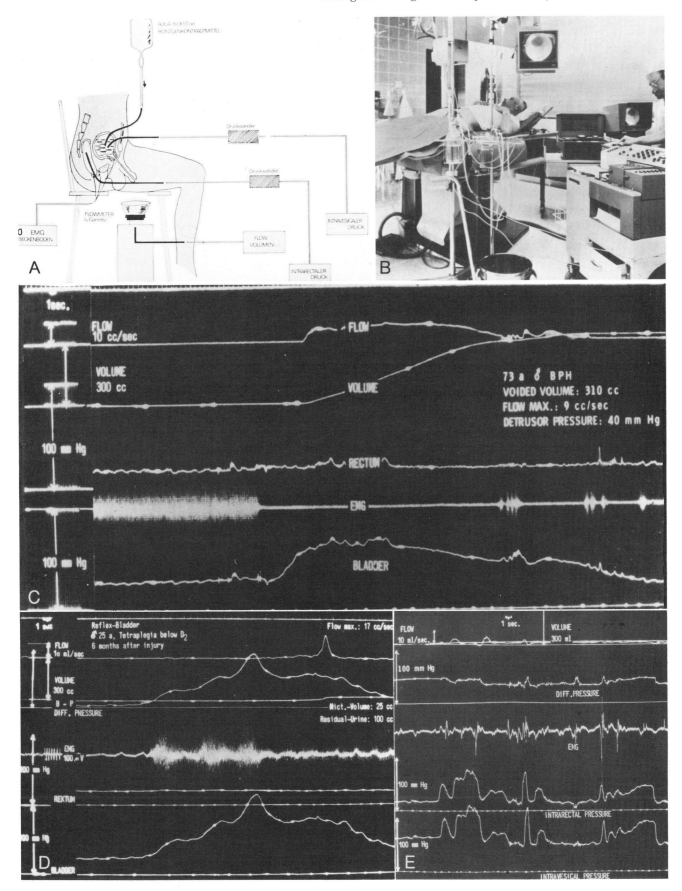

Figure 32.4.

Figure 32.5.

A. Cystoscopic appearance of a trabeculated bladder is shown.

B. Cystoscopic appearance of catheter with incrustations in the bladder is shown.

C. If there is strict indication for an indwelling catheter during the spinal shock phase, the catheter and penis should be lifted and loosely taped to the lower abdomen. This will prevent urethral erosion at the penoscrotal junction.

D. Drainage of bladder with suprapubic catheter.

E. Utensils necessary for intermittent catheterization are prepared in a sterile tray and placed on a treatment table or Mayo stand.

F. The patient is covered with sterile drapes, and the nurse or orderly wears a gown, glove, and cap (not usually done this way in the United States).

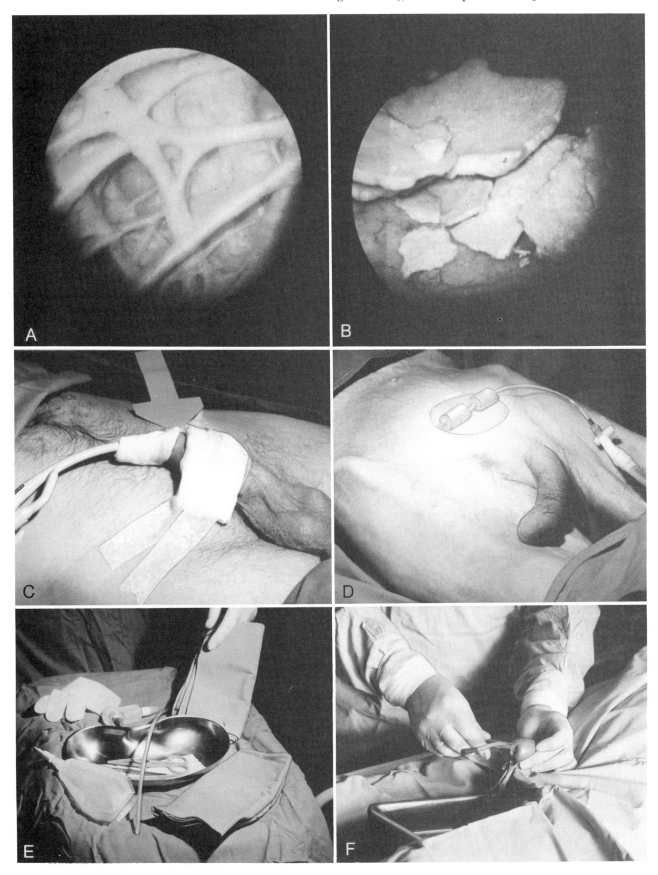

Figure 32.5.

Figure 32.6.

   A. Triggering is done by tapping of suprapubic area with ulnar aspect of the hand.

B–C. Triggering is done by rhythmic compression of the lower abdomen-bladder area with the tips of the extended fingers of one hand. This technique is tiresome, and requires good function; however, it causes less spasm than the tapping with the hand.

D–E. Triggering requires patience and sensitivity, not violence.

   F. Micturition cystourethrogram during passive emptying of the bladder by abdominal straining shows that the bladder and posterior urethra are displaced downward: the section of the urethra that penetrates the pelvic floor muscles is squeezed and elongated.

   G. A radiological view (positive image) of the passive bladder emptying is possible because the urethral segment passing through the pelvic floor is elongated and compressed by muscles, even though they are flaccid. Thus, a functional obstruction is created, and pressure values higher than in the normal become necessary to empty the bladder.

   H. Passive bladder emptying is done by means of the Credé maneuver.

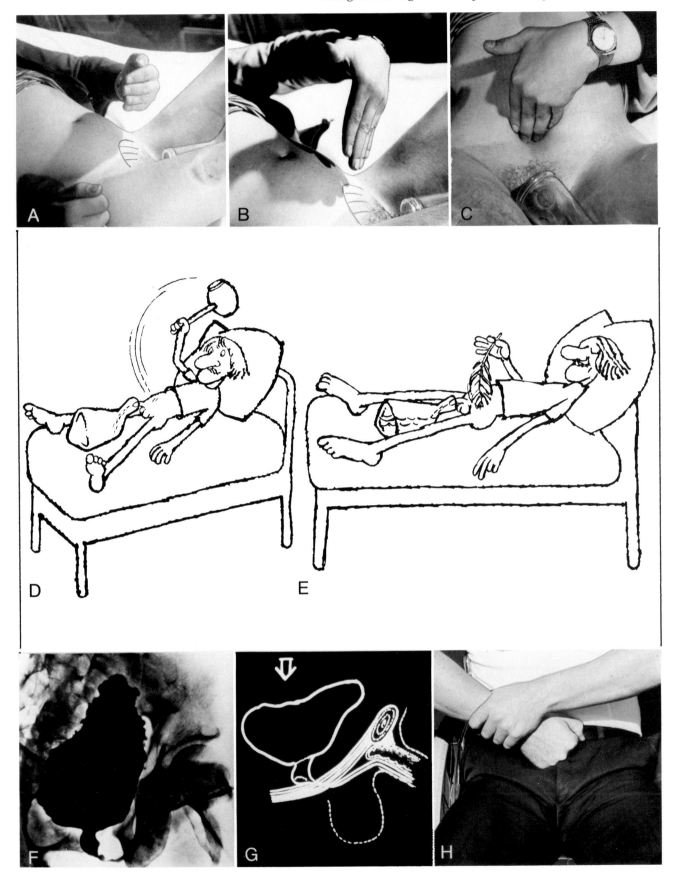

Figure 32.6.

Figure 32.7.

A. A condom collecting device is applied. Medical adhesive is applied over the penis shaft, and the condom is rolled over it.

B. A modified condom urinal is affixed with a double-faced adhesive plastic strip.

C. The technique of application of a double-faced adhesive plastic strip is shown.

D. Schematic drawing of an implanted Scott's hydraulic sphincter shows the sphincter collar positioned around the bladder neck. Pressure on the balloon forces the fluid into the sphincter collar, which in turn compresses the bladder neck and renders the bladder continent. For bladder emptying, the fluid from the sphincter collar is shifted back into the balloon by means of a pump, which is implanted into the scrotum or labia. The direction of the fluid flow is regulated by the "control assembly."

E. Schematic drawing of a Scott's sphincter implanted in a female is shown.

F. An X-ray of an implanted Scott's sphincter clearly shows the sphincter collar around the bladder neck, the pressure balloon, the control assembly, and the pump in the scrotum.

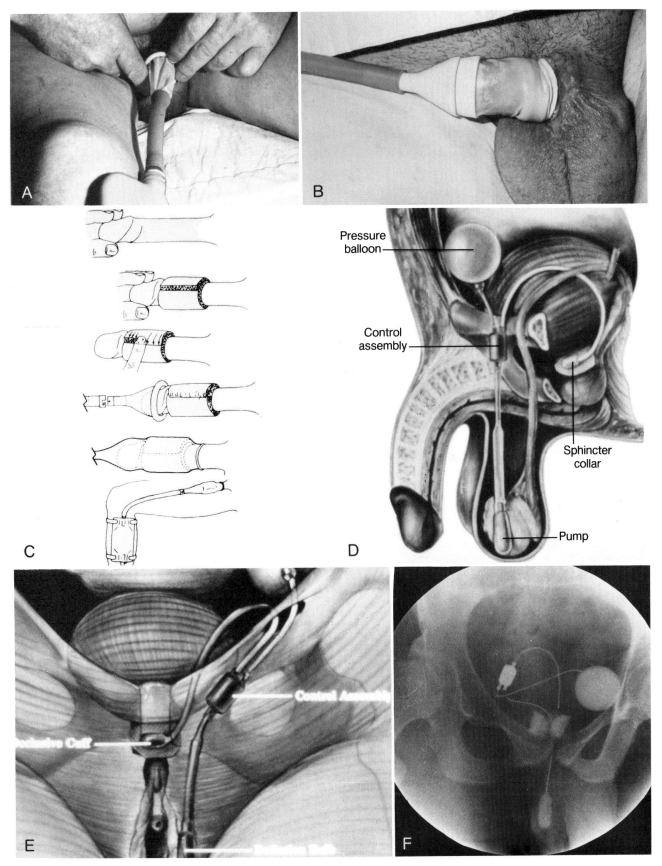

Figure 32.7.

Figure 32.8.

A. Necessary utensils for intermittent self-catheterization include a sterile envelope with a disposable catheter, disinfectants, gauze sponge, scissors, kidney-shaped container, and, for females, a magnifying mirror.

B. Catheterization takes place in a semirecumbent position. The mirror enables the female patient to become oriented to her anatomy; she spreads her labia with her left hand and cleans the urethral orifice with her right one.

C. The catheter is then inserted into the bladder directly from its envelope, thus avoiding contamination by handling the catheter.

D. Complete emptying of the bladder is necessary. To avoid residual urine, the bladder must be compressed at the end of the procedure.

E. For self-catheterization in the male; following the injection of a high-viscosity lubricant, the catheter slides in a well-lubricated cylinder into the bladder.

F. The end of the catheter envelope is cut open: the tip of the catheter exposed and immediately inserted into the distal urethra.

G. The catheter is now advanced into the bladder directly from the envelope.

H. The urine flows through the inserted catheter into the urinal.

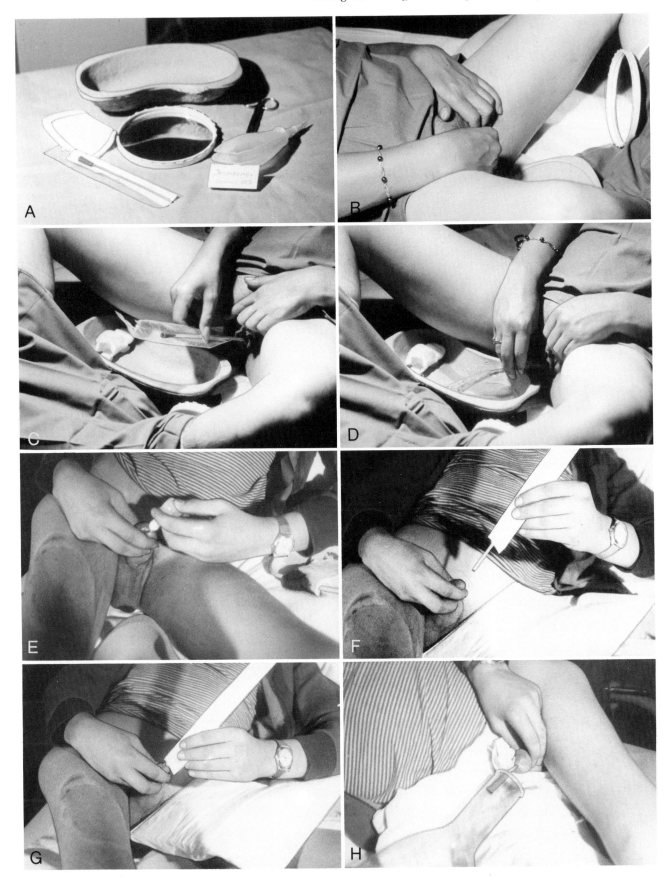

Figure 32.8.

SPECIAL MEDICAL DIAGNOSTIC AND THERAPEUTIC APPROACHES

33

Acupuncture in Amputees

Rudolf Buratti, M.D.

Acupuncture has become an important addition to the wide variety of earlier physical therapy measures for post-surgical treatment of injuries and diseases of the supporting apparatus and the locomotor system.

De La Füye outlined the possibilities of acupuncture in one sentence:

Acupuncture uses insertion of metal needles at precisely determined points on the skin, which can be spontaneously painful or tender to pressure, for diagnosis and therapy of functional reversible diseases.

This therapy is one of the oldest methods of treatment in use today. Apparently, it developed from the relieving effect that was found to result from pressure and mild massage applied to painful areas. This elementary form of acupuncture, the locus-dolendi-puncture, is still used occasionally, e.g., with local muscle spasms in sports medicine and with various local conditions of pain. Especially suitable for treatment by acupuncture are all painful conditions, restricted mobility after long immobilization, swelling tendencies, disturbed circulation, and muscular weakness.

One of the most troublesome, often almost unbearable, sensations of pain is the phantom pain after an amputation. Phantom pain or phantom limb pain is a pain that is localized in a no-longer-present but still experienced limb. The lost extremity is most frequently experienced in the position it was in immediately before its loss or during the injury. Due to the preserved memory of past mobility, voluntary movements of the stump muscles are still possible. The patient can give detailed information about the position of limb, muscular tonicity and skin tension, and, above all, temperature and surface condition.

Unpleasant phantom sensations or autosomatognoses, and phantom limb pain often fail to respond to conventional medical treatment. In such cases, acupuncture has proven to be quite successful in relieving symptoms.

Because of the unique role of acupuncture, stump pain caused by neuromas of the nerve endings must be distinguished from paralgesia, the real phantom pain. The former consists in a high-grade sensibility of the amputation stump to touch or pressure, and its intensity depends very much on weather conditions. Paralgesias are manifested by painful formication, numbness, spasmodic dragging or stinging pain, contusion pain, and feelings of heaviness and tiredness. They do not occur immediately but only after a certain period of time and are mainly projected to the palm and the fingers with upper extremity amputations and to the sole and toes with lower extremity amputations. Paralgesias also depend on weather conditions.

Many attempts have been made to explain the character and development of phantom pain, but all efforts have only disclosed the cause of individual features of this clinical picture, so that the methods developed for treatment have only produced tolerably satisfactory results. Acupuncture is a method that is easily applicable, harmless, can in most cases alleviate pain, and often can make it disappear for months or "indefinitely." Another advantage is the fact that such a treatment safely can be repeated at any time.

The procedure for treating phantom pain involves two steps:

1. Taking important history, including the exact specification of the localization of pain, information about sensitivity to change in the weather, other general conditions of pain, and general nervous overexcitability
2. Inspecting the stump as to shape, skin condition, scars, circulation, temperature, and neuromas

Treatment is given only to the remaining extremity. Treatment is started by pricking needles into the pain areas, which are specified and exactly localized by the disabled. It is necessary that the patient specify the exact localization. In lower limb amputes, these pain areas are mostly the toes, sole, inner or outer edge of the foot, and calcaneal region; in upper limb amputes, the fingers and the metacarpal region are the most common pain areas. In addition to these individual local spots, general pain spots and spots for improvement of circulation should also be punctured.

Several reactions to this treatment can be expected. First, even after a short time, the handicapped patient often experiences an alleviation of pain and an increased tingling sensation or formication in the phantom limb. Second, a sensation of warmth is experienced, so that an absolutely comfortable sensation arises in the phantom limb. The phantom sensation itself remains, but is not experienced as inconvenient. Third, the cramped toes or fingers are frequently relaxed, even after the first puncturing. These spasms are experienced as extremely disagreeable by the patient and are usually combined with a strong sensation of cold.

In case this basic treatment is ineffective, there are still other methods of treatment that can be applied, e.g., Petit Piqure and Grand Piqure, according to Bischko (1978, 1983).

The treatment of bilateral amputees is difficult, especially with bilateral high above-knee amputees, although also in such cases alleviation of pain is sometimes achieved by acupuncture of points on the trunk and the upper extremities, and by ear acupuncture. In most cases, marked stump pain immediately subsides when needles are set in the scar area.

As to the success of treatment and the permanence of success, results can only be assessed by the information given by the patient. Cautious evaluation of this information at the rehabilitation center at Bad Häring in Tirol, Austria shows that a significant improvement can be achieved in 60 to 70% of the cases; from an improvement lasting only for a few days up to an improvement for months and even to complete freedom from pain for a year or more.

Most patients reported that the pain never became as intense as that before treatment. There was hardly any difference between recent and old amputees. The results were usually better with lower limb amputees than with upper limb amputees.

In many cases, acupuncture can bring the disabled patient a true alleviation of existing phantom limb pain and stump complaints. Apart from this, it is also possible to achieve an improvement of circulation, a fact that must not be underrated. Due to the wide range effect of acupuncture in both somatic and psychic respects, a general improvement of the patient's well-being also can be achieved. Figures 33.1 and 33.2 further illustrate the techniques used in acupuncture.

Figure 33.1.

A. The gallbladder meridian contains important acupuncture points for pain control.

B. The bladder meridian is the longest meridian, with 67 points.

C. The colon meridian is shown.

D. The passway of the spleen, pancreas, liver, stomach, gallbladder, and bladder meridians in the anterior, lateral and medial side are shown. On the medial side, the kidney meridian is also marked.

(Reprinted with permission from Ernst Busse and Paul Buss: *Akupunkturfibel*. Richard Pflaum Verlag, Munich, 1954).

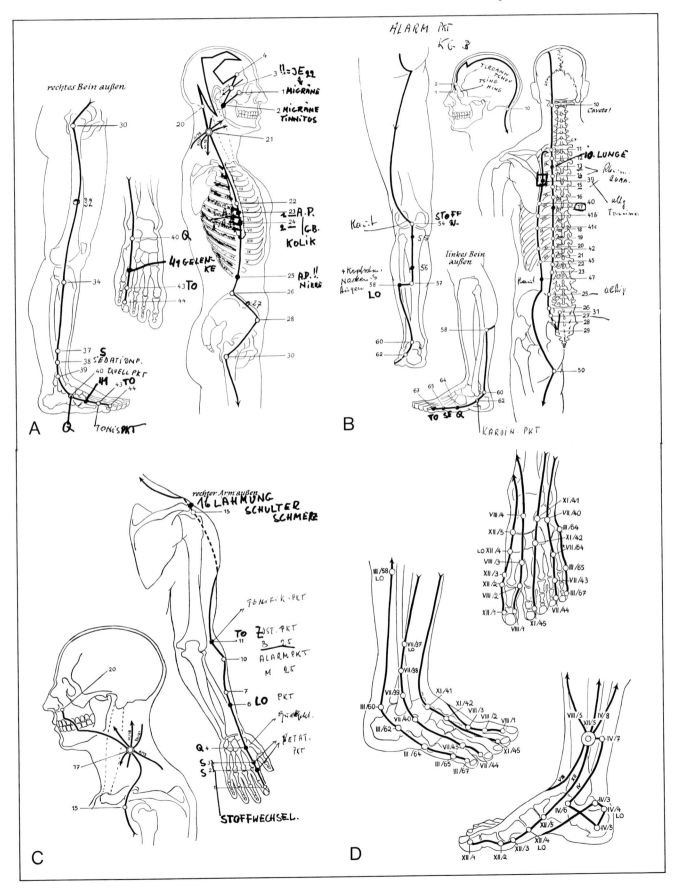

Figure 33.1.

Figure 33.2.

  A. Acupuncture needles of various lengths are made of steel, silver, or gold.

B–C. Location of acupuncture points are made with the point detector (neurolocator).

D–F. Placement of needles on the remaining foot and leg of an amputee are for the relief of phantom pain.

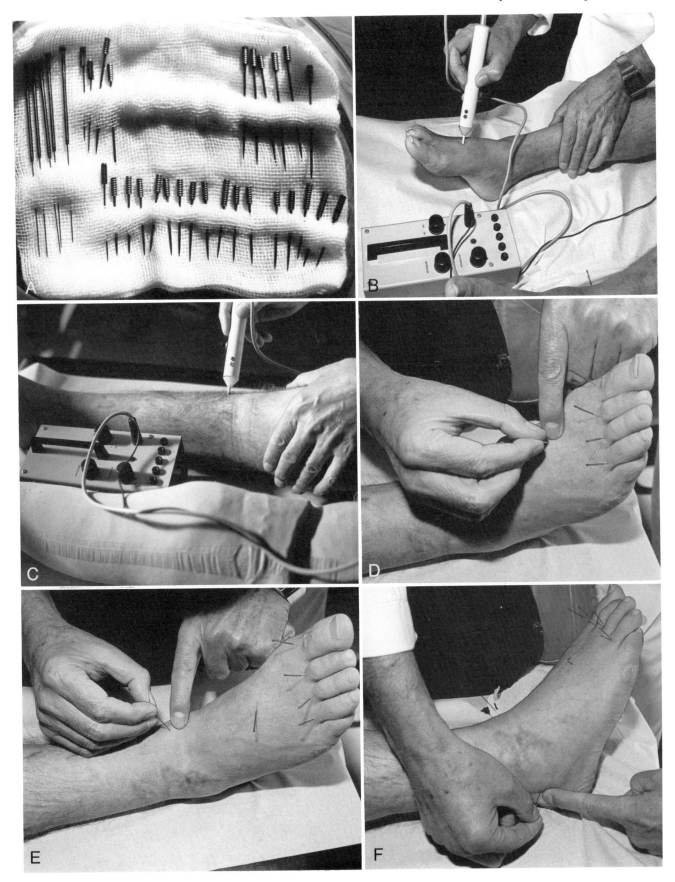

Figure 33.2.

Figure 33.3.

A–C. Positions of needles in the treatment of intermittent claudication are shown.
D–F. Positions of needles in the treatment of shoulder pain are shown.

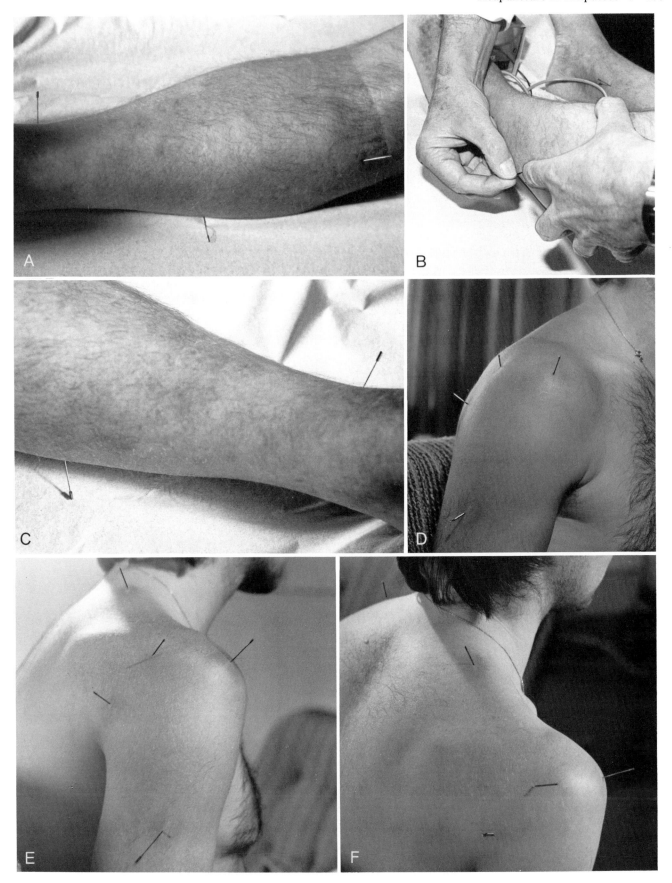

Figure 33.3.

34

Isokinetic Strength Testing

Paul Raether, M.D.

Isokinetic strength testing is a relatively new tool in orthopedic physical therapy. It provides an objective method of quantifying the dynamic strength of a muscle throughout its range of motion (ROM). Prior to the development of the Cybex machine in 1970, muscle strength could be assessed only isometrically or isotonically. Isometric testing measures the maximum force exerted at only one position within the total ROM. Isotonic testing, such as that performed on a weight machine like the Universal Gym, measures dynamic strength by assessing how much weight can be moved through the full range of a joint at one time. A limitation of this method is that the strength measured corresponds to the weakest point in the ROM.

Isokinetic strength testing avoids this by accommodating resistance against a lever moving at a constant angular velocity through the entire ROM. The muscles must contract at the speed of the machine, exerting a torque against the lever arm, which is graphed on a dynamometer, along with the joint angle, which is graphed on an electrogoniometer (see Fig. 34.1).

Parameters of particular importance include the peak torque generated by each muscle group at various speeds (usually from 30 to 240° per sec) and comparisons of agonist and antagonist as well as agonist and contralateral agonist. An endurance curve also is often run at a higher speed, measuring the number of repetitions to 50% torque decrement. One major drawback of isokinetic testing is that most machines do not measure eccentric muscle strength. Many complex extremity movements, including gait, are composed chiefly of coordinated eccentric contractions.

Applications of isokinetics have been primarily in the areas of diagnosis and evaluation; although especially among professional athletes, the machines are used in strength training. The knee is the joint most commonly tested, but the hip, ankles, and shoulder are also often evaluated isokinetically. Specific applications include: as a direct aid to diagnosis; for pre- and postsurgical evaluations; to assess readiness to return to work or athletic competition, and to help determine predilection to injury.

Figure 34.1. This 20-year-old male suffered a left anterior cruciate tear in January, 1983. He had surgical reconstruction in June, 1984, and Cybex testing in January, 1985.

A. Normal quadriceps/hamstring ratio of the right knee is shown.

B. Postoperative quadriceps atrophy is reflected in abnormal quadriceps/hamstring ratio of the left knee. Maximum quadriceps and hamstring torque also are markedly lower than the normal contralateral knee.

C. Endurance curve at 180°/sec. Knee is exercised until a torque drops by 50%.

D–E. Quadriceps testing on the Cybex apparatus is shown. This patient after a skiing accident, had internal derangement of the left knee, including rupture of the anterior cruciate ligament and surgical repair. The therapist encourages the patient to exert maximum effort during the testing period. The same is done during regular exercise sessions.

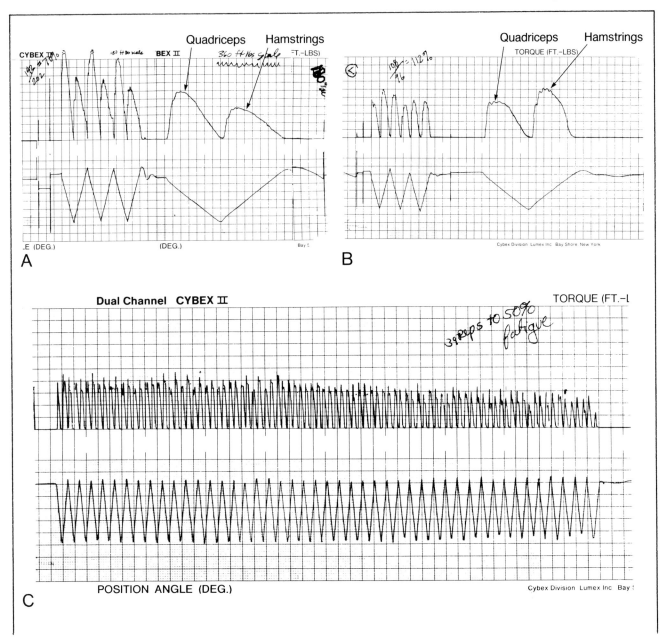

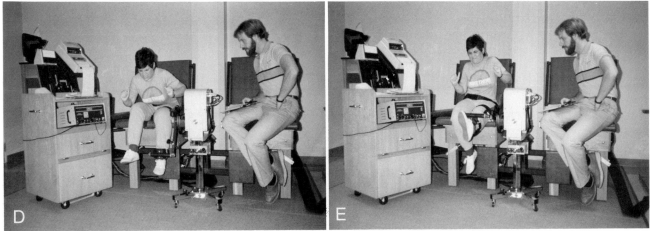

Figure 34.1.

35

Dental Treatment:
Experiences with Handicapped Patients

Axel Pomaroli, D.D.S.

OFFICE EQUIPMENT ADAPTATIONS

For the usual utilization of dental equipment, it is helpful if the handicapped patient can independently transfer from the wheelchair to the dentist's chair. Certain provisions can facilitate this transfer (see Fig. 35.1):

1. The arm rests of the dentist's chair must be very stable and it must be possible to swing them aside
2. Access to the dentist's chair should be possible from both sides. This can be achieved by swinging back the unit for the dentist and the assistant
3. For the transfer from the wheelchair to the dental operating chair, the seat of the wheelchair should be higher than that of the dentist's chair and vice versa as he or she leaves the dental chair (Fig. 35.1). It is much easier for the patient to move from a higher to a lower seat. The use of a sliding board can facilitate this procedure, if this is not prevented by the size of the wheelchair wheel

Additional equipment for the positioning on the dental operating chair will be necessary for patients with high spinal cord lesions, who would be very unstable on the operating chair. The upper part of the body of these patients tends to slide laterally. A broad leather belt (about 30 cm) around their thorax and the back of the chair (with Velcro closures) will avoid this.

A movable footrest with an electric control mounted on the dentist's chair allows adjustment in the longitudinal direction. Mild pressure of the footrest against the soles of the feet will increase the stability of the disabled patient's position, especially in cases when he or she has muscle spasms and is lying on the operating chair with the knee joints in flexion. The counterpressure of the footrest also improves the stability of bilateral amputees fitted with two prostheses. At the same time, this counterpressure gives the patient the impression of not losing the ground beyond his or her feet, especially when the patient is treated in lying position. For pressure relief, the areas at risk should be protected carefully by rolls or fleece.

Balance of the operating dental chair is sufficiently stable for a person with normal physical configuration in the horizontal position, because the load on the foot of the chair by the weight of the lower extremities and on the head of the chair by the upper part of the body is approximately equal. With a bilateral amputee, the whole weight of the patient is shifted towards the head of the operating chair

so that it tends to tip back. The operating chair must therefore be very well secured to the floor.

Additional equipment for the treatment of handicapped patients include a dental mouth-rinsing device mounted on a mobile tube, which greatly facilitates mouth rinsing for the patient.

BEDSIDE TREATMENT

Bedside treatment of patients with severely limited mobility is recommended when (extraction or other analgesic measures) may be necessary to relieve an acute toothache (see Fig. 35.2). Impression for a dental prosthesis or the repair of the prosthesis can also be done at bedside for these patients.

In special cases, the patient's bed can be wheeled into the dentist's surgery room, providing it is large enough. This allows the use of the entire drill assembly, spray, aspiration device, and any other equipment that cannot be moved into the patient's room but is necessary for procedures such as trepanation, preservative treatment, and oral hygiene.

As injured patients are less resistant to psychological stress and have little mobility, it should be possible to carry out simple technical works (repair of prostheses) immediately in the office without recourse to a separate laboratory. The instruments needed for this purpose (steel wire, bending wrench, synthetic material, compressed air, autoclave, polishing device, vibrator, plastic trimmer, etc.) should be available as minimum equipment.

After an accident, the attending physician concentrates his or her attention primarily to the treatment of serious injuries. If the face and jaw are not injured, lost glasses, broken dental prostheses or teeth in need of treatment are frequently overlooked. Unfortunately, the patient does not talk about them either; he or she either is distracted by the pain of the injuries or the patient does not want to bore the doctor or nursing staff with matters that seem less significant. Yet, if such secondary problems are disregarded, additional complications or considerable strain, which could have been avoided by early attention, may develop. It must never be forgotten that the patient is a human being. General rehabilitation should also include sanitation of the masticatory apparatus, in which the dentist can considerably contribute to the general psychological and physical rehabilitation of the patient.

Figure 35.1.

A. A dependent patient is transferred to the treatment chair. Observe sequence of motion from higher to lower seat.

B. Dismantled and removed arm rest of the treatment chair is brought into position after patient is placed in the chair. The footrest is still far away from the distal end of the treatment chair.

C. The spastic-paretic patient is resting with flexed knees on the treatment table. A footrest is pressed against patient's feet, stabilizing the legs to a great extent. A wide leather belt stabilizes the unstable trunk.

D. Conservative treatment is applied to the above patient.

E. The dental chair is brought down to the wheelchair level to enable the patient's independent transfer into the chair.

F. The leg of a bilateral amputee is held in place by the pressure of the adjustable footrest; increasing patient's stability in the treatment chair.

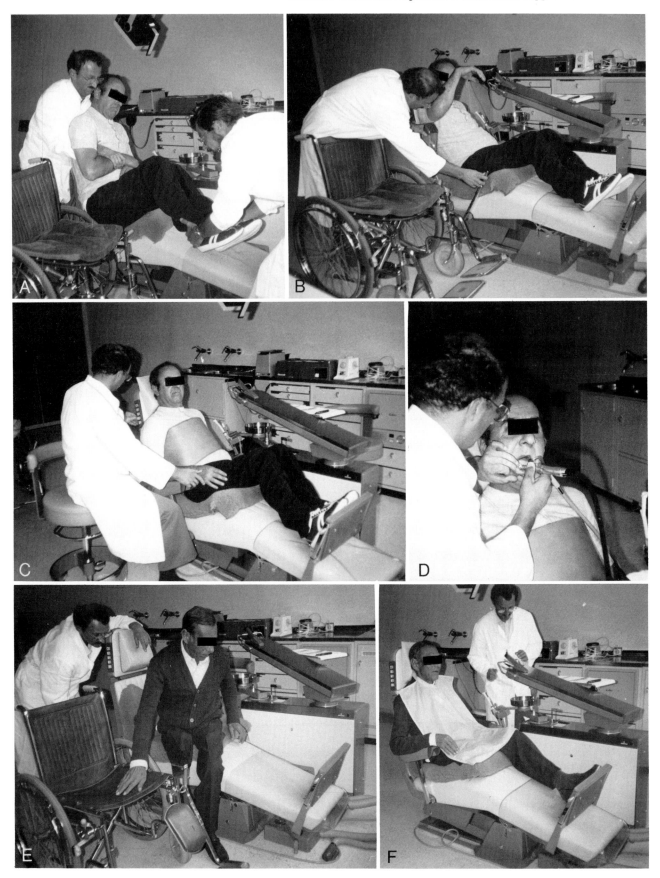

Figure 35.1.

Figure 35.2.

A. Tooth extraction in bed is more difficult as it limits the dentist in his or her freedom of movement. This is partially compensated by special positioning of patient's head.

B. The patient is brought in his or her own bed into the dental treatment room. The X-ray of the teeth is taken.

C. Conservative treatment utilizes all drilling and suction devices of the dental office.

D. In using a local nerve block of the inferior alveolar nerve, there is one caution: transient facial nerve paresis may occur while placing the local anesthetic in supine position. The anesthetic solution might, by gravity, diffuse from the mandibular foramen into the stylomastoid one. The dental assistant stabilizes the lower jaw of the patient.

E–F. Mold is taken for fabrication of denture on a bedridden patient; a halfway recumbant position can facilitate the process.

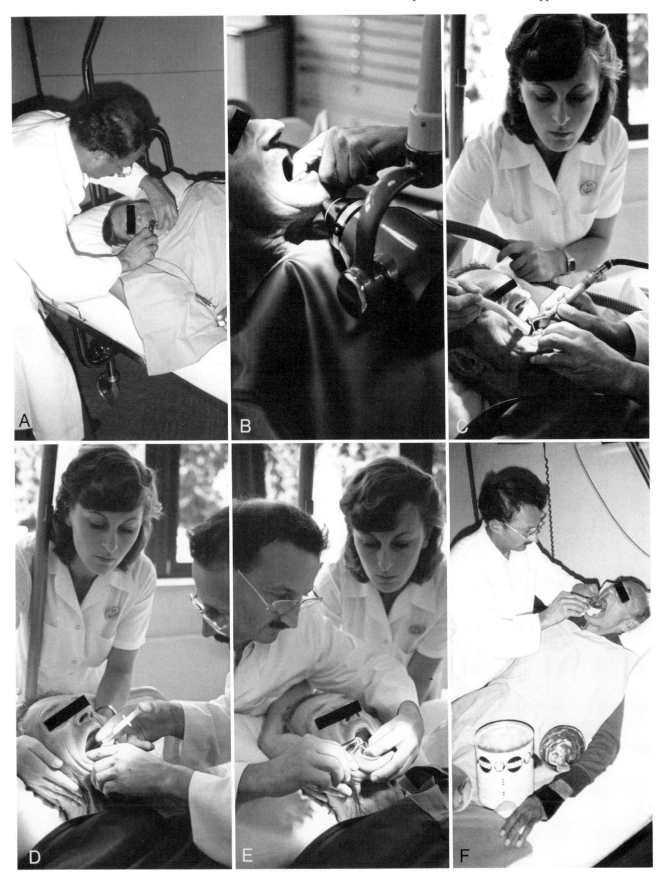

Figure 35.2.

36

Electrodiagnosis and Electromyography

Paul Raether, M.D.

Electrodiagnosis comprises the laboratory method of diagnosis of pathological conditions of the peripheral nervous system. It is dependent on activation, display, and recording of electrical activity of the *motor unit*. The motor unit is composed of the motor nerve cell, its axon, the neuromuscular junction, and the innervated muscle fibers. Electrodiagnosis can, therefore, assist in localizing the lesion along the motor unit, suggest nature of the lesion, and help in prognostication. Electrodiagnosis consists of:

1. *Electromyography (EMG)* Recording of microelectric potentials from within muscles (Fig. 36.1)
2. *Nerve conduction studies (NCS)* Electrical stimulation of peripheral nerve and recording the elicited compound motor action potential or sensory nerve action potential via surface or needle electrodes (Fig. 36.2)

EQUIPMENT

Action potentials are picked up by either a needle or surface electrode and connected to a cathode ray oscilloscope for visual display, an audioamplifier and speaker for acoustic monitoring, and a recorder. For NCS, a stimulator generating rectangular pulses, which triggers the horizontal sweep of the oscilloscope, is required. Equipment is extremely sensitive requiring minimal frequency range of 2 to 10 Hz so as not to distort displayed potentials.

NORMAL EMG

In normal EMG *insertional activity* is the burst of electrical potentials associated with electrode penetration and movement within the muscle. In the absence of pathology, its duration is 300 msec. Endplate activity is the only electrical activity seen in normal muscle at rest. Endplate activity has two components:

1. *Endplate noise:* Monophasic negative potentials equal or less than 50 microvolts, 1–2 msec in duration
2. *Endplate spikes:* Diphasic initial negative potentials up to 300 microvolts, duration less than 4 msec

The *motor unit action potential* consists of diphasic or triphasic potentials with an amplitude of 200 microvolts to 4 millivolts, duration 3 to 15 msec). *Recruitment* is the orderly activation of already firing and new motor units with increasing strength of voluntary contraction. It depends on number of motor units and rate of firing.

The *interference pattern* is the electrical activity recorded during maximum voluntary contraction. Individual motor units are not discernible.

ABNORMAL EMG

Fibrillation potentials are biphasic or triphasic spikes initially positive, with an amplitude of 20 to 200 μv, a duration of less than 5 msec, and a regular firing pattern. *Positive waves* are biphasic potentials with a long positive phase, an amplitude of less than 1 μv, and a duration of 10 to 50 msec; they fire irregularly with slow rates. *Myotonic discharges* are monophasic or biphasic initially positive, duration less than 5 msec and firing at high frequency, waxing and waning with varying amplitude and frequency. *Fasciculation potentials* look like motor units having the same characteristics, but fire spontaneously as single discharge. Large number of fasciculations may produce a rhythmic discharge, which is called *myokymia*. *Bizarre high frequency discharges* (complex repetitive potential) are polyphasic potentials, amplitude 100 μv to 1 millivolt, frequency 10 to 150 Hz with uniform shape and amplitude; they may begin or stop abruptly.

Polyphasic potentials are motor unit potentials with five or more phases. Up to 15% of motor unit potentials may be polyphasic in normal muscle.

NERVE CONDUCTION STUDIES (NCS)

Nerve conduction studies assess peripheral motor and sensory nerve function by recording the evoked response to stimulation of nerve (see Table 36.1). Motor nerve conduction studies involve stimulation of a motor or mixed peripheral nerve while recording from a muscle end organ supplied by that nerve. Superficial electrodes are generally used to record the summated electrical activity of the muscle fibers in the region of the recording electrode. The response is known as the *compound muscle action potential*.

Sensory nerve conduction studies are performed by stimulating a mixed nerve and recording over a sensory nerve, or by stimulating a cutaneous nerve while recording from a mixed or cutaneous nerve. Sensory nerve action potentials can be evoked either orthodromically or antidromically for testing sensory nerve conduction.

With both motor and sensory nerve conduction studies, parameters evaluated include amplitude of the response, latency of the response from the time the stimulus is delivered, and nerve conduction velocity, which is calculated by dividing the distance between stimulation sites by the difference in respective latencies (Table 36.1).

OTHER ELECTRODIAGNOSTIC TECHNIQUES

H Reflex

This is the electrical equivalent of the ankle jerk and is specifically used for evaluation of the S_1 root. The active electrode is placed on gastrocsoleus at midpoint between the knee and medial malleolus. The tibial nerve is stimulated in the popliteal fossa. The H reflex response is seen with submaximal stimulation and disappears with supramaximal stimulation when direct M response starts appearing. Latency is dependent on age and leg length, and must be compared to the contralateral side.

F Wave

This is a late response resulting from antidromic impulses rebounding off the anterior horn cell and orthodromically returning to cause muscle contraction (see Fig. 36.3). It is not a reflex because only motor fibers are stimulated. An F wave can be elicited by placing an active electrode on any muscle and stimulating the appropriate nerve. Intrinsic hand and foot muscles commonly are used.

Cranial Nerve Testing

The trigimenal and facial nerves may be assessed easily via electromyographic techniques in a clinical setting. The facial nerve can be stimulated as any other motor nerve, with recording over the nasalis or other facial muscle. The usual parameters of amplitude and latency are evaluated and compared with the contralateral side.

Excitability Test

The evaluation of facial nerve lesions, e.g., Bell's Palsy, is facilitated by the use of electrophysiological testing (see Fig. 36.4). Standard facial nerve conduction studies have a role; however, the earliest change noted is a change in the threshold current required to produce a minimal contraction on the involved side as compared to the normal side. The facial nerve is stimulated at the tragus with a 1 msec pulse, and the minimal current required for minimal contraction is determined and compared to the opposite side. Clues for impending degeneration are present already 1 to 2 days after insult, while electromyographic signs appear 2 to 3 weeks later. This is too late for consideration of a possible early surgical decompression procedure at the facial canal. If there is Wallerian degeneration, the nerve will become less excitable, requiring a greater current. A difference of 1 or 2 msec between sides is generally considered significant. With neuropraxia lesions, there is no change in excitability.

The blink reflex is composed of an afferent limb mediated by the trigeminal nerve and an efferent limb mediated by the facial nerve with synapses in the brainstem. Electrically, the blink reflex is manifest as two components: the early component (R_1), which is unilateral, and the late component (R_2), which is bilateral. R_1 is mediated via the main sensory nucleus of cranial nerve V on the pons, whereas R_2 is at least partially via the spinal nucleus and tract of the fifth nerve in the medulla, but influenced by structures in the thalamus and cerebral hemispheres.

The blink reflex is recorded by surface electrodes over the orbicularis oculi. The first or second division of the trigeminal nerve may be stimulated. Clinical applications of the blink reflex include lesions of either the trigeminal or facial nerve, brainstem lesions, polyneuropathies, and Parkinsonism.

Traditional Electrodiagnostic Procedures

Traditional electrodiagnostic procedures antedated the development of currently practiced electromyography (Fig. 36.4). They make use of galvanic and faradic current to assess the integrity of the lower motor neuron. Denervated muscle shows a different response to galvanic stimulation at the motor end plate than seen in normally innervated

Table 36.1. Average normal values for nerve conduction

Type of Function	Latency	NCV[a]	
Sensory			
Median	3.2 ± 0.2 msec		
Ulnar	3.2 ± 0.2 msec		
Radial	3.3 ± 0.4 msec		
Sural		> 40 m/sec	
Motor		*Distal*	*Proximal*
Median	3.7 ± 0.3 msec	57 ± 5 m/sec	57 ± 5 m/sec
Ulnar	3.2 ± 0.5 msec	62 ± 5 m/sec	70 ± 7 m/sec
Radial		62 ± 6 m/sec	72 ± 7 m/sec
Deep peroneal	< 6.0 msec	50 ± 6 m/sec	50 ± 6 m/sec
Posterior tibial	5.3 − 5.9 msec ± 0.8 msec	51 ± 6 m/sec	51 ± 6 m/sec
Facial	< 4.0 msec		

[a]NCV, nerve conduction velocity.

muscle. This qualitative change from a brisk contraction to a slow wormlike contraction has been termed the *reaction of degeneration*.

In the *strength duration curve*, the reaction of degeneration response is quantified by plotting the relationship between the intensity and the duration of a stimulus applied to a motor point, which will elicit a minimal contraction.

The *rheobase* is the minimal current below which no response can be elicited regardless of the duration. The *chronaxie* is the minimal duration of a current required to elicit a minimal contraction at twice the rheobase current. When Wallerian degeneration occurs, the entire strength duration curve shifts to the right, usually resulting in an increase in the chronaxie. The strength duration curve has lost popularity because of the length of time required for its determination and the complexity of its interpretation. Changes suggesting degeneration or reinnervation may be appreciated at an earlier stage by strength duration curve testing, but this method is not as sensitive as EMG in determining small or localized areas of denervation and is of no help in differentiating neuropathic processes from myopathy. Conventional electromyography has now replaced the strength duration curve in clinical electrodiagnosis.

Figure 36.1.

A. The EMG needle is inserted into the anterior tibial muscle.

B. The EMG needle is inserted into the deltoid muscle.

C. Fibrillation potential and positive sharp waves (signs of degeneration) are shown.

D. Normal muscle unit action potentials are shown.

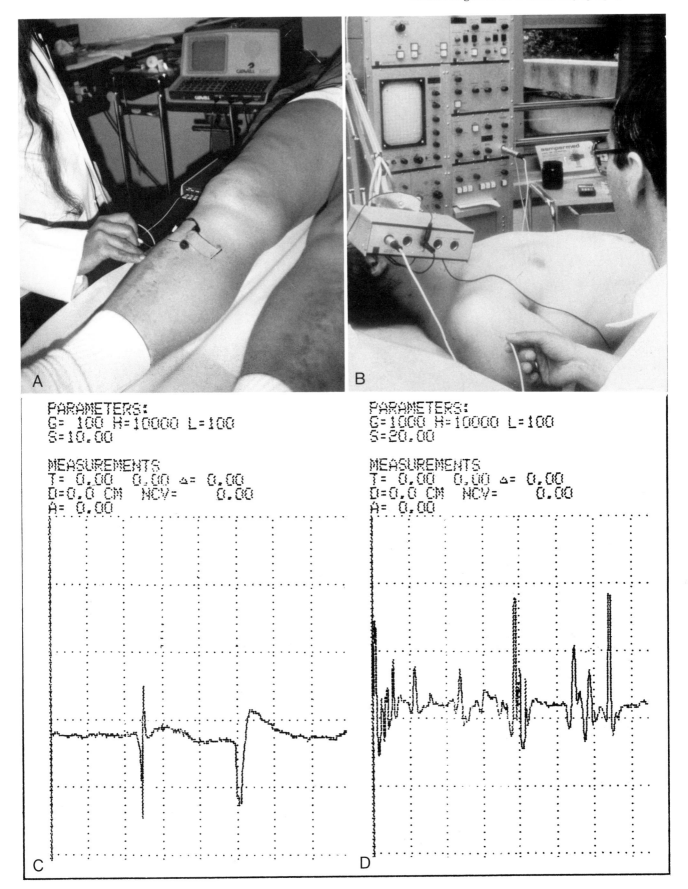

Figure 36.1.

Figure 36.2.

A. Nerve conduction studies involve measuring distance between stimulating and pick-up electrodes.

B. Stimulation of the right median nerve 8 cm proximal to the pick-up electrode on the thenar.

C. The distance between the proximal and distal stimulation point is measured.

D. Stimulation over the left posterior tibial nerve is shown.

E. An example of an antidromic sensory nerve conduction study of the median nerve is shown.

F. An example of a motor nerve conduction study of the median nerve is shown.

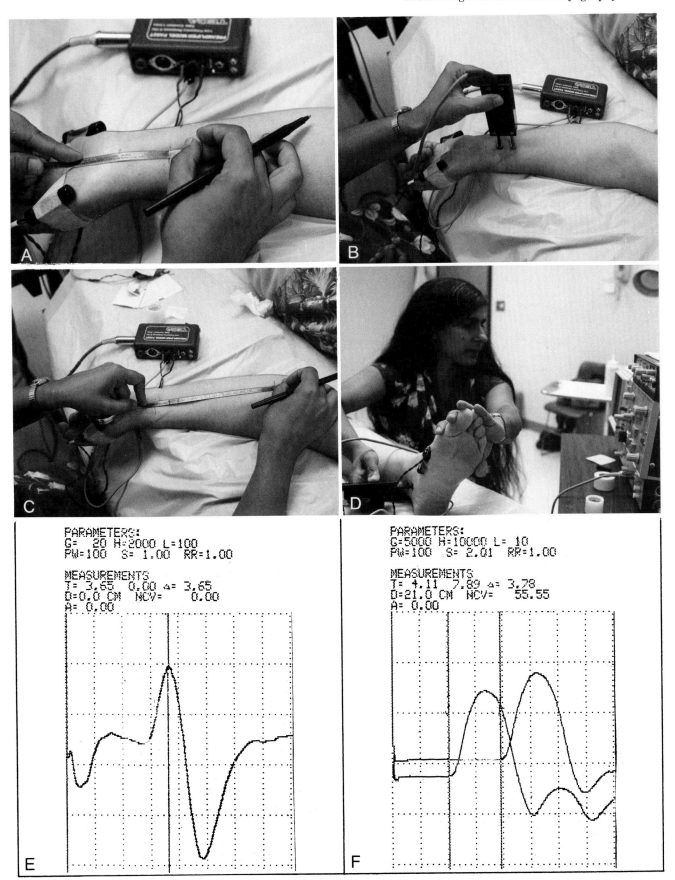

Figure 36.2.

Figure 36.3.

A. F wave from median nerve is shown.

B. The H reflex is recorded over soleus with submaximal stimulation of tibial nerve at popliteal fossa.

C. With increasing stimulus intensity, the H reflex amplitude diminishes and the M wave appears.

D. With supramaximal stimulation, the H reflex has disappeared.

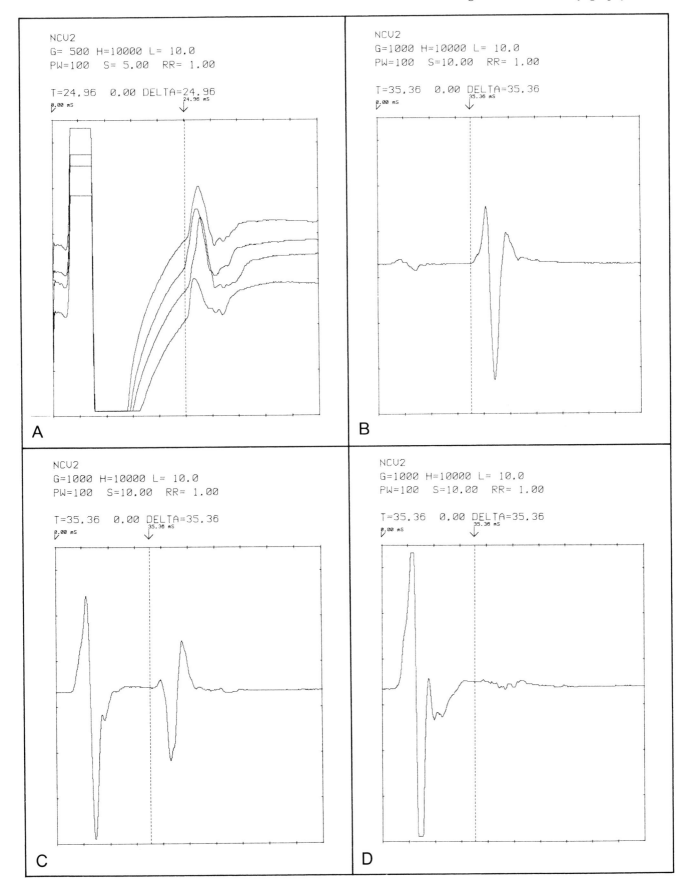

Figure 36.3.

Figure 36.4.

A. This electromyograph has four channels, two scopes, a tape recorder and a printer.
B. Excitability test is done of the right facial nerve.
C. A chronaxie meter is shown.
D. Rheobase and chronaxie are tested.
E. In this strength duration curve diagram, the uninterrupted line is normal. Note shift to the right of the abnormal strength duration curve (interrupted line).

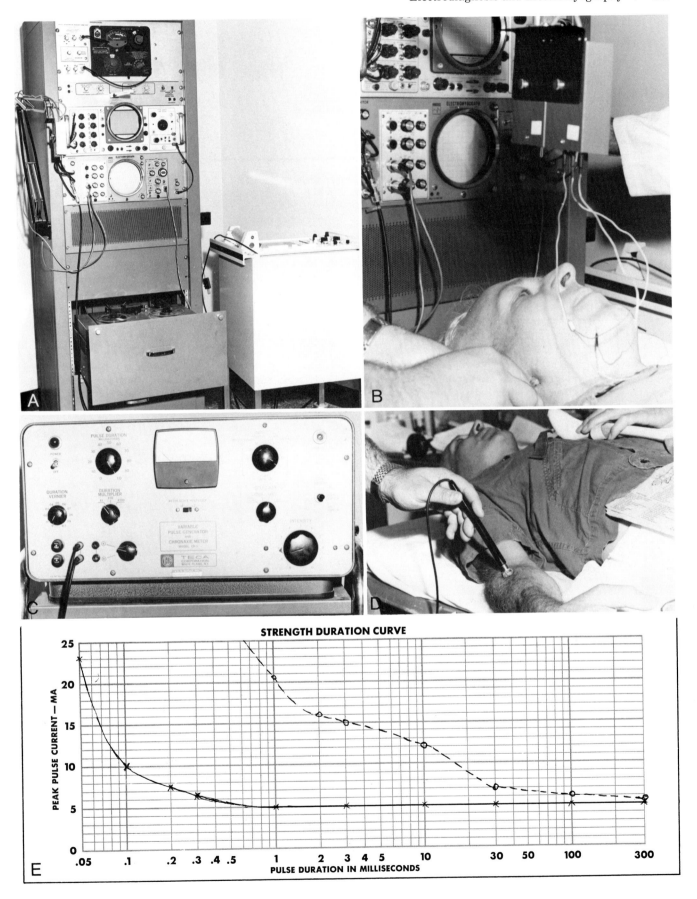

Figure 36.4.

37

Electrostimulation for Pain Control

Marcelo Zurita, M.D.

Sensation of pain and discomfort are often experienced by paraplegics, especially when their lesion is incomplete. Hopelessness, anxiety, depression, stress secondary to sexual problems, and immobility can potentiate pain.

The most common types of pain associated with cord lesions are *localized pain, somatic root pain, visceral pain,* and diffuse pain in areas with sensory loss referred to as *central, sympathetic* or *phantom-limb pain. Causalgia* is associated with cauda equina lesions. The intensity in all of these types of pain is aggravated by many factors, including weather, mental stress, fatigue, infections, bed sores, spasticity, and distention of the bladder or bowel. In each case, local or systemic treatment is warranted,

even though treatment of pain and spasticity with drugs or neurosurgery carry risks of side effects, especially dependency and toxicity.

Electrical stimulation using transcutaneous electrical nerve stimulator (TENS) can be used effectively for treatment of pain (Fig. 37.1). Peripheral nerves such as the radial nerve and branches of the sciatic and femoral nerves, in particular the saphenous nerve, respond favorably to stimulation.

The TENS with specific output current and using defined electrode sizes (anode/cathode ratio) along with proper placement of the electrodes can be used to produce electric nerve blocks.

Figure 37.1.

A. Electronic neurolocators detect areas of lowest skin resistance that correspond to acupuncture and trigger points.

B. Location of the trigger point is shown.

C. Relaxette (TENS) for pain control and electrodes are shown.

D. A patient is trained in the clinic in the use of TENS.

E. The same patient applies TENS at home.

F. A high-voltage (low amperage) muscle stimulator induces effective muscle contraction.

G. In the stimulation electrodes are applied over motor points of the quadriceps muscle. Best results can be achieved when surface electrodes are applied over points of lowest skin resistance. These can be found using a neurolocator. This is an instrument eliciting audio and visual signals over points of low skin resistance.

H. Functional muscle stimulation is used in the clinic to teach the patient for home use. Muscle stimulation must be repeated several times a day for 3 to 5 min to prevent atrophy.

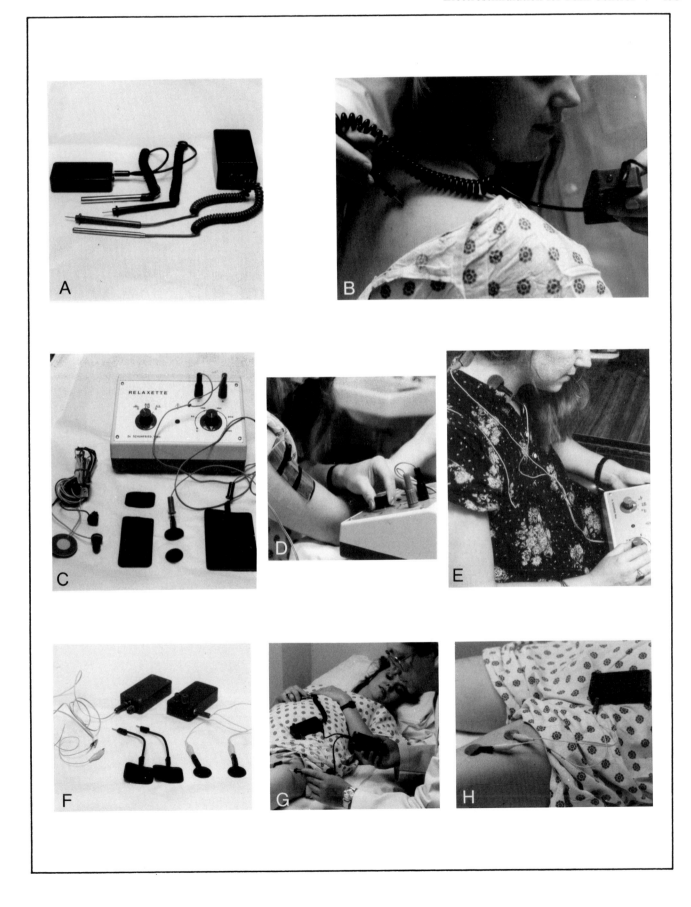

Figure 37.1.

38

Functional Electrostimulation

Marcelo Zurita, M.D.

The idea of a "cure" for spinal cord injury is not a new one; many centers and scientists around the world are working toward this goal. Several reports have considered the use of enzymes, nerve grafts, omentum tissue, laser beam, hypothermia and surgery, nerve growth factors, electrically enhanced regeneration, embryonic grafts, etc. The identification of regeneration inhibitors in the central nervous system and development of methods to counteract them is also being pursued. Meanwhile, the population of chronic spinal cord-injured patients requires a program that will maintain them until an effective treatment becomes available. Functional electrical stimulation (FES) of paralyzed muscles is a way to delay atrophy; it also reduces pain and spasticity (see Fig. 38.1).

Muscle contraction can be achieved by direct stimulation of the muscle or via the motorneuron. In a person with cord transsection, afferent and efferent pathways between the central and peripheral nervous systems are interrupted. To simulate coordinated muscle function, higher control functions must be substituted artificially. This is difficult; for example, in a single step, about 30 muscles are involved to achieve coordinated activity of one leg. Much research and development in the application of interfacing microprocessors are necessary to simulate this intricate mechanism and sequentially activate and inhibit those muscles. However, at the present phase of development, maintenance of muscle activity and prevention of the effects of inactivity on other structures of the body can be provided by simple procedures. The dynamic properties of paralyzed muscles in a paraplegic are almost normal; therefore, the force of contraction and the resistance to fatigue can be enhanced with a training program using simpler electric muscle stimulators.

A muscle stimulator that produces a muscle contraction comparable to the physiological generates a faradic pulse, the optimum frequency being 50 Hz and a variable intensity from 0 to 800 V with minimum amperage (8 to 25 milliamperes).

A complete physical examination will ensure that there will be no danger to the participant in a gradual muscle development. Exercising the paralyzed muscles many times a day improves muscle size, strength, and endurance and diminishes spasticity; it also improves cardiovascular conditioning, bone size and density, and vascular supply to the muscle increases.

The use of a multichannel muscle stimulator permits synchronous contraction of agonist and antagonist muscles. Simultaneous stimulation of the quadriceps and gluteal muscles using surface electrodes can support a paraplegic patient in an upright position when balance is provided by holding to parallel bars or a walker. Rising from a sitting to a standing position is achieved using a FES to stimulate sequentially the hip and knee extensors and plantar flexors (see Figure 38.2). In a paraplegic, as seen in the illustrations, the therapist can achieve gross walking movements of the patient's lower extremities using a manual multichannel FES.

Figure 38.1.

A. Six-channel high voltage (low amperage) muscle stimulator for reciprocal muscle stimulation is used in preparation for possible gait training.

B. Functional electrical stimulation (FES) of the left quadriceps is shown.

C. Functional electrical stimulation (FES) of the right anterior tibial muscle and the quadriceps is shown.

D. Position of electrode for foot dorsiflexion is shown.

E. Foot dorsiflexion using FES is limited secondary to tight heel cords. (Position of foot is not shown due to cropping.)

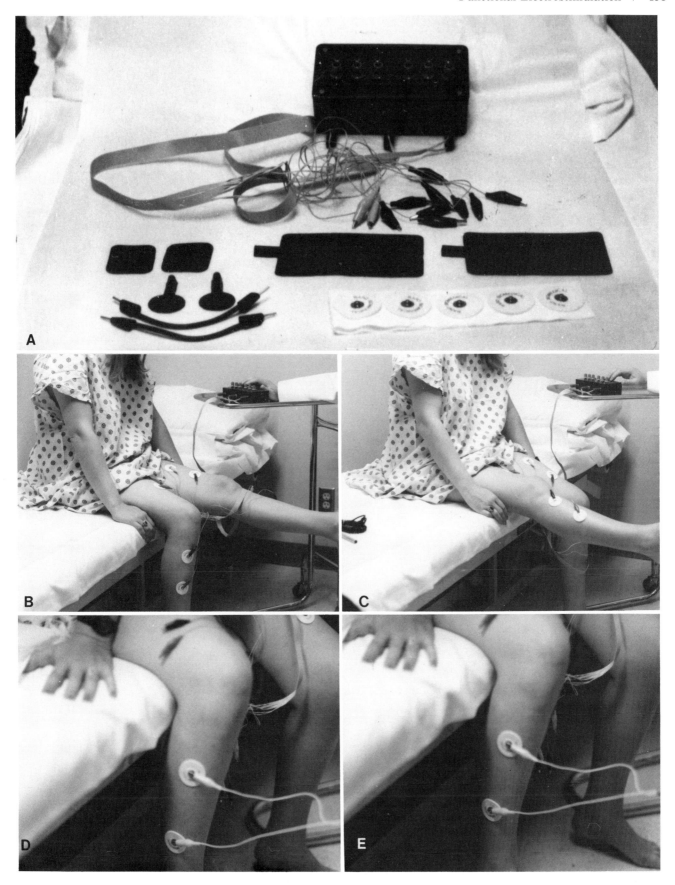

Figure 38.1.

Figure 38.2.

A. Preparation for ambulation. Placement of electrodes over hip flexors, knee extensors and foot dorsiflexors.

B. Knee extension.

C. Knee extension and foot dorsiflexion.

D. Knee extension of both lower extremities.

E. Knee extension and foot dorsiflexion of both lower extremities.

F. Preparation for stimulation between parallel bars.

G. First attempt of standing between parallel bars (patient had no braces). With this 6 channel muscle stimulator, we attempted to provide reciprocal movement of lower extremities while the patient was upright.

H. After right side stimulation for hip flexion, knee extension and foot dorsiflexion, the patient is placing the right foot on the floor.

I. Hip flexion, passive knee flexion and foot dorsiflexion in early swing phase of left lower extremity: knee extension is maintained on the right side while patient supports himself on the parallel bars.

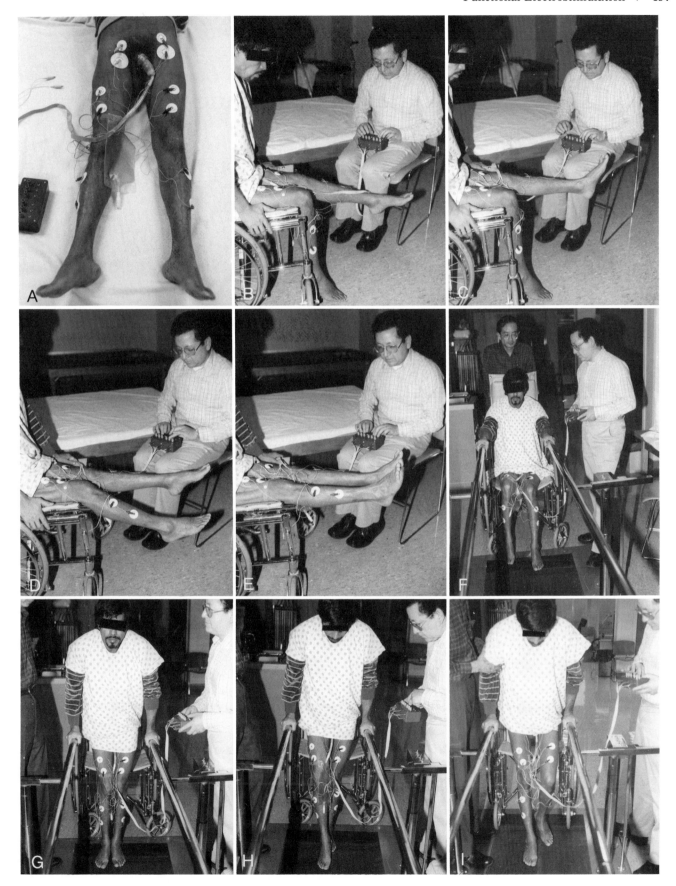

Figure 38.2.

Manual Lymph Drainage Ad Modum Vodder in Physical Medicine and Rehabilitation

Günther Wittlinger, M.D.

The lymphatic system forms part of the circulatory system, combining with the blood vessels to form the complete circulation system. The outward blood flow is through arteries; the return flow, through veins and lymphatics. Arteries and veins are connected by porous capillaries of different patterns specific to the organ in which they are found. At their surface is the exchange of fluids, nutrients, and waste products. A capillary resorption takes place, with lymph obligatory substances (lymph load) not resorbed into the blood capillary but into the lymph capillary (which begins as fingerlike projections in the connective tissue) and flowing back via lymph vessels to the blood system. Thus, the lymph system is part of the circulation; the return flow occurs through veins *and* lymphatics.

Mislin (1972) described how the unique manipulations of manual lymph drainage (MLD) stimulate the lymphatic musculature. Also, Mislin stated that MLD, with its specific movements, stimulates lymph motoricity. Physiological vasomotor lymph drainage results from the autonomic pulsations of the lymphatic sections or series of lymphatic sections. It is likely that MLD has a decisive influence on this drainage system. The process consists of producing rhythmically alternating phases of dilation and contraction in a successive series of metachronously activated lymph sections (Figs. 39.1 and 39.2). This gives rise to a peristaltic wave along the lymphatic vessel. Thus, the dilation-contraction frequency of the lymphatic sections is synchronized, and the resulting pulsations are peristaltically metachronous. Myogenous and nervous control of vascular activities by synergistic receptors in the vessel walls ensure the coordinated transport of lymph. The main physiological stimulations are pressure and temperature. Intravascular stretching across, but also along, the vessels increases the pulse rate of the lymphatic sections. Smooth muscle cells, such as those in the vessel walls, exhibit electrical and mechanical reactions upon passive stretching. Vascular muscles having autonomous, i.e., pacemaker, properties require well-dosed stretching dependent on the momentary intravascular volume in order to ensure regulation of their rhythmical repolarization, which is adapted to the prevailing situation. For all these reasons, MLD, which exerts a physiological (in some respects, inadequate) tensile stimulation, stimulates the vasomotor lymph drainage system.

Extramural lymph drainage, i.e., the action of external mechanical factors on the lymphatic vessels, is due to the fact that certain outside forces not only stimulate the vascular musculature in the manner described above but also exert a mechanical effect on the content of the lymphatic vessels. Foremost among these factors are the movements of the skeletal muscles, the pulsation of the arteries (analogous to functional coupling in the case of the veins), the peristalsis of the intestines, the movements of the diaphragm and other muscles of the respiratory system, and the variations in pressures that arise in the pectoral and abdominal cavities during respiration. This lymph drainage mechanism represents an auxiliary, indirect system that can be enhanced locally or regionally by direct manual lymph drainage.

Extravascular lymph drainage involves lymph formation and extravascular circulation. The higher the content of protein in tissue, the less water can flow out of the tissue via the venous capillaries, because it is bound by protein. By returning protein from the tissue, the lymph system allows more water to drain from the venous capillaries. The lymph capillaries commence as blind fingerlike extensions in interstitial tissue. They lack the basement membrane found in blood capillaries and consist of a single, thin layer of partially overlapping endothelial cells connected radially at one end to stretch-resistant collagen fibers of the connective tissue by extremely fine precollagenous (matrix) filaments. If the connective tissue swells as a result of an increased influx of water, the pressure within the interstitium increases. As a result, the collagen fibers distend, pulling the nonelastic anchor filaments of the lymph capillaries with them. The intercellular spaces in the lymph capillaries thus widen, so that there is an increased flow of water, macromolecules, and large and small particles (sometimes including erythrocytes) into the capillary lumen.

As the lymph capillaries fill, the pressure in the interstitial tissue decreases due to the efflux of water, and the pressure in the lymph capillaries increases due to the influx of water. These pressure changes cause the endothelial cells, which act like flutter valves, to close the intercellular gaps, so that the lymph capillaries are present as filled and closed channels. The anchor filaments have also returned to their initial position because the water content and the pressure in the connective tissue have decreased.

Hauck (1980) and Casley-Smith (1976) described variable prelymphatic tissue and channels in the ground substance of connective tissue, which have the function of returning proteins and fluid relatively quickly to the lymph capillaries. Hauck maintained that the elastic fibers of the connective tissue serve as "guide rails" for the transport of fluids because the flow rate of fluids is faster along the elastic fibers than elsewhere. These channels, which can only be seen under the electron microscope, are far smaller in diameter than the initial lymph capillaries and reveal no wall structure of their own. The beginnings of wall formation can also be identified by darkfield and fluorescent microscopy and recognized as the site of continuous transition to the lymph capillaries. These findings support the view of the lymph system as a converging drainage system open at the periphery. It may be assumed that the lymph capillaries function like suction drains. Such drains are used, for example, in agriculture where they draw water directly from the soil and deliver it to collection drains. Again, the lymph capillaries could be likened to the sap channels in plants, which transport water from the soil up into the leaves and in which similar mechanisms are at work. Complications arise when the lymph system becomes incompetent, such as the result of the extirpation of lymph nodes or their fibrous obliteration by irradiation, so that lymph drainage of whole regions is no longer ensured.

In such cases, MLD attempts to push the lymph against the normal drainage direction via the valveless lymph capillaries and the valved (but, in contrast to the subsequent "transport vessels," still musclefree) "guiding vessels," as found in the superficial network of the skin lymphatics, rerouting it to regions still supplied with sufficient lymph vessels. Transport is against the normal direction of drainage because the lymphatic vessel apparatus no longer functions due to the blockage or absence of regional lymph nodes. It is possible to transport the lymph in the skin lymph vessels deeper into the cutis or subcutis via so-called watersheds and interterritorial anastomoses. It should be borne in mind that the smallest lymphatic vessels of the skin, referred to above as "guiding vessels" and which already possess valves, can be influenced by MLD in such a way that the valves reverse position, and the direction of lymph drainage can be controlled. Furthermore, substances that must be transported via the lymph system can be pushed along in tissue spaces until they reach functional lymphatic vessels. Among the various applications of MLD, chronic cases of inflammation should not be forgotten, these falling in the domain of various disciplines. Inflammation is always accompanied by edema, which is initially situated between fibrils in loose interstitial connective tissue but later also involves the fibrillary structures themselves. When this interstitial edema is mobilized by means of MLD, other lymph-borne substances that sustain the inflammation should, at the same time, be removed. Thus, chronic inflammation is a prime indication for MLD. The massage pressure used in MLD depends on two factors: (a) the pathological tissue condition being treated, (b) the type of tissue being treated.

Thus, in the case of leg ulcers or recent hematomas, the pressure used is markedly different from that employed in the case of severe fibrosis. Also, the thickness and nature of the individual skin layers, especially the subcutis and subcutaneous adipose layer, are important factors, as is the turgor of the skin. In addition, the pressure used depends to a large extent on the regionally variable substrate underlying the skin: bone, cartilage, tendon or aponeurosis, fascia, and ligament. In the most frequent cases, with a firm muscular substrate, muscle tone also plays a key role. The question as to whether and to what extent

the massage pressure can spread laterally also has a considerable influence on the pressure used. In the treatment of edema, the nature of the edema is of importance; namely, its extent, its tension or hardness, and special properties, such as its solgel relation, protein and fiber content, and sensitivity to pain. Under no circumstances can an "optimal" massage pressure be calculated. It can only be learned through many comparative treatments by teacher and student during MLD training and in the subsequent accumulation of experience until a feel for this difficult therapeutic form is gradually developed.

The indications for MLD reach into all domains of medical disciplines. Basically, it can be said that all diseases based on an accumulation of proteins in the loose connective tissue or all diseases that, as a consequence, enrich the connective tissue with proteins, are an indication for MLD. Considering this, MLD is a treatment than can be applied in the field of rehabilitation with great success.

In 1984, a pilot study at the Rehabilitations-Zentrum Bad Häring/Tirol/Austria (medical director, Prim, Dr. Eckhart Reiner), in cooperation with Elpenbad Walchsee, (medical director, Günther Wittlinger), was designed to determine the effects of MLD applied to amputation stumps. It was observed that the treated stumps shrunk more quickly than the untreated ones, so that the patients could be supplied with a prosthesis much earlier. Furthermore, all amputees' phantom pains disappeared, except for those patients who had had previous amputations in the past and were suffering from long-standing phantom pains. The patients were treated daily for half an hour over a period of 20 days.

The theoretical explanation for these findings is the following: The resorption and reflow of the lymph load (so-called lymph obligatory substances) is stimulated by MLD; therefore, the whole area and the scars are revascularized much more quickly. This restores normal metabolism in this area. Normalization results in rapid healing of ulcers (delay of callus formation having been stopped), reduction of pain, and recovery of motility.

Further studies will evaluate the effects of MLD on paraplegias. Stasis in the lymphatic system results in a delay of healing, because lymph load remains in the loose connective tissue and hinders metabolism (i.e., the transit between cell and capillary). By this and the increase of waste products remaining in this area, the disease becomes chronic, or at least there is a considerable delay in healing as can be observed in persons of all ages with lymphedema, especially when they suffer from rheumatic and orthopedic diseases. In such cases, and in all sequelae to trauma, MLD gives rise to decongestion and stimulates lymph flow considerably. Especially after treatment of fractures that require long immobilization, MLD should be started at bedside so that negative consequences, such as swelling, stiffening, muscular atrophy, or circulatory disturbances, can be avoided if possible. In the authors' experience, Sudeck's atrophy can nearly always be improved or even cured. After complicated operations (e.g., orthopedic surgery), exhausting rheumatic diseases, or infections, MLD is an excellent therapy to minimize the excessive use of analgesic drugs and to cut short hospitalization and time of convalescence.

In summary, manual lymph drainage ad modum vodder enhances physical therapy and is recommended for introduction and application in the field of rehabilitation.

Figure 39.1.

A. Manual lymph drainage involves manipulative handgrip for emptying of the terminus.

B. Rotational manipulation on the back.

C. Paravertebral standing circles.

D. Scooping grip at the arm.

E. Pumping grip at the arm.

F. Pumping grip at the elbows.

G. Thumb circling on the dorsum of the hand.

H. Demonstration of dorsal hand edema.

 I. Thumb circling at the palm of the hand.

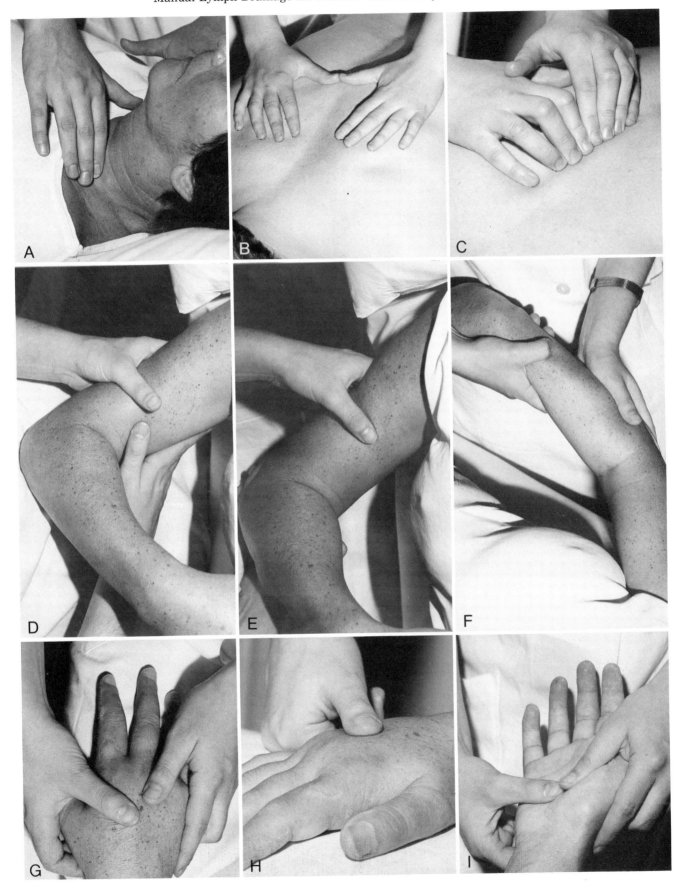

Figure 39.1.

Figure 39.2.

A. Pumping grip at the thigh.
B. Rotational manipulation at the thigh.
C. Rotational manipulation at the thigh.
D. Pumping and pushing up at the leg.
E. Pumping and pushing up at the leg.
F. Thumb circling at the below-knee amputation stump.
G. Pumping and scooping at the noninvolved leg.
H. Edema grip on the above-knee stump.

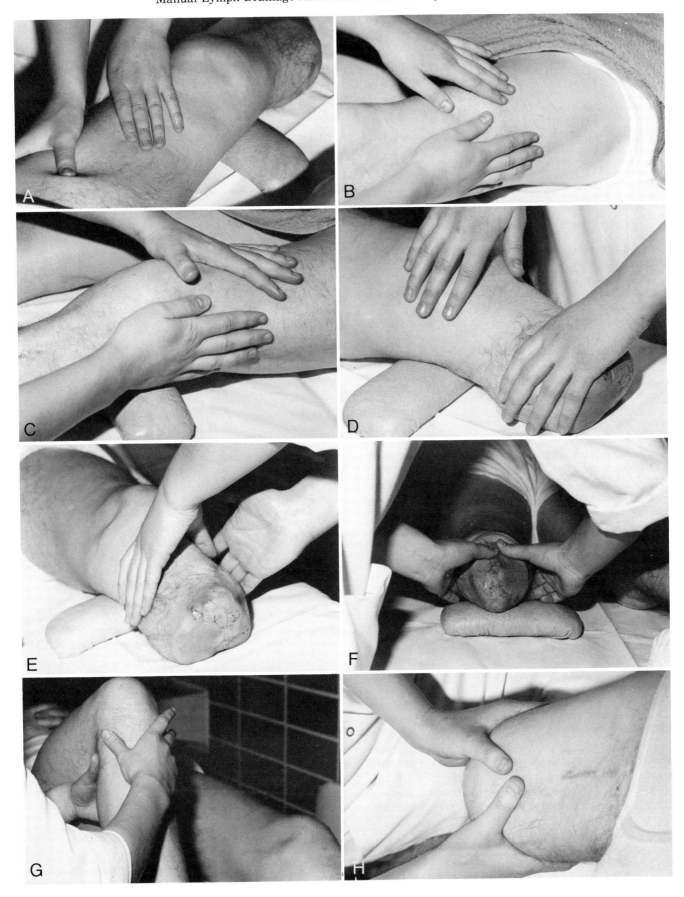

Figure 39.2.

40

Management of Joint Dysfunction by Manual Medicine: Mobilization and Manipulation

John J. Gerhardt, M.D., Lawrence Jones, D.O., Scott Heatherington, D.O., and Richard Koch, D.O.

In dealing with the pathological biomechanics of the musculoskeletal system, frequently one of two problems are encountered: (a) restriction of motion, or (b) excessive motion resulting from relaxation and weakness. Both cause acute and chronic pain syndromes. Trauma can be responsible for either condition, directly or as posttraumatic sequelae. The injury can be sudden and single or may occur as multiple microtraumata, incurred by occupational stress.

Restriction of motion can be caused by "spasm", tightness; reflex bracing and holding which can lead to myofibrositis; adhesions; scarring; contractures; deposition of metabolites; etc. Preexisting asymmetry (e.g., short leg syndrome or an old injury) may intensify the symptoms and make patients more susceptible to injuries. *Excessive motion* can be caused by sprains and strains, subluxations, dislocations, excessive stretch by trauma and muscle imbalance, ligamentous tears, avulsion, inactivity, etc. If there is restriction of motion, mobilization procedures should be used; if there is excessive motion stabilization procedures must be applied. In either case, a daily muscle reeducation program with selective stretching and strengthening must be used concurrently (see Fig. 40.1).

Mobilization is the application of biomechanical principles to restricted structures with the intention of restoring their normal motion (see Fig. 40.2). This accomplishes more than just release of restriction, and has profound biological, metabolic, physiological, and psychological effects. Mobilization can be done by various methods, from simple exercises to elaborate methods used in the discipline of manual medicine. Various techniques have been developed to influence structures in different anatomical-topographical locations and have been applied to different structures in various conditions. Some techniques use direct low amplitude high velocity thrust, reflex and reciprocal inhibition, or active resistance. Various names have been attached to the techniques, including manipulation, muscle energy, and strain and counter strain. Active, passive, or progressive resistive exercises, as well as special forms of traction, such as Goodley's polyaxial cervical mobilization system or Martin's gravity traction, are also used. All are appropriate in certain conditions, and in some of them no other treatment is effective.

The prerequisite for the selection and application of mobilization is an accurate biomechanical and kinesiological diagnosis. An important part of attaining these diagnostic skills is observation and skillful palpation, i.e., "medical feeling." This must be learned and practiced under the supervision of experts in this field. Unfortunately, this modality of treatment is often neglected by schools and practitioners of allopathic medicine. A growing literature and special courses are available. Regular courses, for example, are given at schools of osteopathic medicine such as Michigan State University in Lansing, Michigan, or at the College of Osteopathic Medicine in Kirksville, Missouri, as well as instructional seminars offered by the American Academy of Physical Medicine and Rehabilitation, the American Association of Orthopaedic Medicine, the Foundation of Musculo-skeletal Medicine, the International Rehabilitation Medicine Association, and other national organizations under the auspices of the International Federation of Manual Medicine (FIMM).

STRAIN AND COUNTERSTRAIN

The following is extracted from Lawrence Jones: *Strain and Counterstrain*, The American Academy of Osteopathy, 2630 Airport Road, Colorado Springs, Colorado 80910.

Much of the pain suffered by humans results from one poorly understood dysfunction apparently arising in or around joints. One of the first persons in America to put the study of joint dysfunction on a scientific basis was Andrew Taylor Still, a physician living at the time of the American Civil War. He studied the anatomy of the human body diligently, and by reasoning on a physiological basis, developed manipulative skills, thus greatly improving his capabilities as a physician. Other physicians of his time did not recognize his achievement as beneficial and rejected his ideas concerning the underlying cause of disease. After years of frustration, he founded another school of medicine, which he called osteopathy. The objective of the school was

... to establish a college of osteopathy, the design of which is to improve our present system of surgery, obstetrics and treatment of diseases generally, and place the same on a more rational and scientific basis, and to impart information to the medical profession.

Although the new school served to perpetuate his concepts, it further alienated his contemporaries. Still, he and the graduates of his school, using manipulative methods, were able to relieve patients of conditions where orthodox medical treatment failed. The rivalry that developed served

504

to discredit the efficacy of joint manipulation in the eyes of orthodox physicians until recent years. Today, it is considered to be a treatment of choice at many large rehabilitation centers.

Strain and counterstrain is the process of relieving spinal or other joint pain by passively putting the joint into its position of greatest comfort or relieving pain by reduction and arrest of the continuing inappropriate proprioceptor activity. This is accomplished by markedly shortening the muscle that contains the malfunctioning muscle spindle by applying mild strain to its antagonists, (Figs. 40.3 and 40.4). In other words, the inappropriate strain reflex is inhibited by application of a counterstrain.

Strain and counterstrain is an ongoing process that is useful in the treatment of *somatic joint dysfunction*. The history and course of conditions termed *somatic joint dysfunction* differ from those of most ailments to which the body is subject. Response to traumatic injury generally is resolved in one fashion or another. There may be scarring from burns, lacerations, avulsions, or contusions. Even fractures, given time, heal to be sound and painfree. Joint dysfunction, however, has a singularly everlasting, persisting character. Usually it subsides to a relatively quiescent state without treatment, but it rarely leaves completely. Even in its dormant state, a skilled, deep palpation of the affected area will reveal continuing tenderness and tension and resistance when moved in one direction.

There is something wrong—something active—that is ready to flare up on relatively slight provocation. Yet, even after many years of existence, this dysfunction can be stopped by atraumatic positioning. It can be relieved almost immediately, and, by repeated and adequate treatment, can be maintained in harmonious function until it heals sufficiently, so that its tendency to recur is inhibited indefinitely.

In patients who suffer from chronic pain, the dysfunction can start mildly, then become progressively worse, and continue to wax and wane in intensity but never to cease. Even these patients can be kept functioning normally until they are healed completely and relieved permanently.

This type of onset and course does not suggest static tissue damage, which would be expected to resolve itself and become painfree within a few months. What seems more likely is that the strain, or the body's reaction to it, initiates an ongoing noxious process, which continues to operate inappropriately so as to serve as an ongoing source of irritation. The body may adapt to the continuing dysfunction so that the pain becomes subclinical for a long period of time, but the body is unable to reverse it.

The philosophy of the physician, then, is aimed not just at promoting healing of a lesion, but at stopping a continuing and irritating dysfunction. He or she can rely on the body's healing processes to cure the conditions of inflammation, if the normal function can be maintained long enough for the healing processes to complete their work. Indeed, it is apparent that the only condition with which the body is unable to cope is its own neuromusculoskeletal dysfunction.

MUSCLE ENERGY TECHNIQUE

The muscle energy approach to effective mobilization of restricted range of motion (ROM) in a given articulation

is a safe and effective manipulative technique that is relatively easy to learn and to apply (Fig. 40.5). The most difficult part of effective manipulation is arriving at a correct diagnosis. Soft tissue changes in the paraspinal muscles help to localize restricted motion at a spinal segmental level. Careful motion testing of the spinal segment will reveal the directions in which the involved segment moves easily through a normal range and also in which directions it will not move easily or completely through a normal ROM. A segment that rotates and sidebends easily to the right but is restricted in rotation and sidebending to the left will also be restricted in either flexion or extension.

Identification of the directions of restricted motion is the first and most important step toward successful treatment. The second step is to accurately position the patient so that the involved segment is moved to the point of restriction or barrier. This position usually is not uncomfortable or painful. The patient is then instructed how to use their muscle effort gently and specifically in a direction that will move the restricted segment away from the restriction or barrier.

The third step is for the operator to provide an unyielding counterforce, which prevents movement away from the restriction. The patient's muscle effort should last about 3 to 5 sec. The patient should then be told to relax completely. When relaxation is complete, the operator will find increased motion available in the direction of the restrictive barrier and should then move the segment to the new position of restriction. The patient effort and relaxation is repeated three to five times, and each time the operator should move the segment to the new restrictive barrier. During this entire procedure, the operator should monitor the effectiveness of treatment by palpating over the involved segment. Muscle energy manipulation is nontraumatic, safe, and effective.

PERSONALIZED "SPINAL REHABILITATION PROGRAM"

The purpose of the personalized "spinal rehabilitation program" (Fig. 40.6) is to reduce and, if possible, prevent further progress of an "unbalanced" or "unstable" spine and its complications, such as spondylarthritis and disk degeneration, along with related ailments like fibrosis, contractures, osteoporosis, and pain.

Old injuries, sprains, or various stresses and strains cause many ligaments to weaken and muscles, fascia, and tendons to shorten in certain areas of the spine, resulting in pain, discomfort, tiredness, and "weakness." The normal aging process adds to the problem, and restrictions of normal vertebral motion lead to the impairment of important circulation to nerves and muscles.

The personalized spinal rehabilitation program is specifically designed for each person after a thorough examination, including detailed medical and social history; inspection; palpation; evaluation of conditions of ligaments, tendons and muscles; a dynamic-kinesiological evaluation; and a functional assessment. Standing X-rays of the full spine, anteroposterior, and lateral are imperative for proper evaluation of the spine. The X-ray cassette must be leveled and care taken that patients are properly positioned with feet about 15 cm (6 inches) apart and knees locked. A general medical examination should include laboratory tests, if clinically indicated, to rule out other pathology influencing back pain. The home program should then be designed for each patient and recorded on a specific handout sheet. It includes prescriptions for specific positions using pillows or rolls, traction, stretching and relaxation exercises, isometric exercises, counterresistance, shoe lifts of specific heights, and hip lifts when sitting as well as a listing of allowed or restricted activities, nutritional advice, and medication. Orthopedic devices also are prescribed as indicated. After explanation of the above and practice by patients under supervision, the responsibility for application of the program twice a day is shifted to the patient. Compliance determines results. Rechecks for determining progress and mobilization or stabilization procedures should be made periodically. X-ray rechecks are also done with shoe lifts in place.

All treatments are started at approximately one-tenth of the total time, which is recorded in the patient's home program and then gradually increased over a period of weeks or even months to the maximum specified time. Patients should stay relaxed during the "exercises," which are not strengthening exercises but rather corrective stretching for fibrolysis. Initially, these "exercises" may cause discomfort, some soreness, and stiffness, but most patients report a "good feeling"—never pain. Comfortable tolerance of the "lengthening stretch" is the rule. If soreness persists beyond 2 or 3 days, liniments and ointments, as well as massage and heat (in the form of a heat lamp or moist heat), should be applied. Proper positioning, erect standing, sitting and walking, and good body mechanics always should be observed.

This program has proven very effective over a period of 40 years of the authors' practice. In view of the statistical incidence of traumatic, mechanical, and postural spinal dysfunction, back pain has become one of the major problems in society. It has caused enormous unnecessary expense to patients, employers, and third-party payers and has also caused much suffering. Profound knowledge of anatomy, physiology, pharmacology, and osteopathic evaluation and treatment techniques are necessary not only to understand, but also to successfully treat, these problems.

The personalized spinal rehabilitation program, properly applied by knowledgeable practitioners, is extremely economical to all parties involved and can improve many of the chronic backache syndromes.

Figure 40.1. Evaluation of the spine and joint dysfunction. (Courtesy John Mennell, M.D.)

A. Palpation of lower back muscles is shown.

B. Percussion of spine is shown.

C. Level of posterior superior iliac spines in sitting position is checked.

D. Level of posterior superior iliac spines in prone position is checked.

E–F. Thoracic spine is rotated.

G–H. John Mennell, M.D. demonstrates correct performance of the Straight Leg Raising test and Braggard sign.

I. Joint play and opening of right LS facet joint are checked.

J. Joint play and opening of left LS facet joint are checked.

K. The patient's position is examined before rotation of trunk to left or right to check torsion play of S1 joints.

L. Rotation of trunk to right is done to check for loss of torsion play in the left sacroiliac (SI) joint.

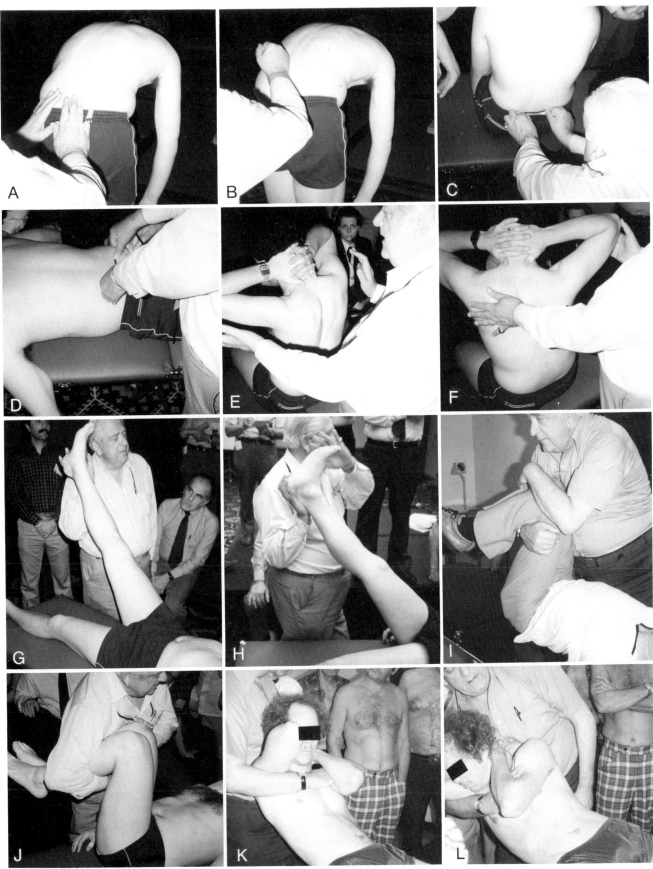

Figure 40.1.

Figure 40.2. Mobilization techniques of the thoracolumbar spine, and evaluation and treatment of sacroiliac dysfunction. (Courtesy Richard Koch, D.O., and Alec Thompson, M.D.)

A–B, F. R and LS1 and lower lumbar posterior vertebral joints are mobilized.

C–E. Postvertebral joints of thoracic spine are mobilized.

G. Demonstration of evaluation of SI joints in prone position, palpation of posterior superior iliac spines.

H. Palpation of symphysis pubis as part of evaluation of integrity of pelvic ring and SI synchondrosis.

I. Correct performance of the so-called "Thompson maneuver," or a "self-reduction" maneuver to restore joint play or reduce subluxation of the R SI synchondrosis, is demonstrated.

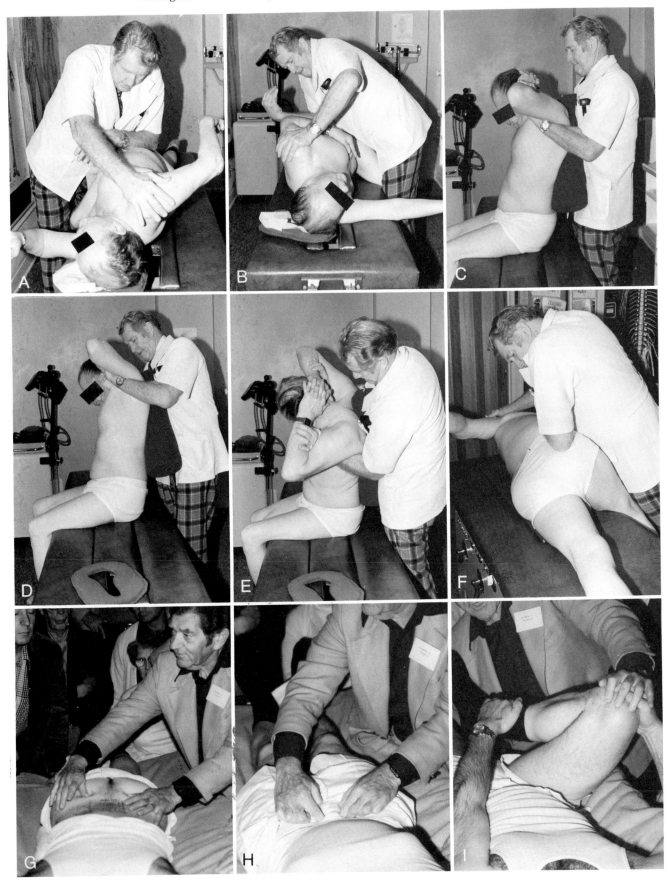

Figure 40.2.

Figure 40.3. Strain-counterstrain techniques (Courtesy Lawrence Jones, D.O.).

A. Shown are: treatment for elevated second rib on the right.
B. Treatment for thoracic strain $T1_1$.
C. Treatment for posterior thoracic strain T_{12}.
D. Treatment for posterior lumbar strain L_3 on the left.
E. Treatment for posterior lumbar strain L_5 on the left.
F. Treatment for anterior lumbar strain L_2 on the right.
G. Treatment for the high ilium on the left.
H. Treatment for medial hamstrings strain on the right.

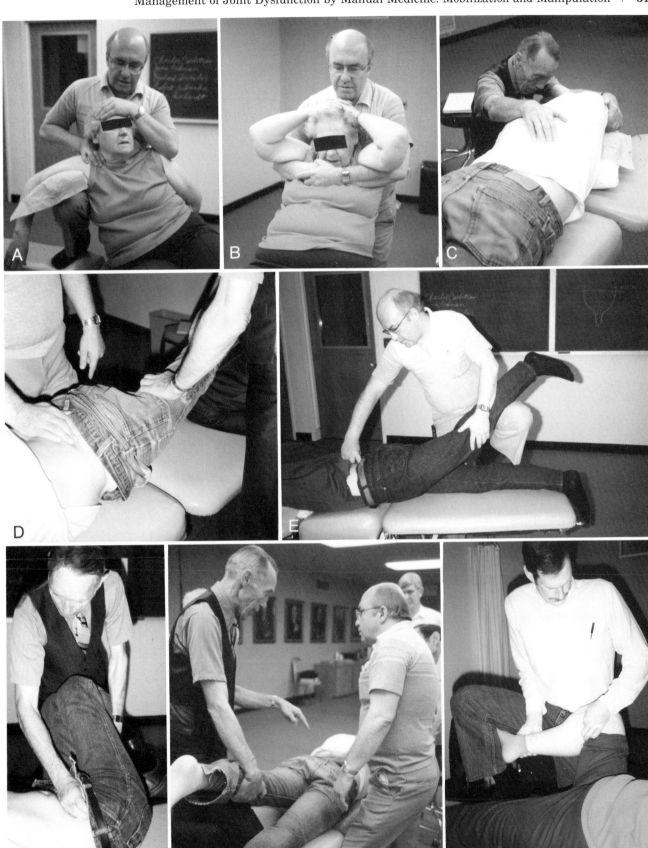

Figure 40.3.

Figure 40.4. Strain-counterstrain techniques (Courtesy Lawrence Jones, D.O.).

A. Piriformis strain syndrome on the right is treated.

B–C. Inguinal ligament strain on the right is treated. Dr. Lawrence Jones teaches proper positioning in which pain and tenderness is eliminated at least 75% (adduction and internal rotation of the hip of the involved side, with good leg crossed over the distal thigh of the involved side). The patient is in late stage of pregnancy and X-rays or other forms of treatment are contraindicated.

D. Temporal canthus is treated.

E. Infraorbital dysfunction is treated.

F. Temporomandibular joint (TMJ) dysfunction (*left*) is treated.

G–I. Dysfunctions of the navicular, dorsal metatarsal, and dorsal cuboid of the left foot are treated.

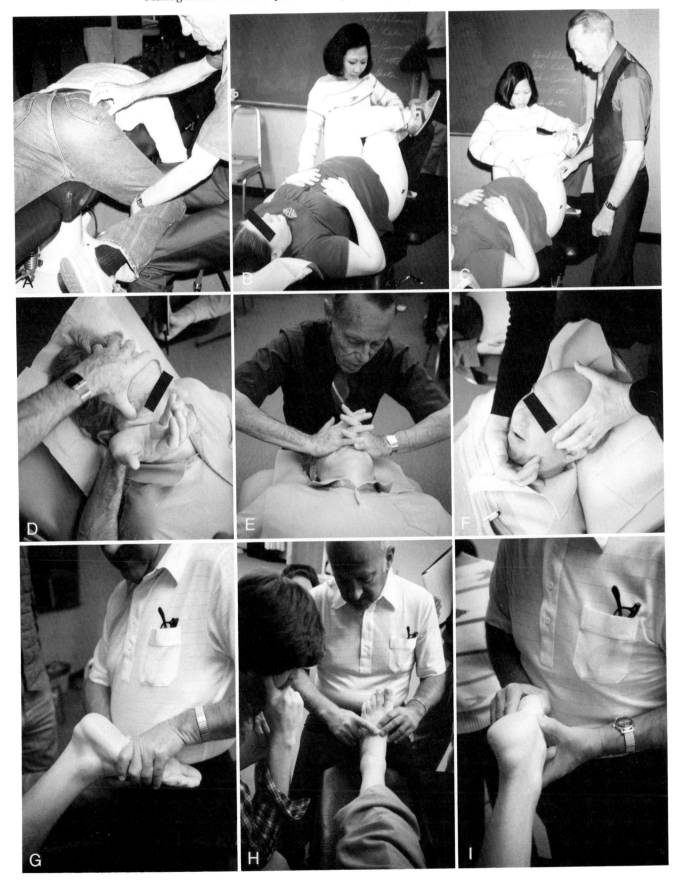

Figure 40.4.

Figure 40.5. Muscle energy technique (Courtesy Scott Haetherington, D.O.).

A. Shown are treatment of atlanto-occipital dysfunction.
B. TMJ dysfunction on the left.
C. Middle cervical spine dysfunction.
D. Upper thoracic spine dysfunction.
E. Lower thoracic spine dysfunction.
F. Depressed rib on the right are shown.
G–I. Maneuvers for treatment of lumbosacral and sacroiliac joint dysfunction are shown.

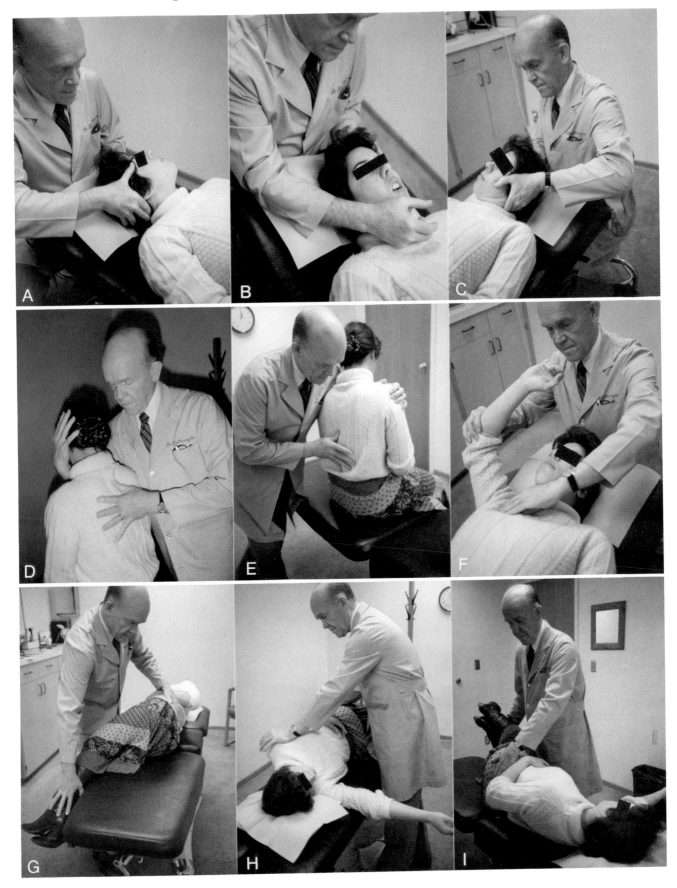

Figure 40.5.

Figure 40.6.   Example of personalized spinal rehabilitation home program (Courtesy Richard Koch, D.O.).

A–B. In this standing X-ray of full spine A-P and lateral on a 65-year-old male, there is dextro-scoliosis of the thoracic spine, levoscoliosis of the lumbar spine, thoracic kyphosis, poor posture, and the left side of the pelvis is about 1/4 inches lower than the right.

  C. Part of the home routine is vertical traction (hanging 5 to 20 sec. on a horizontal bar, which can be easily installed in a door frame).

D–E. Extension of thoracic spine over pillow 3 to 5 min. morning and night. Hip flexion prevents hyperlordosis of lumbar spine. X-ray in lateral view reveals some correction of kyphosis.

F–G. Sidebending to the right using arm support and gravity in sidelying position on the left side; P-A X-ray shows effect of positioning.

 H–I. Pillow roll under right upper rib cage in sidelying position on the right side is shown. The A-P X-ray shows effect. The pillow roll is then applied under the left lumbar area in sidelying position on the left side to influence the levolumbar scoliosis. Even if deformity cannot be corrected at that age, exercises prevent further progression by stretching fibrotic tissue at concavity of curves on the spine and rib cage.

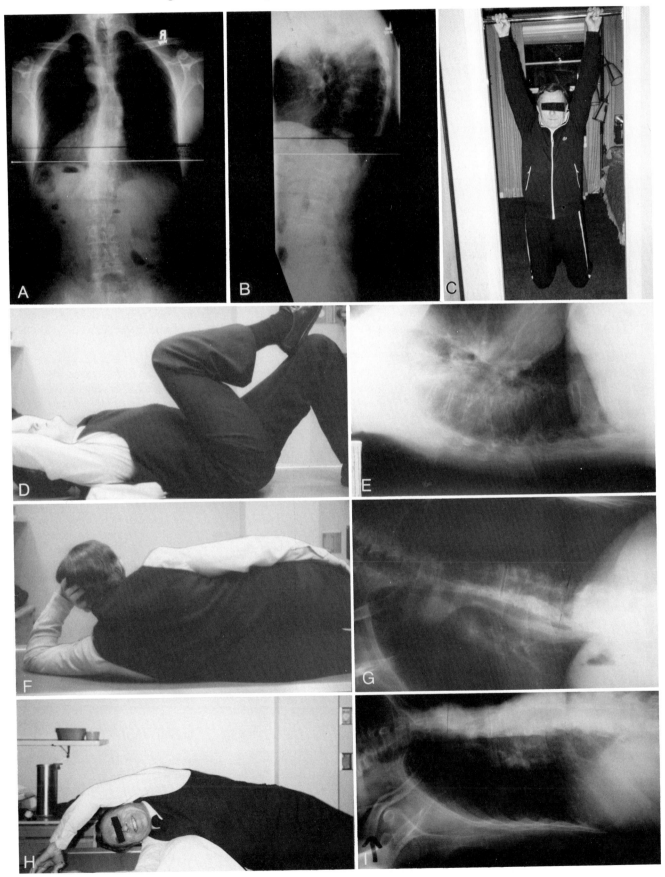

Figure 40.6.

41

Management of Joint Dysfunction by Prolotherapy-Sclerotherapy: Stabilization and Pain Control

John J. Gerhardt, M.D., and Richard Koch, D.O.

Stabilization of joint dysfunction can be accomplished by external devices, surgery, or injection therapy, referred to as prolotherapy-sclerotherapy (Figs. 41.1 to 41.3). Avulsions or partially torn ligaments as well as sprains can be stabilized by external means, such as plaster of paris casts, special splints, or braces. They are only effective if the fixation is done early (within 3 days of trauma), is uninterrupted, and is applied for a sufficiently long period of time i.e., 6 to 12 weeks, depending on age, severity of injury, and anatomical location. Stress X-rays are often necessary to determine the extent of injury and duration of fixation. Surgery can be done primarily or as a delayed procedure where indicated. (Refer to orthopedic literature for specific indications.)

Prolotherapy-sclerotherapy is a very useful method and, in certain conditions, indispensable for restoring function and relief of pain syndromes. It has been known for over 30 years, but has been widely misunderstood, underutilized or used ineffectively by practitioners for the wrong indication, prematurely, or by those who did not learn its exacting technique. This prompted some to call it a highly controversial or experimental procedure. Prolotherapy-sclerotherapy should be used to stabilize or strengthen ligaments and tendons that show dysfunction either secondary to excessive stretch and relaxation, or avulsion at their attachment to the bone. It should be used only after the joint position and muscle balance have been restored to the maximum possible level of normalcy.

The prolotherapy or sclerotherapy is injection of so-called proliferation ("sclerosing") solutions at the ligamentous or tendonous osseous junctions to enhance the healing process (see Figs. 41.1, 41.2, and 41.3). The solutions, which may be hypertonic dextrose solutions from 12½ to 25%, 5% sodium morrhuate, or even sterile pulverized pumice stone suspension, to mention a few, are chemical irritants that produce an inflammatory reaction inducing production of new dense fibrous tissue and bone cells at the site of the injection.

Similar solutions have long been used for varicose vein injections or for selected inguinal hernia cases where production of a fibrous tissue barrier by nonoperative means was considered desirable. Recent studies confirm that the injection produces a flexible, tough fibrous connective tissue rather than nonfunctional scar tissue. This technique is being taught by the Prolotherapy Association, which recently merged with the American Association of Orthopedic Medicine, and the Sclerotherapy Association of Osteopathic Medicine. The results have been excellent. Indications include dysfunction of sacroiliac, sacrospinal, sacrotuberal, iliolumbal, intraspinal ligaments, ligaments in the shoulder area (coracoclavicular, coracoacromial, acromioclavicular, sternoclavicular, etc.), pes anserinus tendonitis, tennis elbow, talofibular ligament and others, as well as transient reducible disk syndromes. The conditions that responded well include low back and neck pain, spondylolisthesis, facet syndromes, tendonitis, epicondylitis, temporomandibular joint (TMJ) dysfunction, posttraumatic syndromes such as whiplash, and the Barrè-Lieou syndrome.

Figure 41.1.

A. The table is set for the prolotherapeutic (sclerotherapeutic) procedure: with merthiolate, betadyne, and alcohol for disinfection; injector for anesthetic and marking injection points; and a syringe with proliferation solution, such as dextrose or sodium morrhuate.

B. The skin is marked and injected with anesthetic (1% carbocaine or similar).

C. The injection site is marked; notice wheals on skin.

D. The needle is inserted into the middle of the wheal.

E. The solution is injected at ligamentous insertion to the bone. No solution should be injected into soft tissue or places not clearly identified.

F. The needle can be partially withdrawn and direction changed to reach different areas of ligamentatous insertion. This avoids repeated skin penetrations.

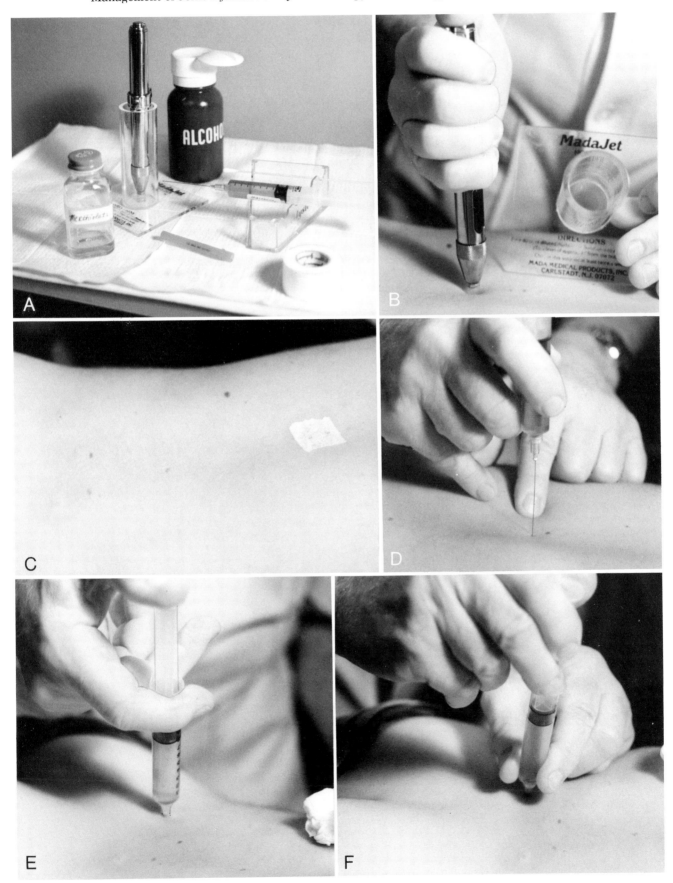

Figure 41.1.

Figure 41.2.

    A. The proliferation solution is injected at ligamentous insertion at lateral aspect of cervical spine in the supine position; sternocleidomastoid muscle and vessels are held anteriorly to prevent inadvertent puncture.

B–C. The right acromioclavicular joint and the right coracoid process are injected. The sternoclavicular joints are treated in the same position.

D–E. The patient is positioned for injections of ligamentous insertions at the occiput, posterior cervical, and thoracic spine, and distal clavicle. Notice pillow under chest and neck flexion; the patient's forehead rests on a mattress; arms are abducted.

    F. The cervical spine is injected.

G–H. The interspinal and supraspinal ligaments are injected.

  I–K. For injections of posterior shoulder, scapular insertions, and costovertebral ligaments, the arm on the injection side is placed at side of the body to abduct and stabilize the scapula. Extreme care should be taken to palpate the bones (ribs, scapula) and not to penetrate the pleura at intercostal spaces or posterior to the clavicle.

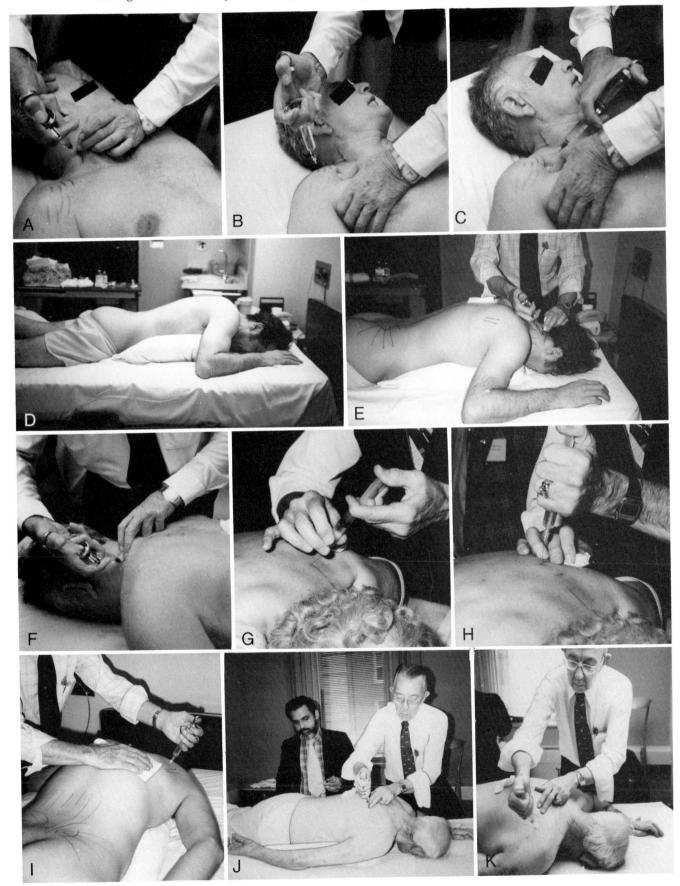

Figure 41.2.

Figure 41.3.

    A. Positioning is done for injection of lower back ligaments, iliolumbar, sacroiliac ligaments, and gluteal insertion.

    B. Dr. Hemwall's method involves marking injection sites with a skin marker.

C–D. The sacroiliac and iliolumbal ligaments are injected.

    E. The patient is shown after multiple injections with 0.5 cc of 12½% dextrose at each site. Multiple injections can be done in the outpatient clinic or same day surgery under sedation (Demerol or Valium i.v.). No general anesthetic is needed (except in children).

F–G. Injections at elbow for epicondylitis or ligamentous insertions on the radius are done. It is often necessary to inject the solution at the radius in supination and pronation of the forearm.

    H. Intraarticular injection of 25% dextrose is done on the right knee.

    I. Injection of 12½% dextrose solution at pes anserinus (for painful pes anserinus tendonitis) is done.

    J. The lateral collateral ligament of left knee is injected.

    K. Injection is done of anterior talofibular ligament at lateral malleolus and neck of the talus in unstable ankle after inversion injury and chronic recurrent inversion subluxation of the talus.

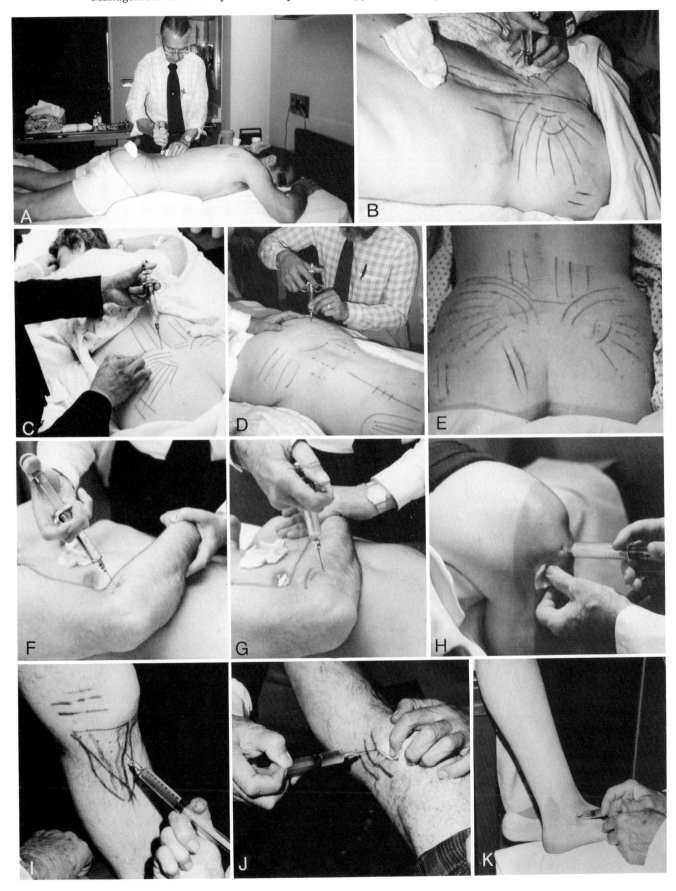

Figure 41.3.

42

Stress and Tension Control

John J. Gerhardt, M.D., Diana Gallardo, C.F.P., and Ken Ravizza, Ph.D.

Tension is an excessive effort state in the muscles as well as in the nervous system that, in turn, affects many other systems and the physiology of the entire body. Stress and tension control can be seen as part of wellness. The concept of wellness is summarized in the following formula by Dr. Stephen Germeroth, professor of health education at the Catonsville Community College Wellness Center near Baltimore, Maryland ("Well" stands for Wellness Evaluation Learning Lab):

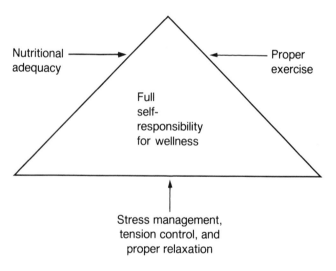

Wellness is a chosen way of life, a dynamic state of full and effective living, a proactive attitude. Beneficial effects of nutrition and exercises are available to most in our society. Stress and tension control, however, is not practiced on a broad basis. It is also known that persons who are physically fit and practice relaxation, if they are involved in accidents, have better healing, a shorter course of recovery, and markedly fewer so-called posttraumatic syndromes that manifest themselves in muscle tension, "spasms," holding, and reflex bracing. This phenomena leads to pain in a vicious cycle. Autonomic nervous system disturbances or dysfunctions are also related to it. An example is the Lieou-Barrè syndrome as sequelae to whiplash injuries secondary to rear-end automobile collisions.

There are many approaches to tension control. Among the most important are Jacobson's progressive physical relaxation, Alexander's learning method, Feldenkrais' awareness through movement and functional integration biofeedback (Fig. 42.1), autogenic training, and relaxation response. In passive relaxation, hypnotherapy also is used.

The progressive physical relaxation approach is a physiological technique that produces a state of rest and relaxation in specific muscles, muscle group, and the entire body. It also has a profound effect on the entire nervous system, including the autonomic. The method teaches the patient how to "listen" and recognize signals within his or her muscles and to constantly monitor the tension state of these muscles. It requires self-responsibility, prolonged learning, and practice with considerable investment of time. It is one of the basic techniques for tension control. Jacobson validated his approach by tedious measuring and recording muscle responses to tension states electromyographically. The training procedure involves tensing the muscle or "shortening" it without moving the joint. This is followed by relaxing or "lengthening" the same muscle. While doing this, the patient tries to perceive signals or sensations from muscles elicited during contraction. This allows him or her to monitor the tension state, and through awareness and focusing on the neuromuscular control, which "resides" in the muscle spindles, affect the tension state. In progressive lectures, relaxation of arm, leg, trunk, shoulder, neck, forehead, eyelids, and, finally, eyes is learned. Dr. Jacobson's research confirmed the previous perception that in every form of a mental act there is a specific but changing neuromuscular response. In turn, muscles can be the primary source of tension states, including emotional tension. With control of eye movement and speech, tension, including emotional tension, is also reduced.

The Alexander learning method teaches efficient movement patterns and better alignment of the body. It facilitates awareness of sensations associated with new movement patterns that had not been experienced previously. In other words, it brings proprioceptive feedback mainly from tendons and joints into a conscious level. With repeated application of these new movements and patterns, old habitual ones are inhibited and tension is released.

The Feldenkrais method (Fig. 42.2) was introduced and perfected by the late Moshe Feldenkrais, a mechanical and electrical engineer who became fascinated with body mechanics of the human and its integration and relationship with the brain cortex and the sensori-motor connections with other parts of the brain and the spinal cord. The integration regulates the tone and movement of muscles by facilitating, inhibiting, or modifying impulses or by reflexes. This, in turn, affects posture and functioning. Feldenkrais developed specific lessons, which can be taught

524

and learned and which can help individuals to become aware of those movements. The more awareness developed the more the brain will be activated. The activated regions stimulate adjacent areas. The more the patient is aware of what he or she is doing, the more he or she can do. This is true for the so-called healthy individual as well as the person with disease or injury. Amazing things have been seen to happen in regard to function, for example, in patients after severe craniocerebral injuries that cannot yet be explained fully (see Chapter 3).

As the great anatomist H. Stieve (personal communication) used to say in his lectures:

Obscura res cerebrum humanum
Obscuriores morbi
Obscurissime functiones

This translates that there is a dark thing about the human brain; darker are its diseases; and darkest, its functions. The Feldenkrais method mobilizes the person's ability for releasing tension, and introduces relaxation as well as instructs the body to move in ways that through internal biofeedback and integration, will instruct the brain to permit the body (and hence, itself) to function at a level much closer to its full human potential. Feldenkrais said:

Through awareness, we can learn to move with astonishing lightness and freedom at almost any age and thereby improve our living circumstances, not only physically but also emotionally, intellectually and spiritually (D. Gallardo, personal communication).

Biofeedback and autogenic training have been described in Chapter 15.

Hypnotherapy in tension control usually combines other techniques, such as Jacobson's progressive physical relaxation, with direct or indirect hypnotic or posthypnotic suggestions or self-hypnosis. Guided imagery can also be used. Hypnosis is a rather passive process and an active learning process is preferable for increasing awareness and controlling through awareness.

STRESS MANAGEMENT FOR RECOVERY FROM TRAUMA OR SURGERY

Stress is a normal part of everyone's life. A certain amount of stress is necessary for a person to perform at his or her fullest potential. Good stress management does not eliminate stress but teaches methods of managing stress effectively by increasing or decreasing the person's arousal level, as needed. Thus, stress management requires the abiilty to recognize what adjustments need to be made.

Appropriate stress levels may depend upon the amount of stressors that confront persons at different points in their lives. Two well-known cardiologists, Holmes and Rahe (1967), found that certain life events, such as the death of a loved one, divorce, illness and injury were all situations that contributed to medical dysfunction. Personal injury or illness ranked seventh highest on this list. For this reason, physicians should emphasize that the patient needs to recover physically and simulta-

neously should recognize that emotional vulnerability and high levels of stress also play a part in the healing process. The emotional aspects of recovery are frequently manifested by feelings of being overwhelmed, loss of patience, and emotional control. For example, a parent may have had no significant problems coping with young children before trauma (or surgery), but following trauma and the return home from the hospital, may lack patience.

In order to effectively manage the stress following trauma or surgery, the patient needs to recognize what situations or persons tend to produce a physical or emotional response. This will allow him or her to prepare for these situations so that the patient is fully focused and prepared to deal with the situation from a balanced, centered perspective.

After acknowledging stressors and preparing for the situation, the patient needs to recognize which part of the body tightens up first. For example, under prolonged stress, does he or she tend to tighten the shoulder muscles or the lower back? How does his or her behavior change to respond to the stressor? Does the person get angry, tired, or revert to forgotten negative habit patterns, like smoking or drinking? The final area to monitor is how the patient's thoughts are affected; does he or she forget or lose things, like keys, or bump into things more often?

These physical, behavioral, and cognitive manifestations need to be monitored just like a biofeedback machine monitors physiological changes. The essential point is for the person to learn to recognize, as soon as possible, when he or she is being pulled off-center so the tension does not build to the point where the person becomes out of control. By recognizing it sooner, the recovering patient can do something to intervene and get him- or herself back on track. When a person is recovering from an injury, stress tolerance levels often are lower than usual. As a result, it is more important to monitor physical, behavioral, and cognitive processes so the person can employ appropriate intervening measures, thereby avoiding unnecessary stress that might hinder recovery.

In addition, a person's confidence level often becomes lower when the person is adjusting to a major assault on his or her body and is learning to cope with physical limitations imposed by surgery. This lack of confidence often leads to frustration for the patient because activities of daily living to which he or she may never have given much thought, now require greater effort or even assistance from others. Imagery is a specific technique that has been used with a variety of patients to help them gain a feeling of control over themselves and their illness. This allows the individual to feel more responsible for enhancing or accelerating the healing process. In working with athletes, the author often has had them do imagery focused on healing the injured area.

Another major point in reducing frustration is to focus on where the patient is now in his or her immediate situation. Often the patient reflects on what was possible previously, before the trauma or surgery, and this simply focuses on behavior that cannot be achieved at the present time. The attention should be focused on what is possible today; if a comparison needs to be made, it should be made to the previous day or week so that the energy is focused on progress being made and not the frustration of the limitations imposed by the illness.

Relaxation training and practice are very helpful during the recovery period. The physiological response to relaxation lowers heart rate, blood pressure, and body temperature. Also, control of emotional levels provides a sense of confidence.

In summary, acknowledgment of stressors, learning the unique ways persons experience tension, and learning specific methods to adjust stress levels allows for a more productive use of the healing and recovery period.

Figure 42.1. Biofeedback and Relaxation Techniques

- **A.** Biofeedback-self application: patient is engaged in relaxation training on biofeedback apparatus using audiovisual clues to monitor his progress.
- **B.** Imagery technique: Patient listens to tape utilized in imagery technique. Biofeedback device monitors skin temperature changes.
- **C–F.** Various monitoring devices use color changes, temperature changes, digital displays and sound signals as indicators for responses: bracelet with color display monitoring temperature changes (C); skin thermometer (D); skin thermometer with digital readout (E); and auditory biofeedback instrument (F).
- **G.** Two patients practice progressive relaxation according to E. Jacobson technique under supervision of physical therapist M. Showers at Bess Kaiser Medical Center, Portland, Oregon.
- **H.** Physical therapist teaching relaxation uses the "autogenic training" technique.
- **I.** A progressive relaxation lesson is demonstrated in a class of school children during a course at the University of Sussex, Brighton, England in 1983.
- **J.** B. Fredrick, Ph.D., physical educator checks the response of relaxation during his lesson on one of the pupils.

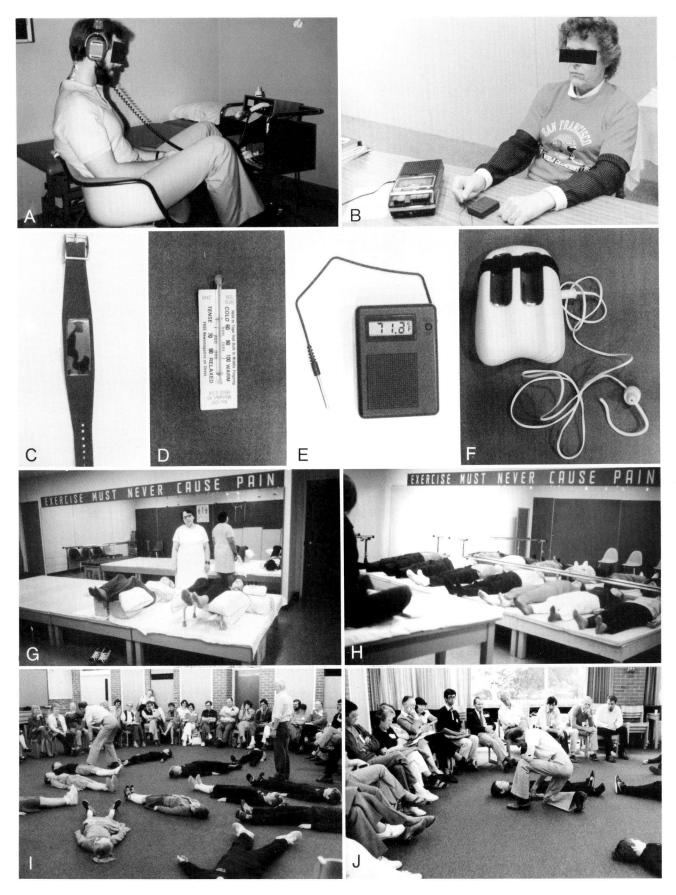

Figure 42.1.

Figure 42.2. Feldenkrais Method.

    A. Gallardo works on functional integration in the Feldenkrais approach on a patient with a "frozen shoulder". The technique of making a patient aware of "feeling" his own weight is demonstrated.

B–D. Gallardo working with same patient (frozen shoulder) on head-upper back, head-neck relationships, and functional integration of the back extensors.

    E. Gallardo treating a participant of the course in the Feldenkrais technique held in Portland, Oregon in 1985, while others are watching the original Feldenkrais teaching videotape.

F–G. "Awareness through movement" lesson is conducted in a group practice session.

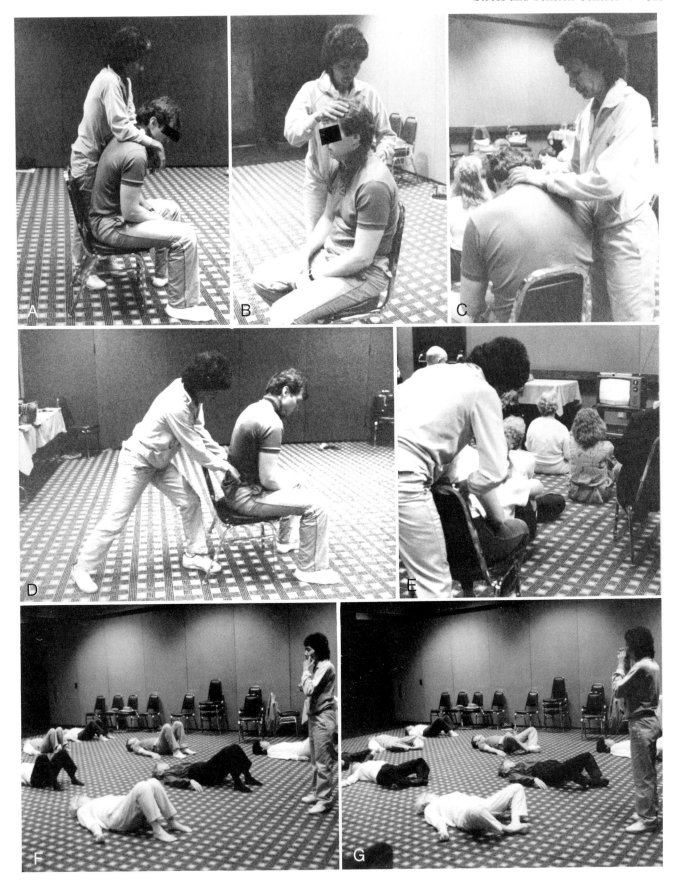

Figure 42.2.

43

Thermography in Trauma

Paul H. Goodley, M.D.

Medicine aims to objectify abnormalities, which is not difficult with gross musculoskeletal trauma. However, persisting complaints, unvalidated by X-ray or by other traditional tests and unaccompanied by signs that clinicians customarily seek, are a common cause for consternation.

The problem is the training of physicians. Most view traditional clinical examinations as inherently complete, and the disadvantages of overdedication to X-rays are generally not appreciated. What is not found becomes "subjective." The "soft signs" that early on accompany common segmental articular dysfunctions and other soft tissue injuries are invisible to those techniques.

Musculoskeletal thermography challenges orthodoxy by objectifying vital but previously unappreciated processes and, therein, its ultimate value may be as a hone on which diagnosticians may sharpen their clinical skills. Thermography has become an instant visualization methodology in both black/white and color (Fig. 43.1). Both are important. Heat distribution is modulated through vascular flow by the sympathetic nervous system and, in health,

Figure 43.1.

A. The author is viewing the black/white monitor. The color module is to its *left*. Note the patient's gown is taped along her chest, completely exposing the neck and back. It is tucked between her legs for frontal lower extremity views. Male patients are completely disrobed for lumbar studies.

B. The patient must be carefully monitored during preparation and the examination. Skin surface must be examined for visible varicosities and lesions, which have a distinctive appearance, regardless.

C. *Black/white thermograph* of a 56-year-old female with lower back pain. Note the *horizontal scale (bottom)* ranging from white to black. In AGA equipment, the color in the *lower right* denotes relative heat. In this exam, black is hot. At times, the reverse is more easily visualized. (Note the bulbous relative increase in the vascular heat emission pattern (VHEP) from which a subtle linear elongation extends down and to the right in the area of the L5 root and also, unusually, the increase along the medial aspect of the right gluteal fold. This relative heat represents the pattern of local tissue response to the injury.

D. The view of the dorsal legs reveals one of the disadvantages of black-and-white photos in this area. Isothermic (color) views would have more clearly delineated the relative decrease of the "VHEP" on the right, seen here as a *higher line of demarcation* from grey to black. This is a "consistent pattern," i.e., relative increased heat in the vertebral area, and relative coolness, due to vasoconstriction, along the sympathetic course of the nerves involved.

E. The same patient experienced nonradiculopathic pain along the right medial scapular border, associated with positive "soft signs": cutaneous hyperalgesia, and scapulothoracic dysreflexia (i.e., reflexic medial muscular tightness and inability to mobilize the scapula). The thermographic examination correlates with it.

F–G. A 67-year-old female, 1 day preop., with massive herniation of the L5 disc, on CT scan, entrapping the right S1 root, exclusively. (Note bilateral extensions of the VHEP and the considerably cooler right calf.) (White is hot.)

H–I. The same patient is seen, 2 days later, totally asymptomatic, ambulatory, and discharged from hospital. (Note the broad VHEP (surgical), the absence of the "tails" and the improved temperature balance in the calves. A remarkable surgical result!

J–K. A 54-year-old asymptomatic woman is seen with broad VHEP and elongations and a relatively cooler left ankle. On history, she has been pain-free for 1½ years on light activities. Lifting 50 pounds predictably causes pain.

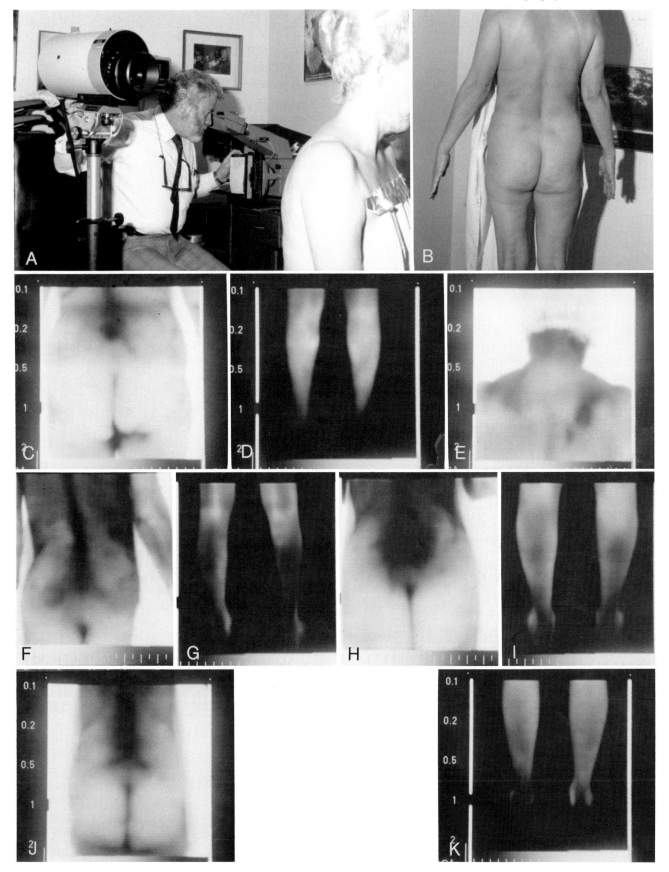

Figure 43.1.

is essentially symmetric. This system is ubiquitous and variability is the rule; therefore, exact and predictable patterns are not expected. However, persistent pathology in one individual reveals reliably duplicatable pictures over prolonged periods. The hues may be subtle and, like electromyography, reveal process, not diagnosis. Anything that changes temperature becomes visible: abscess, occlusion, immersion, varicosity, etc.

In studying vertebrogenic pain, the normal pattern is a relatively thin line of heat, the "vascular heat emission pattern" (VHEP), which follows the midline, fades at the lumbosacral area, and reappears in the gluteal cleft. Small mild focal increases are usually seen over the sacroiliac joints. Through the lower extremities, the sympathetic distribution is followed where, excepting other pathology, the prepared patient demonstrates a gently symmetric descending temperature gradient, usually seen as obliqued changes below the knees.

With lower back injury, a local asymmetric increased temperature may be seen, usually surrounded with a rather intense gradient line. Root irritation may be accompanied by a linear extension. Superficial muscular injury is usually seen as a diffuse pattern of medium intensity, lacking focal increases. When the sympathetics are irritated, they produce relative vasoconstriction, therefore cooling along their individualistic distributions. If it is intense, overflow is the rule. When paravertebral inflammation accompanies ipsilateral peripheral relative cooling, a "consistent pattern" is present, and it is "crossed" when it occurs on the contralateral side. A rapid trend toward symmetry seems to suggest a better prognosis, and persistence, despite apparent normalcy, may be a warning, but its use as a routine "fingerprint" is to be condemned.

Thermography is most potentially valuable as a validator of cryptic injury. When it, alone, supports the complaint, the wise clinician continues to seek.

44

Treatment of Myofascial Pain and Dysfunction

Edgar DeMar, M.D.

Techniques for treating myofascial pain and dysfunction are described in detail by Travell and Simons (1983). The authors highly recommend this approach to assist in proper diagnosis and treatment of posttraumatic syndromes and soft tissue injuries.

A myofascial trigger point is a hyperirritable spot in the muscle. It usually is found within a taut band of skeletal muscle, and/or sometimes in the muscle's fascia. The tender point is painful on compression. It can give rise to referred pain and tenderness. A local twitch response is unequivocal evidence of the presence of a myofascial trigger point (TP), either active or latent. Active TPs of muscles cause pain; latent TPs do not. An active TP causes referred pain, even when inactive, and is a specific referred pain pattern for a specific muscle. Myofascial pain due to TPs is the most common source of musculoskeletal pain and is easily missed if not suspected by the examiner. Furthermore, the pain cycle from these trigger areas can continue almost indefinitely if not properly recognized and treated.

The treatment involves the recognition of TPs of pain within traumatized muscle tissue that can be influenced or extinguished by stretching and spraying the muscle with a vapocoolant to effect an interruption of the neutral pathway of pain and its reflex muscle spasm.

The stretch-and-spray procedure, which involves steady, passive stretch of the involved muscle during unidirectional, brief application of a vapocoolant spray, is one of the most effective methods of inactivating a myofascial TP.

The technique has to be learned and applied correctly to be effective. The authors again refer to Travell and Simons for details.

Alternative methods can be used to treat TPs. They can be injected with small amounts of 0.5% procaine using a 22- or 25-gauge needle, according to the muscle injected. Sterile technique is used. The patient should be placed in a recumbent position for relaxation and protection. The precise injection technique needs to be learned and practiced. Precautions to be observed are the same as for any injection (e.g., allergy).

Superficial TP may be inactivated by ischemic compression or myotherapy. Sustained and slowly increasing pressure is applied long enough to inactivate the TP. It can be done in one treatment or in a succession of several treatments.

Other methods include massage, ultrasound, rhythmic stabilization, heat, ice, drugs, and biofeedback. Transcutaneous nerve stimulation (TNS) also has been used with varying success.

"Shiatzu" ("Shiatsu,") and acupressure are terms used to describe a pressure version of acupuncture in which the operator applies digital compression in a manner similar to that described for ischemic compression or myotherapy. The spot for compression, however, is selected not for TP tenderness, but because of its location on an acupuncture chart. The acupressure results are said to be comparable to those obtained by acupuncture at corresponding points. To the extent that the Shiatzu points are located where there is a tender TP, the Shiatzu treatment should yield results comparable to those of ischemic compression. Shiatzu is philosophically quite different from the authors' concept of myofascial TPs, but in practice, the treatments may seem similar.

Like any other mode of treatment, the spray-and-stretch technique may be rendered ineffective or less effective by mechanic or systemic perpetuating factors that may be present, and therefore it is most important to be aware of them and to treat them also. Perpetuating factors include leg length differences; repeated pressure on muscles by clothing straps, luggage, or purse straps; vitamin deficiencies; thyroid deficiency; hypoglycemia; infections, and psychological problems, such as depression, anxiety, and tension.

Recently, the technique of patient postisometric relaxation (Fig. 44.1) described by Lewit and Simons (1984) is being used successfully for control of pain caused by myofascial TPs. In this method, the patient is placed in supported relaxed position, the muscle is stretched slightly to take up the slack using one hand of the physician or therapist, and the patient is then asked to contract the muscle against resistance given by the other hand. The contraction is held 5 sec, and the patient asked to relax the muscle completely. While he or she relaxes, the practitioner takes up the slack of the muscle and stretches the muscle slightly more. This process is repeated until the muscle reaches its maximal length, and then it is moved three times through its newly achieved full range.

Figures 44.2 to 44.4 show other methods for treating myofascial pain and dysfunction.

533

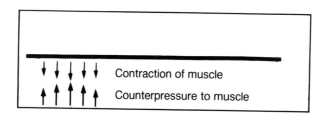

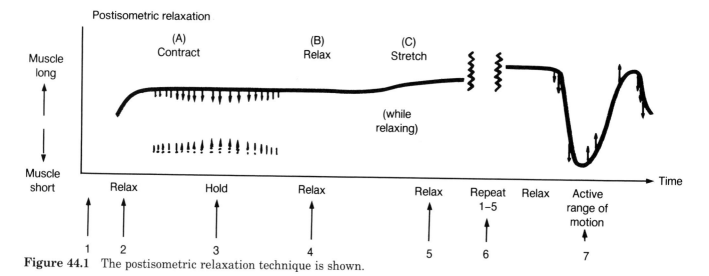

Figure 44.1 The postisometric relaxation technique is shown.

Figure 44.2.

A. The apparent relation of the trigger point (*X*) to factors that clinically can activate it and to its pain reference zone is shown. The *triple arrows* (*A*) from the trigger point to the spinal cord represent the multiplicity of effects originating at the trigger point. The *arrow* returning to the trigger point (*B*) completes a feedback loop that is evidenced by the self-sustaining nature of many trigger points. The *long arrow* (*C*) to the pain reference zone represents the appearance of referred pain in neurologically distant sites that may be several segments removed from the trigger point. *Arrow D* indicates the influence on the trigger point of the vapocoolant-stretch procedure applied to the reference zone. *Arrow E* signifies the activating effect of indirect stimuli on the trigger point; *dashed arrow F* denotes effects of TPs on visceral function (after David Simons, 1984, personal communications).

B–C. Schematic drawing shows taut bands, myofascial trigger points (dark spots), and a local twitch response seen in longitudinal view of the muscle (light spots). In *B* the palpation of a taut band (*straight lines*) among normally slack, relaxed muscle fibers (*wavy lines*) is shown. The density of *stippling* corresponds to the degree of tenderness of the taut band to pressure. The trigger point is the most tender spot in the band. In *C*, rolling the band quickly under the fingertip (snapping palpation) at the trigger point often produces a local twitch response that is most clearly seen toward the end of the muscle, close to its attachment.

D. *Cross-sectional schematic drawing* shows flat palpation of a taut band (*ring*) and its trigger point (*spot*). Flat palpation is used for muscles (light) that are accessible only from one direction, such as the infraspinatus. The skin is pushed to one side to begin palpation. The fingertip slides across muscle fibers to feel the cord-like texture of the taut band rolling beneath it. The skin is pushed to the other side at the completion of snapping palpation.

E. *Cross-sectional schematic drawing* shows pincer palpation of a taut band (*ring*) at a trigger point (spot). Pincer palpation is used for muscles (light) that can be picked up between the digits, such as the sternocleidomastoid, pectoralis major, and latissimus dorsi. Muscle fibers are surrounded by the thumb and fingers in a pincer grip. The hardness of the taut band is felt clearly as it is rolled between the digits. The change in the angle of the distal phalanges produces a rocking motion that improves discrimination of fine detail. The edge of the taut band is sharply defined as it escapes from between the fingertips, often with a local twitch response.

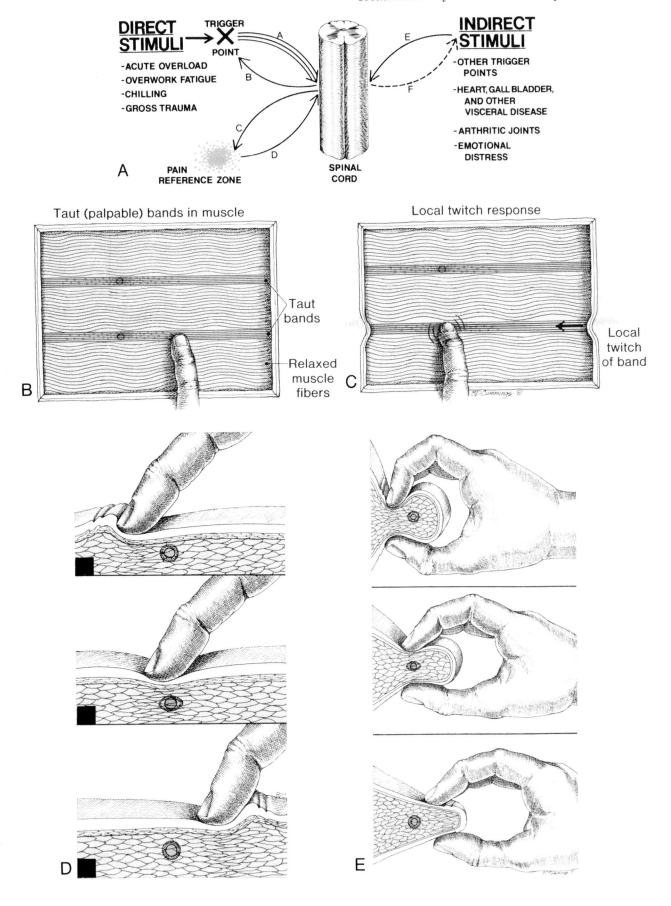

Figure 44.2.

Figure 44.3.

A. Sequence of steps when stretching and spraying any muscle for myofascial trigger points, as applied to the upper trapezius is shown. 1. The patient is supported in a comfortable relaxed position. 2. One end of the muscle (light) is anchored. 3. The skin is sprayed with repeated parallel sweeps of the vapocoolant over the length of the muscle in the direction of pain pattern (dark dots). All of the muscle is covered. 4. Immediately after the first sweep of spray, pressure is applied to stretch the muscle and is continued as the spray is applied. 5. Sweeps of the spray are continued to cover the referred pain pattern of that muscle. 6. Sweeps of the spray are continued to cover the referred pain pattern of that muscle. 6. *Steps 3, 4 and 5* repeated only two or three times, or fewer times if the passive range of motion becomes maximal. Hot pack and then several cycles of full active range of motion follow (see Fig. 44.8 for details of the spray technique).

B. In this schematic representation, neural pathways that can account for the effectiveness of vapocoolant applied to skin overlying an active myofascial trigger point (dark). The sudden cold and touch stimuli of the spray inhibit the pain and reflex spasm that would otherwise prevent passive stretching of the muscle. The *black bar* in the dorsal horn of the spinal cord represents this inhibition.

C. *Schematic drawing* shows how the jet stream of vapocoolant is applied. Unidirectional sweeps cover, first, parallel lines of skin over those muscle fibers that are stretched the tightest, then over the rest of the muscle and its pain pattern. The lines of spray follow the direction of the muscle fibers (*solid area*) progressing toward the referred pain zones (*stippled area*). The spray bottle is held at an acute angle, approximately 45 cm (18 inches) from the skin, as the spray sweeps over the skin at a rate of about 10 cm (4 inches) per second.

D. Stretch position and spray pattern (*arrow*) for trigger points (*xs*) in the posterior cervical muscles, primarily on the right side, is shown. 1. Upper cervical stretch for the semispinalis capitis muscles bilaterally, using straight flexion with an upsweep pattern, is shown. 2. The lower posterior cervical and upper thoracic longissimus stretch bilaterally with the down-pattern of spray application. 3. Stretch of the 'v' diagonal muscles (*right*) and the diagonal fibers (*left*) is done by firmly flexing the head and neck while applying gentle side pressure and turning the face to the left. The skin over the muscles being stretched is covered with an up-pattern of the vapocoolant. 4. Passive stretch, primarily of the right diagonal and left v diagonal muscles are done by strongly flexing the head and neck while turning the face toward the right and pulling the neck post gently to the left.

E. Supine stretch-position, usual location of trigger point (x), and vapocoolant spray pattern for the latissimus dorsi muscle are shown.

F. Side-lying stretch position, usual location of trigger point (x), and vapocoolant spray pattern (*arrows*) for the latissimus dorsi muscle are shown.

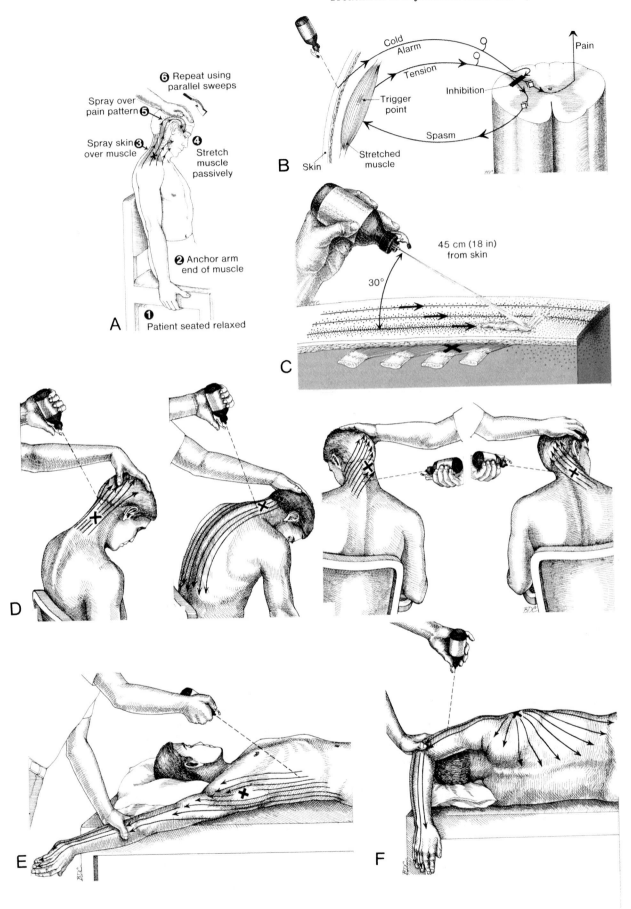

Figure 44.3.

Figure 44.4.

A. *Cross-sectional schematic drawing* shows flat palpation to localize the taut band (*oval*) and fix the trigger point (*dark spot*) for injection. 1–2. Use of alternating pressure between two fingers confirms the location of a taut band. 3. The band is positioned halfway between the fingers for injection of the trigger point that lies within the band.

B. *Schematic top view* of two approaches to the flat injection of a trigger point area (*spot encircled in black*) in a taut band (*closely spaced black lines*) is shown. 1. Injection is done away from fingers, which have pinned down the trigger point so it cannot slide away from the needle. *Dotted outline* indicates additional probing to explore for a cluster of trigger points. The fingers are pressing downward and apart to maintain pressure for hemostasis. 2. Injection is done toward the fingers with similar finger pressure. Additional trigger points are often found in the immediate vicinity by probing with the needle.

C. Technique for applying ischemic compression to trigger points in the right extensor carpi radialis brevis muscle is shown. Pressure is gradually increased over a period of 30 to 60 sec until TP tenderness is eliminated.

D. Patient position and injection technique for trigger points in the left trapezius muscle are shown. In *trigger point 1*, the patient lies supine for the anterior approach to the upper trapezius, to avoid penetrating the apex of the lung. In *trigger point 2*, the patient lies on the right side for the posterior approach to the left upper trapezius, with the muscle lifted off the apex of the lung. In *trigger point 3*, in the lateral border of the lower trapezius, the patient is on the opposite side. The needle is aimed at a rib to avoid penetrating an intercostal space. In *trigger point 5*, in the middle trapezius close to the medial end of the muscle fibers, the patient is on the opposite side (optional).

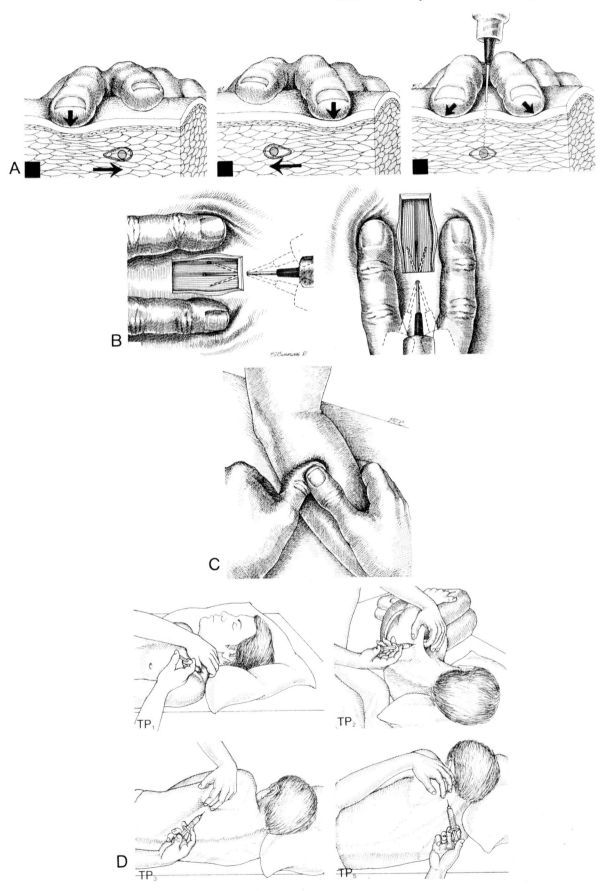

Figure 44.4.

45

Treatment of Cervical Syndromes

Fritz Jenkner, M.D.

Soft tissue injuries, such as extension-flexion (whiplash injuries) seen after a rear-end automobile collisions, may heal spontaneously, but they usually must be treated properly to prevent long-term posttraumatic syndromes or permanent disability. The injuries consist of disc lesions resulting in a malposition or malalignment of the cervical spine and cause pain.

X-rays are indispensable for the diagnosis and must be correlated with an exact history and physical findings prior to initiation of any treatment. For example, widening of the intervertebral space points to discogenic injury (swelling, edema); vertebral shift in extension of flexion, to ligamentous and/or disc injury; and straightening of the spine with loss of physiological lordosis, to muscle bracing. Anterior or posterior angulation (reversed curvature) indicates combined soft tissue injury. Figure 45.1 shows unique X-rays taken just before and after an automobile accident.

A questionnaire designed by the author is filled out by patients to determine subjective symptoms. The questionnaire correlates these symptoms with the patient's level of lesion (Fig. 45.1). It helps an even less experienced practitioner to reach a better diagnosis, including determination of the level of lesion of somatoradicular origin, or to recognize autonomic, sympathetic, or vascular syndromes (e.g., Barre Lieou syndrome). If the patient marks with a cross an excessive number of squares, depression should be suspected.

Figure 45.2 shows Jenkner demonstrating his technique of mobilizing the spine. Cervical exercises are shown in Figure 45.3.

Figure 45.1.

A–D. Dr. Jenkner demonstrates his technique of mobilization of the cervical spine to correct reverse curvature and malalignment on a female patient involved in a motor vehicle accident (rear-end collision extension-flexion injury).

E–F. Position of hands during mobilization procedure is shown.

G. This X-ray of the cervical spine of an 18-year-old male was taken before treatment. (Note reversed curve and acute angulation at C2–3 level, anterior sliding (C3–4, C5–6.)

H. X-ray of the cervical spine of the same patient was taken after completion of treatment.

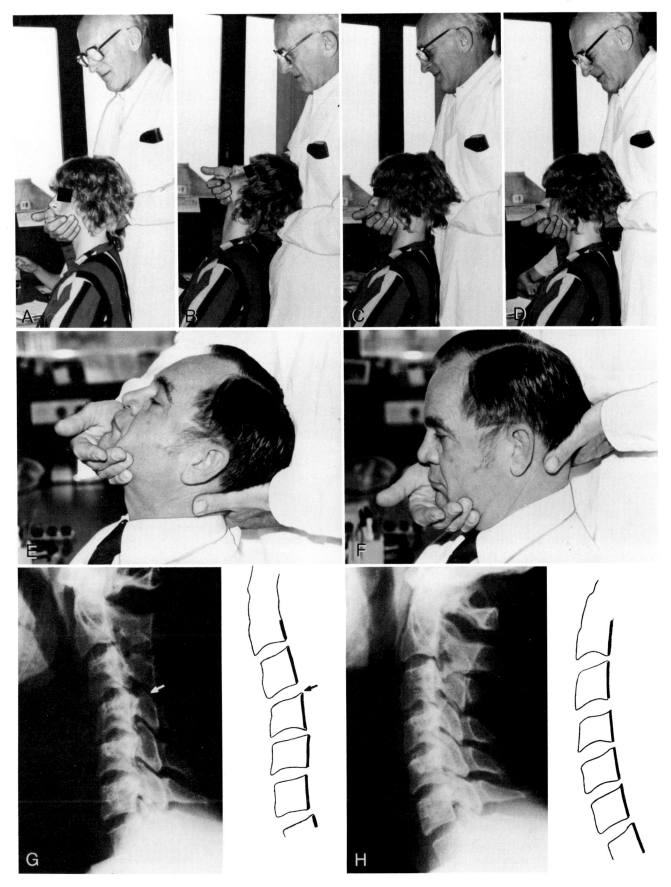

Figure 45.1.

Figure 45.2.

A–B. Acute angulation and reversed curve as direct cause of rear-end collision injury is demonstrated. This 45-year-old female was in the radiology institute for a routine x-ray of the cervical spine. After the x-ray was taken, the patient left the institute, and while driving out in her sedan, was rear-ended by a bus. She immediately returned to the institute where just minutes after the accident another x-ray of her cervical spine was taken, under the same conditions, the same technician, and using the same techniques and views.

X-ray "A" taken immediately after the injury shows a reversed curvature (kyphotic "kink") and slight anterior sliding of C_4 over C_5, while X-ray "B," taken few minutes before the accident, shows normal physiological lordosis and alignment.

C. This X-ray is of the cervical spine of a 20-year-old female before treatment.

D. The same case is shown after treatment.

E. Jenkner's cervical syndrome questionnaire (self-assessment form), is completed by the patient prior to evaluation by the physician.

Pictures reproduced from: Jenkner F., *Das Cervicalsyndrom*, Springer Verlag Wien, New York, 1982 (pp. 68–69 and 96–97).

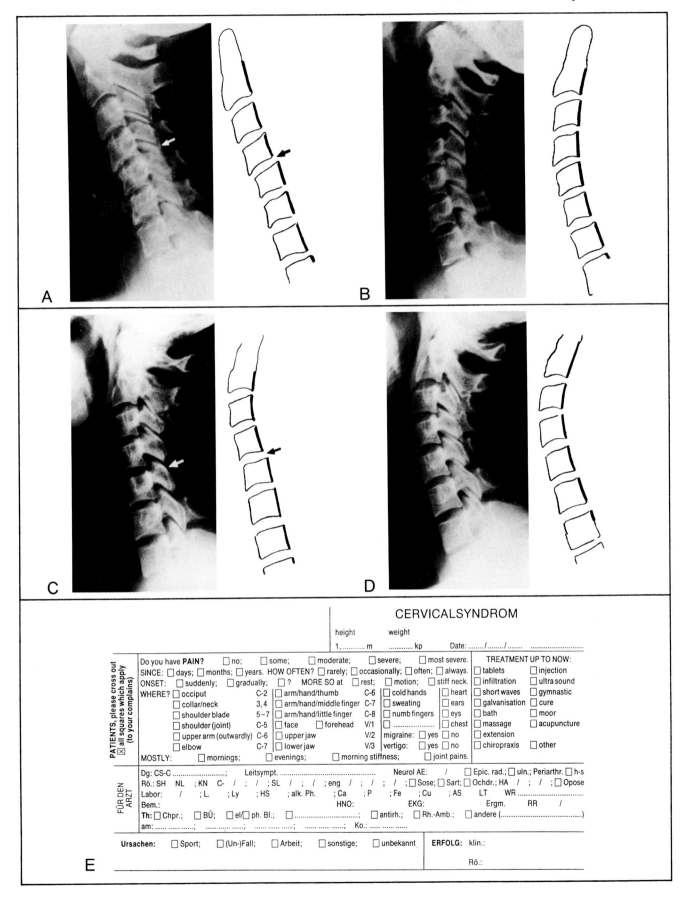

Figure 45.2.

Figure 45.3. Cervical exercises are recorded on a handout sheet.

Appointment for: ....
(In case of cancellation please call ....
in advance)

EXERCISES FOR CERVICAL SPINE

I. Head in Neutral Position

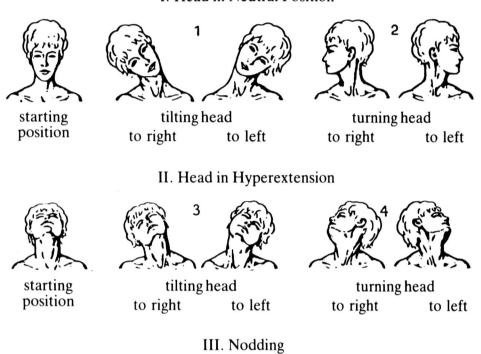

starting position   tilting head   turning head
to right   to left   to right   to left

II. Head in Hyperextension

starting position   tilting head   turning head
to right   to left   to right   to left

III. Nodding

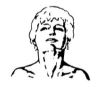

ATTENTION PLEASE to the following advises:
1. Each exercise should be done 5 times mornings and evenings; as relaxed as possible and not as forceful or extensive as possible.
2. During course of treatment (and not thereafter) please avoid all combined motions of head involving turning and bending at the same intention. Avoid during work and sportive activities (such as golfing, tennis, skiing, bowling − these are not to be done during treatment course). For certain jobs work may have to be interrupted for two weeks, such as in case of auto mechanics. When driving do not turn head, use mirror only for rear view. In house hold chores, bedding, kitchen work or care for small children, attend to avoiding combined movements as indicated above!
3. After end of treatment, as well as during same, do not circle your head (as is done frequently during gymnastics) and do not lie or sleep on your stomach (flat, neither during sun bathing). Due regard is advised for full recovery and lasting well being.

Figure 45.3.

Figure 45.4. Acceptable sleeping positions.

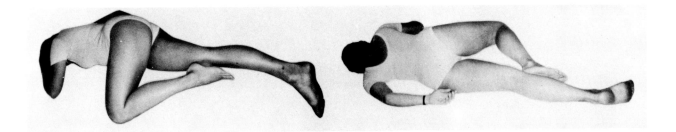

SECTION

6

APPENDICES

Appendix 1

Establishing a Trauma Department and a Minirehabilitation Service in an Acute Care Hospital

John J. Gerhardt, M.D., Friedrich Russe, M.D., Kay Schweickart, R.N., Martha Rushing, O.T.R., Gerhard Peter, C.P.O., Sherry Kleier, R.N., M.S., and Gerhard Schicht, Dipl. Ing. Architect.

ESTABLISHING A TRAUMA DEPARTMENT IN AN ACUTE HOSPITAL

Justification

A trauma department should be established in an acute hospital because it can provide the following advantages:

1. A highly organized and, therefore, efficient management of all trauma at a specially designed, equipped, and staffed facility on an in- and outpatient basis
2. Immediate access for evaluation and treatment 24 hours per day, 7 days per week
3. A facility in which the rehabilitation process is started immediately and short- and long-term planning is instituted on a consistent basis
4. The most efficient treatment and management of industrial injuries (avoiding the tendency to prolonged morbidity and disability)
5. Effective access and treatment of athletic and sport injuries
6. Immediate definition and treatment of traffic and motor vehicle accidents
7. A center for management of pediatric injuries
8. A superior center for management of growing numbers of geriatric injuries
9. A training center in trauma for interested physicians, technicians, and nurses
10. A training program for house staff.

The benefits of such a department include: (a) superior, more efficient treatment and management of trauma, (b) a shorter period of acute care hospitalization, (c) reduction of short- and long-term disability, (d) reduction of treatment and rehabilitation time and increased function of patients with permanent disability, and (e) savings in overall expense to hospitals as well as third-party payers.

Facilities and Staff

Several facilities are needed to accommodate trauma care. One floor should be dedicated to the evaluation, admission, and outpatient treatment of injuries (Fig. A1.1). Two operating rooms and an X-ray department should be dedicated to trauma. Also, there should be one wing for inpatient care, with specially trained orderlies and nursing personnel and traction beds. The facility should be located close to freeways and have easy access. The trauma department should be integrated with other surgical departments, such as orthopaedics, general surgery, vascular surgery, ENT, and neurosurgery, within the same facility. The department should be small enough to facilitate superior management and care, and large enough to justify around-the-clock staff; the facility must also be cost effective. There should be a well-equipped stockroom. A mini-rehabilitation center should be attached to the facility so that the rehabilitation process can begin on admission. Also, there should be a helicopter pad.

The number of personnel should be determined by the number of hospital beds dedicated to trauma and the number of outpatients to be treated in the facility. The chief and assistant chief of the center should be traumatologists. The rest of the staff could be composed of interested orthopaedists (on a rotational basis), general surgeons, trauma clinic physicians, interns, and residents. There should be a specially trained nursing staff, two X-ray technicians, and two cast room technicians available. Physical therapy, occupational therapy, speech and language pathology, medical social work, and prosthetics orthotics also should be represented at the Center.

PLANNING A TRAUMATOLOGY DEPARTMENT IN AN ACUTE HOSPITAL

The traumatology department plan presented in this chapter is designed to be integrated within an acute general hospital or a university hospital. The department is architecturally connected to the general hospital, so specific areas or facilties (such as operating rooms, recovery rooms, sterilization, kitchen, and cafeteria) can be used jointly or shared.

Although general surgeons should participate in staffing the trauma department, a chief must be in full authority in regard to the organization of the department, staffing, and independent medicosurgical decisions. The X-ray service should be under the direction of the chief of traumatology rather than part of the centralized X-ray department. It should be properly equipped and have sufficient staff to provide independently full management of patients with injuries of all degrees of severity 24 hours a day and 7 days a week.

The department presented in this appendix is designed for treatment of 15,000 to 20,000 patients a year, with the ratio of outpatients to inpatients 3:1. Space is needed for:

1. Reception
2. Initial evaluation
3. Shock treatment
4. Minor surgery and treatment
5. X-ray service
6. Casting
7. Follow-up (reevaluation)
8. Physical medicine and early rehabilitation (see Fig. A1.2)
9. Operating (major surgery)
10. Wards for inpatients.

Space is also necessary for waiting rooms; male and female staff rooms for night duty; a conference room; a consultation room; offices for chief of the department, head nurse, secretary, and administration; restrooms; showers and bathrooms for patients and personnel; utility rooms; storage (including space for wheelchairs; stretchers; and beds).

Distribution of space should be carefully planned. The following distribution is suggested:

Entrance

Entrance for ambulatory patients and visitors: 4 × 8 m
Two staircases, 4 × 8 (include two telephones)
Two elevators for visitors and personnel: 2 × 2 × 3 m
Information: 4 × 4.5 m
Phones and radio communication room: 4 × 3.5 m

Reception

Patient reception (two desks or windows for first admission and recheck visits): 4 × 4 m
Room for Xerography and a printout machine such as the BANDA Hospital records multiform copying machine (used in the trauma hospital in Vienna) and archives for initial evaluation records: 4 × 7 m

Initial Evaluation

Desks for physician, typist-stenographer, and nurse
Two examination areas, divided by curtains, with two examination tables that are easily accessible from three sides: 8 × 7 m
One elevator that can be reached from the hallway as well as from initial evaluation area: 7 × 3
Staff room for initial evaulation: 4 × 5 m
Waiting room for initial evaluation and castroom: 10 × 3.5 m

Minor Surgery Room

Two operating tables, desk for night admissions, ministerilizer: 7.5 × 7 m
Waiting room for minor surgery patients: 8 × 3.5 m
Staff and night duty room for surgical nurses: 6 × 3.5 m
Restrooms for patients and staff: 1.5 × 3.5 m (each)

Cast Rooms

Cast rooms with 2 tables for out- and inpatients: 8 × 7 m
Cast room with general anesthesia capability, overhead suspension rail, and traction devices for spinal reduction: 6 × 7 m

Cast-drying and recovery room: 4 × 7 m
Cast storage room: 4 × 3.5 m
Cast technicians' staff and night duty room: 4 × 3.5 m

X-Ray Area

Two X-ray rooms: 4.5 × 7 m each
X-ray reception: 3.5 × 4 m
Darkroom: 3.5 × 3 m
X-ray archives and workroom: 5 × 7 m and 3 × 3 m
Waiting room for X-ray: 10 × 3.5 m, including a bed elevator: 3 × 2.5 m
X-ray personnel, staff, and night duty room: 4 × 5 m

Ambulance Entrance

Covered entrances for ambulances: 14 × 5 m
Entry for bed-patients (stretchers): 4 × 7 m
Stretcher parking area: 6 × 3.5 m
Shock room with X-ray (C-arm): 8 × 7 m
Angiography room: 6 × 7 m

Surgery

Two operating rooms: 7 × 7 m each
Two preparation rooms: 4 × 4.5 m each
Two washrooms: 4 × 2.5 m each
Recovery room: 7 × 4 m
Stretcher parking area: 4 × 4.5 m
Bed storage area: 11 × 5 m
Sterilization: 8 × 4.5 m
Surgery staff room: 5.5 × 3.5 m
Dressing room with restroom for males: 3 × 4 m
Dressing room and restrooms for females: 4 × 4 m
Surgical clean-up room: 3 × 2 m

Outpatient Department

Two reevaluation rooms (each with desks for one physician, one typist-stenographer, and one nurse, and 1 free-standing examination table): 7 × 5.5 m
Consultation room (for patient, physician, and family): 5 × 5 m
Waiting area for outpatients: 12 × 3.5 m
Restrooms for patients, male and female: 4 × 3.5 each
Restroom for staff: 2 × 2.5 m
Clean-up room: 2 × 3.5 m

Administration

Room: 16 × 7 m
Cashier: 5 × 3.5 m
Storage: 7.5 × 7 m

Physical Medicine and Early Rehabilitation

Pool and hydrotherapy: 15 × 7.5 m
Dressing and restrooms, lockers for males and females: 7.5 × 3 m each
Physical therapy: 6 × 7.5 m
Occupational and ergotherapy: 6 × 7.5 m
Gymnasium: 8 × 18 m; equipment room: 7.5 × 3 m; dressing and restrooms for males and females: 7.5 × 3 m each

Chief of physical medicine and chief of rehabilitation office: 7.5 × 3 m
Staff room: 7.5 × 5 m
Exit to outdoor exercise and training areas
Chief traumatology office: 7.5 × 5 m
Secretary to the chief of the department: 7.5 × 4 m
Head nurse office: 5 × 5 m
Physicians-on-duty (four rooms): 7.5 × 4 m each
Staff restrooms and showers (two): 7.5 × 5 m each
X-ray conference room: 7.5 × 5 m
Record office: 7.5 × 5 m

There also should be a conveyor belt in three sections, with access to the receptionist and the initial evaluation, minor surgery, X-ray reception, reevaluation, and follow-up treatment rooms. Wards should be designated for mens aseptic, womens aseptic; septic ward and isolation, attached to it septic surgery, recovery and waiting; rooms for outpatients and intensive care.

Each nursing station should have an office for the head nurse, a staff room with a kitchenette, an examining room, a cloak room, a utility room, storage space, a bath and restroom, a sink and bedpan cleaning area, patients' rooms with restrooms and telephones, and a solarium.

Rooms that are shared by general surgery and orthopaedics include: central sterilization, a kitchen and dining room, additional septic elective surgery rooms, plaster of paris and garbage disposal, laundry, a pharmacy, laboratories, central X-ray, nuclear medicine, and pathology. Social service, respiratory therapy, speech-language pathology, diet service, pharmacy, central supply, housekeeping, and other services should be integrated with the general hospital. Room or office space can be assigned close to the trauma department or the minirehabilitation center, if available.

For the prosthetic-orthotic shop and amputee training center (see Fig. A1.3), the size will depend upon needs, the size of the hospital or department, geographical area, etc. It can be accommodated in an available space or built as an addition. The courtyard can be adapted for outdoor exercise, gait training, and handicapped sports.

ESTABLISHING A MINIREHABILITATION UNIT IN AN ACUTE CARE HOSPITAL

In a very real sense, rehabilitation begins the day the patient is admitted for acute care. The physician should assess the patient's status and mobilize the rehabilitation team. Each team member should take the physician's information and orders and should incorporate his or her own treatment plan into the overall plan. Often, team members in the acute care setting are separated geographically. Therefore, there must be a strong commitment to an interdisciplinary philosophy. This commitment brings about integration or coordination of services, in spite of the geographical separation, and insures that the patient will receive quality care. Team members should meet on a regular basis to discuss short- and long-term goals and specific treatment plans for each patient (see Fig. A1.4). This communication is of paramount importance not only in acute care but also in extended care.

In the acute care setting, rehabilitation begins with the basics. The team may deal with positioning and rotation to prevent decubiti, sensory stimulation, reality orientation, feeding and swallowing evaluation and training, and splinting to prevent deformities. These issues and others can be dealt with effectively by evaluation, treatment planning, and coordinated implementation. The progress is monitored steadily by individual team members and periodic team meetings.

Each specialty represented on the rehabilitation team will have certain space and equipment needs that can be integrated into the acute rehabilitation setting with the commitment of all involved, including the hospital administration. Some of the existing space may be converted for rehabilitation purposes, such as the prosthetic-orthotic service, model kitchen, living room, and bedroom for occupational therapy. A small therapeutic pool may be integrated into the physical therapy area. Ingenuity and improvisation might enable this to be done without excessive expense or extensive remodeling and additions. Figure A1.5 shows examples of such an implementation.

With this quality care from each team member, the patient may move to the next phase of his rehabilitation, which may be in a rehabilitation center, an extended or skilled care facility, a home health program, or outpatient follow-up care.

ESTABLISHING A REHABILITATION SERVICE IN AN ACUTE CARE HOSPITAL

The establishment of a rehabilitation service in an acute care setting follows procedures similar to the establishment of any new service (see Figs. A1.6 and A1.7). Basic guidelines for the development of such a program include: assessment of need, determining the goal or outcome, planning for the necessary resources, implementing the plan, and evaluating the service.

As with any new service, the work that needs to be done to undertake the development of the program calls for a strong commitment by the key players. Administration, medical staff, and the governing body should share a common belief in the value of the service. Agreement on philosophy as to how the care should be developed is essential, as this will guide many of the underlying assumptions of the planning effort.

The following basic program elements are fundamental to any consideration of new program development. There may be either resources or constraints into such considerations.

Physical Space Criteria

Space must currently be available or obtainable with minimal impact on other services.
Such structural needs as adequate plumbing, power, and engineering support must be available.
Projected space must be in proximity to related services.
Provision should be made for flexibility to expand this new service as demand increases.
Access to the service should be convenient for both consumer and visitors.

Human Resource Criteria

Skill level to provide the service must be available or assurances made that these skills can be acquired at a reasonable cost. Congruency with organizational values of the health care team must be considered.

Consumer Criteria

The new service should be viewed as desirable and/or necessary by its potential users.
A balance must be maintained between consistency with organizational and community values and consumer demand.

Legal and Regulatory Criteria

Adherence to laws, rules and regulations governing construction and delivery of services will be maintained.

Fiscal Criteria

All direct and indirect costs, including amortized expense of capital buildings and equipment as well as amortized and start-up costs will break even 5 years after the beginning of the service. Direct operating costs will break even in 1 year.

Impact on Existing Services Criteria

Unless specifically planned to supplement or replace an existing service, any new service should have acceptable and manageable impact on current services.
Evaluation must be made of what existing services could be eliminated when a new service is introduced.

Quality of Care Criteria

Level of demand for a new service must be such that acceptable standards for performance can be met.
The diversion or development of resources to provide a new service should not adversely affect the quality of existing programs. Resources must be available to meet demand.

The key to successful development of a rehabilitation program is the selection of top-notch staff who are prepared academically and experientially to deliver the service required. Providing a core team with guidelines and general parameters for program planning and allowing them to develop the service based upon professional judgments are appropriate ways to assure success.

THE ROLE OF THE INTERDISCIPLINARY TEAM IN THE ACUTE CARE SETTING

The acute rehabilitation team functions to assess needs and to deliver rehabilitation services in the acute care setting.

Team Membership

The rehabilitation assessment planning team should include the following members: (a) primary physician, (b) physiatrist, (c) primary nurse, (d) physical therapist, (e) occupational therapist, (f) speech pathologist, (g) social worker, and (h) dietitian. Other health care providers, such as the neurosurgeon, orthopaedist, psychiatrist, psychologist, respiratory therapist, prosthetist-orthotist (see Fig. A1.8), and home health referral coordinator, may also be included as needed.

Functions

Several key functions are performed by the team:

Case Finding

Referrals of neurologically impaired patients may be initiated by the primary physician or by any health team member after consultation with the primary physician. Early detection of rehabilitation candidates is a primary activity of the team in order to promote cost-effective utilization of acute care services.

Assessment

Upon referral to the interdisciplinary team, each team member is responsible for documentation of patients assessment in the medical record within 48 hr.

Coordinated Care Planning

Weekly rehabilitation assessment/planning team meetings should be held to identify actual or potential problems, coordinate care of professional and ancillary services and establish short- and long-term goals consistent with the needs of the patient and family. Communication between team members, the patient, and the family should be facilitated and all activities coordinated.

Posthospital Discharge Planning

Recommendations for appropriate rehabilitation follow-up and posthospital care should be made by the team. In many cases the patient/family conference with the team is arranged in order to match needs and goals with available services and resources.

Figure A1.1. Physical therapy is shown in the hydrotherapy area

    A. At the Kaiser Sunnyside Medical Center.
    B. A therapeutic pool is used during group therapy session.
    C. A lift is used for nonambulatory patients.
    D. Mixed group therapy in the pool.
E–F. Individual pool therapy may use the Ragaz Ring method.
G–H. In hydrotherapy, various whirlpools, including a Hubbard tank are used.

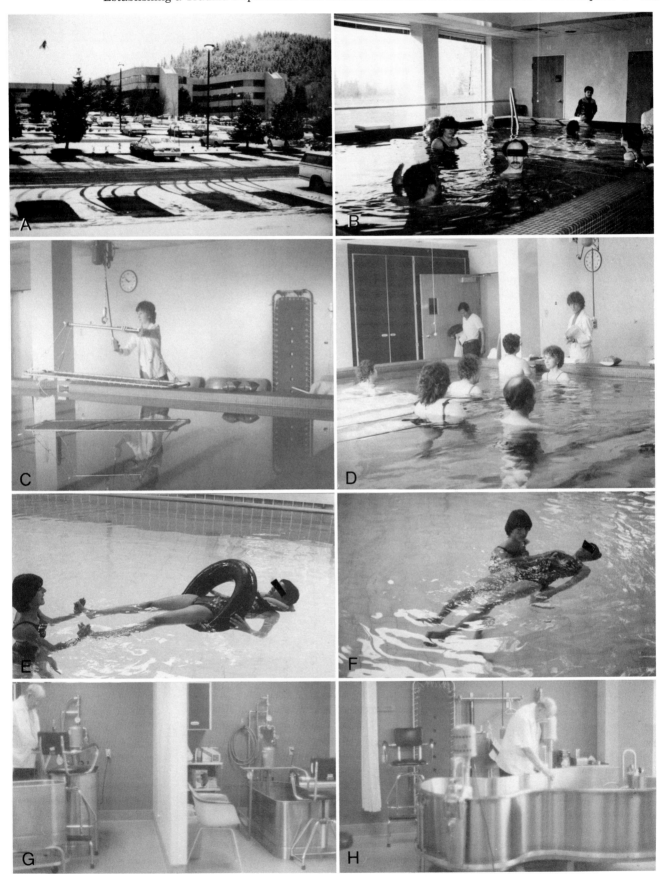

Figure A1.1.

Figure A1.2. Physical therapy techniques include:

A. A workout on the stationary bicycle

B. Strengthing leg exercises, and

C. A Sayre's cervical traction, which can be assembled quickly and attached to a door for use in the patient's home

D–E. A general physical therapy area is shown.

F–G. Cybex-isokinetic stress testing and exercises are shown.

H. In the individual treatment area, the physical therapist adjusts intermittent cervical traction.

I. Simple devices used in group therapy sessions include clubs, redaptor sticks, and balls.

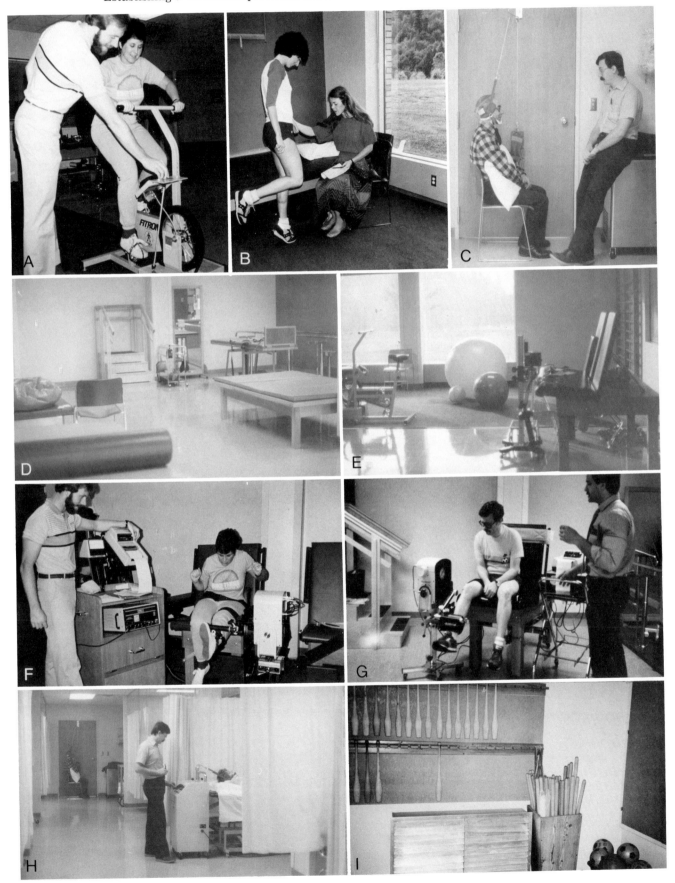

Figure A1.2.

Figure A1.3. The plan of a trauma department and minirehabilitation area in an acute hospital was designed for a specific hospital in which this wing could be dedicated to trauma. The only addition was the covered ambulance entrance, the prosthetic-orthotic and amputee training center area. The arrangement can, of course, be different and even vertical using one or two floors above or below the main area as long as the basic rooms are in proximity to allow for functional patient flow.

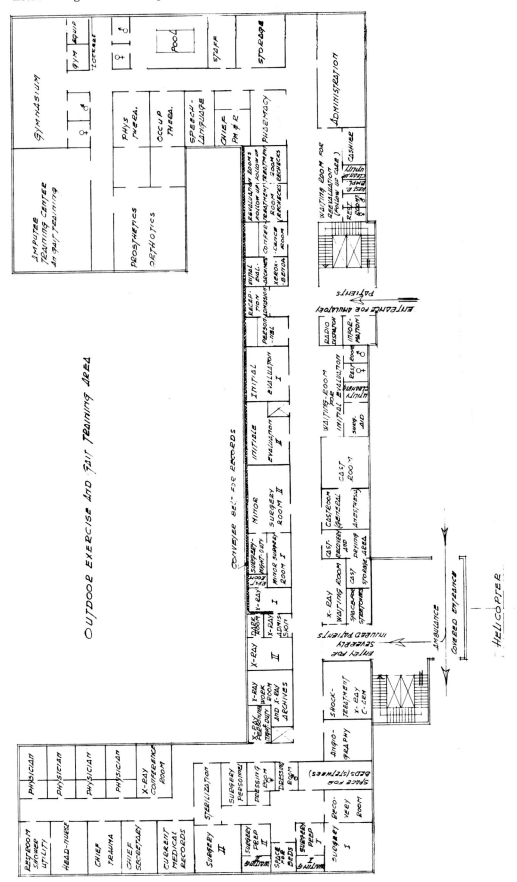

Figure A1.4. A patient flow sheet includes all information from admission to discharge.

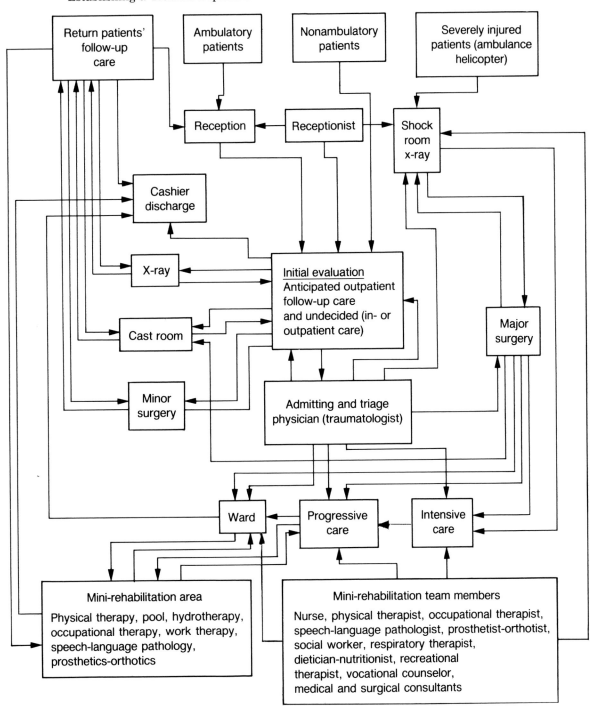

Figure A1.4.

Figure A1.5. In the occupational therapy, respiratory therapy and speech-language pathology areas, there are

A. A training kitchen and

B. An improvised bedroom, with an easily movable bed for access from different angles to simulate home situation.

C. Computer technology is applied to occupational therapy for the brain-injured patient.

D. General view of the individual treatment area in the occupational therapy department is shown.

E. Blood is drawn from a radial artery for determination of arterial blood gases by respiratory therapist.

F. Postural drainage is done.

G. A speech-language pathologist evaluates a trauma patient.

H. A patient group education and instruction room doubles as a conference and lecture room for staff.

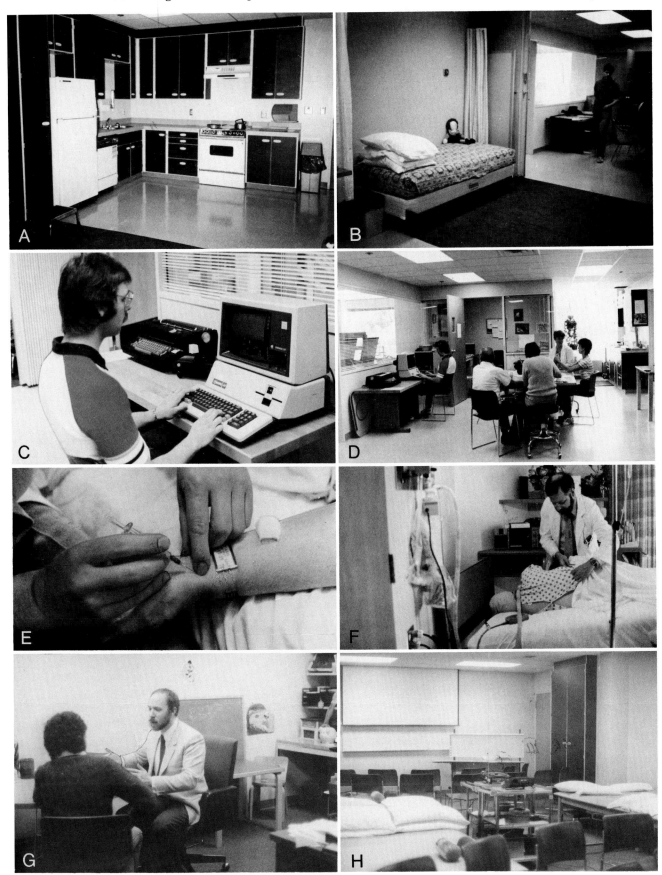

Figure A1.5.

Figure A1.6. The physical and occupational therapy areas at the Kaiser Sunnyside Medical Center are shown. Speech and language pathology and respiratory therapy areas are located in different rooms nearby.

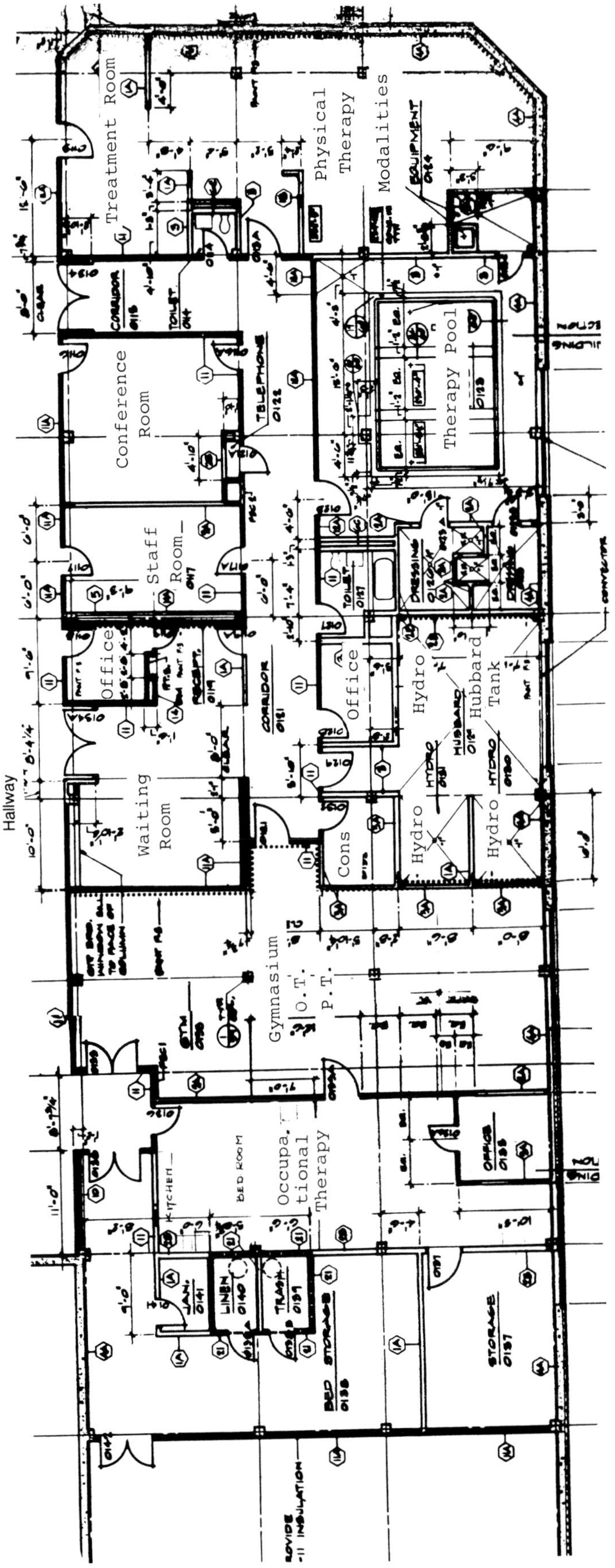
Treatment Room
Physical Therapy Modalities
Conference Room
Therapy Pool
Staff Room
Office
Office
Hydro
Hubbard Tank
Hallway
Waiting Room
Cons
Hydro
Hydro
Gymnasium
O.T.
P.T.
Occupational Therapy
KITCHEN
BED ROOM
TELEPHONE
CORRIDOR
STORAGE
BED STORAGE
LINEN
TRASH
JAN.

Figure A1.6.

Figure A1.7. The prosthetics-orthotic service at the Kaiser Sunnyside Medical Center is temporarily located in three different spaces; it will be consolidated into one area as soon as the space is vacated according to the plan shown.

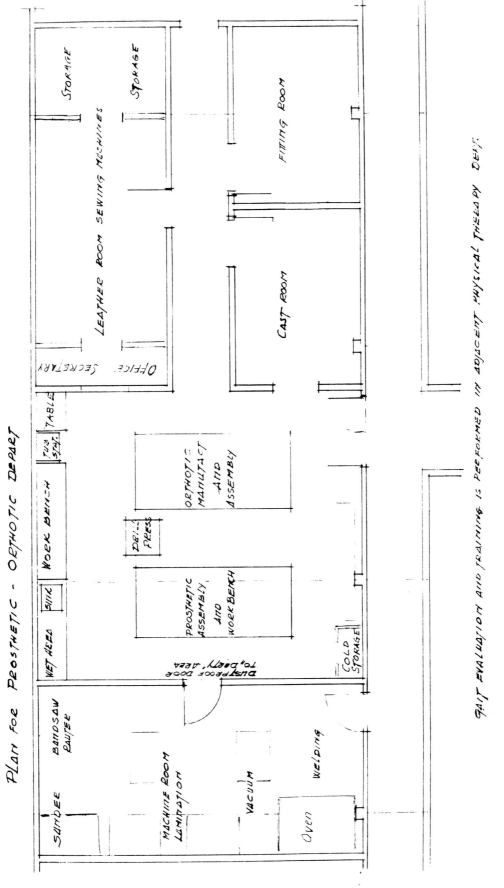

PLAN FOR PROSTHETIC - ORTHOTIC DEPART

GAIT EVALUATION AND TRAINING IS PERFORMED IN ADJACENT PHYSICAL THERAPY DEPT.

Figure A1.7.

Figure A1.8. The *prosthetic-orthotic service* was temporarily placed in three different available spaces; one room was used for sewing machines and leather work, another room as fitting and cast room; and the machine shop and oven were placed in part of a welding room and storage area.

A. The orthotist takes plaster molds for orthotics in the fitting and plaster room.

B. A thermoplastic body jacket is being fabricated for a child with juvenile scoliosis.

C. Vacuum forming of an ankle-foot orthosis (AFO) is shown.

D. A polypropylene AFO is constructed.

E. Work takes place on the grinder and belt sander.

F. An assembly bench is shown.

G. Sewing and leather work areas are shown.

H. Gait training takes place with an amputee with a new below-knee prosthesis.

I. Two newly fabricated short leg braces (AFOs) are evaluated. The patient walks between parallel bars in an adjacent physical therapy department.

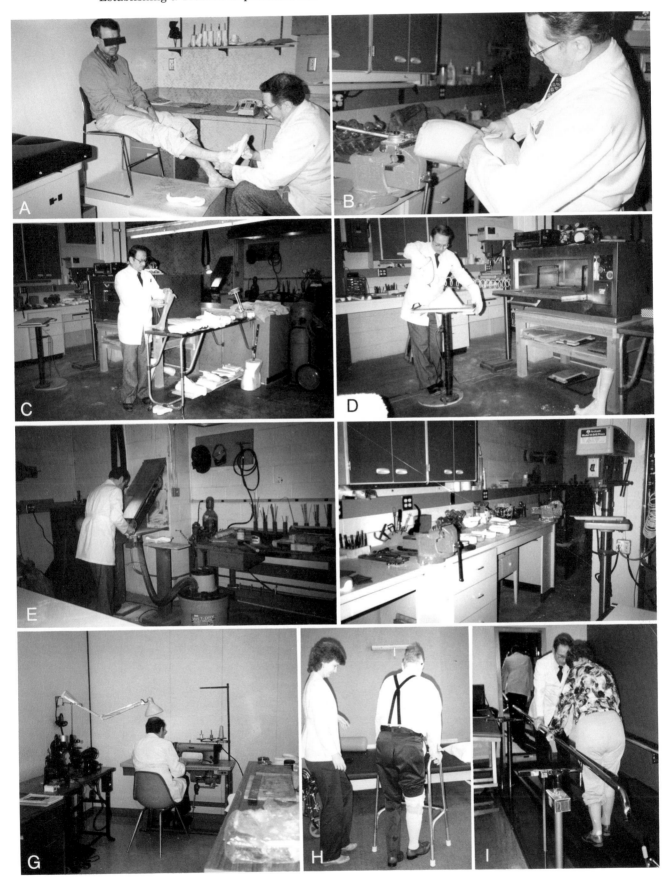

Figure A1.8.

Appendix 2

Medicolegal Aspects of Rehabilitation

Roger Miyaji, M.A., J.D.

Medicolegal issues in a rehabilitation center are similar to those for other health care delivery systems, but include additional concerns, such as approval and use of prosthetic devices.

Rehabilitation centers must comply with all federal, state, and local laws, with special attention to licensing regulations of personnel, facilities, and services. The U.S. Food and Drug Administration also governs the use of some prosthetic devices and specialized equipment.

All personnel must be especially careful about protecting patient confidentiality, avoiding or reducing malpractice risks, and making sure patients have given adequate informed consents.

Personnel should be trained to deal with release of information, informed consent, proper and complete documentation of injuries or accidents (all incidents should be reported, even those which occur in parking lots or on property belonging to the rehabilitation center), and the importance of medical records. Medical records are legal documents that cannot be changed, modified, or altered. Late entries can be added if the reasons are given and some changes can be made if the original entry is still visible and the change is dated and signed.

If a problem arises that may result in litigation, second opinions, write-off of accounts receivable, or payment of some expenses may help prevent a lawsuit. In most cases, prompt notification to the insurance carrier may be needed to insure coverage.

It is essential that internal policies are followed or promptly modified if obsolete. A professional code of ethics is also important. Violation of a code of ethics can result in a complaint to a state agency or can be used to discredit testimony during a medical malpractice trial.

Rehabilitation centers are especially vulnerable to lawsuits over abandonment. The long-term nature of rehabilitation and the uncertainties regarding the point in time when a patient reaches an optimal or final stage of rehabilitation mean that there is theoretically always something more that could be done that might help the patient. At some point, however, additional care may not be appropriate. If treatment is terminated without attention to certain legal issues, the patient may bring a charge of abandonment. Rehabilitation centers must be careful not to guarantee or even imply a guarantee of results but must explain carefully what they hope to achieve and some reasonable time frame or target dates.

If treatment is being terminated, and patient or family wants additional treatment that the center or its physicians feel is inappropriate, the center must offer its assistance in referring or transferring the patient to another center or health care provider. The transfer must be accomplished in a safe and reasonable manner. Any waivers of liability must be explained and carefully worded and should not just be incorporated in a large unrelated document.

Detailed information about medicolegal aspects and suggestions for avoiding or preventing lawsuits is available in the literature or can be obtained from hospital administrators, risk management departments, and hospital attorneys, as well as state and local medical societies.

Appendix 3

Measuring and Recording Joint Motion and Position: Longitudinal and Circumferential

John J. Gerhardt, M.D.

Clinical measurements are of great value only if they can be recorded, understood, and read by others in the same way. To facilitate national and international communication and exchange of data, standardization of measurements *and* recording is urgently needed. The neutral-zero method of measurements adopted worldwide by the Orthopedic-Traumatologic and Hand Surgery associations at the SICOT (Société Internationale de Chirurgie Orthopédique et de Traumatologie) meeting in Mexico City in 1969 is most suitable for this purpose. The recording, however, is done in haphazard manner by different practitioners and therefore cannot be read by others in the same way. There is additional confusion secondary to language and terminology. The SFTR (S = sagittal, F = frontal, T = transversal, R = rotation) method allows for the first time a standardized and truly international recording of joint motion and position in the neutral-zero method.

Every investigator or examiner can use his own national language and terminology but records the measurements in the standardized SFTR method. It then can be understood and read by everyone in the same way regardless of the different language and terminology of the reader. The recording is short, precise and therefore suitable for computer use. The standards are contained in five basic rules. I suggest that the reader takes a sheet of paper and a pencil and follows the development of the recording. In our example we would like to record the abduction and adduction of both shoulders, extension and flexion of both elbows and external and internal rotation of the cervical spine (head).

RULE 1: THE SFTR RULE

To avoid confusion of terminology, all motions are reduced into motions in three basic planes. S = sagittal plane, F = frontal plane, and T = transverse plane. The rotations can take place in any of the three planes and are recorded as R. The planes relate always to the body's anatomical position, regardless whether the subject is standing, sitting, prone, or supine.

In the author's example, the abduction and adduction of the shoulder takes place in the *frontal plane* and will therefore be designated F. The extension and flexion of the elbow takes place in the sagittal plane and will be designated "S" and the rotation of the cervical spine is "R":

Example:

Shoulder:	Right	Left
F:		
Elbow:	Right	Left
S:		
Cervic. spine (head)		
R:		

RULE 2: STARTING POSITION

All motions begin at defined starting anatomical positions with the exception of rotations of extremities. The anatomical position is the upright position with feet straight forward, the arms at the side of the body, and the palms of the hands facing anteriorly. The standard starting position for rotation of the hip: hip and knee in 90 degrees flexion—the leg indicates motion. Rotation of the shoulder: arm in 90 degrees abduction, elbow in 90 degrees flexion; the forearm indicates motion. Supination and pronation of the forearm: arm at side of the body, elbow in 90 degrees flexion, palm parallel to the sagittal plane (thumb up); the extended thumb indicates motion. When using the plurimeter (Dr. Rippstein, La Conversion, Switzerland), the hand grasps the arm of the instrument and the values are directly read on the scale.

The starting position in physiological conditions is always "0" and is recorded as a reference point in the middle –0–. In pathological conditions, the motion can start in a position other than the anatomical position, and accordingly, the number in the middle will be different than zero. This calls immediate attention to the pathological condition.

RULE 3: SEQUENCE OF MOTION

All motions are recorded with three numbers. All motions leading generally away from the middle of the body are recorded on the left side of the starting position, for example, abduction, external rotation, supination, and extension. Motions of the head and spine to the left are also recorded on the left side. Motions which generally

From *International Rehabilitation Medicine: Official Journal of the International Rehabilitation Medicine Association.* Basel, Switzerland, Eular Publishers, 1985.

Table A3.1. Example of Conventional Recording of Joint Measurements in the Neutral Zero Position Method

		Left	Right
Shoulder	Forward flexion	170	70
	Horizontal flexion	100	Horizontal flexion and horizontal extension cannot be measured because of limitation of shoulder abduction
	Horizontal extension	30	Horizontal flexion and horizontal extension cannot be measured because of limitation of shoulder abduction
	Backward extension	50	20
	Abduction	170	70
	Passive	170	80
	Adduction	75	30
	Passive	75	30
	Rotation:		
	Arm at side:		
	Internal rotation	70	30
	External rotation	60	20
	Arm in abduction (90 degrees):		
	Internal rotation	50	Internal and external rotation of the shoulder with arm in 90 degrees abduction cannot be measured due to limited abduction
	External rotation	60	Internal and external rotation of the shoulder with arm in 90 degrees abduction cannot be measured due to limited abduction
Elbow	Flexion	150	The right elbow has a flexion deformity of 30 degrees with further flexion to 90 degrees
Forearm	Hyperextension	5	0
	Pronation	80	0
	Supination	90	The forearm cannot be brought into neutral position; the motion starts at 10 degrees of supination with further supination to 30 degrees. Total forearm motion is 20 degrees

Table A3.2. Example of SFTR recording

			Left			Right
Shoulder		S	50–0–170		S	20– 0–70
		F	170–0– 75		F	70– 0–30
	Passive	F	170–0– 75		F	80– 0–30
		T	30–0–100		T	0
		R (F–0)	60–0– 70		R (F–0)	20– 0–30
		R (F90–0)	60–0– 50		R (F90–0)	0
Elbow		S	5–0–150		S	0–30–90
Forearm		R	90–0– 80		R	30–10– 0

All information described in the conventional recording is contained in the SFTR recording with avoidance of lengthy description and confusion in a short, concise format.

lead towards the middle of the body, such as flexion, adduction, internal rotation, and motions of the head and the spine to the right are recorded on the right side of the starting position. This rule is crucial as it allows a third person to understand and read the recorded message in one way only. For example shoulder abduction of 180 degrees and adduction of 30 degrees would be recorded: F: 180–0–30, and abduction of 180 degrees and adduction of 45 degrees would be F: 180–0–45. Pathological flexion deformity of the elbow of 30 degrees with further flexion to 90 degrees would be recorded: S: 0–30–90. Starting position (recorded in the middle) is not "0" but 30 degrees; there is "0" extension (recorded on the left side of the starting position) and there is further flexion to 90 degrees (recorded on the right side of the starting position).

In our example, we record:

Rt. shoulder: F: 180–0–30   Lt. shoulder: F: 180–0–45
Rt. elbow: S: 0–30–90   Lt. elbow: S: 0–0–145
Cerv. spine   R: 45–0–30
  (head)

In our example, we measure:

Abduction of rt. shoulder of 180 degrees ⎫
Abduction of lt. shoulder of 180 degrees ⎬ F Plane
Abduction of rt. shoulder of 30 degrees ⎪
Abduction of lt. shoulder of 45 degrees ⎭

Flexion deformity of rt. elbow of 30 degrees
with further flexion to 90 degrees; lack of full   S plane
extension of 30 degrees – total range of motion
30 degrees–90 degrees

Average normal range of motion of
left elbow (145 degrees flexion)
Rotation of cervical spine to the left 45 degrees
Rotation of cervical spine to the right 30 degrees

The SFTR recording containing all above information is
as follows:

	Right	*Left*
Shoulder:	F: 180–0–30	F: 180–0–145
Elbow:	S: 0–30–90	S: 0–0–145
Cervical spine:		R: 45–0–30

The international terminology recording is

	Dext.	*Sin.*
Artic. hum.	F: 180–0–30	F: 180–0–45
Artic. cubiti	S: 0–30–90	S: 0–0–45
Artic. vert. cervic.		R: 45–0–30

RULE 4: POSITIONS

Positions are recorded with two numbers, the degree of
the position and the "0" starting position as the reference
point. The degrees of the position which is within the range
of motions recorded on the left side of the starting position
are placed on the left side of "0." The degrees of position
within the range of motion recorded on the right side of

the starting positions are placed to the right of "0." For
example, position of the right hip in 45 degrees of abduction is recorded: Rt. hip: F: 45–0. Position of the right hip
in 25 degrees of adduction is recorded: Rt. hip: F: 0–25.
Position in a different plane than the three basic planes
can also be recorded. For example, arthrodesis of the Rt.
shoulder in 60 degrees abduction, and 30 degrees horizontal flexion is clearly identified as follows: F: 60–0, T: 0–
30. The SFTR method also allows brief recording of the
strength of agonists and antagonists by using standardized
numbers 0–5. The numbers are placed above and below
the directional vectors which indicate direction of motion
from and to the zero starting position. For example: full
strength of the flexors of the right elbow and poor strength
of elbow extensors with free range of motion would be
recorded:

$$\begin{matrix} 5 \\ S: 0–0 \rightleftarrows 145 \\ 3 \end{matrix}$$

RULE 5: DESIGNATION OF THE JOINT AND THE SIDE FOR INTERNATIONAL USE

The joint and side are designated in Latin according to
the already standardized *Nomina Anatomica* (1977).

Example:
  Artic. hum. dext. (Articulatio humeri dextra)
    = right shoulder
  Artic. hum. sin. (Articulatio humeri sinistra)
    = left shoulder
  Artic. cubiti dext. (Articulatio cubiti dextra)
    = right elbow
  Artic. cubiti sin. (Articulatio cubiti sinistra)
    = left elbow
  Artic. vert. cervic. (Articulationes vertebrae cervicales)
    = cervical spine

Further detailed explanation of the application of SFTR
recording is contained in Gerhardt J. and Russe O. (1975):
*International SFTR Method of Measuring and Recording
Joint Motion.* Hans Huber, Berne, 1985.

Table A3.3.

Plane	Motion (in degrees)	Starting position	Motion (in degrees)
S:	Extension, hyperextension, dorsiflexion	–0–	Flexion, palmar and a plantar flexion
F:	Abduction, elevation, radial deviation, lateral bending to the left (spine)	–0–	Adduction, depression, ulnar deviation, lateral bending to the right (spine)
T:	Horizontal extension of shoulder, abduction of hip in 90 degrees flexion	–0–	Horizontal flexion of shoulder, adduction of hip in 90 degrees flexion
R:	External rotation, supination, eversion, rotation of head and trunk to the left	–0–	Internal rotation, pronation, inversion, rotation of head and trunk to the right

Figure A3.1.

A. Measuring of backward extension and forward flexion (called also posterior and anterior elevation) is performed in the sagittal plane and recorded simply as S: 45–0–180.

B. Measuring of abduction and adduction (called also lateral and medial elevation) is performed in the frontal plane and recorded F: 180–0–45.

C. Measuring of the horizontal motion described as horizontal extension and horizontal flexion is performed in the transverse plane and recorded as T: 45–0–135.

D. Most *rotations* take place in the transverse plane, but some in the frontal or sagittal plane. Therefore, all rotations are recorded as ‹R› and not in the planes in which they are actually taking place. Supination and pronation as well as eversion and inversion are also recorded as ‹R›.

In the above illustration, the rotation of the left shoulder in 90-degree abduction is measured with the forearm as indicator (S plane).

The rotation of the right hip in 90-degree flexion is measured with the lower leg as indicator (F plane).

The rotation of the left hip with extended knee and hip is measured with the foot as indicator (T plane).

The rotation of the right shoulder with the arm close to the body is also measured with the forearm as indicator (T plane).

E–F. The three basic planes are shown with patient in upright and supine position: The planes are always in reference to the body, regardless whether the examined person is standing, sitting or lying down. In other words, the frontal plane, when the person is standing, does not become a transverse plane when the person is supine, but remains frontal in relation to the person.

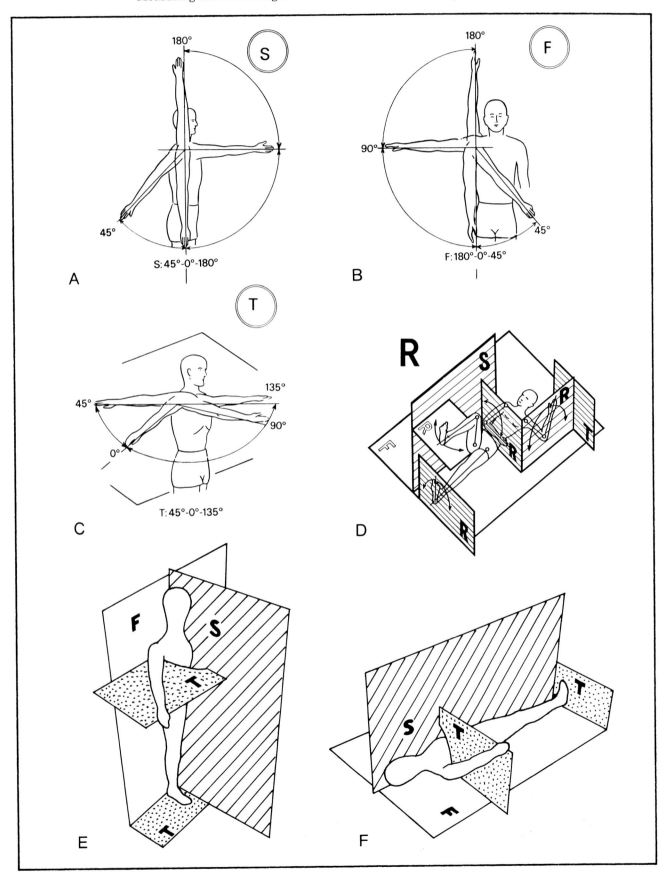

Figure A3.1.

Figure A3.2.

A–B. All joint motions in the three basic planes are measured from a defined neutral 0 position. The position is the anatomical position of the body when the examined person is standing with body upright, arms at side of the body and palms facing anteriorly. When the person is sitting or lying down, the starting position is referred to as the standard anatomical standing position. The neutral 0 starting position of rotations is the midposition between external and internal rotation and for supination and pronation it is also the midposition.

The starting position for measurement of the horizontal extension and flexion of the upper extremity is with the extended arm in abduction of 90 degrees, and of the lower extremity with the hip and knee in 90 degree flexion.

C. The Neutral-0-Starting Position is recorded in the middle, between the range of motion values of the agonists and antagonists. The recording is S: 180–0–45 (abduction of 180 degrees—Neutral 0—and adduction of 45 degrees).

D. Normal range of motion of the elbow with natural motion in one direction from 0 point is noted S: 0–0–145 (since there is no natural extension). Abnormal motion of 10 degrees in the other direction from 0-degree starting point is called hyperextension and is noted S: 10–0–145.

E. Limitation of elbow motion may be expressed the following ways:
   a. the elbow lacks 30-degree extension and flexes to 90 degrees.
   b. there is flexion deformity of 30 degrees with further flexion to 90 degrees.
   c. the angle of greatest flexion (AGF) is 90 degrees. Lack of extension is 30 degrees. Total joint motion is 60 degrees.

   SFTR recording is S: 0–30–90. (From *Joint Motion, Method of Measuring and Recording,* published by American Academy of Orthopedic Surgeons, 1965, Carter R. Rowe, M.D., Boston, Massachusetts.)

F. Abduction of the hip is examined in supine position. The pelvis must be stabilized by an assistant. In this example there is an abduction deformity: there is no adduction, the motion starts at 10 degrees of abduction and there is further abduction to 45 degrees. Recording: F: 45–10–0

G. In testing adduction of one extremity, the other must be lifted out of the way and supported passively. Abduction is always recorded first, and adduction last. In example above, there is no abduction, the motion start at neutral 0, and there is adduction to 25 degrees. Recording: F: 0–0–25

H. Abduction and adduction of the hip in 90 degrees of hip flexion takes place in the transverse plane (in relation to the body) and is recorded as «T». Recording: T: 50–0–10

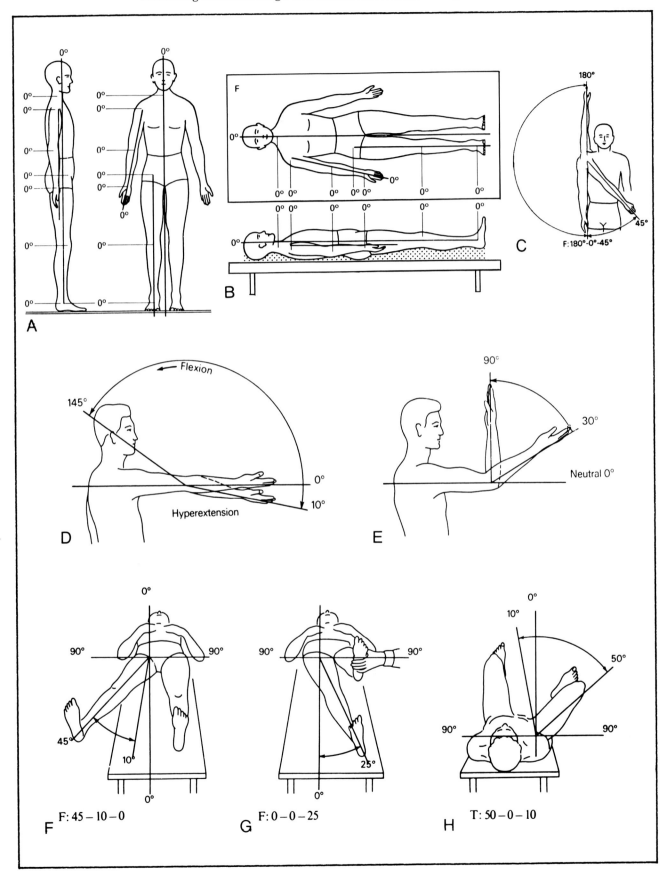

Figure A3.2.

Figure A3.3. Circumferential Measurements at Different Levels

A. Anterior view

B. Lateral view

C. Posterior view

Identification of labels:
1   at greater trochanters;
1a trochanter to perineum;
2   between iliac crest and trochanter (trochanteric space);
3   at iliac crest;
4   at waist;
5   site of measurement to be governed by height of back uprights;
6   at axilla;
7   neck;
8   occiput to chin;
9   head to brow;

Important landmarks:
M manubrium sterni;
X xyphoid process;
U umbilicus;
S symphysis pubica;
A spinous process, C7;
B midpoint spine of scapula;
C inferior angle of scapula;
D lumbosacral joint;
E sacrococcygeal joint.

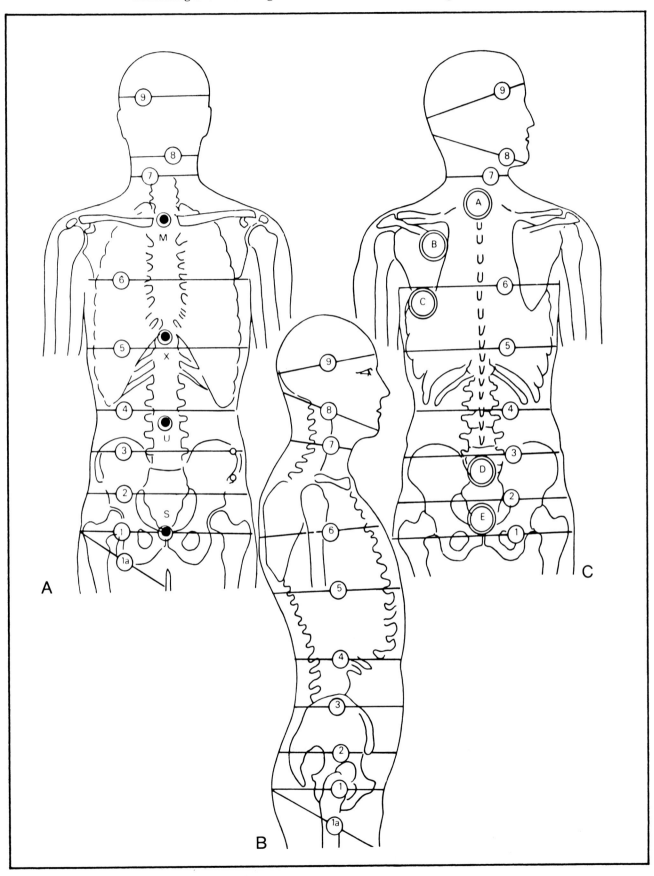

Figure A3.3.

Figure A3.4. Girth Measurements and Anatomical Landmarks of Upper Extremities

A. Length measurements of upper extremity

    A   tip of middle finger to olecranon
    B   tip of olecranon to axilla

B. Circumferential measurements of upper extremity

    1   over shoulder
    2   arm at axilla
    3   over biceps
    4   above elbow
    5   elbow joint line
    6   below elbow (maximum circumference)
    7   mid-forearm
    8   above wrist (minimum circumference)
    9   wrist at styloid process
    10   hand at knuckles (exact level to be indicated on tracing)

C–D. Important landmarks on upper extremity

    A   acromion
    B   tuberculum majus (greater tubercle)
    C   epicondylus radialis (lateral epicondyle)
    D   processus styloideus radii (radial styloid process)
    E   tip of middle finger
    F   fracture
    G   olecranon
    H   processus styloideus ulnae (ulnar styloid process)
    I   biceps (maximum)
    K   forearm (maximum)
    R   rasceta (distal skin crease on volar aspect of wrist)
    RE   length of hand (rasceta to tip of third finger)

E. Finger lengths

    1   distal phalanx
    2   middle phalanx
    3   proximal phalanx
    4   distal phalanx of thumb
    5   proximal phalanx of thumb

F. Shoulder girdle measurements

    A   width to be specified (according to appliance desired)
    B   height to be specified (according to appliance desired)
    1   circumference, axilla over base neck
    2   circumference, axilla over opposite acromion
    3   circumference of chest at level of axillae
    4   circumference of chest at level governed by height of chest strap (see width measurement A)
    5   circumference, arm at axilla
    6   circumference, arm over biceps

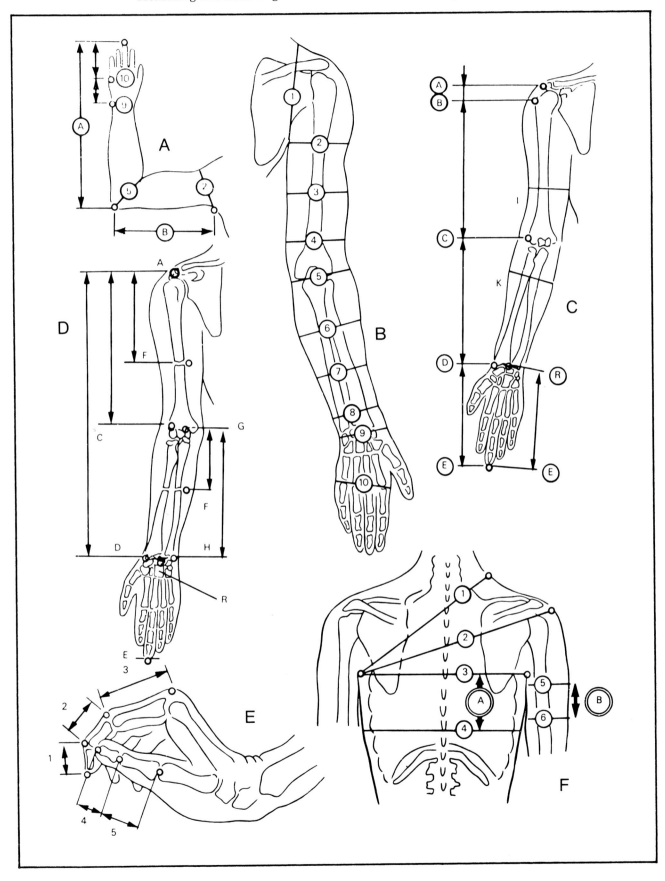

Figure A3.4.

Figure A3.5. Lower Extremity Measurements

A. TS   distance from trochanter to sole
    IS   distance from ischium to sole
    KS distance from knee joint line to sole
    AS distance from ankle joint line to sole
    1   trochanter to perineum
    2   thigh to perineum
    3   mid-thigh
    4   lower thigh
    5   femoral condyle
    6   knee joint line
    7   tibial condyle
    8   calf (maximum)
    9   lower leg
    10   above ankle (minimum)
    11   ankle at malleoli
    12   tuber calcanei (floor)

Circumferential and leg measurements, exact level to be indicated on tracing

B. U   umbilicus
    S   anterior superior iliac spine
    T   trochanter major
    E   lateral femoral epicondyle
    C   medial tibial condyle
    X   fracture
    H   heel
    D   toe tip
    6   knee joint line
    8   maximum calf
    10   minimum above ankle
    IM anterior superior iliac spine to medial malleolus
    IH   anterior superior iliac spine to tuber calcanei
    UM umbilicus to medial malleolus
    UH umbilicus to tuber calcanei
    TF ischial tuberosity to floor (heel)
    TX distance trochanter to fracture
    TE distance trochanter to lateral femoral epicondyle
    CX distance medial tibial condyle to fracture
    CM distance medial tibial condyle to medial malleolus
    HD distance tuber calcanei to tip of longest toe

C. 1   circumference of ankle at malleoli
    2   circumference of heel (apex of instep to heel)
    3   circumference of instep (level of cuboid)
    4   circumference of waist (proximal to ball)
    5   circumference of ball of foot (beneath ball over metatarso-phalangeal joints I, V)
    6   maximum width of sole
    7   length metatarsal heads to heel
    8   length of sole of foot

Measurement redrawn partially from *Orthopedic Appliance Atlas* (Mr. J.J. Ufheil), copyright 1952, American Academy of Orthopedic Surgeons, published by J.W. Edwards, Ann Arbor, Michigan.

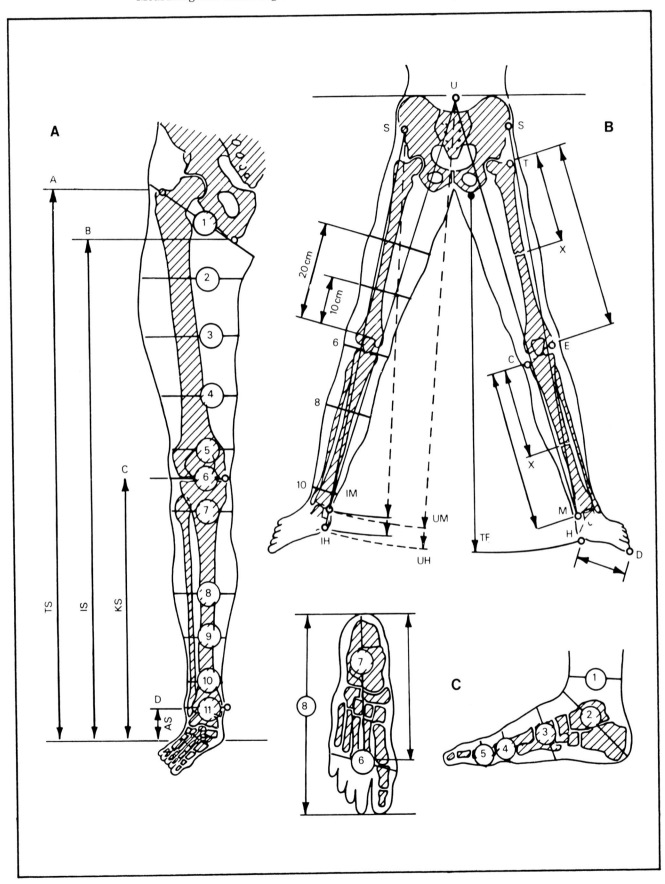

Figure A3.5.

Appendix 4

Measuring Instruments

John J. Gerhardt, M.D., and Jules Rippstein, M.D.

MULTISTRESS DEVICE
(Patent Pending)

General Information

A thorough examination of a ligamentous lesion requires an X-ray examination under stress. It is the most certain procedure to diagnose a ligament tear. The Multistress is a new device specially designed for the knee and the ankle, but may also be used for the fingers, the elbows, etc.

This product consists of three principal elements: one, which applies the force of traction, and the two counterstress pieces; one standard and one adjustable to which accessories can be fitted. These three pieces are provided with suction cups operated by a lever, which permits easy fixation anywhere on the X-ray examination table. The strain applied is regulated in a progressive and simple manner. For convave examining tables, a base plate (A.MS.04) is available (upon special order) to affix the suction cups.

Advice on General Use

Before the first examination of a patient, it is advisable to try one or two experimental examinations to become familiar with the Multistress. If the surface available on the examining table is insufficient, place the limb on the diagonal. At the beginning of the examination, the traction element must be *completely* unlocked (position "Start"). *Before placing the suction cups, press on them to void the air between them and the table.* The lock handle is specially designed to augment the pressure in a progressive manner. When the desired pressure is attained, ask the patient to relax completely to judge if there is a diminution of pressure. If there is a diminution of pressure, recommence, augmentating the pressure until the desired tension is attained.

Advice on Care

The electronic pressure indicates functions on four standard 1.5 V batteries (very inexpensive), which are sold everywhere. Two sets of batteries permit about 1000 examinations. To replace the batteries, unlock the two screws located on the left side of the apparatus (opposite the digital display), and open the top. The right side contains the electronic circuit and must not be opened except by a trained technician.

The Multistress suction cups must be stored in the "off" position, avoiding warm places and high humidity.

Use for Stress X-Ray Positioning

Clinical evaluations of sprained and ruptured ligaments are not sufficient to establish an accurate diagnosis or reproducible data.

Stress X-rays are indispensable to determine the extent of ligamentous sprains or ruptures and thus the degree of joint instability. Only with availability of this additional data can a proper therapeutic approach be planned.

Stress X-rays are taken in a forced extreme joint position simulating the mechanism of trauma, e.g., forced inversion of the ankle for injury to the talo fibular ligament, forced abduction of the knee for injury to the medial collateral ligament, etc.

The best previously available instrument was developed by Dr. Scheuba and manufactured by TELOS (GmbH, D 6103 Griesheim, Friedrich-Ebert-str 25, Germany).

It is rather massive and heavy, difficult to handle and to store. Some patients with ankle injuries complain of pain because the holding plate of the instrument exerts its pressure over the injured ligament. The Multistress apparatus was developed to alleviate these shortcomings of the available instruments.

The advantages of the Multistress apparatus can be summarized as follows:

1. The modular construction allows not only stress X-rays at the knee and ankle joints, but also the elbow, thumb, fingers, etc.
2. The Multistress is sturdy and durable, yet lightweight and handy and requires only small storage space.
3. The applied force can be easily read on a large digital display. The values can thus be recorded.
4. The applied force can be objectively reproduced by other investigators or practitioners.
5. The force is transmitted in such a way that no pain is elicited and troublesome interfering muscle contractions are prevented.
6. A small electrometer can be built into the main element which could allow the patient to adjust the maximum tolerable force slowly and smoothly. This is very helpful in fearful and anxious patients.
7. The practitioners and X-ray technicians are protected from direct and indirect radiation exposure.

It is suggested that a tension of 15 kg be applied for X-rays of the ankles or knees (according to international

584

standards). This permits precise comparison between different examinations and different practitioners.

A light tension, of 4 to 8 kilos should be applied while the counterstresses are put in place; and should be increased progressively to 15 kg. This is done by turning the button "T." *Caution: Before starting an examination, the traction system should be completely undone (i.e., position "START").*

Knee Joint

In order to obtain a firm immobilization of the thigh, a special accessory (A.MS.03) is available. The diagnosis of an instability is easily obtained in comparing the X-ray with the healthy side. This accessory is placed onto the polyvalent counterstress, and firmly tightened on the thigh above the femoral condyles. The diagnosis is easily obtained in comparing the x-ray with one of the healthy side.

The knee joint laxity is pathological if a difference of more than 2 mm is found compared to the healthy knee (made under the same stress conditions). Make sure the polyvalent counterstress is on a level with the knee; then, slide the cassette under the adjustable part.

In case of an opening of the joint surfaces of more than 10 to 15 degrees, a stress X-ray of the other knee joint is suggested. (A difference of more than 2 mm must be considered as pathological.) The three points of pressure of the Multistress must be at an equal distance (20 cm, for instance).

Finger Joint

Use any available counterstress, such as a handle, or the authors' special accessory (A.MS.02), which is particularly useful for the thumb. Fix it onto the polyvalent counterstress. Then, grip the hand between the special accessory and the standard counterstress.

Ankle Joint

More than 10 mm displacement of the talus in anterior direction is pathological. For a displacement between 5 and 10 mm, a comparative X-ray should be made. Apply the polyvalent counterstress 2 to 3 cm above the inner part of the ankle; slide the cassette underneath to adjust the X-ray position. The foot should be turned inward (20 degrees) and the knee slightly raised on a foam cushion. *Make sure the loop is carried out correctly according to which foot is being examined—the right or the left. Traction should be parallel with the table.*

GONIOMETERS

The International Standard Goniometer is a very useful measuring device for clinic or hospital use due to its large dimensions which enable the examiner to take accurate measurements and readings. It contains scales: 0 to 180 degrees, 0 to 90 degrees, and 180 to 360 degrees, as well as linear scales in inches and centimeters.

The arms of the goniometer are applied as close as possible and in the line with the functional or mechanical axes of the limbs or body parts which define the angle of the joint to be measured. True axes of rotation of joints often change in different positions of the joint and are difficult to determine. Therefore, placement of the rotational axis of the goniometer can only be approximate and the examiner must concentrate on accurate application of the arms of the goniometer. The standard pocket goniometer is a handy yet precise measuring device to facilitate the SFTR standard measurements. The arms of the goniometer are placed over or parallel to the long mechanical axes of the structures which define the angle of the joint. The values are generally indicated by the black (large) arrow. Motions of the shoulder are read at the black triangle, and those of the ankle joint at the red (small) arrow.

THE PLURIMETER

The plurimeter is a new precision measuring instrument designed and developed by Dr. Rippstein (CH–1093 La Conversion, Switzerland).

The main component of the plurimeter is a container with a precision indicator which maintains constant vertical position. The container is filled with silicon oil which lubricates the axis of the indicator and dampens its oscillations.

The precision-mechanism is manufactured by a Swiss clock factory and the indicator reacts readily to minimum rotations of 0.1%. The housing of the container can be rotated 360 degrees, but locks automatically at 90 degree intervals by virtue of a snap-in mechanism. This makes this instrument suitable for easy measurements in the SFTR neutral zero method.

The combination of the main component of the goniometer and a special caliper with two gliding parts, one of which glides horizontally along the long arm of the caliper, whereas the other moves vertically. It allows not only measurements of joint motion in various body positions but also measurements of length, inclinations, torsion, pronation-supination, diameters, verticality, levels, scoliosis, kyphosis, heights of rib humps and others.

Its construction permits it to be held in one hand, freeing the other hand of the examiner to move the joint to be measured.

Figure A4.1.

A. Multistress is applied to ankle, simulating inversion injury.

B. Drawing shows manual application of forced inversion producing subluxation of talus due to rupture of talo fibular ligament. A lateral view should also be taken while applying anterior traction to heel and counterpressure on the antero-distal aspect of the tibia.

C. The Multistress is applied to demonstrate injury to the medial side of the knee. Note that there is no pressure over the injured ligament.

D. Drawing shows manual forced abduction of the knee and the medial gap between femur and tibia due to ruptured medial collateral ligament.

E. The Multistress is applied to demonstrate internal derangement injury of the knee.

F. Drawing shows positive "drawer sign" as result of injury to the anterior crucial ligament.

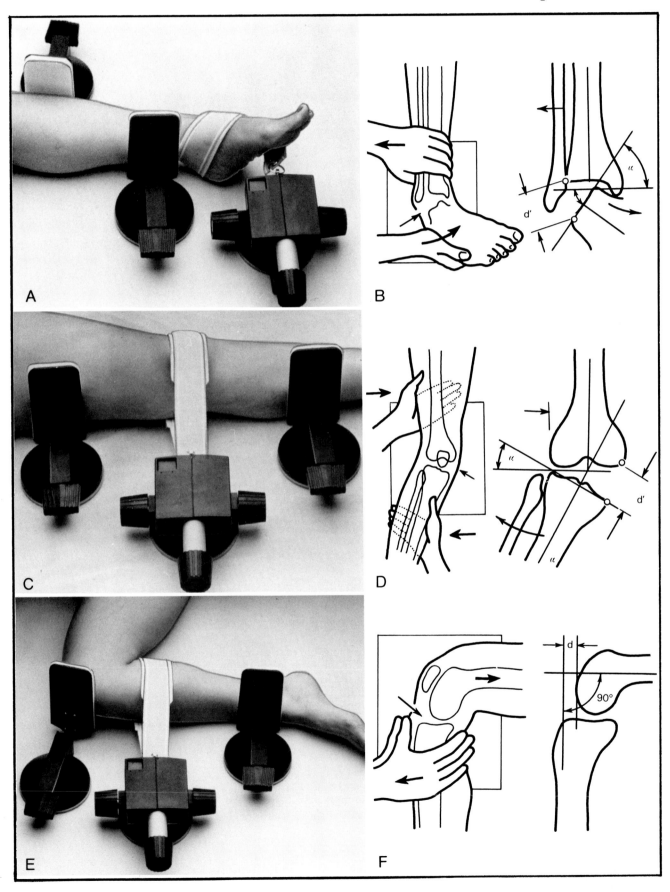

Figure A4.1.

Figure A4.2.

A. The International Standard SFTR Goniometer. Numbers on the outside and inside circles the goniometer are printed red.
OEC Bourbon, Indiana, Cat. No. 238

The International Standard Goniometer is a very useful measuring device for clinic or hospital use due to its large dimensions which enable the examiner to take accurate measurements and readings. It contains scales: 0 to 180 degrees, 0 to 90 degrees, and 180 to 360 degrees, as well as linear scales in inches and centimeters.

Application of the goniometer

The arms of the goniometer are applied as close as possible and in line with the functional or mechanical axes of the limbs or body parts which define the angle of the joint to be measured. True axes of rotation of joints are often varying in different positions of the joint and are difficult to determine. Therefore, placement of the rotational axis of the goniometer can only be approximate and the examiner must concentrate on accurate application of the arms of the goniometer.

B. The international standard pocket goniometer. Numbers on the inner-circle of the goniometer and the small black arrow are printed red.
OEC Bourbon, Indiana, Cat. No. 240

The Standard Pocket Goniometer is a handy yet precise measuring device to facilitate the SFTR standard measurements. The arms of the goniometer are placed over or parallel to the long mechanical axes of the structures which define the angle of the joint. The values are generally indicated by the black arrow. Motions of the shoulder are read at the black triangle, and those of the ankle joint at the red arrow.

The information regarding the SFTR Recording Method and the SFTR Goniometers are reprinted with permission from: Russe, Gerhardt, King: *An Atlas of Examination, Standard Measurements and Diagnosis in Orthopedics and Traumatology*, 2nd Ed. Hans Huber Publ, Berne, 1976; and Gerhardt et al: *Immediate and Early Prosthetic Management, Rehabilitation Aspects*, Hans Huber Publ, Toronto, 1986 (2nd Edition of *Amputations*).

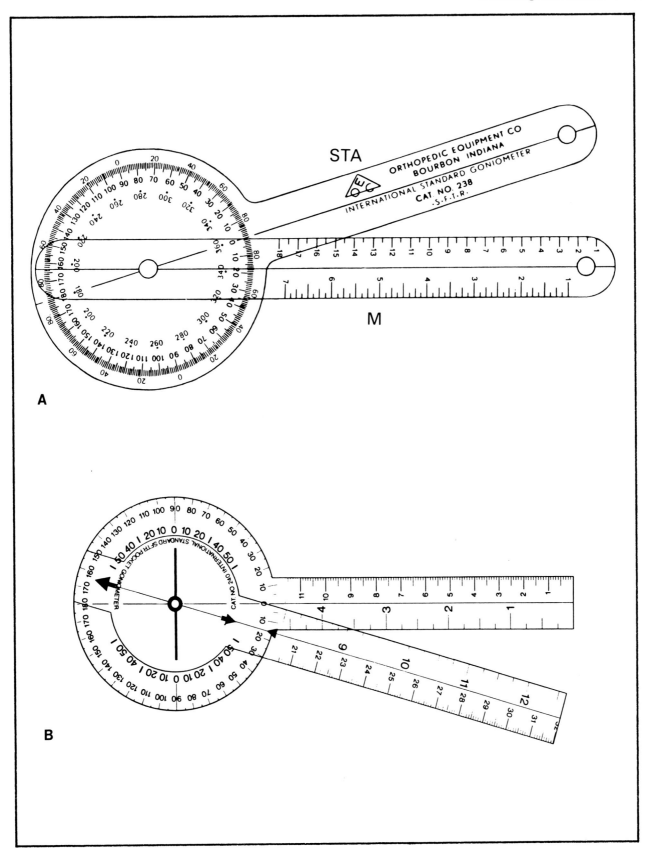

Figure A4.2.

Figure A4.3. Application of the goniometer. Fixed arm or line connecting 0 points and axis is applied in neutral 0 position. The long part of movable arm of the goniometer follows the motion of the long axis of the distal joint component or the vector indicating joint motion, e.g., forearm indicating shoulder rotation. The short part of the movable arm serves as the indicator for reading. The axis is placed as close as possible to the approximate axis of rotation (functional axis) of the joint (or its projection). To facilitate application of goniometer in certain joints, use red numbers (line connecting red 0 with axis in neutral 0 position.

S-motion
A. Extension and flexion of shoulder
B. Flexion of elbow
C. Extension (dorsiflexion) and flexion of wrist
D. Flexion of hip
E. Flexion of knee
F. Extension (dorsiflexion) and flexion of ankle
G. Extension and flexion of head (cervical spine)
F-motion
H. Lateral bend of head (cervical spine)
I. Abduction of shoulder
J. Valgus of elbow
K. Radial and ulnar deviation of wrist
L. Lateral bend of spine (trunk to left and right)
M. Abduction of hip
N. Neutral position of knee
S. Elevation and depression of shoulder girdle
T. Inversion and eversion of hind part of foot (passive motion)
T-motion
R. Flexion (forward) and extension (backward) of shoulder girdle
R-motion
O. Eversion and inversion of ankle
P. Rotation of lower leg (with knee in 90° flexion)
Q. Rotation of head (cervical spine)

In original goniometers the printout is in two colors (black and red) to facilitate correct application and reading.

From *Joint Motion, Method of Measuring and Recording*, published by American Academy of Orthopedic Surgeons, 1965, Carter R. Rowe, M.D., Boston, MA.

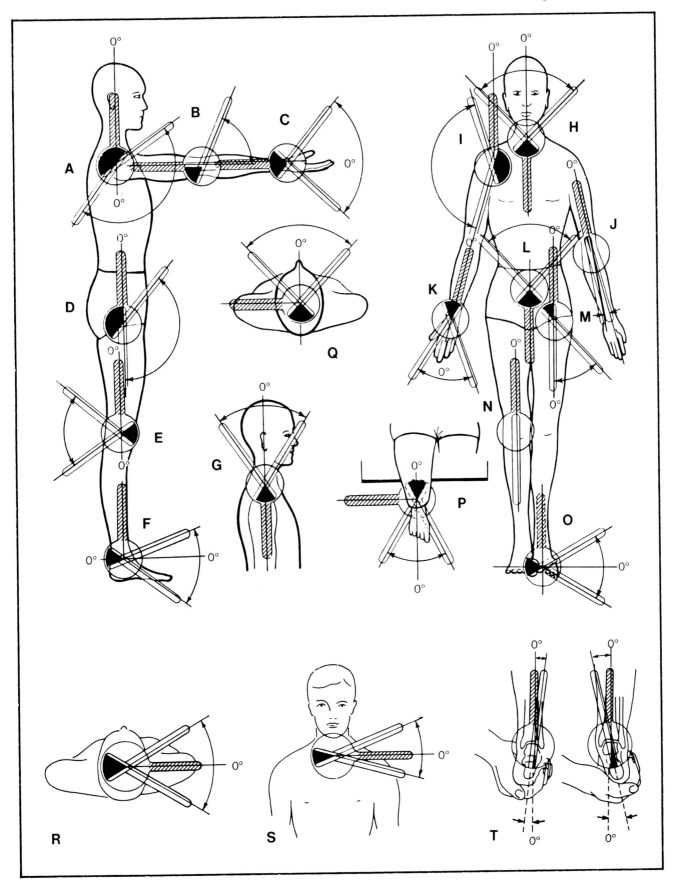

Figure A4.3.

Figure A4.4. Application of the goniometer.

S-motion:
D. Extension of hip.

F-motion, T-motion:
E. Abduction and adduction of hip in 90 degree flexion
B. Horizontal extension and horizontal flexion of shoulder.

R-motion:
A. Rotation of shoulder in 90 degree abduction
C. Supination and pronation of forearm
F. Rotation of hip with extended hip and knee
G. External and internal rotation of shoulder with arm at side of body
H. External and internal rotation of hip with hip and knee flexed 90 degrees (patients supine)
I. External and internal rotation of hip, with hip extended and with knee flexed 90 degrees (patient prone).

In original goniometers the printout is in two colors (black and red) to facilitate application and reading.

From *Joint Motion of Measuring and Recording*, published by American Academy of Orthopedic Surgeon, 1965, Carter R. Rowe, M.D., Boston, MA.

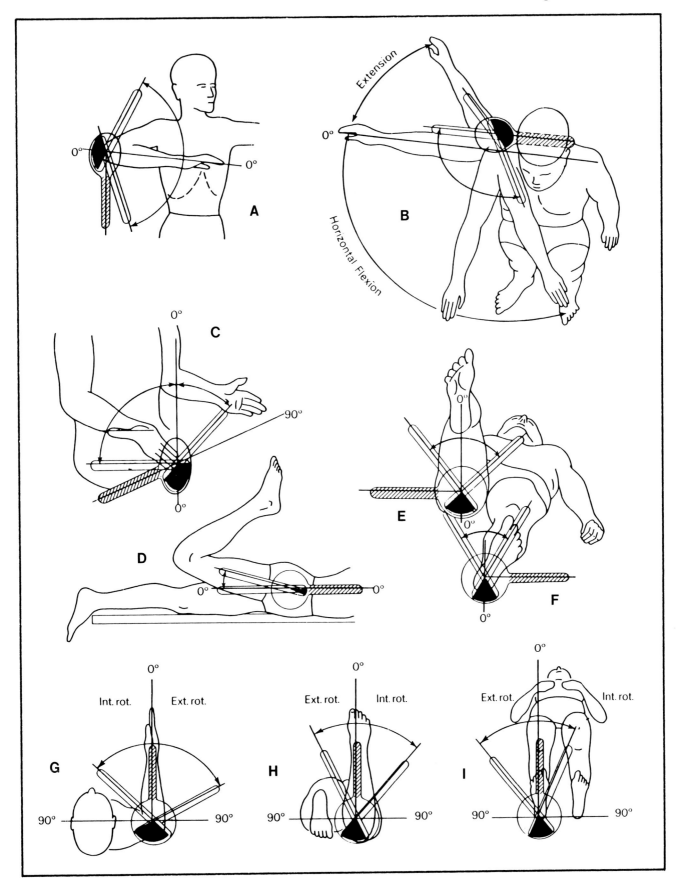

Figure A4.4.

Figure A4.5. Application of the Plurimeter.

    A. The plurimeter with the caliper attached

B–J. Application of the plurimeter:
    The arm of the plurimeter is aligned with the long axis of the distal joint component or
    the vector indicating joint motion in the neutral position. The scale on the plurimeter
    is then set to "0" by rotating the housing. When the joint is moved through its range,
    direct readings can be taken on the scale. When using the caliper, the scale of the
    plurimeter is set and kept at "0". This assures the level of the caliper and reading of
    the distance differences on the scale at the movable part of the caliper. Various other
    applications of the caliper are shown.

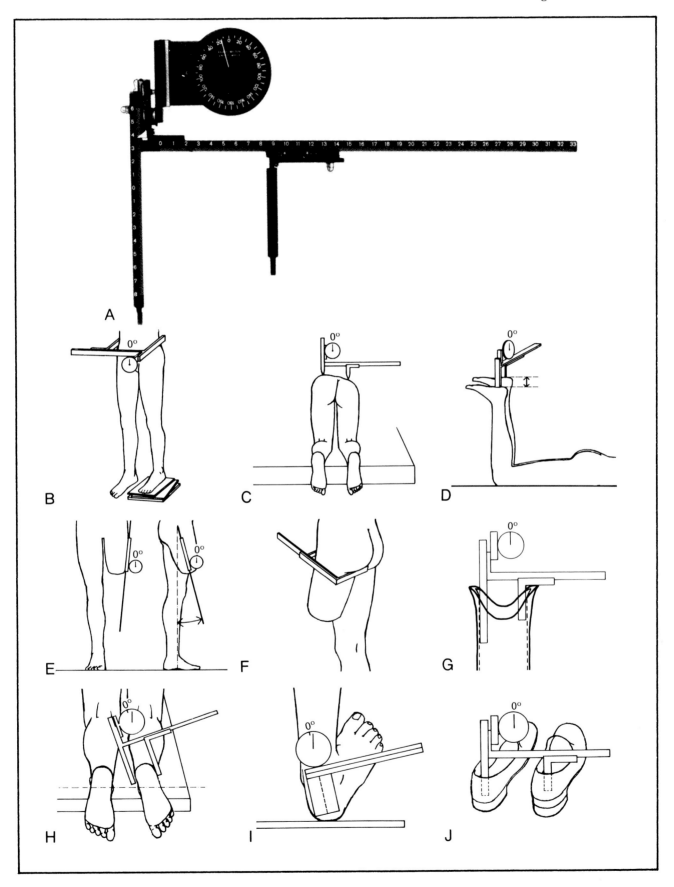

Figure A4.5.

Figure A4.6. Other Applications of the Plurimeter

A. Lumbar spine: lateral bend.

B. Pelvic motion of 50 degrees.

C. Pelvic and lumbar spine motion combined of 95 degrees. Combined pelvic and lumbar spine motion less pelvic motion indicates motion of lumbar spine proper: 95 degrees − 50 degrees = 45 degrees.

Deformities of the spine

D. Kyphosis (standing).

E. Kyphosis (prone-sphinx position to detect early Scheuermann's disease).

F. Scoliosis angle on X-ray.

G. Height of rib hump or lumbar bulge.

H. Pelvic inclination or tilt.

I. Cervical spine, rotation, patient supine.

J. Shoulder rotation.

K. Pronation-supination of forearm.

L. Forefoot supination (eversion–inversion). Patient sitting.

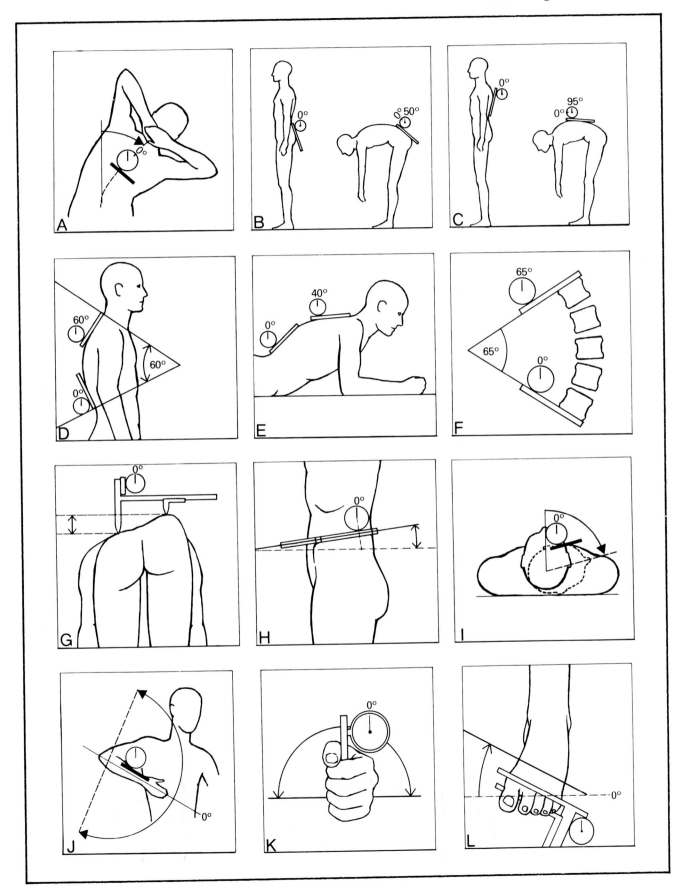

Figure A4.6.

Appendix 5

Planning Data for the Construction of an Accident Victim's Rehabilitation Center

Eckhart Reiner, M.D.

Before final planning for a rehabilitation center, the first step is to examine certain major criteria:

1. *The legal bases.* Most countries have their own laws and agencies for assistance for trauma victims. These must be considered in all further stages of planning.
2. *Previously existing installations.* These must be analyzed to determine whether a new rehabilitation center will be necessary. Not only the capacity, but also the medical programs of the existing centers must be considered. The regional organization and location of the existing units and the proposed new center should be included in the evaluation.

The results of detailed studies and analyses from the fields of traffic technology, landscaping, meteorology, crop sciences, geology, energy technology, and earth radiation also should be taken into account. After evaluation of these many factors, planning for the special center can begin. Very important are cost estimates, both for construction and for later operation.

The next step is to consider allocation of space, including *treatment blocks* and *treatment clinic areas*.

Treatment blocks are projections that are necessary as they relate to the types of patients who will be treated in the rehabilitation center. One possible distribution, for example, might be:

One unit for paraplegics
One unit for amputees
One unit for other accident patients with average nursing requirements
One unit for self-supporting patients

For paraplegics, more space about the bed is required than for the other patients.

Each unit should be divided into two parts, one for acute patients and one for the more mobile. Adequate bathrooms and sufficient storage space are extremely important. The unit for amputees and the other two units can be planned smaller because they will have fewer wheelchair patients.

Treatment clinic areas should include units for occupational therapy, physical therapy, speech-language pathology, orthopaedic engineering, social work, and examining and treatment rooms for the consultant physicians. For the urologist, there should be a larger unit, including an operating theater.

In the rehabilitation center, there should be a septic and an aseptic operating room, a room for central supply and sterilization, a central X-ray room, a cast room, a medical laboratory, and a pharmacy.

The treatment block presented in this chapter is based on the "Weißer Hof" project.

TREATMENT BLOCK FOR PARAPLEGICS

This treatment block requires a patient area of approximately 1,151 m² and a nursing/therapy area of approximately 727 m², totaling 1,878 m².

The patient area is divided into:

Two single-bed rooms, 26 m² each, with sanitary groups (consisting of washroom, WC, and shower) of 10.5 m² each:	73.0 m²
Six two-bed rooms of 42 m² each, with sanitary groups of 11.5 m² each:	321.0 m²
12 three-bed rooms of 42 m² each and sanitary groups of 11.5 m² each:	642.0 m²
Anterooms to the rooms:	115.0 m²
Total:	1,151.0 m²

The nursing/therapy area is divided into:

Supervisor's room/nurses' duty room:	19.5 m²
Scullery:	22.0 m²
Nurses' restroom:	22.0 m²
Storage (medication store, splints):	39.5 m²
Examination rooms and recording positions 27.8/33.5 m²:	61.3 m²
Conference room:	28.5 m²
Two exercise baths of 16.7 m² each:	33.4 m²
Three bathrooms with tubs/therapy of 27.8 m² each:	83.4 m²
Two laundry rooms for severely dirty linen of 22 m² each:	44.0 m²
Day rooms for smokers/nonsmokers of 74.6 m² each:	149.2 m²
Bathroom groups ladies/men 25/27.5 m²:	52.5 m²
Therapy room:	44.5 m²
Bed changing locations:	44.0 m²
Rooms for cleaning equipment, clean and dirty linen storage, aseptor, storage for devices:	83.0 m²
Total:	727.0 m²

598

TREATMENT BLOCK FOR AMPUTEES

The treatment block for amputees and patients to be treated orthopaedically (level 3) is for the treatment of patients with amputations that need to be fitted with prostheses and should also serve as accommodation for other injured patients that need special or orthopaedic treatment. It is to be supplied with support equipment, extenders, splints, etc. It is also planned with 50 beds. This block also must be adapted for the rehabilitation of children. Patients who suffer from weakness of limbs and need supports also should be treated here. This block will also handle hemiplegics needing special orthopaedic-technical care, e.g., walking aids or wheelchairs.

This treatment block is divided into a patient area of approximately 1151 m² and a nursing/therapy area of approximately 681 m², totaling approximately 1,832 m².

The patient area is divided into:

Two single-bed rooms of 26 m² each, with sanitary groups of 10.5 m² each:	73.0 m²
Six two-bed rooms of 42 m² each and sanitary groups of 11.5 m² each:	321.0 m²
12 three-bed rooms of 42 m² each and sanitary groups of 11.5 m² each:	642.0 m²
Anterooms ot the rooms:	115.0 m²
Total:	1,151.0 m²

The nursing/therapy area is divided into:

Supervisor's room/nurses duty room:	19.5 m²
Scullery:	22.0 m²
Nurses' restroom:	22.0 m²
Storage (medication store, splints):	39.5 m²
Examination rooms and recording positions 27.8/33.5 m²:	61.3 m²
Two bathrooms with tubs/therapy of 27.8 m² each:	55.6 m²
Conference room:	44.5 m²
Two laundry rooms for severely dirty linen of 22 m² each:	44.0 m²
Day rooms smokers/nonsmokers of 74.6 m² each:	149.2 m²
Bathroom groups ladies/men 25/27.5 m²:	52.5 m²
Multifunctional room/therapy:	44.0 m²
Workrooms:	47.5 m²
Rooms for cleaning equipment, clean and dirty linen storage, and storage for devices:	80.0 m²
Total:	681.0 m²

TREATMENT BLOCK FOR OTHER ACCIDENT VICTIMS

The treatment block for patients with average nursing requirements, including craniocerebral patients (level 4), like the two previously mentioned treatment blocks, also is outfitted with 50 beds (for men, women, and children). This block is to treat patients suffering from various medium-grade injuries of the locomotor and support system. Additionally, patients suffering from medium-degree craniocerebral injuries are treated here.

This treatment block requires a patient area of approximately 1146 m² and a nursing/therapy area of approximately 665 m², totaling approximately 1811 m².

In the "Weißer Hoff" project, the patient area is divided into:

Two single-bed rooms of 26 m² each, with sanitary groups consisting of washroom, toilet, and shower of 10.5 m² each:	73.0 m²
Six two-bed rooms of 42 m² each, with four sanitary groups of 11.5 m² each and two sanitary groups of 9.3 m² each:	316.0 m²
12 three-bed rooms of 42 m² each, with sanitary groups of 11.5 m² each:	642.0 m²
Anterooms to the rooms:	115.0 m²
Total:	1,146.0 m²

The nursing/therapy area is divided into:

Supervisor's room/nurses' duty room:	19.5 m²
Scullery:	22.0 m²
Nurses' restroom:	22.0 m²
Storage (medication store, splints:	39.5 m²
Examination rooms and recording positions 27.8/33.5 m²:	61.3 m²
Conference room:	44.5 m²
Two bathrooms with tubs/therapy of 27.8 m² each:	55.6 m²
Two laundry rooms for severely dirty linen:	44.0 m²
Day rooms smokers/nonsmokers of 74.6 m² each:	149.2 m²
Bathroom groups ladies/men 25/27.5 m²:	52.5 m²
Multifunctional room/therapy:	44.0 m²
Rooms for cleaning equipment, clean and dirty linen storage, reserve storage space, intermediate passage, and storage for devices:	80.0 m²
Two workrooms:	31.5 m²
Total:	665.0 m²

TREATMENT BLOCK FOR SELF-SUPPORTING PATIENTS

In the treatment block for self-supporting patients (level 5), a large number of accident patients achieve major recovery. It is therefore meaningful to install a so-called self-supporting, or self-service, unit. Self-supporters are patients still requiring intensive physio- and ergotherapy, as well as various measures of vocational and social rehabilitation, so as to speed their reintegration into their home and social environment. There is no longer any extensive medical nursing requirement.

This block also contains 50 beds and requires a patient area of approximately 855 m² and a nursing/therapy area of approximately 611 m², totaling 1,466 m².

The patient area is divided into:

Two two-bed rooms of 26 m² each, with sanitary groups of 10.5 m² each:	73.0 m²
Six three-bed rooms of 42 m² each, with four sanitary groups of 11.5 m² each and two sanitary groups of 9.3 m² each:	319.0 m²
Seven four-bed rooms of 42 m² each, with sanitary groups of 11.5 m² each:	374.5 m²
Anterooms to the rooms:	88.5 m²
Total:	855.0 m²

The nursing/therapy area is divided into:

Supervisor's room/nurses' duty room:	19.5 m²
Scullery:	22.0 m²
Nurses' restroom:	22.0 m²

Storage (medication store, splints): 39.5 m²
Examination rooms and recording positions 27.8/33.5 m²:
    61.3 m²
Conference room: 44.5 m²
Six bathrooms with tubs/therapy of 10.5 m² each: 63.0 m²
Wet workroom: 16.5 m²
Day rooms smokers/nonsmokers of 74.6 m² each: 149.2 m²
Bathroom groups ladies/men 22/27.5 m²: 49.5 m²
Multifunctional room/therapy: 44.0 m²
Workroom: 14.0 m²
Rooms for cleaning equipment, clean and dirty linen, storage,
laundry storage, storage room, storage for devices: 66.0 m²
Total: 611.0 m²

TREATMENT INSTALLATIONS

The following spectrum of therapy installation is to be
available for medical rehabilitation:

Medical coordination (level 1) (integrated medical services):
    approximately 135.0 m²

Occupational Therapy

Approximately 22% of patients in rehabilitation participate in occupational therapy. Occupational therapy, including ergotherapy, teaches the patient the necessary
activities of daily life as a means of self-sufficiency and
produces additional aids for self-aid. Such occupational
therapy as weaving, plaiting, braiding, working with clay
and the like combine a functional training of the injured
region of the body with a stimulation of the patient's creativity.

The following treatment and accessory rooms should be
available for ergotherapy:

Training workshop: 205.0 m²
Raw and small material room: 33.0 m²
Training room/kitchen: 22.0 m²
Plastics processing room: 22.0 m²
Gripping and prosthesis training: 22.0 m²
Individual therapy room: 22.0 m²
Storage room: 22.0 m²
Room allocated to the therapist: 22.0 m²
Sanitary group (therapist): 10.0 m²
Sanitary group (patients): 18.5 m²
Quiet workroom/workroom: 22.5 m²
Speech and writing training: 34.0 m²
Storage room: 10.5 m²
Total: 465.5 m²

Work therapies can include woodworking, metalworking, electrical engineering and electronics, sound and photo
studio, and gardening. These will assure the realization
of a general occupational therapy. Together with vocational counseling, these therapies also play a role in vocational guidance and serve as a stimulant for creative
spare-time activity.

Space for these therapies are divided into the following

Woodworking (level 0)
Training workshop—wood: 172.0 m²
Training machine shop: 64.5 m²

Wood- and working material storage rooms: 75.0 m²
Painting, spraying, and enameling room: 33.5 m²
Total: 345.0 m²

Metalworking (level 0)
Training metal workshop: 146.0 m²
Smithy chimney room: 22.0 m²
Grinding and polishing room: 22.0 m²
Welding room: 22.0 m²
Lock chamber: 11.0 m²
Gas container room/storage: 11.0 m²
Storage rooms/stock rooms 22/4 × 10.5 m²: 64.0 m²
Total: 298.0 m²

Electrical engineering (level 0)
Training workshop—electrical: 33.5 m²
Drawing shop: 22.0 m²
Storage room: 11.0 m²
Total: 66.5 m²

Sound studio (level 0)
2 workrooms of 16.5 m² each: 33.0 m²
Anteroom, storage rooms: 15.5 m²
Total 48.5 m²

Photo studio (level 0)
Shooting room: 16.5 m²
Workroom: 16.5 m²
Anteroom, two darkrooms: 15.0 m²
Total: 48.0 m²

Day room for the therapist: 25.0 m²
Sanitary groups for therapists and patients: 47.0 m²
Storage room, wheelchairs: 43.0 m²
Total: 115.0 m²

Horticultural unit (level −1)
Glass house: 66.0 m²
Preparation room: 53.0 m²
Material storage room: 21.0 m²
Planting room: 21.0 m²
Gardening tools: 10.0 m²
Sanitary group for personnel and patients: 20.0 m²
Total 191.0 m²

Physical Therapy

Approximately 78% of patients in rehabilitation participate in various types of physical therapy, including hydrotherapy (10%), balneotherapy (10%), electrotherapy
(10%), and gymnastics (48%). Space for these therapies is
divided into the following components.

*Hydrotherapy (level 1)—walking exercises in water, underwater
massage, swimming training to loosen up the spine, and the like*
Swimming hall (sports pool, therapy course,
water passage): 935.0 m²
Supervisory area: 8.5 m²
Equipment room: 8.5 m²
Observation room: 43.0 m²
Sauna area (sauna room, Kneipp cure room, restroom): 78.5 m²
Cloakroom ladies/men: 81.5 m²

Shower, bathrooms ladies/men:	46.0 m²
Fresh air area and diving pool (outside):	
Total:	1201 m²

Balneotherapy (level 1)—used for the treatment of injury sequelae, i.e., swellings, reduced mobility, and reduced circulation; improves circulation and mobilizes; paraffin packs, medical baths, massage, fango packs, etc. are used; Cryotherapy, a special form of balneotherapy, applies medicinal ice to treat local damage, such as swellings

Room for baths of parts of the body:	41.0 m²
Room for fango baths:	42.0 m²
Room for clean and dirty linen:	14.5 m²
Medicinal bath:	28.5 m²
Butterfly bath:	28.0 m²
Two rooms for underwater treatment of 16.6 m² each:	33.2 m²
Restroom:	25.0 m²
Room for dry massage:	24.5 m²
Supervisor's room:	11.5 m²
Therapist's room:	22.0 m²
Sanitary rooms for personnel:	10.0 m²
Sanitary rooms for patients:	38.0 m²
Storage rooms:	21.0 m²
Total:	339.0 m²

Electrotherapy (level 1)—particularly indicated with nerve injuries and for treatment of painful states; Diadynamics and magnetic field irradiation used for quicker wound healing with slow-healing fractures and pressure sores; Further therapy components: irradiation with short- or microwaves, rhythmic extensions, treatment with stimulating current, etc.

Electrotherapy rooms and respective booths for irradiation, including short waves, microwaves with stimulating currents and biodynamics:	185.0 m²
Biocheck station:	64.0 m²
Room for therapists:	22.0 m²
Sanitary rooms for personnel:	10.0 m²
Sanitary rooms for patients:	18.5 m²
Total:	300.0 m²

Gymnastics (level 0)—can be done individually or in groups; belt ergometers serve as controls, for telemetric studies, etc.

Gymnastics hall:	531.0 m²
Equipment room:	32.5 m²
Four group gymnastics rooms of 34 m² each:	136.0 m²
Two condition training rooms of 34 m² each:	68.0 m²
Walking school with various surfaces and stump gymnastic training:	144.0 m²
Changing, sanitary, and bathrooms for ladies/men:	100.0 m²
Total:	1011.5 m²

Orthopaedic Engineering (Level 0)

Orthopaedic engineering fits patients with prostheses, splints, supporting apparatus, walking aids, corsets, and stabilizing dressings. Space is divided into the following components:

Prosthesis workshop (including research):	90.0 m²
Room for work with casting and artificial resin:	34.0 m²
Office:	11.0 m²
Room for plaster casting:	29.0 m²
Waiting zone:	22.5 m²

Machine room:	34.0 m²
Workshop for myoelectric devices:	17.0 m²
Storage and stowing rooms:	31.0 m²
Bathrooms for patients:	18.5 m²
Total:	287.0 m²

For patients who are involved jointly in orthopaedic engineering and gymnastics:

Day room:	22.0 m²
Sanitary rooms:	10.0 m²
Total:	32.0 m²

MEDICAL TREATMENT

Urology (Level 2)

This area deals with the development of findings and important clinical follow-up studies of neurogenically disturbed bladders and their treatment. Space is divided into the following components:

Room for urological diagnosis and treatment (linked with the septic operating area for X-ray, endoscopy, and gynecology):	
	48.5 m²
Preparation room:	17.5 m²
Switch room:	9.5 m²
Electrostimulation room:	67.5 m²
Room for urological examinations:	33.0 m²
Storage room:	5.0 m²
Bathroom for patients (wheelchair-suitable):	5.0 m²
Total:	186.0 m²

Septic Treatment (Level 2)

Surgical problems posed in the septic area of operations are: operation on fistulae in soft tissue, removal of foreign bodies, operation of pressure sores with paraplegics, and urological operations for infections of the urinary tract, e.g., suprapubic drainages, operations of diverticula, and operations of urethric fistulae. Space is divided into the following components:

Septic operating room:	47.5 m²
Room for preparations:	22.0 m²
Recovery room:	19.5 m²
Washroom:	11.0 m²
Wet workroom:	14.5 m²
Personnel room (jointly with urology):	14.0 m²
Changing rooms and sanitary group:	35.0 m²
Total:	163.5 m²

Aseptic Treatment (Level 2)

The aseptic operating area is planned for the execution of absolutely necessary interventions during rehabilitation treatment, such as operations on bone and bone marrow; removal of osteosynthesis material, such as intramedullary pins, plates, screws, and drilling wires; execution of tenodeses, tenolyses, arthrodeses and arthrolyses; invasive use of diagnostics, e.g., bronchoscopy; neurosurgical operations that involve the implantation of epidural electrodes for the treatment of pain; penis prostheses; artificial digital joints; and execution of stump corrections. Space is divided into the following components:

Aseptic operating room:	47.0 m²
Room for preparations:	22.0 m²
Washroom:	11.0 m²
Wet workroom, including aseptor:	14.0 m²
Recovery room:	19.5 m²
Personnel room:	14.0 m²
Storage and equipment room, waste removal:	49.0 m²
Changing rooms and sanitary group:	35.0 m²
Total:	211.5 m²

Consultant Physicians (Level 2)

Room for neurology, EEG, and EMG:	42.0 m²
Room for acupuncture:	33.0 m²
Room for psychologists and social workers:	51.0 m²
Room for ENT and ophthalmologist:	42.0 m²
Room for internal medicine, including EKG and ergometrics:	
	42.0 m²
Room for dental physician:	33.5 m²
Office (consultant room without designation):	34.5 m²
Total:	278.0 m²

Central Sterilization (Level 2)

Room for central sterilization clean:	29.0 m²
Room for central sterilization unclean:	42.0 m²
Equipment room:	11.0 m²
Instrument sterilization:	24.0 m²
Changing room/bathroom, storage room:	12.0 m²
Issuing and collecting room, 11 m² each:	22.0 m²
Total:	140.0 m²

Central X-ray, including Plaster Cast Room (Level 2)

Two X-ray rooms of 31 m² each:	62.0 m²
Registration office:	17.0 m²
X-ray developing room:	17.0 m²
X-ray reference archive:	16.0 m²
Equipment room:	10.5 m²
Presentation room and recording position:	42.0 m²
Four changing booths of 3.4 m² each:	13.6 m²
Bathroom for patients:	5.5 m²
Office (reserve) and storage room:	51.0 m²
Plaster cast room:	38.5 m²
Total:	273.0 m²

Medical Laboratory (Level 2)

The medical laboratory will undertake photometric, electrophoretic, and all other routine lab examinations.

Blood-sampling room:	6.0 m²
Laboratory:	54.0 m²
Personnel room (jointly with X-ray section):	25.0 m²
Bathroom for patients:	4.5 m²
Bathroom ladies/men of 18 m² each:	36.0 m²
Total:	125.5 m²

Medication Store (Level 0)

Medication storage:	44.5 m²
Storage room for medication, dressings, etc.:	47.5 m²
Counter room for issuing:	48.5 m²
Total:	140.5 m²

Mortuary (Level 0)

Laying out room:	21.5 m²
Cold storage box:	5.5 m²
Storage room:	5.0 m²
Total:	32.0 m²

MEDICAL AND NURSING MANAGEMENT
Nursing Management (Level 2)

Head nurse/duty room:	41.5 m²
Bathroom/washroom:	7.5 m²
Total:	49.0 m²

Medical Management (Level 2)

Duty room for medical director:	42.0 m²
Bathroom/shower:	7.5 m²
Conference room:	51.0 m²
Examination room:	42.0 m²
Secretariat:	25.0 m²
Medical library and conference room:	56.0 m²
Scullery:	13.5 m²
Sanitary groups ladies/men:	23.0 m²
Total:	260.0 m²

Physicians (Level 5)

10 physicians' duty rooms of 18 m² each:	180.0 m²
Four sanitary groups of 11.2 m² each and one sanitary group of 9.3 m²:	54.0 m²
Five anterooms of 10 m² each:	50.0 m²
Clubroom (physicians' duty room):	32.0 m²
Storage room/cleaning material room:	16.0 m²
Total:	332.0 m²

Medical Records Office (Level 2)

Central office, 6 working positions:	34.0 m²
Working archive, copier location:	20.0 m²
Central archives, tape archives (anamneses, X-rays):	87.5 m²
Total:	142.0 m²

Waiting Zones in the Medical Area (Level 2)

Four waiting zones, total:	400.0 m²

Installations for Vocational and Social Rehabilitation (Level 1)

Room for psychologist:	34.0 m²
Three rooms for social counselors of 34 m² each:	102.0 m²
Room for teacher:	19.0 m²
Room for teaching aids:	18.0 m²
Teaching room:	33.5 m²
Conference room (team, officials):	29.0 m²

Conference room:	60.0 m²
Exhibit room:	44.5 m²
Storage rooms 12/10.5/10.5 m²:	33.0 m²
Sanitary groups ladies/men:	34.0 m²
Total:	407.0 m²

ADMINISTRATION

Administrative Management (Level 1)

Office of administration manager:	34.0 m²
Secretariat:	22.0 m²
Office manager:	16.5 m²
Cashier's office:	16.5 m²
Accountant's office:	42.0 m²
Mail office:	11.0 m²
Copying room and paper store:	22.0 m²
Telex room:	10.5 m²
Scullery:	10.5 m²
Sanitary group for personnel:	20.0 m²
Office of shop steward:	16.5 m²
Storage room:	10.5 m²
Room for chauffeurs/visitors:	28.0 m²
Porter's area (luggage room, porter's lodge, fire alarm center):	
	27.0 m²
Total:	287.0 m²

Technical Services (Level 0)

Foreman's office:	22.5 m²
Electro-workshop/storage 22/11 m²:	33.0 m²
Technical control center:	22.0 m²
Glazier's workshop/storage 22/11 m²:	33.0 m²
Joiner's workshop:	67.5 m²
Locksmith's and plumber's workshop:	87.5 m²
Room for outside technicians:	22.0 m²
Workshop/storage:	56.5 m²
Sanitary group for personnel:	28.0 m²
Total:	372.0 m²

Material Administration (Levels 0 and 1)

Office of material manager:	22.5 m²
Duty room material administration:	44.5 m²
Small components storage:	22.0 m²
Large components storage:	97.5 m²
Storage for office and cleaning materials:	88.0 m²
Administration of archives and storages:	100.0 m²
Furniture storage 80/121.5 m²:	201.5 m²
Storage therapy/reserve:	131.5 m²
Building components depot (level 1):	162.0 m²
Total:	870.0 m²

In-House Services

Reception for dirty linen (level 1):	63.0 m²
Storage and issue area/clean linen (level 0):	206.0 m²
Linen sewing room with changing booth (level 0):	22.5 m²
Storage material room (level 1):	3.9 m²
Storage minigolf (level 1):	11.1 m²
Central disinfecting area (level 1):	192.0 m²
Total:	516.0 m²

Catering (Level 0)

Office kitchen manager:	8.5 m²
Kitchen:	419.0 m²
Refrigerating rooms:	83.0 m²
Beverage store:	81.0 m²
Washrooms:	103.5 m²
Storage rooms:	97.0 m²
Manipulation zone:	70.0 m²
Dining room:	25.0 m²
Cloakroom ladies/men clean/unclean:	36.0 m²
Sanitary installations ladies/men:	30.0 m²
Total:	953.0 m²

Central Cloakroom (Level 0)

Nursing Personnel

Cloakroom ladies:	43.0 m²
Sanitary group ladies:	19.0 m²
Cloakroom men:	43.0 m²
Sanitary group men:	19.0 m²

Technical Personnel

Cloakroom:	43.0 m²
Sanitary group:	19.0 m²

Administration

Cloakroom ladies:	10.5 m²
Sanitary group ladies:	10.0 m²
Cloakroom men:	10.5 m²
Sanitary group men:	10.0 m²
Cloakroom outside personnel:	10.5 m²
Sanitary group:	10.0 m²

Day Room Personnel: *65.0   m²*

Total:	312.5 m²

Garages/Parking Deck (Level 0)

Garage for transport fleet:	170.0 m²
Storage for road-sanding material:	22.5 m²
Car components storage:	34.5 m²
Parking deck for 16 vehicles:	500.0 m²
Total:	727.0 m²

COMMUNAL INSTALLATIONS (LEVEL 1)

Entry hall:	141.0 m²
Sanitary groups ladies/men:	52.5 m²
Library:	32.5 m²
Telephone booths:	9.0 m²
Tape cassette listening room:	50.5 m²
Games room/automats:	50.5 m²
Music room:	50.5 m²
Club room and billiards room:	140.0 m²
Chapel (ecumenical):	120.0 m²
Sacristy:	30.0 m²
Discussion room:	19.0 m²
Exhibit cases:	15.0 m²

Lecture hall (for 200 persons, partly in wheelchairs or bed; subdivisible, including stage):	583.0 m²	Dining room patients (including food issuing area):	317.0 m²
Stage depot:	23.0 m²	Dining room personnel (including food issuing area):	241.0 m²
Chair depot:	38.0 m²	Sanitary group ladies:	19.0 m²
Cloakroom, sanitary group, storage room:	73.5 m²	Bowling alley:	158.5 m²
Projectionist's room, passage:	24.0 m²	Canteen (including storage):	138.0 m²
Sales booth (including storage):	39.0 m²	Room for table tennis:	240.0 m²
Cafeteria:	118.5 m²	Sanitary groups ladies/men:	37.0 m²
Hairdresser:	22.0 m²	Two model flats of 83 m² each:	166.0 m²
		Total:	2948.0 m²

Figure A5.1. Overview of the main entrance, reception, waiting rooms, administration, dining rooms and communal services in the new Accident Victim's Rehabilitation Center "Weisser Hof." Area "C" is the auditorium, it is marked "H" in Figure A5.3.

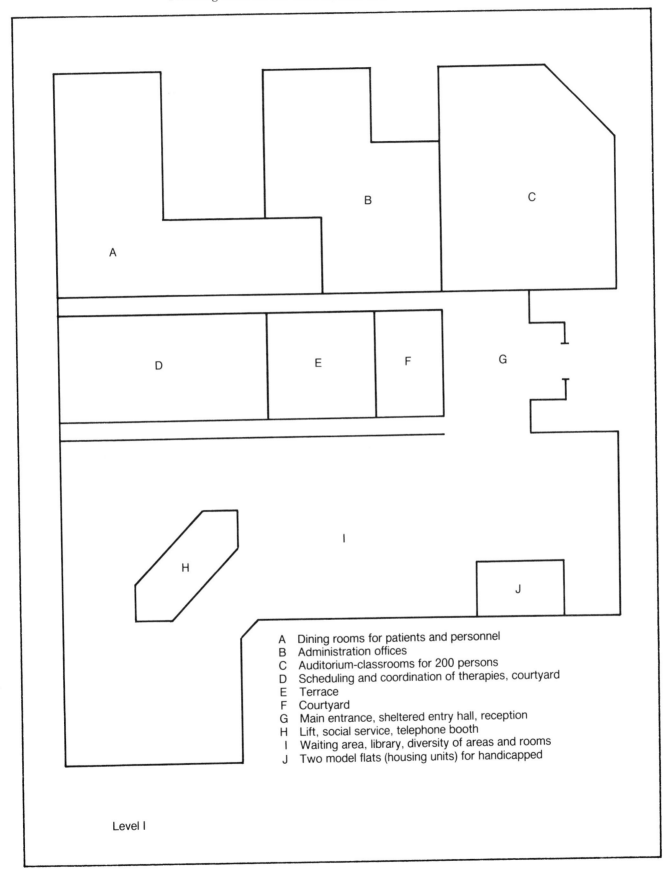

A   Dining rooms for patients and personnel
B   Administration offices
C   Auditorium-classrooms for 200 persons
D   Scheduling and coordination of therapies, courtyard
E   Terrace
F   Courtyard
G   Main entrance, sheltered entry hall, reception
H   Lift, social service, telephone booth
I   Waiting area, library, diversity of areas and rooms
J   Two model flats (housing units) for handicapped

Level I

Figure A5.1.

Figure A5.2. Blueprint showing two adjacent three-bed ward-rooms, which open onto a terrace, that is large enough to accommodate beds and wheelchairs. On the other end there is access to the "wet area," and the nursing support floor. The wet area is large and specifically designed for wheelchair use, featuring, separate tubs, showers, sink, toilet and dressing areas.

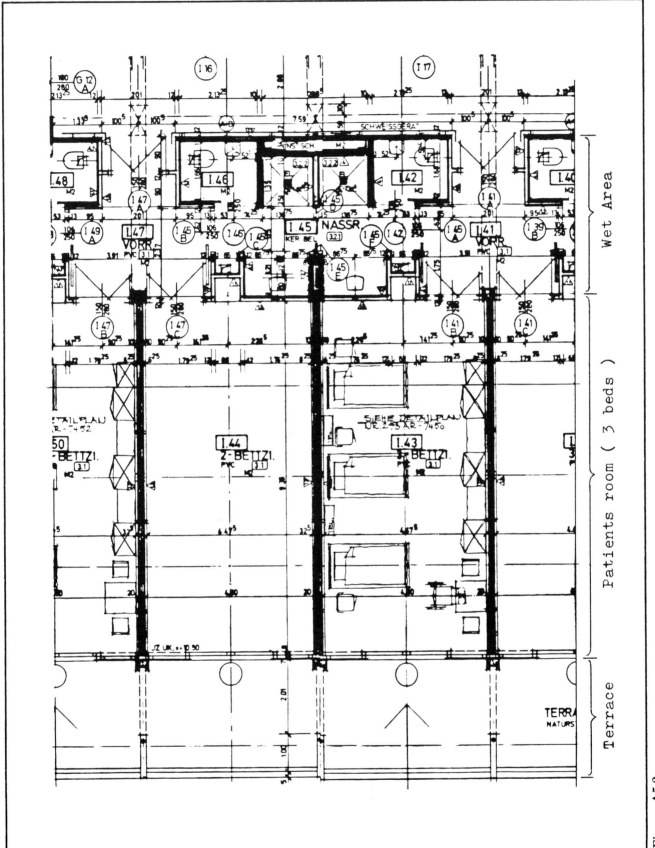

Figure A5.2.

Figure A5.3. Architect's drawing of the new Accident Victim's Rehabilitation Center "Weisser Hof" in Korneuburg near Vienna, Austria.

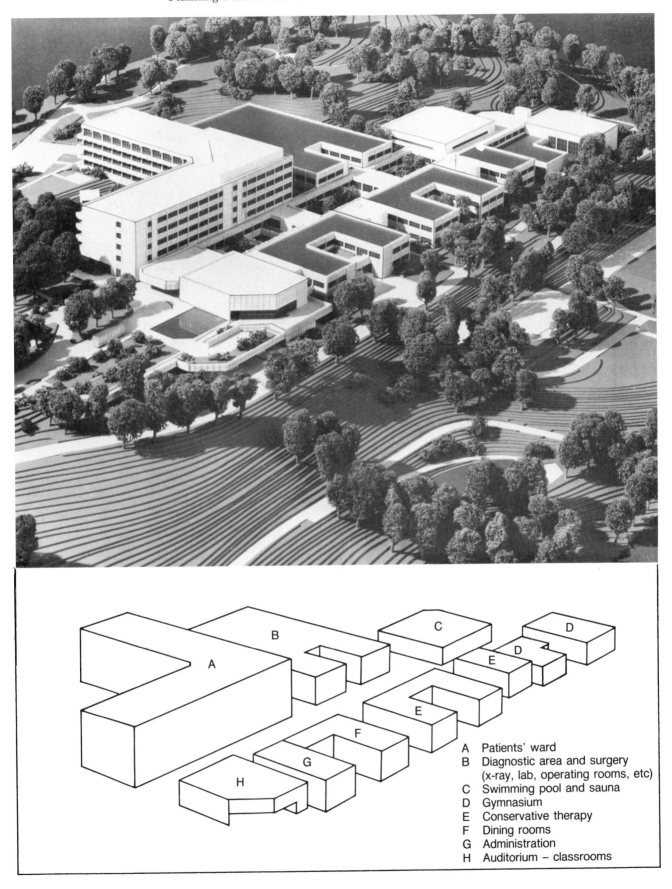

Figure A5.3.

Bibliography

Chapter 4. Administration in a Rehabilitation Center

Fowlks E.W.: Personal experiences; 39 years as chief of the Department of P.M.&R. VA Medical Center, Portland, OR; 25 years Professor in P.M.&R. Oregon Health Sciences University, Portland, Oregon.

Kristiansen K: Sunnaas hospital 25 years. The story of a rehabilitaton center. *J. Oslo City Hosp* 29:23–36, 1979.

Chapter 5. Rehabilitation in the Acute Care Hospital

Böhler L: *Die Technik Der Knochenbruchbehandlung.* Vienna, Verlag Wilhelm Maudrich, 1951.

Gögler E: *Chirurgie der Gegenwart.* vol IV, Munich, Urban & Schwarzenberg, 1978.

Jahna H, Wittich H: *Konservative Methoden in der Frakturbehandlung.* Vienna-Munich-Baltimore, Urban & Schwarzenberg, 1985.

Russe O: *An Atlas of Operations for Trauma.* Wien-Bonn, Wilhelm Maudrich, 1955.

Chapter 6. Rehabilitation of Pediatric Traumatic Injuries

Gnutz RR: Accidental injury in childhood: A literature review on pediatric trauma. *J Trauma* 19:55, 1970.

Hallen JA: Newer concepts in emergency care of children with major injuries. *Md State Med J* 22:65, 1973.

Hallen JA: Problems in children's trauma. *J Trauma* 10:269, 1970.

Ramenofsky ML, Morse TS: Standards of care for the critically injured pediatric patient. *J Trauma* 22:921–33, 1982.

Tachdjian MO: *Pediatric Orthopedics.* Philadelphia-London-Toronto, WB Saunders Co., 1972.

Chapter 7. The Rehabilitation Team

Burri C: *Unfallchirurgie.* Berlin-Heidelberg, Springer Verlag, 1982.

Granitzka S: *Der Aerztliche Notdienst.* Stuttgart-New York, G Thieme Verlag, 1981.

Pashley J, Wahlstrom ML: Polytrauma: the patient, the family, the nurse, and the health team. *Nurs Clin North Am* 16:721–27, 1981.

Chapter 8. The Organization of Therapy

Reiner E: Original contribution, Medical Director Rehabilitation Center Bad Häring, Tirol, Austria.

Chapter 9. Nursing

Derscheid G: Rehabilitation of common orthopedic problems. *Nurs Clin North Am* 16:709–20, 1981.

Fowler R, Fordyce W: Adapting care for the brain damaged patient, 2 part. *Am J Nursing* Oct-Nov, 1972.

Henderson V: *The Nature of Nursing.* New York, Macmillan, 1978.

Niles B: The nurse makes rehabilitation really happen. *Occup Health SAF* 46:14–16, 1977.

Sayles SM (Ed): *Rehabilitation Nursing: Concept and Practice.* Rehabilitation Nursing Institute, Evanston, IL, 1981.

Wilkinson AW: Major Trauma—an intensive problem from site of accident to rehabilitation. *South Am Nursing J* 42:12–14, 1975.

Chapter 10. Nutrition and Diet: Nutritional Considerations of Trauma Patients

Blackburn GL, Bistrian BR: Nutritional care of the injured and/or septic patient. *Surg Clin North Am* 56:1195–1224, 1976.

Blackburn GL, Bothe A, Bistrian BR: Advances in hyperalimentation a practical approach. CME course Sep 18–20, 1985. New England Deaconess Hospital, Harvard Medical School, 1985.

Feman FJ: *Clinical Nutrition and Dietetics.* Lexington, MA, The Callamore Press, DC Heath & Co, 1983.

Food and Nutrition Board, National Research Council: *Recommended Dietary Allowances*, ed 9. Washington DC, National Academy of Sciences, 1980.

Goodhart RS, Shils ME: *Modern Nutrition in Health and Disease.* Philadelphia, Lea & Febiger, 1973.

Halpern LS: *Quick Reference to Clinical Nutrition.* Philadelphia, J.B. Lippincott Co. 1979.

Handbook of Clinical Dietetics. The American Dietetic Association. New Haven, London, Yale University Press, 1981.

Long GL, Birkhahn RH, Geiger JW, Blakemore WS: Contribution of skeletal muscle protein in elevated rates of whole body protein catabolism in trauma patients. *Am J Clin Nutr* 34:1087–93, 1981.

Long GL, Schaffel N, Geiger JW, et al: Metabolic response to injury and illness: Estimation of energy and protein needs from indirect calorimetry and nitrogen balance. *JPEN* 3:452–56, 1979.

Wallie AW, Hendricks KM: *Manual of Pediatric Nutrition.* Philadelphia, W.B. Saunders Co. 1985.

Zeman FJ: *Clinical Nutrition and Dietetics.* Lexington, MA, The Callamore Press, D.C. Heath & Co. 1983.

Chapter 11. Occupational Therapy

Brattstrom M: *Gelenkschutz und Rehabilitation bei chron. polyarthritis.* Stuttgart, Fischer-Verlag, 1984.

Eggers O: *Ergotherapie bei Hemiplegie.* Heidelberg, Springer, 1982.

Eggers O: *Occupational Therapy in the Treatment of Adult Hemiplegia.* Rockville, MD, Aspen Systems Corporation, 1984.

Hasselblatt A: *Ergotherapie in der Orthopadie.* Munich, Bardtenschlager-Verlag, 1985.

Jentschura G, Janz HW: *Beschaftigungstherapie.* Stuttgart, Thieme, 1979.

O'Conell AL: *Understanding the Scientific Basis for Human Movement.* Baltimore, Williams & Wilkins, 1972.

Pfenninger B: *Ergotherapie bei Erkrankungen und Verletzunge der Hand.* Heidelberg, Springer, 1984.

Turner A: *The Practice of Occupational Therapy.* Edinburgh, Churchill-Livingstone, 1981.

Chapter 12. Physical Therapy

Berg D: An approach to the rehabilitation of the injured. *Papua New Guinea Med J* 19:212–219, 1976.

Cotta H, Heiperz W, Huter-Becker, Rompe: *Krankengymnastik, Taschenlehrbuch in Bänden.* Stuttgart, Thieme-Verlag, 1982.

Dirschauer: *Physikalische Therapie in Klinik und Praxis.* Stuttgart, Kohlhammer-Verlag, 1985.

Gillmann H: *Physikalische Therapie.* Stuttgart, Thieme-Verlag, 1981.

Gunther R, Jantsch H: *Physikalische Medizin.* Heidelberg, Springer, 1982.

Hickok RJ: *Physical Therapy Administration and Management.* Baltimore, Williams & Wilkins, 1983.

Paeslack S: *Physiotherapie in der Rehabilitation Querschnittgelahmter.* Berlin, Heidelberg, New York, Springer-Verlag, 1980, p. 185.

Chapter 13. Prosthetics and Orthotics

Burgess EM, Romano RL, Zettl JH: The management of lower extremity amputations. TR 10–6, Washington, DC, Veterans Administration, 1969.

Gerhardt JJ, King PS, Zettl JA: *Immediate and Early Prosthetic Management—Rehabilitation Aspects.* Hans Huber Publishers, Toronto, 1986.

Hohmann D, Uhlig R: *Orthopadische Technik.* ed 7, Stuttgart, Ferdinand Enke Verlag, 1982.

Kristen H, Reiner E, Hiebler W, Muller S: *Prothesen Fur Die Untere Extremitat.* Vienna, Munich, Berne, Verlag Wilhelm Maudrich, 1983.

Marquardt von E, Trauth J: Criteria for the supply of children with hand and arm prostheses. *Orthop Technik,* 8:524–29, 1985.

Marquardt E, Roesler H: Prothesen und Prothesenversorgungen der oberen Extremitat. In: *Orthopadie in Praxis und Klinik.* hrsg. von A N Witt, H Rettig, F K Schlegel, M Hackenbroch, W Hupfauer, Bd. II, Allgemeine Orthopadie, S. 16.1–16.39, Stuttgart, New York, Georg Thieme Verlag, 1981.

Marquardt E: Prothetische Versorgung nach Amputationen. *Der Chirurg* 55:311–317, 1984.

Mazet R Jr, Chupurdia R: Pylons and peg legs. *Clin Orthop* 57:117, 1968.

Russe OA, Gerhardt JJ, et al: *Atlas of Orthopedic Diseases.* Berne, Hans Huber, 1964.

Wilson AB Jr: Limb prosthetics—1967. *Artif Limbs,* 2:1, 1967.

Chapter 14. The Prosthetic-Orthotic Laboratory

Design Shriners Hospital for Crippled Children, Portland unit, Oregon, 1984.

Chapter 15. Psychology

Brewin CR, Robson MJ, Shapiro DA: Social and psychological determinants of recovery from industrial injuries. *Injury* 14:451–455, 1983.

Homes TH, Rahe RH: The social adjustment rating scale. *J Psychosom Res* 11:213–218, 1900.

Ince LP: *Behavioral Psychology in Rehabilitation Medicine: Clinical Applications.* Baltimore, Williams & Wilkins, 1980.

Kerson TS, Kerson LA: *Understanding Chronic Illness.* New York, The Free Press, 1980.

Lyman HB: *Test Scores and What They Mean.* Englewood Cliffs, NJ, Prentice-Hall, 1963.

Chapter 16. Radiology in Trauma

Department of Traumatology: Original contribution, University Hospital, Innsbruck, Austria.

Chapter 17. Recreational Therapy

Kraus R: *Therapeutic Recreational Services—Principles and Practice.* Philadelphia, W B Sanders, Chap 7, 1978.

Peterson CN, Gunn SL: *Therapeutic Recreation Program Design—Principles and Procedures,* ed 2. Englewood Cliffs, NJ, Prentice Hall, 1984.

Weiss C: Recreation leadership for quadriplegic patients in a treatment center. *Therap Recreat J* second quarter, 1968, pp. 32–37.

Chapter 18. Respiratory Therapy

Burton G, Hodgkin J: *Respiratory Care, A Guide to Clinical Practice.* Philadelphia, J.P. Lippincott, 1977.

Fraunfelter D: *Chest Physical Therapy and Pulmonary Rehabilitation.* Chicago, Year Book Medical, 1978.

Gaskell DV, Webster BA: *The Brompton Hospital Guide to Chest Physiotherapy.* Oxford, Blackwell Scientific Publications, 1979.

Chapter 19. Sexuality in Trauma

Ayrault EW: *Sex, Love and the Physically Handicapped.* New York, Continuum Publishing Co., 1981.

Becker E: *Female Sexuality Following Spinal Cord Injury.* Bloomington, IL, Accent of Living: Special Publications, Cheever Publishing Co., 1978.

Comfort A: *Sexual Consequences of Disability.* Philadelphia, George F. Stockley Co., 1978.

Heslinga K, Scheller A, Verkuyl A: *Not Made of Stone: The Sexual Problem of Handicapped People.* Springfield, IL, Charles C Thomas, 1974.

Shakid A: *Sexual Functioning Following Spinal Cord Injury.* Baltimore, Williams & Wilkins, 1981.

Chapter 20. Social Work: Vocational and Social Rehabilitation of Traumatized Patients

Palmer S, et al: Psychosocial services in rehabilitation medicine: An interdisciplinary approach. *Arch Phys Med Rehab* 66:690–692, 1985.

Puryear D: *Helping People in Crisis.* San Francisco, Josey-Bass, 1979.

Chapter 21. Speech and Language Pathology: Treatment of Trauma Patients with Communication and Swallowing Disorders

Adamovich BB, Henderson J: Treatment of communication deficits resulting from traumatic head injury. In Perkins DW (ed), *Current Therapy of Communication Disorders.* New York, Thieme-Stratton, 1983.

Adamovich B, Henderson J, Auerbach S: *Cognitive Rehabilitation of Closed Head Injured Patients; A Dynamic Approach.* San Diego, College Hill Press, 1985.

Johns DF: *Clinical Management of Neurogenic Communication Disorders.* Boston, Little, Brown & Co., 1985.

Heilman KM, Safron A, Geschwind N: Closed head trauma and aphasia. *J Neurol Neurosurg Psychiatry* 34:265–69, 1971.

Holland AL: *Language Disorders in Adults.* San Diego, College Hill Press, 1984.

Lezak M: *Neuropsychological Assessment.* New York, Oxford University Press, 1983.

Logemann J: *Evaluation and Treatment of Swallowing Disorders.* San Diego, College Hill Press, 1983.

Scharf B: The Physician's Guide to Better Communication. Glenview, IL, Scott Foresman, 1900.

Chapter 22. Sports for the Disabled

Allgemeines Sozialversicherungsgesetz (Schriftenreihe des Osterreichischen Gewerkschaftsbundes) Abenteuer Rehabilitation von Ger Tudolf, Verlag Jugend und Volk.

Chapter 23. Sports Prosthetics

Zettl J: Original contribution. Assistant Professor Rehabilitation Medicine, University of Washington, Seattle, WA.

Chapter 24. Vocational Rehabilitation

Workman EL: Vocational rehabilitation in the private, profit-making sector. *Annu Rev Rehabil* 3: 292–320, 1983.

Chapter 25. Wheelchairs

Reiner E: Original contribution. Medical Director, Rehabilitation Center, Bad Häring, Tirol, Austria.

Chapter 26. Amputations

Aitken GT: The child amputee. *Orthop Clin North Am* 3:447, 1972.

Aitken GT, Franz CH: The juvenile amputee. *J Bone Joint Surg* 35–A:659, 1953.

Banerjee SN: *Rehabilitation Management of Amputees.* Baltimore, Williams & Wilkins, 1982.

Baumgartner R: *Die orthopadietechnische Versorgung des Fusses.* Stuttgart, Georg Thieme Verlag, 1972.

Berlemont M: Nore experience de l'apperaillage precose des ampute des mebres inferieurs aux Etabilssements Helio-Marins de Berck. *Ann Med Physique* 4:45, 1961.

Burgess EM, Romano RL, Zettl JH: The management of lower extremity amputations. TR 10–6, Washington, DC, Veterans Administration, 1969.

Burgess EM, Romano RL: Immediate postsurgical prosthetic fitting in children and adolescents following lower-extremity amputations. *Inter-Clin Inform Bull* 7:1, 1967.

Burgess EM: Sites of amputation election according to modern practice. *Clin Orthop* 37:17, 1964.

Callander CL: Tendinoplastic amputation through femur at knee; further studies, *JAMA* 110:113, 1938.

Childress DS, et al: Myoelectric immediate postsurgical procedure: A concept for fitting the upper-extremity amputees. *Artif Limbs* 13:Autumn, 1969.

Compere CL, Thompson RG: The role of the orthopaedic surgeon in the treatment of amputees. *Clin Orthop* 37:11, 1964.

Dederich R: *Amputationen der unteren Extremitat.* Stuttgart, Georg Thieme Verlag, 1970.

Edmonson AS, Crenshaw AH: *Campbell's Operative Orthopaedics.* ed 6, vol 1, pp 821–872 and 869–872, St. Louis, CV Mosby Co., 1980.

Gerhardt JJ, King PS, Zettl JH: *Amputations: Immediate and Early Prosthetic Management.* Berne, Stuttgart, Vienna, Hans Huber Publishers, 1982.

Gerhardt JJ, Peirson PS, Fowlks GA, Altman DC: Immediate post-surgical prosthetics: Rehabilitation aspects. *Am J Phys Med* 49:3–105, 1970.

Gerhardt JJ, King PS, Fowlks EW, Usselman LB, Pfeiffer EA: A device to control ambulation pressure with immediate postoperative prosthetic fitting. *Bull Prosthet Res* 10–16: 153–160, 1971.

Hohmann D, Uhlig R: *Orthopadische Technik,* ed 7. Stuttgart, Ferdinand Enke Verlag, 1982.

Lambert CN: Amputation surgery in the child. *Orthop Clin North Am* 3:473, 1972.

Marquardt E, Heyne S: Beratung von Amputierten der oberen Gliedmaben. *Die Rehabilitation* 22:56–61, 1983.

Marquardt E, Martini AK: Die Krukenberg-Plastik in der Modifikation von E. Marquardt. From: Handchirurgie, Mikrochirurgie, Plastische Chirurgie 17, 117–121, Hippokrates Verlag GmbH, 1985.

Marquardt E: Fruhversorgungen von Amputationen der oberen Extremitat. *Orthop Technik Heft* 7, 1970, pp 171–177.

Rogers SP: Amputation of the knee joint. *J Bone Joint Surg* 44A:1697, 1962.

Romano RL, Burgess EM: Level selection in lower extremity amputations. *Clin Orthop* 74:177, 1971.

Russek AS: Immediate postsurgical fitting of the lower extremity amputee: research experience with 175 cases. *Med Clin North Am* 53:665–676, 1969.

Sarmiento A: A modified surgical-prosthetic approach to the Syme's amputation: A follow-up report. *Clin Orthop* 85:11, 1972.

Vitali M, Harris EE: Prosthetic management of the elderly lower limb amputee: Part I Surgical management. *Clin Orthop* 37:61, 1964.

Vitali M, Harris EE: Prosthetic management of the elderly lower limb amputee: Part II Rehabilitation after operation. *Clin Orthop* 37:68, 1964.

Weiss M, et al: Physiologic amputation Immediate prosthetics and early ambulation. *Prosthet Internat* 3:38–44, Kopenhagen, 1969.

Chapter 27. Burns

Artz, Moncrief, Pruitt: *Burns: A Team Approach.* Philadelphia, WB Saunders Co., 1979.

Helm P: Rehabilitation management in burn injury. *Arch Phys Med Rehab* vol 63, Jan, 1982.

Jensen L, Parshley PF: Post burnscar contracture: Histology and effects of pressure treatment. *J Burn Care Rehabil* 2:119–123, 1984.

Larson D, Aston LS, Evans: Splints and traction. In Polc HC, Stone HH *Contemporary Burn Management.* Boston, Little Brown & Co., 1971.

Larson D, Aston LS, Evans, et al: Techniques for decreasing scar formation and contractures in burn patient. *J Trauma* 11:807, 1971.

Malik M: *Manual or Static Hand Splinting.* Pittsburgh Hamarville Rehabilitation Center, 1972.

Salisbury RE, Major MC, Pruitt BA: *Burns of the Upper Extremity.* Philadelphia, London, Toronto, WB Saunders, 1976.

Wagner MM: *Care of the Burned-Injured Patient. Multidisciplinary Involvement.* RSG Publishing Co., 1981.

Chapter 28. Rehabilitation of Cardiopulmonary Injuries

Ciesla N, Klemic N, Imle PC: chest physical therapy to the patient with multiple trauma. Two case studies. *Phys Ther* 61:202–205, 1981.

Fletcher GF: *Exercise and Exercise Testing: Heart and Lung.* Jan, 1984.

Greenland P, Briody ME: Rehabilitation of the MI Survivor. *Postgrad Med* Jan, 1984.

Gill W, Long WB: *Shock Trauma Manual.* Baltimore, Williams & Wilkins, 1979.

Moore EE, Eiseman B, VanWay CW III: *Critical Decisions in Trauma.* St. Louis, Toronto, CV Mosby Co., 1984.

Parmley LF, Matlingly TW, Manion WC, Jahnke EJ: Nonpenetrating traumatic injury of the aorta. *Circulation* 17:1086, 1958.

Shires GT: *Care of the Trauma Patient.* McGraw Hill Book Company.

Trinkle JK, Glover FL: *The Management of Thoracic Trauma Victims.* Philadelphia, JB Lippincott Co., 1980, pp 39–46.

Wenger NK, Hellerstein HK: *Rehabilitation of Coronary Patient.* John Wiley & Sons, A Wiley Medical Publication, 1978.

Wilson PK, Winga Er, Edgett JW, Gushiken TL: *Cardiac Rehabilitation Program.* Philadelphia, Lea & Febiger, 1978.

Chapter 29. Rehabilitation of Craniocerebral Injuries

Adamovich B, Henderson J, Auerbach S: *Cognitive Rehabilitation of Closed Head Injured Patients; A Dynamic Approach.* San Diego, College Hill Press, 1985.

Bach-y-Rita P: *Recovery of Function: Theoretical Considerations for Brain Injury Rehabilitation.* Baltimore, University Park Press, 1980.

Bhatt K: Head injury rehabilitation. *Fam Pract* 8:29–32, 1982.

Bickford RG, Klass DW: Acute and chronic EEG findings after head injury. In Cavennes WF, Walker AE (Eds.) *Head Injury.* Philadelphia, JB Lippincott, 1966, pp 63–88.

Bobath B: *Abnorme Haltüigs—reflexe bei gehim schäden.* 3rd ed, G. Thieme, Stuttgart, 1976.

Bobath B: *Adult Hemiplegia: Evaluation and Treatment.* London, William Heinemann, 1978.

Bond MR: Assessment of psychosocial outcome after severe head injury. *CIBA Symposium,* 34:141–157, 1975.

Carlsson C, et al: Factors affecting the clinical course of patients with severe head injuries. *J Neurosurg* 9:29–45, 1968.

Carpenter MB, Sutin J: *Human Neuroanatomy,* ed 8. Baltimore, London, Williams & Wilkins, 1983.

Committee on Trauma, American College of Surgeons: *Advanced Life Support; Instructors Manual.* American College of Surgeons, 1984, p. 205.

Cowley RA, Dunham CM: *Shock Trauma Critical Care Medicine—Initial Assessment and Management.* Baltimore, University Park Press, 1981.

Dresser, et al: Gainful employment following head injury—Prognostic factors. *Arch Neurol* 29:106–116, 1973.

Fowler R, Fordyce W: Adapting care for the brain damaged patient. 2 part. *Am J Nursing* Oct-Nov, 1972.

Gill W, Long W: *Shock Trauma Manual.* Baltimore, Williams & Wilkins, 1979.

Illis LS, Sedgwick EM, Glanville HJ: *Rehabilitation of the Neurological Patient.* Oxford, London, Edinburgh, Boston, Melbourne, Blackwell Scientific Publications, 1982.

Jennett B, Teasdale G: Prognosis after severe head injury. In: *CIBA Symposium on Outcome of Severe Damage to the CNS,* 1975.

Menkes JH, Batz U: Postnatal trauma and injuries by physical agents. In Merritt HH (Ed):. *A Textbook of Neurology,* ed 5. Philadelphia, Lea & Febiger, Chap 8, 1973.

Mitchell, Rosenthal M, Griffith ER, Bond MR, Miller JD: *Rehabilitation of the Head Injured Adult.* Philadelphia, FA Davis, 1983.

Moore EE, Eiseman B, VanWay III CW: *Critical Decisions in Trauma.* St. Louis, CV Mosby Co., 1982.

Russe O: *An Atlas of Operations for Trauma.* Vienna, Bonn, Wilhelm Maudrich, 1955.

Russel WR: *The Traumatic Amnesias.* London, Oxford University Press, 1971.

Saunders MG, Westmoreland BF: The EEG in evaluation of disorders affecting the brain diffusely. In Klass DW, Daly DD (Eds). *Current Practice of Clinical Electroencephalography.* New York, Raven Press, 1979.

Zinn WM, *The Place of the Spa in Modern Rheumatology.* The Halliwick Mc Millan Method of Pool Therapy. Practical Use of Hydrotherapy in Rehabilitation. Merkblatt Nr. 194/1968/1978, pp 2–3 and 7–8.

Zinn, WM: Orienterung uber die Medizinische Abteilung Bad Ragaz und die Bäderklinik Valens. Medizinische Abteilung Thermalbäder Bad Ragaz. *Bäderklinik Valens Interkantonales Rheuma und Rehabilitationszentrum.* Merkblatt Nr. 253, 1983, pp 1–4.

Chapter 30. Rehabilitation of Hand Injuries: A Case History in Team Approach

Kilgore ES, Graham WP: *The Hand,* Philadelphia, Lea & Febiger, 1977, pp 6–35, 261–278.

Nickel VL: *Rehabilitation of the Hand.* St. Louis, CV Mosby, 1978, pp 655–659.

Parry WCB: *Rehabilitation of the Hand.* Butterworths, 1973, pp 243–246.

Chapter 31. Rehabilitation of Spinal Cord Injuries

Burke DC, Murray DD: *Die Behandlung Rückenmarkverletzter.* Berlin, Heidelberg, New York, 1979.

Flesch JR, et al: Harrington instrumentation and spine fusion for instable fractures and fracture dislocations of the thoracic and lumbar spine. *J Bone Joint Surg* 59A:143, 1977.

Hardy AG, Rossier AB: *Spinal Cord Injuries—Orthopedic and Neurological Aspects.* Stuttgart, Thieme, 1975.

Harrington PR: The history and development of Harrington instrumentation. *Clin Orthop* 93:110, 1973.

Katthagen BD, Muller-Farber J: Langzeitergebnisse der funktionellen Wirbelbruchbehandlung. *Zbl Chir* 106:1480, 1981.

Ludolph E, Hierholzer G: Funktionelle Behandlung der Frakturen an der Brust-und Lendenwirbelsäule. *Der Orthopäde,* 12:136, 1983.

Magerl F: Operative Frühbehandlung bei traumatischer Querschnittslahmung. *Der Orthopäde* 9:34, 1980.

Morscher E: Operative Korrektur post-traumatischer Wirbelsäulendeformitäten. *H Unfallheilk* 163:138, 1984.

Murray DD, Burke DC: *Handbook of Spinal Cord Medicine.* London, Basingstoke, Macmillan Press Limited, 1975.

Roy-Camille R, Saillant G, Berteaux D, Marie-Anne S: Early management of spinal injuries. In: *Recent Advances in Orthopedics.* Edinburgh, London, McKibbin, Churchill-Livingstone, 1979.

Roy-Camille R, Saillant G, Marie-Anne S, Mamoudy P: Behandlung von Wirbelfrakturen und-luxationen am thorako-lumbalen Ubergang. *Der Orthopäde* 9:63, 1980.

Staufer SE: Current concept reviews: Internal fixation of fractures of the thoraco-lumbar spine. *J Bone Joint Surg* 66A:1136, 1984.

Chapter 32. Urological Management of Spinal Cord Injured Patients: Diagnostic and Therapeutic Aspects

Madersbacher H: Probleme bei der harnableitung frischer querschnittspatienten. *Monatschir Unfallheilk* 76:461–466, 1973.

Madersbacher H: Urinary flow and flow pattern in paraplegics. *Paraplegia* 13:95–100, 1975.

Madersbacher H: The twelve o'clock sphincterotomy—Technique, indications, results. *Paraplegia* 13:261–267, 1976.

Madersbacher H: Combined pressure, flow, EMG and X-ray studies for the evaluation of neurogenic bladder disturbance: Technique. *Urol Int* 32:176–183, 1977.

Madersbacher H: The neuropathic urethra: Urethrogram and pathophysiologic aspects. *Eur Urol* 3:321–332, 1977.

Madersbacher H: Urologische behandlungsprinzipien, in *Urologie für Rückenmarkverletzte.* Vienna, Springer-Verlag, 1979, p. 136–150.

Madersbacher H: Rehabilitation of micturition by transurethral electrostimulation of the bladder in patients with incomplete spinal cord lesions. *Paraplegia* 20:191–195, 1982.

Madersbacher H: Urodynamic practice in neuro-urological patients: Techniques and clinical value. *Paraplegia* 22:145–156, 1984.

Madersbacher H: Management of striated sphincter dyssynergia. *Neuro-urol Urodyn* 5:307–315, 1986.

Chapter 33. Acupuncture in Amputees

Bischko J: *Einfuhrung in die Akupunktur,* ed 13. Heidelberg, Haug Verlag, 1983.

Bischko J: *An Introduction to Acupuncture.* Heidelberg, Haug Verlag, 1978.

Bischko J: *Akupunktur fur mäBig Fortgeschrittene* ed 3, Heidelberg, Haug Verlag 1981.

Busse E, Busse P: *Akupunkturfibel.* München, Richard Pflaum, 1954.

Chapter 34. Isokinetic Strength Testing

Davis GJ: Compendium of Isokinetics in *Clinical Usage and Rehabilitation Techniques,* ed 2, La Crosse, S & S Pub, 1985.

Chapter 35. Dental Treatment: Experiences with Handicapped Patients

Pomaroli A: Original contribution and personal communications. Rehabilitation Center, Bad Häring, Tirol, Austria, 1985.

Chapter 36. Electrodiagnosis and Electromyography

Dawson DM, Hallett M, Millender LH: *Entrapment Neuropathies.* Boston, Toronto, Little Brown & Co., 1983.

Delagi EF, Perotto A, Iazzetti J, Morrison D: *Anatomic Guide for the Electromyographer: The Limbs* ed 2. Springfield, Charles C Thomas, 1980.

Goodgold J: *Anatomical Correlates of Clinical Electromyography.* Baltimore, Williams & Wilkins, 1974.

Kimura J: *Electrodiagnosis in Diseases of Nerve and Muscle: Principles and Practice.* Philadelphia, FA Davis, 1983.

Chapter 37. Electrostimulation for Pain Control

Campbell JA: A critical appraisal of the electrical output characteristics of ten transcutaneous nerve stimulators. *Clin Phys Physiol Meas* 3:141–150, 1982.

Gersh MR, et al: Applications of transcutaneous electrical nerve stimulation in the management of patients with pain. State-of-the-art update. *Phys Ther* 65:314–336, 1985.

Jenkner FL: *Transcutaneous Electric Nerve Block.* Vienna, New York, Springer-Verlag, 1986.

Long DM: Stimulation of the peripheral nervous system for pain control. *Clin Neurosurg* 31:323–343, 1983.

Naidu KR: Transcutaneous electrical stimulation in the management of phantom limb pain. *J Assoc Physicians India* 30:309–310, 1982.

Patterson MM, Kesner RP: *Electrical Stimulation Research Techniques.* New York, Academic Press, 1981.

Waisbrod H, et al: Direct nerve stimulation for painful peripheral neuropathies. *J Bone Joint Surg* 67B:470–472, 1985.

Chapter 38. Functional Electrostimulation

Brandell BR: Development of a universal control unit for functional electrical stimulation (FES). *Am J Phys Med* 61:279–301, 1982.

Currier DP, et al: Muscular strength development by electrical stimulation in healthy individuals. *Phys Ther* 63:915–921, 1983.

Eichhorn KF, et al: Maintenance training and functional use of denervated muscles. *J Biomed Eng* 6:205–211, 1984.

Eriksson E, et al: Effect of electrical stimulation on human skeletal muscle. *Int J Sports Med* 2:18–22, 1981.

Gruner JA, et al: A system for evaluation and exercise-conditioning of paralysed leg muscles. *J Rehab R&D* 10–38:21–30, 1983.

Jackson KM, et al: A battery powered constant current stimulator. *J Biomed Eng* 5:165–166, 1983.

Kralj A, et al: Gait restoration in paraplegic patients: A feasibility demonstration using multichannel surface electrode FES. *J Rehab R&D* 10–38:3–20, 1983.

McMiken DF, et al: Strengthening of human quadriceps muscles by cutaneous electrical stimulation. *Scand J Rehabil Med* 15:25–28, 1983.

Moorthy CV, et al: Muscular training through localized in vivo electrical stimulations. *Ind J Physiol Pharmacol* 25:229–236, 1981.

Chapter 39. Manual Lymph Drainage Ad Modum Vodder in Physical Medicine and Rehabilitation

Vodder E: Drainage de lymphatique, une nouvelle methode therapeutique. *Revue de Hygiene Individuelle,* April, 1936.

Vodder E: Technische Grundlagen der Manuellen Lymphdrainage. *Z Phys Ther* 1, 1983.

Chapter 40. Management of Joint Dysfunction by Manual Medicine: Mobilization and Manipulation

Jones L: *Strain and Counterstrain.* Colorado Springs, CO, American Academy of Osteopathy, 1980.

Lewit K: Muskelfazilitations- und Inhibitionstechniken in der Manuellen Medizin. Teile II & III. Postisometrische Muskelrelaxation *Manuelle Medizin* 19:12–22, 40–43, 1981.

Mitchell FL, Moran PS, Pruzzo NA: *Evaluation and Treatment Manual of Osteopathic Muscle Energy Procedures.* Valley Park, Mo, Mitchell, Moran and Pruzzo Associates, 1979.

Travell J, Travell W: Technic for reduction and ambulatory treatment of sacroiliac dysplacement. *Arch Phys Ther* 23:222–232, 1942.

Dvorak J, Dvorak V: *Manuelle Medizin.* Stuttgart, New York, Georg Thieme Verlag, 1983.

Chapter 41. Management of Joint Dysfunction by Prolotherapy-Sclerotherapy: Stabilization and Pain Control

Hackett GS: *Ligament and tendon relaxation treated by Prolotherapy,* ed 3. Springfield, IL, Charles C Thomas, 1958.

Hackett GS, Huang TC: Prolotherapy for sciatica from weak pelvic ligaments and bone dystrophy. *Clin Med* 8:12, 1961.

Kayfetz DO: Occipito-cervical (whiplash) injuries treated by prolotherapy. *Med Trial Tech Quart* Mundelein, IL, Callahan & Co., reprinted from June, 1963.

Kayfetz DO, Blumenthal LS, Hackett GS, Hemwall GA, Neff FE: Whiplash injury and other ligamentous headache—its management with prolotherapy. Reprint from *Headache* 3:1, 1963.

Leedy RF: Basic techniques of sclerotherapy. *Osteopath Med* 1977, pp 15–113.

Leedy RF: Basic techniques of sclerotherapy. *Osteopath Med* 1977, pp 79–97.

Liu YK, Tipton CM, Mathes RD, Bedford TG, Maynard JA, Walmer HC: An in-situ study of the influence of a sclerosing solution in rabbit medial collateral ligaments and its junction strength. *Connec Tissue Res* 2:95–102, 1983.

Myers A: Prolotherapy treatment of low back pain and sciatica. Reprinted from *Bull Hospital Joint Dis* 22:1, 1961.

Naeim F, Froetscher L, Hirschberg GG: Treatment of the chronic iliolumbar syndrome by infiltration of the iliolumbar ligament. *West J Med* 136:372–374, 1982.

Peterson TH: Injection treatment for low back pain. *Am J Orthop* 5:320–325, 1963.

Pomeroy KL, Sawtell J: *Prolotherapy: A Historical Review and Present State of the Art.* (a personal search and review of the literature), Phoenix, AZ, 1978.

Chapter 42. Stress and Tension Control

Benson H: *Relaxation Response.* New York, William Morrow & Co, 1975.

Feldenkrais M: *Awareness Through Movement.* Harper Row Publ, New York, 1972.

Feldenkrais, M: Eshkol N: Faculty of Fine Arts, Twenty-five Lessons. Tel Aviv University, 1977.

Feldenkrais M: *The Elusive Obvious or Basic Feldenkrais.* Meta Publications, 1981.

Germeroth SR: Wellness evaluation learning laboratory, program guide. The Cottonsville Community College, 1984.

Holmes TH, Rahe RH: The social readjustment rating scale. *J Psychosom Res* 11:213–218, 1967.

International Stress and Tension Control Society. Regional Conferences and Proceedings, 1985.

Jacobson E. *Tension Control for Businessmen.* Whitehall Co., 1963.

Jacobson E: Self operation's control, National Foundation for Progressive Relaxation, 1964.

Jacobson E: *You Must Relax.* McGraw-Hill Book Co., 1962.

Mathews DB: *Relaxation Training.* South Carolina State College, Phi Delta Kappa Newsletter 3, 1, 3, 1982.

McGuigan SG: *Calm Down, a Guide to Stress and Tension Control.* Englewood Cliffs, NJ, Prentice Hall, 1981.

Selye H: *Stress Without Distress.* Philadelphia, New York, JB Lippincott, 1974.

Truch S: *Teacher Burnout.* Academic Therapy Publication, 1980.

Tubesing NC, Tubesing DA: *Structured Exercises in Stress Management* vol I. Whole Person Press, 1983.

Chapter 43. Thermography in Trauma

Goodley PH: Musculoskeletal pain and thermography. *Acta Thermograf* 5:1–3, 1980.

Goodley PH: A comprehensive objective assessment of pain: A seminar on chronic pain syndromes in medical practice: Expanded options. Proc Eisenhower Medical Center Arthritis Foundation, 1980, pp 73–77.

Goodley PH: Thermography. *JAMA Letters*, 249:1003–1004, 1983.

Chapter 44. Treatment of Myofascial Pain and Dysfunction

Lewit K, Simons DG: Myofascial pain: Relief by post-isometric relaxation. *Arch Phys Med Rehabil* 65:452–456, 1984.

Travell JG, Simons DG: *Myofascial Pain and Dysfunction; The Trigger Point Manual.* Baltimore, London, Williams & Wilkins, 1983.

Travell J, Rinzler SH: The myofascial genesis of pain. *Grad Med* 5, May, 1952.

Chapter 45. Treatment of Cervical Syndromes

Blumenthal LS: Injury to the cervical spine as a cause of headache. *Postgrad Med* 5:147–152, 1974.

Jenkner FL: *Das Cervical syndrom Manuelle und Elektrische Therapie.* Wien, New York, Springer-Verlag, 1982.

Kayfetz DO, Blumenthal LS, Hackett GS, Hemwall GA, Neff FE: Whiplash injury and other ligamentous headache. It's management with prolotherapy. *Headache* 3, 1963.

Kayfetz DO: Occipito-cervical (whiplash) injuries treated by prolotherapy. *Med Trial Tech Quart* June, 1963.

Appendix 1. Establishing a Trauma Department and a Minirehabilitation Service in an Acute Care Hospital

Russe F: Original contribution. Unfallkrankenhaus, Vienna 12, Austria.

Appendix 2. Medicolegal Aspects of Rehabilitation

Rozovsky FA: *Consent to Treatment: A Practical Guide.* Boston, Little, Brown & Co. 1984.

Sharf BF: *The Physicians Guide to Better Communication.* Glenview, IL, Scott Foresman & Co.

Social Insurance Law. S 172/2 (Suppl 32), 1977.

The Defense Research Institute: *The Expert Witness in Litigation.* vol 3 DRI, 1983.

Appendix 3. Measuring and Recording Joint Motion and Position: Longitudinal and Circumferential

Gerhardt JJ, Russe OA: *International SFTR Method of Measuring and Recording Joint Motion.* Hans Huber, Berne, 1975.

Gerhardt JJ: *International Standard Orthopedic Measurements (Wall Chart).* SFTR Recording of Joint Motion and Position in the Neutral-O-Method. Bourbon, Indiana, Orthopedic Equipment, 1964.

Russe OA, Gerhardt JJ et al: *An Atlas of Examination, Standard Measurements and Diagnosis in Orthopedics and Traumatology.* Berne, Hans Huber, 1972.

Gerhardt JJ: Measurement of Joint Motion and Position in the Neutral-O-Method and SFTR Recording. J. International Rehabilitation Medicine, Euler Verlag, 1985.

Appendix 4. Measuring Instruments

Rippstein J: Original Contribution, La Conversion, Switzerland.

Gerhardt JJ, King P, Zettl J: *Immediate and Early Prosthetic Management: Rehabilitation Aspects.* Berne, Toronto, New York, Hans Huber, 1986.

Appendix 5. Planning Data for the Construction of an Accident Victim's Rehabilitation Center

Reiner E: Original contribution with use of plans of the Trauma Rehabilitation Center "Weisser Hof" of the Allgemeine Unfallversicherungsanstalt, Vienna 2, Austria.

Index